KU-280-987

Vaccinology

Principles and Practice

Vaccinology

Principles and Practice

EDITED BY

W. John W. Morrow, PhD, DSc, FRCPath
Seattle, WA, USA

Nadeem A. Sheikh, PhD
Dendreon Corporation
Seattle, WA, USA

Clint S. Schmidt, PhD
NovaDigm Therapeutics, Inc.
Grand Forks, ND, USA

D. Huw Davies, PhD
University of California at Irvine
Irvine, CA, USA

WILEY-BLACKWELL

A John Wiley & Sons, Ltd., Publication

ALISTAIR MACKENZIE LIBRARY
Barcode
Class no.

ALISTAIR MACKENZIE LIBRARY
Barcode: 3690289864
Class no: QW 805 MOR

This edition first published 2012, © 2012 by Blackwell Publishing Ltd.

Blackwell Publishing was acquired by John Wiley & Sons in February 2007. Blackwell's publishing program has been merged with Wiley's global Scientific, Technical and Medical business to form Wiley-Blackwell.

Registered office: John Wiley & Sons, Ltd, The Atrium, Southern Gate, Chichester, West Sussex, PO19 8SQ, UK

Editorial offices: 9600 Garsington Road, Oxford, OX4 2DQ, UK
The Atrium, Southern Gate, Chichester, West Sussex, PO19 8SQ, UK
350 Main Street, Malden, MA 02148-5020, USA

For details of our global editorial offices, for customer services and for information about how to apply for permission to reuse the copyright material in this book please see our website at www.wiley.com/wiley-blackwell

The right of the author to be identified as the author of this work has been asserted in accordance with the UK Copyright, Designs and Patents Act 1988.

All rights reserved. No part of this publication may be reproduced, stored in a retrieval system, or transmitted, in any form or by any means, electronic, mechanical, photocopying, recording or otherwise, except as permitted by the UK Copyright, Designs and Patents Act 1988, without the prior permission of the publisher.

Designations used by companies to distinguish their products are often claimed as trademarks. All brand names and product names used in this book are trade names, service marks, trademarks or registered trademarks of their respective owners. The publisher is not associated with any product or vendor mentioned in this book. This publication is designed to provide accurate and authoritative information in regard to the subject matter covered. It is sold on the understanding that the publisher is not engaged in rendering professional services. If professional advice or other expert assistance is required, the services of a competent professional should be sought.

The contents of this work are intended to further general scientific research, understanding, and discussion only and are not intended and should not be relied upon as recommending or promoting a specific method, diagnosis, or treatment by physicians for any particular patient. The publisher and the author make no representations or warranties with respect to the accuracy or completeness of the contents of this work and specifically disclaim all warranties, including without limitation any implied warranties of fitness for a particular purpose. In view of ongoing research, equipment modifications, changes in governmental regulations, and the constant flow of information relating to the use of medicines, equipment, and devices, the reader is urged to review and evaluate the information provided in the package insert or instructions for each medicine, equipment, or device for, among other things, any changes in the instructions or indication of usage and for added warnings and precautions. Readers should consult with a specialist where appropriate. The fact that an organization or Website is referred to in this work as a citation and/or a potential source of further information does not mean that the author or the publisher endorses the information the organization or Website may provide or recommendations it may make. Further, readers should be aware that Internet Websites listed in this work may have changed or disappeared between when this work was written and when it is read. No warranty may be created or extended by any promotional statements for this work. Neither the publisher nor the author shall be liable for any damages arising herefrom.

Library of Congress Cataloging-in-Publication Data

Vaccinology : principles and practice / edited by W. John W. Morrow . . . [et al.].
     p. ; cm.
  Includes bibliographical references and index.
  ISBN 978-1-4051-8574-5 (hardback : alk. paper)
  I. Morrow, John, 1949–
  [DNLM: 1. Vaccines.   2. Drug Design.   3. Vaccination–methods.   QW 805]
  615.3′72–dc23

                                                                2012002555

A catalogue record for this book is available from the British Library.

Wiley also publishes its books in a variety of electronic formats. Some content that appears in print may not be available in electronic books.

Set in 9/12pt Meridien by Aptara® Inc., New Delhi, India
Printed and bound in Singapore by Markono Print Media Pte Ltd

1   2012

Contents

Alistair Mackenzie
Wishaw General
50 Netherton Street
Wishaw
ML2 0DP

Part 7 Evaluating Vaccine Efficacy

Part 8 Implementing Immunizations/Therapies

List of Contributors

Murrium Ahmad, PhD
The John van Geest Cancer Research Centre, School of Science and Technology, Nottingham Trent University, Nottingham, UK

Sir Roy M. Anderson, FRS, FMedSci
Chair in Infectious Disease Epidemiology
Division of Epidemiology, Public Health and Primary Care, School of Public Health, London, UK

Antony N. Antoniou, PhD
Senior Research Fellow Department of Infection and Immunity/Centre of Rheumatology, University College London, London, UK

Victor Appay
INSERM UMR S 945, Infections and Immunity, Avenir Group, Université Pierre et Marie Curie (UPMC), Sorbonne Universités, and Hôpital Pitié-Salpétrière, Paris, France

Carolina Arancibia-Cárcamo, PhD
Translational Gastroenterology Unit, Nuffield Department of Clinical Medicine, University of Oxford, Oxford, UK

Helen S. Atkins, BSc, PhD
Department of Biomedical Sciences, Defence Science and Technology Laboratory, Porton Down, UK

R. Bruce Aylward, MD, MPH
Assistant Director-General, Polio, Emergencies and Country Collaboration, World Health Organization, Geneva, Switzerland

Lorne A. Babiuk, OC, SOM, PhD, DSc, FRSC
Office of Vice President Research, University of Alberta, Edmonton, Canada

Graham Ball
The John van Geest Cancer Research Centre, School of Science and Technology, Nottingham Trent University, and CompanDX Ltd, Nottingham, UK

Janine Bilsborough, PhD
Inflammation Research, Amgen, Thousand Oaks, CA, USA

Marie-Claude Boily, PhD
Senior Lecturer in Infectious Disease Ecology
Division of Epidemiology, Public Health and Primary Care, School of Public Health, London, UK

Diane L. Bolton
Vaccine Research Center, National Institute of Allergy and Infectious Diseases (NIAID), National Institutes of Health (NIH), Bethesda, MD, USA

Catharine M. Bosio, PhD
Rocky Mountain Laboratories, National Institute of Allergy and Infectious Diseases, National Institutes of Health, Hamilton, MT, USA

Marc Brisson, PhD
Unité de Recherche en Santé des Populations, Centre de Recherche Fonds de la Recherche en Santé du Québec du Centre Hospitalier affilié Universitaire de Québec, Canada

Victoria Byers
NJM European Economic & Management Consultants Ltd, Gosforth, Newcastle Upon Tyne, UK

Claudio Carini, MD, PhD
Boston Biotech Clinical Research, Cambridge, MA, USA

Miles W. Carroll, PhD
Microbiology Division, Health Protection Agency, Porton Down, UK

Darrick Carter, PhD
Protein Advances, Inc., Seattle, WA, and Infectious Disease Research Institute, Seattle, WA, USA

Bryce Chackerian, PhD
Department of Molecular Genetics and Microbiology, University of New Mexico School of Medicine, Albuquerque, NM, USA

Dipshikha Chakravortty, PhD
Department of Microbiology and Cell Biology, Center for Infectious Disease Research and Biosafety Laboratories, Indian Institute of Science, Bangalore, India

Robert T. Chen, MD, MA
Division of HIV/AIDS Prevention, National Center for
HIV/AIDS, Viral Hepatitis, STD, and TB Prevention, Centers
for Disease Control and Prevention (CDC), Atlanta, GA, USA

Zhengrong Cui
Pharmaceutics Division, College of Pharmacy, University of
Texas-Austin, Austin, USA

Julie M. Curtsinger, PhD
Department of Laboratory Medicine & Pathology, Center for
Immunology, University of Minnesota, Minneapolis,
MN, USA

Priyanka Das
Department of Microbiology and Cell Biology, Center for
Infectious Disease Research and Biosafety Laboratories,
Indian Institute of Science, Bangalore, India

Nelson Cesar Di Paolo, PhD
Department of Medicine, Division of Medical Genetics,
University of Washington, Seattle, WA, USA

Candida Fratazzi, MD
Boston Biotech Clinical Research, Cambridge, MA, USA

Volker Gerdts, DVM
Vaccine & Infectious Disease Organization, Saskatoon;
Department of Veterinary Microbiology, University of
Saskatchewan, Saskatoon, SK, Canada

Jane Gidudu MD, MPH
Immunization Safety Office, Division of Healthcare Quality
Promotion, National Center for Emerging and Zoonotic
Infectious Diseases, Centers for Disease Control and
Prevention (CDC), Atlanta, GA, USA

Gregory M. Glenn
Intercell USA, Inc., Gaithersburg, MD, USA

David B. Guiliano
Division of Infection and Immunity/Centre for
Rheumatology, Windeyer Institute of Medical Science,
University College London, London, UK

Patrick Guirnalda, PhD
Department of Microbiology, University of Pennsylvania,
Philadelphia, PA, USA

Yper Hall, BSc
Microbiology Division, Health Protection Agency, Porton
Down, UK

David L. Heymann, MD, DTM&H
Professor and Chair, Infectious Disease Epidemiology,
London School of Hygiene and Tropical Medicine,
London, UK

Maria Candela Iglesias
INSERM UMR S 945, Infections and Immunity, Avenir
Group, Université Pierre et Marie Curie (UPMC), Sorbonne
Universités, and Hôpital Pitié-Salpétrière, Paris, France

John Iskander, MD, MPH
Office of the Associate Director for Science, Centers for
Disease Control and Prevention (CDC), Atlanta, GA, USA

Camilla Jandus, MD, PhD
Division of Clinical Onco-Immunology, Ludwig Institute for
Cancer Research, Lausanne, Switzerland

Sylvia Janetzki, MD
Zellnet Consulting, Inc., Fort Lee, NJ, USA

Ross M. Kedl, PhD
Department of Immunology, University of Colorado Denver,
Denver, CO, USA

Amit Lahiri
Department of Microbiology and Cell Biology, Center for
Infectious Disease Research and Biosafety Laboratories,
Indian Institute of Science, Bangalore, India

Stephen M. Laidlaw
Department of Virology, Imperial College London Faculty of
Medicine, London, UK

Yvette Latchman, PhD
The Puget Sound Blood Center, Seattle, WA, USA

Ed C. Lavelle, PhD
Adjuvant Research Group, School of Biochemistry and
Immunology, Trinity Biomedical Sciences Institute, Trinity
College, Dublin, Ireland

Stephanie Laversin
The John van Geest Cancer Research Centre, School of
Science and Technology, Nottingham Trent University,
Nottingham, UK

F. Eun-Hyung Lee, MD
Emory University Department of Medicine, Division of
Pulmonary, Allergy, and Critical Care Medicine, Atlanta, GA,
USA

Izabela Lenart
Division of Infection and Immunity/Centre for
Rheumatology, Windeyer Institute of Medical Science,
University College London, London, UK

André Lieber, MD, PhD
Department of Medicine, Division of Medical Genetics, and
Department of Pathology, University of Washington, Seattle,
WA, USA

Margaret A. Liu, MD
ProTherImmune, Lafayette, CA, USA

Amit A. Lugade, PhD
Department of Immunology, Roswell Park Cancer Institute,
Buffalo, NY, USA

Megan MacLeod, PhD
Integrated Department of Immunology, Howard Hughes
Medical Institute, National Jewish Health, Denver, CO, USA

Philippa Marrack, PhD
Integrated Department of Immunology, Howard Hughes
Medical Institute, National Jewish Health, Denver, CO, USA

Preston A. Marx Jr, PhD
Tulane National Primate Research Center, Tulane University,
Covington, LA, USA

Matthew F. Mescher, PhD
Department of Laboratory Medicine & Pathology, Center for
Immunology, University of Minnesota, Minneapolis, MN,
USA

Benoit Mâsse, PhD
Public Health Sciences Division, Biostatistics, Fred
Hutchinson Cancer Research Center, Seattle, Washington,
USA

Arnaud Moris
INSERM UMR S 945, Infections and Immunity, Avenir
Group, Université Pierre et Marie Curie (UPMC), Sorbonne
Universités, and Hôpital Pitié-Salpêtrière, Paris, France

Cliff Murray, PhD
Source BioScience, Nottingham, UK

George K. Mutwiri, DVM, PhD
Vaccine & Infectious Disease Organization, Saskatoon;
School of Public Health, University of Saskatchewan,
Saskatoon, SK, Canada

Scott Napper, PhD
Vaccine & Infectious Disease Organization, Saskatoon;
Department of Biochemistry, University of Saskatchewan,
Saskatoon, SK, Canada

Derek T. O'Hagan, PhD
Global Head, Vaccine Delivery and Formulation, Novartis
Vaccines and Diagnostics, Inc., Cambridge, MA, USA

Yvonne Paterson, PhD
Department of Microbiology, University of Pennsylvania,
Philadelphia, PA, USA

Andrew A. Potter, PhD, FCAHS
Vaccine & Infectious Disease Organization, Saskatoon;
Department of Veterinary Microbiology, University of
Saskatchewan, Saskatoon, SK, Canada

Simon J. Powis, PhD
School of Medicine, University of St Andrews, St Andrews,
Fife, UK

Robert Rees
The John van Geest Cancer Research Centre, School of
Science and Technology, Nottingham Trent University,
Nottingham, and CompandX Ltd, Nottingham, UK

Mario Roederer, PhD
Vaccine Research Center, National Institute of Allergy and
Infectious Diseases (NIAID), National Institutes of Health
(NIH), Bethesda, MD, USA

Pedro Romero
Division of Clinical Onco-Immunology, Ludwig Institute for
Cancer Research, Lausanne, Switzerland

Iñaki Sanz, MD
Division of Allergy, Immunology, and Rheumatology,
University of Rochester Medical Center, Rochester, NY,
USA

Aaron K. Sato, PhD
OncoMed Pharmaceuticals, Redwood City, CA, USA

John T. Schiller, PhD
Laboratory of Cellular Oncology, National Cancer Institute,
Bethesda, MD, USA

Matthew Seavey, PhD
Department of Microbiology, University of Pennsylvania,
Philadelphia, PA, USA

Robert C. Seid Jr
Intercell USA, Inc., Gaithersburg, MD, USA

Fiona A. Sharp, PhD
Fahmy Research Group, Department of Biomedical
Engineering, School of Engineering and Applied Science,
Yale University, New Haven, CT, USA

Dmitry Shayakhmetov, PhD
Department of Medicine, Division of Medical Genetics,
University of Washington, Seattle, WA, USA

Michael A. Skinner
Department of Virology, Imperial College London Faculty of
Medicine, London, UK

Brian R. Sloat
Pharmaceutics Division, College of Pharmacy, University of Texas-Austin, Austin, USA

Kalathil Suresh, PhD
Department of Immunology, Roswell Park Cancer Institute, Buffalo, NY, USA

Rudolf H. Tangermann, MD
Global Polio Eradication Initiative, World Health Organization, Geneva, Switzerland

Yasmin Thanavala, PhD
Department of Immunology, Roswell Park Cancer Institute, Buffalo, NY, USA

Richard W. Titball, BSc, PhD, DSc, FRCPath
School of Biosciences, University of Exeter, Exeter, UK

Hugh Townsend, DVM, MSc
Vaccine & Infectious Disease Organization, Saskatoon; Department of Large Animal Clinical Sciences, University of Saskatchewan, Saskatoon, SK, Canada

Hoi K. Tran
Department of Pharmaceutical Sciences, College of Pharmacy, Oregon State University, Corvallis, OR, USA

Sylvia van Drunen Littel-van den Hurk, PhD
Vaccine & Infectious Disease Organization, Saskatoon; Department of Microbiology and Immunology, University of Saskatchewan, Saskatoon, SK, Canada

Claudia Vellozzi, MD, MPH
Division of Healthcare Quality Promotion, National Center for Emerging and Zoonotic Infectious Diseases, Centers for Disease Control and Prevention (CDC), Atlanta, GA, USA

Joanne L. Viney, PhD
Inflammation Research, Amgen, Thousand Oaks, CA, USA

Alexander F. Voevodin, MD, PhD, DSc, FRCPath
Vir&Gen, Toronto, ON, Canada

Andreas Wack
Division of Immunoregulation, National Institute for Medical Research, London, UK

Britta Wahren, MD, PhD
Department of Virology, Karolinska Institutet and Swedish Institute for Infectious Disease Control, Stockholm, Sweden

Heather L. Wilson, PhD
Vaccine & Infectious Disease Organization, Saskatoon; Department of Biochemistry, University of Saskatchewan, Saskatoon, SK, Canada

Peter Wilson, PhD, MBA, LLB
NJM European Economic & Management Consultants Ltd, Gosforth, Newcastle Upon Tyne, UK

Laurence Wood, PhD
Department of Microbiology, University of Pennsylvania, Philadelphia, PA, USA

Preface

"Vaccinology" is a term that encompasses the whole process of producing vaccines – from basic research and preclinical demonstration of efficacy, to approval and clinical trial in humans. While there are many excellent books that detail the various steps, such as antigen discovery or delivery systems, there are fewer that also cover so called "downstream development," such as the design of clinical trials, or their regulation in the United States and the European Union. In this book we have aimed to fill this gap by providing the reader with a comprehensive and authoritative reference that describes the design and construction of vaccines from first principles to implementation. We hope it will appeal both to scientists engaged in vaccine research and development, and to clinicians, or indeed anyone, with an interest in the opportunities and challenges facing the development of new vaccines.

To tackle this vast subject we have organized the chapters into sections. We start with an examination of the concept and scope of modern vaccines. We follow this with the basic tenets of the immune system that govern our thinking about vaccines, with chapters on innate immunity, antigen processing and presentation, mucosal immunity, immunological memory in T and B cells, and the utility of mouse and nonhuman primate models for testing vaccine efficacy. In the following section we explore antigen discovery in the postgenomic era, during which there has been remarkable progress in proteomic mining for potential vaccine antigens, and powerful predictive algorithms and high-throughput assay and display technologies. Together these offer unprecedented opportunities for the rapid development of new vaccines. This is then followed by a selection of chapters on antigen engineering and delivery: attenuated microbe vaccines, virus-like particles, recombinant viruses (orthopox, avipox, lentivirus, and adenovirus) and bacteria, DNA vaccines, and artificial cells. In parallel we explore methods for antigen delivery, with chapters on transcutaneous vaccination, needle-free jet delivery, and oral vaccines. The need to potentiate otherwise inert proteins is the subject of the next section, with chapters on designing adjuvants, particulate delivery systems such as PLGs and microspheres, co-administration of co-stimulatory moieties, and the role of TLR signaling in adjuvanticity. We then transition from basic research to vaccine implementation. The first of these sections discusses regulatory considerations, with chapters on working with the US Food and Drug Administration (FDA) and the European Medicines Agency (EMA), developmental pipelines, the design of clinical trials, immune monitoring and biomarkers, and vaccine safety. This is followed by chapters on mass immunization strategies, and mathematical models and epidemiological monitoring.

This book would not be possible without the impressive array of experts who have contributed chapters. We wish to thank every one of you for making this possible and bearing with us on this ambitious project. Finally we wish to thank the production team at John Wiley, especially Julie Elliott, Maria Khan, and Michael Bevan. This has been a team effort, but ultimately any omissions or errors are the responsibility of the editors. We welcome comments and feedback for future editions of this book.

W. John W. Morrow
Nadeem A. Sheikh
Clint S. Schmidt
D. Huw Davies

PART 1
Introduction

CHAPTER 1

Concept and Scope of Modern Vaccines

D. Huw Davies[1], Clint S. Schmidt[2], & Nadeem A. Sheikh[3]
[1]School of Medicine, University of California at Irvine, Irvine CA, USA
[2]NovaDigm Therapeutics, Inc., Grand Forks, ND, USA
[3]Clinical Immunology, Research, Dendreon Corporation, Seattle, WA, USA

Introduction

Historically, vaccination has probably had the greatest impact on human health of any medical intervention technique. Immunization is the only cost effective solution that can arrest and even eradicate infectious diseases. The science of vaccinology can be traced to the ancient Chinese, who protected against smallpox by the process of variolation, in which small quantities of scabs from a lesion of an infected person were intranasally inoculated [1]. This process was revived in the early 18th century when Lady Mary Montagu, who had observed variolation being practiced in Turkey, advocated its use to prevent smallpox. Modern vaccinology started as a proper scientific endeavor by Edward Jenner's findings that cowpox pustules would prevent smallpox infection [2]. His work was the first to be evaluated scientifically and established the scientific basis for using a related but less dangerous pathogen to engender immune responses that are cross-protective against the more virulent pathogen [3]. The seminal work and findings of Jenner lay unexploited for nearly a century until Louis Pasteur demonstrated that chickens could be protected from cholera by inoculation with attenuated bacteria [4]. Similar experiments also showed that sheep could be protected from anthrax [5]. This concept of weakening a pathogen to invoke the immune system to produce a response forms the basis of immunity elicited by the Bacille Calmette-Guérin (BCG) tuberculosis vaccine, first administered in 1921 [6] and still in wide use today.

Vaccines are defined as immunogenic preparations of a pathogen that evoke an immune response without causing disease. While attenuation and inactivation of pathogens are conventional approaches, and are still used, modern vaccines also exploit recent developments in immunology, genomics, bioinformatics, and structural and protein chemistry. At the heart of all vaccines is antigen – the ligand of the receptors of T and B lymphocytes. Lymphocytes are the effector cells of the adaptive immune system that mediate immunologic memory responses – the very hallmark of vaccination – which set vaccination apart from other forms of modern immune system manipulation, such as broad-spectrum immunopotentiators, cytokine therapy, or passive transfer of specific hyperimmune globulins derived from human plasma.

The scope of modern and future vaccines has widened considerably since the empirical approaches of the pre-genomic era. Vaccines can now be designed rationally, even customized to individual needs. Developments in many areas of vaccinology, from adjuvants, proteomics, expression library immunizations (ELI), and sub-unit vaccines, to innovative funding and philanthropy, continue to reach new milestones. However, there are challenges in the road ahead. The vaccines that have not yet been made either exceed the limits of

Vaccinology: Principles and Practice, First Edition. Edited by W. John W. Morrow, Nadeem A. Sheikh, Clint S. Schmidt and D. Huw Davies.
© 2012 Blackwell Publishing Ltd. Published 2012 by Blackwell Publishing Ltd.

current technology or there is a lack of incentive. Here we outline the limitations of current vaccine technology and, through the following chapters, identify technologies that may help the field of vaccinology to advance.

Triumphs and limitations of current vaccination

After access to affordable nutrition, clean drinking water, and sanitation, low cost vaccines are the single most cost effective healthcare measure that can be taken to protect human health. This is highlighted by the fact that mass immunization programs have directly resulted in the control of several infectious diseases. For example, rates of incidence of diphtheria, measles, mumps, pertussis, and a number of other common diseases have been reduced by over 99% in the United States (Table 1.1). In the case of smallpox, global eradication was achieved through a concerted effort led by the World Health Organization (WHO). For polio, a concerted eradication program has reduced the incidence year after year from approximately 35 000 cases annually to fewer than 4000 in 1996 (Figure 1.1). Similarly, as the number of immunizations against measles has risen over the past two decades, the number of reported measles infections has fallen (Figure 1.2).

In addition, by controlling infections, vaccines reduce expenditure on future treatment (Table 1.2). Such costs are highlighted by the Centers for Disease Control (CDC) [8], which estimates that for every dollar invested in immunization, between $2 and $29 are saved. In addition the entire cost of the global smallpox eradication program, approximately $32 million, is returned every 20 days in not having to vaccinate travelers. A specific case in point is made by the combined measles, mumps, and rubella (MMR) vaccine. Immunization with this combined MMR vaccine was estimated to provide $5.1 billion direct and indirect cost savings in the USA for 1992 alone [9].

Despite the impact of vaccines on childhood infectious diseases such as measles, diphtheria, polio, and meningitis, there are many infectious diseases that continue to thwart vaccination programs, particularly in resource-poor countries, such as malaria, salmonellosis, and tuberculosis. There are several reasons why we lack vaccines to these diseases:

• *Genetic instability*. A major roadblock to vaccination against many pathogens is unpredictable antigenic variation. Antigenic variation per se is not an insurmountable challenge: current vaccine technology already protects us from pathogens with relatively small numbers of serotypes, for example polio (three serotypes) and rotavirus (four serotypes), and in principle scaling to dozens or even hundreds of strains of a pathogen, such as *Streptococcus pneumoniae* (ninety known serotypes), is possible. It is well known that an individual can become immune

Table 1.1 Incidence of disease and the year of peak rate in the USA prior to and after mass immunization programs were initiated.

| Disease | Peak incidence (year) | Incidence | | Percentage change 1997 |
		1996	1997	
Diphtheria	206 939 (1921)	2	5	−99.9976
Measles	894 134 (1941)	508	135	−99.9849
Mumps	152 209 (1968)	751	612	−99.9959
Pertussis	265 269 (1934)	7796	5519	−99.9791
Polio, paralytic (wild poliovirus)	21 269 (1952)	0	0	−100.000
Rubella (German measles)	57 686 (1969)	238	161	−99.9972
Rubella, congenital syndrome	20 000 (1964–5)	4	4	−99.9998

Adapted from [7] for 1996 statistics and from *Vaccine and Immunization News*, No. 6, March 1998.

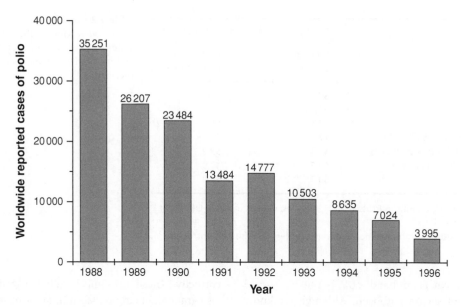

Figure 1.1 Impact of polio eradication program upon cases of polio infection worldwide. Each year there has been a gradual decrease in the numbers of polio cases reported. Adapted from *Vaccine & Immunization News* No. 5, 1997 (WHO Publications).

to a formidable number of strains of a particular pathogen, as evidenced by the acquisition of immunity to malaria or the common cold over the course of two or three decades of natural exposure. This could be replicated in a compressed time frame with the appropriate vaccine. The real challenge is to provide pre-existing immunity to pathogens or strains of pathogens that do not yet exist. While the pre-existing repertoire of the adaptive immune system clearly has the capacity to respond to and retain immunologic memory of any antigen, current vaccine production methods require these antigens

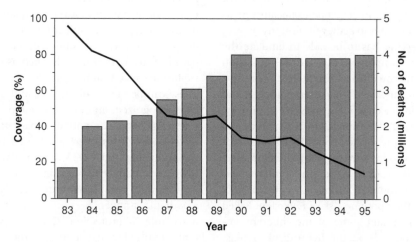

Figure 1.2 Impact of measles eradication program upon cases of measles infection worldwide. Shaded bars, coverage; line, number of deaths. Each year there has been a gradual decrease in the numbers of deaths due to measles. Adapted from *Vaccine & Immunization News* No. 4, 1997 (WHO Publications).

	Savings per "vaccine dollar" invested	
Vaccine	Direct medical savings	Direct and indirect savings
DTP	$6.0	$29.1
MMR	$15.3	$21.3
OPV	$3.4	$6.1
Integrated (DTP, MMR, OPV)	$7.4	$25.5
Haemophilus influenza type b	$1.4	$2.2
Hepatitis B (perinatal/infant)	$0.5	$2.0
Varicella	$0.9	$5.4

Table 1.2 Cost effectiveness of childhood vaccines in the United States and the estimated returned savings, both direct and indirect, from vaccination.

DTP, diphtheria, tetanus, pertussis; MMR, measles, mumps, rubella; OPV, oral polio vaccine.
Data from National Immunization Program, Centers for Disease Control and Prevention.

to be known beforehand. HIV is the worst-case scenario of such a pathogen. Although we know antibodies to gp120 can confer protection, the ability of the virus to generate a seemingly infinite number of antigenically distinct molecules as it replicates has thwarted most attempts to develop a vaccine. This intractable problem remains a major hurdle to development of vaccines against organisms with unpredictable antigenic variation.

• *Complexity.* This generally goes hand-in-hand with the size of the genome of a pathogen and the number of distinct stages in its life cycle. Most successful vaccines are against viruses, much fewer are against bacteria, and few are in development against parasites or fungi. In order to achieve immunity by vaccination, a vaccine has to be able to emulate the immunogenic components of natural infection without causing the disease. Attenuated organisms lack the pathogenicity of the parent pathogen and retain the ability to engender protective immunity. Often only a single immunization is required, and immunity is frequently life long. Using these criteria, the best vaccines are arguably therefore live, attenuated organisms. However, the trend today is toward the development of killed or subunit vaccines because they pose no risk of reversion. Killed organisms may retain some of the inherent immunogenic properties of the live organism (e.g., components in the cell wall) although such vaccines may contain live organisms if not prepared

correctly. These risks mean killed organisms are also gradually being replaced in favor of safer subunit or recombinant protein-based vaccines or nucleic acid vaccination. Unfortunately, recombinant protein vaccines face the greatest challenges, particularly those aimed against bacteria or parasites. Unless pathogenicity is mediated by a single component (such as an exotoxin, which can be protected against using a simple toxoid vaccine) protective immunity appears to be mediated by responses to multiple antigens. To date, single recombinant protein vaccines have performed poorly in providing protection against bacteria.

• *Correlates of protection.* A related roadblock is a lack of knowledge of the antigen(s) required to engender protection. We measure immune responses to a pathogen using *in vitro* tools, such as ELISAs, neutralization assays, and γ-interferon release assays. These can be very sophisticated and map the antigens recognized, and even the epitopes within, in fine detail. The assumption is made that these detectable responses overlap, at least in part, with the antibodies and T cells that mediate protection. However, many may be immunologically irrelevant. Simply because we can detect a response to a particular antigen does not always connote a primary role in protection. Conversely, an antigen that is critical for engendering a protective response may not be detected by our *in vitro* assays. Thus the antigen(s) used for a vaccine do not necessarily have to be particularly immunogenic in natural infection. The overlap between the measurable "reactome" and the "protectome" is a largely unexplored area.

• *Adjuvants*. Expectations of modern vaccines can sometimes be unrealistic. Current vaccines are prophylactic and are administered to healthy individuals. Therefore any safety issues have to be weighed carefully against the benefit. While subunit vaccines are the safest of all our options, the gain in safety is a tradeoff in efficacy. Most subunit vaccines and recombinant protein vaccines lack the inherent proinflammatory properties of attenuated organisms, which have to be replaced by the inclusion of an adjuvant. For reasons that are still not fully understood, immunity generated by proteins formulated in adjuvants decays more rapidly than that generated from live organisms, thereby requiring booster immunizations. Swelling, aching, and fever – the very proinflammatory properties required of a good adjuvant – are considered unacceptable side effects. (The stress suffered by a parent when their child has a fever will serve as a reminder of this.) These are trivial compared to the disease itself, yet relatively few adjuvants are approved for human use, and those that have been approved are all mild. Ultimately it may be impossible to engender complete immunity by vaccination without causing "disease" of some sort, and the best vaccines are likely to be a compromise.

Modern approaches that impact vaccine design

Genomics

In the pre-genomic era, vaccines were made from animal pathogens, or human pathogens either attenuated by abnormal growth conditions or killed by chemical inactivation. Many successful vaccines were developed using this empirical approach. This gave way to extracts of pathogens – or subunit vaccines – where components of the pathogen were used in place of the whole organism. In the post-genomic era, the production of subunit vaccines has become more rational and the preparations of antigens more precisely controlled.

Despite their drawbacks, recombinant protein vaccines have had, and will continue to have, a major impact on diseases caused by simple pathogens, especially viruses, where a single antigen is often enough to provide immunity (e.g., human papilloma virus, HPV). Even for more complex pathogens such as bacteria and parasites, there is still the expectation that recombinant protein vaccines can provide protection, particularly if adjuvanted cocktails of protective antigens are used. Continued progress in this area has been hampered by the identification of candidate antigens. The problem has been the sheer size of the genome and the number of potential antigens available, and until recently the discovery of potential subunit vaccine antigens have been piecemeal and nonsystematic.

Modern high throughput approaches to proteome-wide expression and screening technologies promise to revolutionize the discovery of new vaccine antigens for old diseases. A recent antibody profiling study of acquired immunity to malaria in the Gambia, for example, identified antibodies to several antigens present in children with acquired immunity that are absent from children who were still undergoing seasonal bouts of malaria [10]. These antigens would be considered prime targets for vaccine development. Importantly, the same study revealed the antigens currently being evaluated in clinical trials were not among these discriminatory antigens. The conclusion from studies like this is that non-biased screening approaches may lead to the discovery of different antigen sets than conventional "intuitive" approaches. It remains to be determined whether these new antigens lead to better vaccines, and Part 3 of this book focuses on these new technologies.

Improved delivery systems and adjuvants

Recombinant proteins are, for the most part, poorly immunogenic and require delivery in an immunogenic package. The most successful delivery systems for recombinant proteins are often based on macromolecular assembles of one sort or another, and can take the form of immune stimulating complexes (ISCOMs), liposomes, or virus-like particles. Suspensions of antigen bound to inorganic particles such as alum are also immunogenic. It seems dendritic cells are particularly efficient at ingesting and responding to insoluble, particulate antigens, but less so to soluble proteins.

Other steps can be taken to improve the immunogenicity of existing vaccines. For example, peptide vaccines suffer from short half life *in vivo*, which can be improved by chemical modification to improve stability. Nucleic acid vaccines, although showing great promise in animal models, currently have had less developmental success in humans. The reasons are still unclear but their efficacy can be improved by using live vectors to boost them. The immunogenicity of recombinant vectors such as vaccinia or adenovirus is blunted by pre-existing immunity. This can be overcome by using animal viruses as vectors, such as fowlpox, where pre-existing immunity does not exist. These examples and other antigen engineering technologies are examined in Part 4.

Therapeutic vaccination

Currently none of the licensed traditional vaccines for use in humans are therapeutic, but instead are prophylactic and depend on antibodies to block initial infection. A vaccine administered after infection in order to treat (not prevent) disease is a realistic goal of modern vaccination. Once a pathogen has established an infection, the type of immune response required to eliminate the infection depends largely on whether the pathogen remains extracellular or gains entry into cells, where it becomes inaccessible to antibody. The optimism for therapeutic vaccines comes from great strides in the 1980s and 1990s in understanding T-cell recognition and antigen processing/presentation, and the realization that vaccines specifically targeting cell-mediated immunity could engender protection against pathogens that reside within cells. Both CD8 and CD4 T cells can mediate killing of cells harboring intracellular pathogens, particularly viruses (CD8) and bacteria that reside in endosomal compartments (CD4). Many model systems in animals have shown proof-of-principle of therapeutic vaccination. The bottleneck to translating this to

vaccine development is, as with antibody vaccines, the size of the pathogen genome. Uniquely with T cells, the problem is amplified if synthetic peptides are desired for vaccination. Again, high throughput proteomic screening platforms and ever improving predictive algorithms promise to define the antigens needed, while carefully selected delivery vehicles or adjuvants will ensure the correct T cell subset(s) is stimulated.

Although the field of therapeutic vaccination is still developing for infectious disease, some promising inroads have been made in the cancer immunotherapy field. These technologies are based on the *ex vivo* activation [11] and amplification of the specific cellular immune response, followed by re-infusion of immune cells to the patient, as opposed to the *in vivo* activation hopefully achieved by traditional vaccines. The oncology targets for this approach are many. However, the field is gaining momentum with the FDA approval of Dendreon Corporation's Provenge™ (sipuleucel-T) for asymptomatic, or minimally symptomatic metastatic, androgen-independent prostate adenocarcinoma [12].

A return to attenuated organisms?

With the notable exception of toxoids, the disappointing previous performances of single recombinant protein subunit vaccines against complex pathogens (bacteria, fungi, and parasites) compel us to continue the development of live attenuated vaccines alongside subunit vaccine development, to ensure the highest probability of discovering a successful vaccine against any particular pathogen. Live attenuated vaccines have many advantages over killed or subunit vaccines, although the safety requirements are more stringent owing to the risk of reversion to a pathogenic phenotype. Attenuated live bacterial vaccines currently licensed for human use include *Mycobacterium bovis* strain Bacille Calmette-Guérin (developed in the 1920s), *Salmonella typhi* Ty21a (1970s), and *Vibrio cholerae* CVD 103-HgR (1980s) [13]. The latter was derived by site-directed mutagenesis of the cholera toxin A gene (*ctxA*), and in some respects it represents the flipside of the traditional cholera toxoid vaccine. Although "low hanging fruit" for an attenuated vaccine, it points toward the rational way in which such vaccines may be made in the future. For most bacteria, multiple virulence factors are linked to pathogenesis. Traditional approaches to attenuation, such as forced adaptation to unusual culture conditions or radiation/chemical mutagenesis, are too "hit and miss" for modern rational approaches. With increasingly rapid annotation of sequenced pathogens comes the potential for systematic identification of virulence factors and their targeting for mutagenesis or deletion. Technologies for screening large numbers of mutants for attenuation and immunogenicity need to be developed, and will likely involve *in vitro* models.

Allied to this are vaccines based on animal pathogens – the "Jennerian" approach. The smallpox vaccine is often described as the prototype of all vaccines, and the only vaccine to have approached the eradication of a human disease. The principle of the original smallpox vaccine (which was cowpox) is somewhat different to the attenuated and killed vaccines that have followed. Cowpox is not an attenuated version of the human pathogen, but a closely related, less pathogenic, species of orthopoxvirus. The origins of vaccinia are not clear but modern phylogenetic analyses indicate it is a "domesticated" version of cowpox. Although vaccines based on animal pathogens are less pathogenic, attenuated strains are preferable. Replication-competent smallpox vaccines are being replaced by attenuated vaccinia strains such as MVA. The attenuated *Mycobacterium bovis* strain BCG, first produced as a vaccine against *M. tuberculosis* in the 1920s, also works on this Jennerian principle. More recent examples include the human-animal "reassortant" rotavirus vaccines that have been developed using animal rotaviruses engineered to contain antigens from the human rotavirus [14].

Improve existing vaccines and vaccine uptake

Most attenuated live organisms have limited efficacy, in part because the attenuation is so severe.

Attempts to improve existing vaccines, such as with more potent adjuvants or adjuvant combinations, or improved manufacturing methods, is therefore another approach upon which modern technologies can be brought to bear. Basic research in immunologic processes will undoubtedly continue to reveal novel approaches to improving the immunogenicity of existing vaccines. The discovery of the role of Toll-like receptors [15,16] and the application of contemporary immunologic techniques [17] have helped our understanding of the basis of adjuvanticity. Likewise, our understanding of antigen processing pathways and different regulatory and effector T cell subsets has revealed the importance of antigen delivery in the type of immune response elicited. In the future, immunomodulators that switch off suppressive pathways and promote proinflammatory pathways, or ligands that target antigens to specific cells and tissues of the immune system, may be routinely engineered into vaccines. It is likely that our understanding of other critical processes, such as immunologic memory and immunodominance, will also become clearer in the near future and influence our design of vaccines and the adjuvants used.

It is worth remembering we do not need to discover new vaccines to make an impact on global health. The WHO estimates that 2.7 million children die annually from diseases that could be prevented with existing vaccines, almost half of which are caused by rotavirus and *Streptococcus pneumoniae* [18]. The majority of these are in resource-poor countries. The WHO's Expanded Programme on Immunization (EPI), first introduced in 1974, aims to bring vaccination to children throughout the world. The scheme was recently expanded to cover the world's poorest nations through the Global Alliance for Vaccines and Immunisation (GAVI) (www.gavialliance.org). Complacency and misinformation are problems in developing countries, and threaten to undermine vaccine-induced protection. Simply because a disease is no longer as common as it once was creates the illusion it is eradicated, allowing re-emergence if vaccination is not maintained. Clearly, mandatory childhood vaccination is important but remains essentially optional in most countries. Regardless of whether or not one believes there is a role for the MMR vaccine in the development of autism, the reduction in uptake of the MMR vaccine in response to the recent hysteria had a direct effect on the rise in cases of childhood measles [19].

Hurdles and challenges for the future

Non-infectious diseases as targets for modern vaccines

The identification of autoantigens associated specifically with cancer and autoimmune disease has opened up new opportunities for vaccination. These are predominantly "therapeutic" T cell-based vaccines administered to individuals who already have disease. This considerably extends the concept of a "vaccine" beyond the traditional immunogenic preparation of a pathogenic microorganism, and indeed the recently approved HPV vaccines are a significant advance in the prophylactic vaccination against a virus-associated cancer [20].

Transition from research to trial

The pages of vaccine journals (and indeed this very book) are full of novel and ingenious vaccines, delivery systems, adjuvants, vectors, and scientific methods. Yet only the simplest and safest vaccines are ever considered for clinical trial. The realities of obtaining necessary approvals, producing a vaccine to current good manufacturing practice (cGMP) standards, and finding funding are far removed from most academic laboratories where basic vaccine research is conducted. Even if a candidate is evaluated in Phase I or II clinical studies, the investment required to enter Phase III trial is beyond the scope of most government funding agencies and requires the involvement of industry. For example, it is estimated that the research and development costs of bringing Gardisil™, an HPV vaccine comprising four recombinant proteins, to market was in excess of $1 billion. There have been several attempts to overcome the economic barrier against the development of less lucrative vaccines and diagnostics, such as with tax incentives and guaranteed government purchases. Additionally, non-profit organizations, such as the Wellcome Trust, and more recently the Bill & Melinda Gates Foundation, have become pivotal drivers for vaccine development. Thus, with the cooperation between scientific, industrial, non-profit, and political entities, the field of vaccinology will continue to advance, meeting the world's unmet medical needs.

References

1 Fenner F, Henderson DA, Arrita L, Jezek Z, Ladnyi ID. *Smallpox and its Eradication*. World Health Organization, Geneva, 1988, p. 4.

2 Jenner E. *On the Origin of the Vaccine Inoculation*. Printed by D. N. Shury, London, 1801.

3 Jenner E. An inquiry into the causes and effects of the variolae vaccinae, a disease discovered in some of the western counties of England, particularly Gloucestershire, and known by the name of the cow pox, London 1798. In CNB Camac (Ed.) *Classics of Medicine and Surgery*. Dover Press, London, 1959, pp. 213–40.

4 Pasteur L, Chamberland CE, Roux E. Sur la vaccination charbonneuse. *CR Acad Sci Paris* 1881;**92**: 1378–83.

5 Pasteur L. Une statistique au sujet de la vaccination préventive contre le charbon portant sur quatre-vingt-cinq-mille animaux. *CR Acad Sci Paris* 1882;**95**:1250–52.

6 Calmette A. *La Vaccination préventive contre la tuberculose par le BCG*. Masson, Paris, 1927.

7 Saldarini RJ. For vaccines, the future is now. *Nat Med* 1998;**4**:485–91.

8 Bloom BR, Widdus R. Vaccine visions and their global impact. *Nat Med* 1998;**4**:480–84.

9 Hatziendru EJ, Brown RF, Halpern MT. *Report to the Centers for Disease Control and Prevention. Cost benefit analysis of the measles-mumps-rubella (MMR) vaccine*. Batelle, Arlington, VA, 1994.

10 Crompton PD, Kayala MA, Traore B, *et al*. A prospective analysis of the Ab response to *Plasmodium falciparum* before and after a malaria season by protein microarray. *Proc Natl Acad Sci U S A* 2010;**107**: 6958–63.

11 Schmidt CS, Morrow WJW, Sheikh NA. Smart adjuvants. *Expert Rev Vaccines* 2007;**6**:391–400.

12 Wesley JD, Whitmore JB, Trager JB, Sheikh NA. An overview of sipuleucel-T: autologous cellular immunotherapy for prostate cancer. *Hum Vaccin Immunother* 2012;**8**(4).

13 Levine MM, Kaper JB, Herrington D, *et al.* Safety, immunogenicity, and efficacy of recombinant live oral cholera vaccines, CVD 103 and CVD 103-HgR. *Lancet* 1988;**2**:467–70.

14 Dennehy PH. Rotavirus vaccines: an overview. *Clin Microbiol Rev* 2008;**21**:198–208.

15 Lemaitre B, Nicolas E, Michaut L, Reichhart JM, Hoffmann JA. The dorsoventral regulatory gene cassette spatzle/Toll/cactus controls the potent antifungal response in Drosophila adults. *Cell* 1996;**86**(6):973–83.

16 Medzhitov R, Preston-Hurlburt P, Janeway CA, Jr. A human homologue of the Drosophila Toll protein signals activation of adaptive immunity. *Nature* 1997;**388**:394–7.

17 Marrack P, McKee AS, Munks MW. Towards an understanding of the adjuvant action of aluminium. *Nat Rev Immunol* 2009;**9**:339–48.

18 *Immunization Summary: The 2007 Edition.* Geneva: United Nations Children's Fund & World Health Organization, Geneva, 2007.

19 Eaton L. Measles cases in England and Wales rise sharply in 2008. *BMJ* 2009;**338**:b533.

20 Hariri S, Unger ER, Powell SE, *et al.* The HPV vaccine impact monitoring project (HPV-IMPACT): assessing early evidence of vaccination impact on HPV-associated cervical cancer precursor lesions. *Cancer Causes Control.* 2011, Nov 23 [Epub ahead of print].

PART 2

Principles of Vaccine Design

CHAPTER 2

Strategies to Stimulate Innate Immunity for Designing Effective Vaccine Adjuvants

*Heather L. Wilson[1,2], Scott Napper[1,2], George K. Mutwiri[1,3],
Sylvia van Drunen Littel-van den Hurk[1,4], Hugh Townsend[1,7], Lorne A. Babiuk[5],
Andrew A. Potter[1,6], & Volker Gerdts[1,6]*

[1]Vaccine & Infectious Disease Organization, Saskatoon, Canada
[2]Department of Biochemistry, University of Saskatchewan, Saskatoon, Canada
[3]School of Public Health, University of Saskatchewan, Saskatoon, Canada
[4]Department of Microbiology and Immunology, University of Saskatchewan, Saskatoon, Canada
[5]Office of Vice President Research, University of Alberta, Edmonton, Canada
[6]Department of Veterinary Microbiology, University of Saskatchewan, Saskatoon, Canada
[7]Department of Large Animal Clinical Sciences, University of Saskatchewan, Canada

Principles of vaccine design: stimulation of innate immunity

Stimulation of innate immunity is an important requirement for the induction of effective immune responses following vaccination. The majority of today's vaccines contain adjuvants that were added for the purpose of enhancing the magnitude, type, onset, and duration of the acquired immune response. The recognition of the role and importance of adjuvants in the stimulation of innate immunity and the relationship between innate and acquired immunity are more recent.

Innate and acquired immunity are intimately linked through antigen-presenting cells (APCs), in particular macrophages and dendritic cells (DCs). In an immature stage, these cells specialize in uptake of antigens and are equipped with a variety of pattern recognition receptors (PRRs), which facilitate the recognition of highly conserved pathogen-associated molecular patterns (PAMPs) such as

bacterial and viral DNA, lipopolysaccharide (LPS), and flagellin (Table 2.1)[1]. Signaling through PRRs results in activation of multiple signaling pathways and the subsequent increase in expression of a plethora of effector molecules, including major histocompatibility complex (MHC), co-stimulatory molecules, and proinflammatory chemokines and cytokines (see Chapter 26 for more detail). Once activated, DCs begin to mature and home to the draining lymph node, where they present the antigen to naïve lymphocytes as part of the specific or acquired immune response (Figure 2.1). This maturation process is characterized by a loss of endocytic and phagocytic capacities and an increase in the surface expression of co-stimulatory molecules such as CD80, CD86, and CD40 [2,3]. With maturation, DCs also change expression of chemokine receptors (CCR) from those that are expressed in the peripheral tissues (CCR1, CCR2, CCR5, and CCR6) toward expression of CCR7, which recognizes CCL19 and CCL21. These two chemokines

Vaccinology: Principles and Practice, First Edition. Edited by W. John W. Morrow, Nadeem A. Sheikh, Clint S. Schmidt and D. Huw Davies.
© 2012 Blackwell Publishing Ltd. Published 2012 by Blackwell Publishing Ltd.

Table 2.1 PRRs and their activating PAMPs.

PRR	Class of PRR	Agonists	Signaling event(s)
TLR1/TLR2	TLR	Triacyl lipopeptides lipoarabinomannan from mycobacterium, yeast/zymosan, glycosylphosphatidyl inositol-linked proteins	Promotes proinflammatory cytokine expression
TLR2	TLR	Zymosan, lipoteichoic acid, peptidoglycan(?)	Expressed most abundantly in peripheral blood leukocytes
			Promotes proinflammatory cytokine expression via NF-κB and MAPK signaling cascades
			May promote apoptosis in response to lipoproteins
TLR3	TLR	dsRNA	Expressed in placenta and pancreas, and dendritic cells
			Recognizes dsRNA associated with viral infection, and induces the activation of NF-κB and the production of type I interferons
			Promotes proinflammatory cytokine expression via NF-κB and MAPK signaling cascades
TLR4	TLR	LPS, taxol	Most abundantly expressed in placenta, and in myelomonocytic cells and B cells
			Induced by LPS found in most Gram-negative bacteria
			Promotes proinflammatory cytokine expression via NF-κB and MAPK signaling cascades
TLR5	TLR	Flagellin	Expressed in myelomonocytic cells
			Recognizes bacterial flagellin
			Promotes proinflammatory cytokine expression via NF-κB and MAPK signaling cascades
TLR6/TLR2	TLR	Di-acyl lipopeptides, lipoteichoic acid, yeast/zymosan, glycosylphosphatidyl inositol-linked proteins	Cooperatively with TLR2
			Promotes proinflammatory cytokine expression via NF-κB and MAPK signaling cascades
TLR7	TLR	Imidazoquinoline, loxoribine, ssRNA	Expressed in lung, placenta, and spleen
			Promotes proinflammatory cytokine expression via NF-κB and MAPK signaling cascades
TLR8	TLR	ssRNA	Expressed in lung and peripheral blood leukocytes
			Promotes proinflammatory cytokine expression via NF-κB and MAPK signaling cascades
TLR9	TLR	Non-methylated CpG-containing DNA	Expressed in spleen, lymph node, bone marrow, and peripheral blood leukocytes
			Mediates cellular response to unmethylated CpG dinucleotides in bacterial DNA
			Promotes proinflammatory cytokine expression via NF-κB and MAPK signaling cascades

Table 2.1 PRRs and their activating PAMPs. (*Continued*)

PRR	Class of PRR	Agonists	Signaling event(s)
TLR10	TLR	Unknown	Highly expressed in lymphoid tissues such as spleen, lymph node, thymus, and tonsil
			Exact function is not known
TLR11	TLR	Uropathogenic bacteria	–
TLR12	TLR	Unknown	–
TLR13	TLR	Unknown	–
TLR15	TLR	Unknown	–
NOD1	NOD	GM-TriDAP	Induces NF-κB activity via RIPK2
			Promotes proinflammatory cytokine expression via NF-κB and MAPK signaling cascades
NOD2	NOD	MDP (GM-Di), M-TriLys	Induces NF-κB activity via RIPK2
			Promotes proinflammatory cytokine expression via NF-κB and MAPK signaling cascades
Nalp1	NLR	Anthrax LT	Activation of caspase 1 inflammasome
IPAF	NLR	Flagellin	Activation of caspase 1 inflammasome
Cryopyrin	NLR	LPS, MDP, uric acid	Activation of caspase 1 inflammasome
RIG-1	RLR	dsRNA	Expressed on intestinal epithelial cells
			Associates with melanoma differentiation-associated gene 5 (MDA5)
			Activates the IFN-stimulated response element (ISRE) and NF-κB driven transcription
			Antiviral effects in virus-infected cells
Cathepsin G	Neutrophil serine protease	–	Cytokine processing and degradation, cleavage of adhesion molecules
			Activates proteinase-activated receptor 2 (PAR2) expressed on epithelial cells leading to IL8 and CCL2 expression
			Calcium flux, MAPK activation leading to cytoskeletal rearrangement
Neutrophil elastase	Neutrophil serine protease	–	Cytokine processing and degradation, cleavage of adhesion molecules
			Activates PAR2 expressed on epithelial cells leading to IL8 and CCL2 expression
Proteinase-3	Neutrophil serine protease	–	Cytokine processing and degradation, cleavage of adhesion molecules
			Activates PAR2 expressed on epithelial cells leading to IL8 and CCL2 expression.
			May act via TLR4 to promote IL8 expression
Mannose receptor	C-type lectin	Wide range of endogenous and exogenous ligands	Primarily expressed on macrophages and dendritic cells
			Essential for pro- and anti-inflammatory cytokine expression
			Role in antigen processing and presentation, cell migration, and intracellular signaling

Table 2.1 PRRs and their activating PAMPs. (*Continued*)

PRR	Class of PRR	Agonists	Signaling event(s)
Dectin-1	C-type lectin	Fungal β-glucans	Role in killing of fungi via phagocytosis
			Promotes proinflammatory cytokine expression
DC-SIGN	C-type lectin	ICAM3	Expressed on macrophages and dendritic cells
			Binds to mannose-type carbohydrates, and activates phagocytosis
			Mediates dendritic cell rolling and lymphocyte interactions
			Modulates TLR-induced activation

are constitutively expressed in T-cell zones of secondary lymphoid organs and facilitate the migration of mature DCs into the lymph nodes for antigen presentation to T cells [4–6].

Effective antigen presentation is mediated by a sequence of signals, the first being the antigen itself. The second and third signals are provided by co-stimulatory molecules and secreted cytokines, which ultimately determine the nature of the acquired immune response. Co-stimulatory molecules have both positive and negative modulatory effects on T- and B-cell activation and include members of the B7/CD28 family, tumor necrosis factor (TNF) superfamily, and the signaling lymphocyte activation molecule family (see Chapter 25). Depending on the nature of the maturation stimulus, the subset of dendritic cells, and the local environment in which antigen is recognized, dendritic cells are able to prime naïve T cells and then induce clonal expansion and differentiation into T helper 1 (Th1), Th2, or Th17 cells, all of which are distinguishable on the basis of their receptors and subsequent cytokine production profile [7,8]. Dendritic cells that induce a proinflammatory immune response are referred to as DC1 or DC2. These are the cells that ultimately induce Th1-type or Th2-type immune responses, respectively. Conversely, tolerogenic dendritic cells, referred to as DC0, are required for induction of tolerance and immune suppression and are characterized by expression of CD154. Thus, it is the nature of the danger signal at the initial site of infection that provides the immune system with the necessary information regarding the nature of the antigen and instructs the type of immune response needed to control the infection.

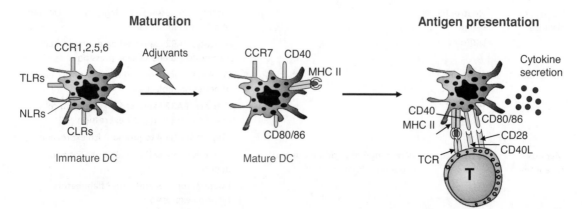

Figure 2.1 Activation and maturation of dendritic cells. CCR, C-chemokine receptor; TLR, Toll-like receptor; CLR, C-type lectin receptor; NLR, NOD-like receptor; MHC II, type II major histocompatibility complex; TCR, T cell receptor.

In the absence of inflammation or infection, dendritic cells are considered quiescent, not fully mature, and present self-antigens or non-immunogenic proteins leading to T cell deletion, anergy, or differentiation into regulatory cells [9]. This important immunologic process is designed to purge the peripheral T-cell repertoire of autoreactive T cells that have escaped thymic depletion and could potentially give rise to autoimmunity.

Innate immune stimulators

The stimuli involved in the activation and maturation of dendritic cells can act either independently or synergistically to promote cytokine secretion as well as upregulation of PRR expression. Integration of the host response to several PAMPs or damage-associated molecular patterns (DAMPs) allows for a highly tailored immune response [10,11]. Most pathogens contain several PAMPs that are recognized by the host cell PRRs, suggesting that the immune responses do not act in isolation but instead act in concert to elicit protective immune responses. Therefore, it is logical to design vaccines with multiple PAMPs/DAMPs to stimulate complementary and/or redundant PRR signaling pathways to mimic what occurs in nature. Vaccine components should instruct dendritic cells at the site of vaccination as to the type of immune response required to establish effective immunity and immunologic memory to combat subsequent, natural infection. Here we will review Toll-like receptors (TLRs) and non-TLRs for their potential use as vaccine adjuvants, alone and in combination, and describe how activation of their corresponding innate immune receptors may contribute to instruction of adaptive immunity and/or vaccine efficacy.

Toll-like receptors

TLRs are germline encoded PRRs that recognize a variety of PAMPs associated with bacteria, viruses, parasites, and fungi to initiate innate immune responses and to instruct adaptive immunity [12,13] (see Chapter 26). TLRs are highly conserved type I integral membrane proteins that share a conserved Toll/interleukin 1 (IL1) receptor (TIR) domain with IL1 receptors [14]. The ligand-binding domain con-

sists primarily of a repeating pattern of a leucine-rich repeat (LRR) motif, which provides an adaptable structural matrix for biomolecular interactions with a variety of distinct ligands [15,16].

Signaling through TLRs involves an intracellular cascade that includes the myeloid differentiation primary response gene 88 (*MyD88*), IL1 receptor activated kinase (IRAK), TIR-associated-protein (TIRAP), Toll receptor-associated activator of interferon (TRIF), Toll receptor-associated molecule (TRAM), and TNF receptor-associated factor 6 (TRAF6), leading to activation of NF-κB [12] (Figure 2.2). NF-κB activation results in a proinflammatory response through the induction of proinflammatory cytokines, and induction of MHC molecules and co-stimulatory signals that provide a link from pathogen recognition by the innate immune system to activation of the adaptive immune system (see Chapters 3 and 4) [17]. Some of the specific mechanisms by which activation of the TLR system promotes adaptive immune responses include: (i) antigen internalization and maturation of DCs [18]; (ii) influencing migration of DCs [19]; (iii) promoting Th1 responses [20]; (iv) cross-priming and -presentation [21,22]; (v) reversal of tolerance [23–26]; and (vi) upregulation of MHC and co-stimulatory molecules [27,28] (see Chapter 26). Comparative evaluation of various TLR ligands as adjuvants must consider the appropriateness of the resulting responses as well as properties of the ligand, such as stability and ease of production.

TLR1/2/4/6 agonists

The bacterial outer-surface lipoprotein (OspA) has been shown to possess adjuvant activity in a manner that is dependent upon the presence of TLR1 in humans, and both TLR1 and TLR2 in mice [29]. In humans, the efficacy of an induced response correlates with levels of TLR1 expression [29]. In mice, a tri-palmitoyl-*S*-glyceryl-cysteine (Pam$_3$Cys)-modified OspA vaccine offered protection even in TLR2$^{-/-}$ mice, indicating the potential presence of additional adjuvants [30]. Similarly, *Haemophilus influenzae* type b (Hib) outer membrane protein complex (OMPC) vaccine-induced proinflammatory cytokines, but not antigen-specific IgG titers, were also TLR2-dependent, indicating that other adjuvant factors

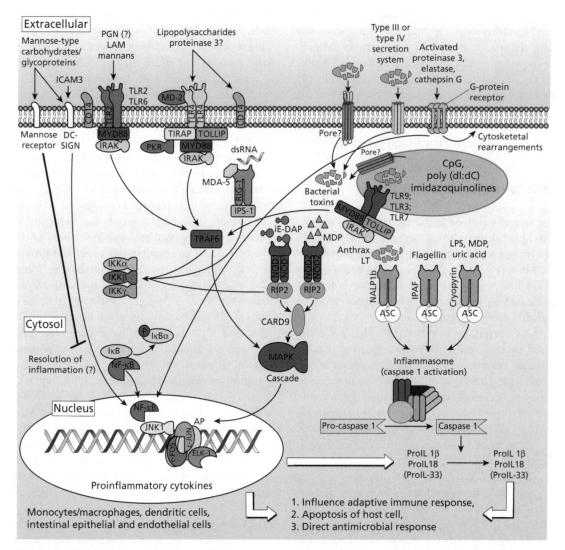

Figure 2.2 PRR signaling events lead to production and maturation of proinflammatory cytokines. The innate immune response responds in a general manner to factors present in invading pathogens.
Pathogen-associate patterns activate the innate immune response, trigger an inflammatory response, and ultimately stimulate antigen-specific immunity. Both ligands and simplified pathways are shown. Adapted from Biocarta (www.biocarta.com/pathfiles/h_tollPathway.asp) with permission.

may be present in this vaccine formulation [31]. Two bacterial membrane components, macrophage-activating lipopeptide 2 (MALP-2) of *Mycoplasma* spp. and a synthetic bacterial lipopeptide PAM3CSK4, are potent adjuvants [32,33] recognized by TLR2/6 and TLR2/1 heterodimers, respectively [34,35].

TLR3 agonists

TLR3 plays a critical antiviral role through recognition of viral double-stranded RNA (dsRNA) as well as nucleic acid intermediates of viral replication. A synthetic analog of dsRNA, polyinosinic:polycytidylic acid (poly I:C), has been investigated as a therapeutic agent in patients for treatment of leukemia [36]. Poly I:C, in combination with chitin microparticles, offers protective immunity against pathogenic strains of influenza virus [37]. Mechanistically, the ability of dsRNA to promote maturation of CD8α^+ DCs and induction of CD4$^+$ and CD8$^+$ T cell responses through interferon-mediated cross-priming is thought to be critical to the ability of TLR3 to function as an effective target for adjuvants [21].

TLR4 agonists

LPS, the ligand of TLR4, has been shown to be a potent vaccine adjuvant (see Chapter 23) [38,39]. LPS has been modified to monophosphoryl lipid A (MPL), which is much less toxic and has been used as a vaccine adjuvant in human clinical studies [40, 41]. An aqueous formulation of MPL1 and alum, AS04^{TM} (GlaxoSmithKline), achieves higher antibody titers with fewer injections and was employed as an adjuvant for a licensed hepatitis B (HBV) vaccine (Fendrix1). Other TLR4 agonists, such as lipid A mimetics (termed the aminoalkyl glucosaminide phosphates [39], glucopyranosyl lipid A [GLA] and E6020), induced immune responses compatible with their application as adjuvants [42].

TLR5 agonists

Recombinants of the TLR5 agonist flagellin exert potent adjuvant activity that enhances protection from *Listeria monocytogenes* (p60 and listeriolysin O) and influenza (matrix 2 proteins, M2e [43]).

TLR7 and 8 agonists

Viral single-stranded RNA (ssRNA) and synthetic imidazoquinolins are potent ligands for TLR7 and TLR7/8 in mice and humans, respectively, for induction of type I interferons (IFNs) and for the promotion of cellular immune responses [44,45]. The distinct pattern of expression of TLR7 and TLR8 in humans (where TLR7, but not TLR8, is highly expressed in plasmacytoid DCs, and TLR8, but not TLR7, is highly expressed in monocytes) explains the differential responses of particular cells to these ligands. Activation of plasmacytoid DCs through TLR7 results in production of type I IFNs,

while activation of monocytes through TLR8 induces synthesis of proinflammatory cytokines [46]. TLR7 agonists, such as imiquimod, have been used as immunotherapeutics for treatment of a variety of disorders such as genital warts, actinic keratosis, hepatitis B/C, and cancer [41,47–49]. TLR7/8 agonists enhance the generation of Th1 responses and CD8 T cell proliferation when used as adjuvants with HIV Gag protein vaccine [50].

TLR9 agonists

Toll-like receptor 9 has been the focus of considerable research for the ability to modulate its activity, and subsequent innate immune responses, through DNA-based immunotherapeutics. The immunostimulatory action of bacterial DNA can be effectively mimicked with synthetic, single-stranded oligodeoxynucleotides (ODNs) that are typically 24–30 nucleotides in length. These ODNs are attractive as therapeutics because of their low cost, chemical stability, and ease of production. In macrophages, dendritic cells, and B cells, CpG ODNs induce production of proinflammatory cytokines and chemokines to shift the host's immune response to favor a Th1 response, accounting for their action as vaccine adjuvants for a variety of bacterial and viral antigens in a large number of species [51].

Non-Toll-like receptors

Neutrophil serine proteases

Neutrophils are the first cells recruited to the site of infection whereupon they can directly initiate an attack against the invading pathogens or modify the local environment to promote increased immune cell recruitment. To kill pathogens, neutrophils phagocytose and sequester pathogens into the phagolysosome, where they release large quantities of reactive oxygen species (ROS), antimicrobial peptides, and serine proteases such as cathepsin G, neutrophil elastase, and proteinase 3 [52]. Upon activation, these zymogens are released through exocytosis to assist in extracellular killing. Upon cleavage by serine proteases, CCR1 ligands show up to 1000-fold increase in monocyte recruitment

[53]. Similarly, cleavage of chemerin by cathepsin G and elastase triggers increased dendritic cell recruitment [54]. Neutrophils release granule proteins and chromatin, which together form extracellular traps (NETS) that bind bacteria within minutes of activation and release [55]. These localized areas are exposed to a high concentration of serine protease, which degrades virulence factors and kills Gram-positive and Gram-negative bacteria [55]. The importance of these proteases is evident in experiments in which mice with normal superoxide production but deficient in neutrophil-granule proteases such as cathepsin G and elastase cannot effectively combat and clear staphylococcal and candida infections [56,57]. Serine proteases provide the host with a mechanism to control and/or fine tune the immune response, making these proteins very attractive as vaccine adjuvants [54].

NOD-like receptors

NOD-like receptors (NLRs) are PRRs comprised of three domains: an N-terminal effector binding region (such as caspase recruitment domain [CARD], pyrin domain [PYD], and baculovirus IAP [inhibitor of apoptosis protein] repeat [BIR]), which mediate protein-protein interactions; a NOD domain, which is responsible for nucleotide binding and self-oligomerization; and a C-terminal leucine rich repeat (LRR), which detects conserved microbial patterns and modulates NLR activity (reviewed in [58]). Upon ligand binding, these receptors undergo oligomerization, associate with accessory proteins, and ultimately induce NF-κB and MAPK signaling. NOD1 is an NLR that is present in a variety of cell types, but NOD2 appears to be restricted to macrophages, DCs, Paneth cells, keratinocytes, and epithelial cells [58]. NOD1 recognizes the peptidoglycan fragments FK156 and meso-DAP (iE-DAP) [59] whereas NOD2 recognizes muramyl dipeptide (MDP) [60], a component of Freund's Complete Adjuvant (FCA) [61]. When used in conjunction with lipophilic carrier systems such as liposomes, oil-in-water emulsions, or some lipophilic derivatives, MDP induces strong cellular immunity (reviewed in [62]). MDP is too pyrogenic and arthritogenic to be used as an adjuvant in humans.

The inflammasome

Members of the NLR family such as Nalp1, Ipaf, and cryopyrin respond to damage and inflammatory signals by complexing with caspase 1 and an adaptor protein ASC (apoptosis-associated speck-like protein containing a CARD domain) to form the inflammasome, which mediates activation of caspase 1 [63–65]. Activation of the inflammasome requires DAMPs such as ATP, toxins, HMGB1, crystals, or membrane-damaging molecules. Ligands for Ipaf include flagellin from *Salmonella typhimurium*, *Legionella pneumonia*, and *Pseudomonas aeruginosa*, which are delivered by the type III or type IV secretion system into the cytosol [66–68]. Cryopyrin inflammasomes may respond to changes in cellular potassium, MDP [69], LPS [70], and uric acid [71]. Activated caspase 1 processes immature proinflammatory cytokines pro-IL1β, pro-IL18, and pro-IL33 into active proteins. IL1β and IL18 in turn recruit inflammatory cells to sites of infection, and IL33 promotes Th2-biased immunity [72,73]. Thus, IL1β, one of the key players in the innate immune response, requires TLR signaling through various PAMPs for production and secretion, but it requires DAMP-dependent activation of the inflammasome to become activated. Inflammasome agonists should be regarded as useful components of vaccines and immunostimulators.

One of the most recognized inflammasome agonists is alum, an adjuvant that has been used in humans for over 50 years. However, its mechanism of action has only recently been discovered. Alum was originally thought to assist in the depot effect of the vaccine; that is, to cause the antigen and other vaccine components to reside for an extended period of time at the site of injection. It has since been shown to increase antigen uptake by dendritic cells *in vitro* [74], and to induce myeloid cell migration to mouse spleen, where the myeloid cells may play a role in priming and expansion of antigen-specific B cells [75]. Intraperitoneal injection of alum induces monocyte recruitment and migration to local lymph nodes, where they differentiate into inflammatory dendritic cells capable of priming T cells

[76]. Alum has been shown to synergize with TLR agonists to enhance both cellular and humoral immune responses compared to each adjuvant alone [77]. Recent studies have shown that alum is phagocytosed by macrophages and is responsible for activation of the capase 1 inflammasome [78,79].

RIG-1-like receptors

dsRNA generated during viral replication is recognized by the cytoplasmic RNA helicases retinoic acid-inducible gene I (RIG-I) and melanoma differentiation-associated gene 5 (MDA5), which associate with interferon-β promoter stimulator 1 (IPS-1) and signal through NF-κB signaling cascade and IFN regulatory factor 3 (IRF3) in a caspase 8 and caspase 10 dependent pathway [80]. Activation of caspase 8 and caspase 10 induces inflammatory cytokine expression [80,81], inhibition of translation and viral replication [82], and direct activation of DCs and natural killer (NK) cells, which subsequently promote the survival and effector functions of T and B cells [83,84]. Understanding how these viral sensors mediate immunity will be vital to the development of designer vaccines.

C-type lectin receptors

C-type lectin-like receptors are cell-surface receptors that bind carbohydrate structures and facilitate uptake of pathogens into dendritic cells. Examples of these lectin-like receptors are dectin-1, the dendritic cell-specific ICAM3-grabbing nonintegrin (DC-SIGN), and mannose receptor (MR). MR plays a role in phagocytosis, cellular migration, intracellular signaling (such as IFN-γ production, NF-κB production, etc.), and MHC class II presentation, and it may play a role in resolution of inflammation [85–87]. DC-SIGN can activate NF-κB directly to induce proinflammatory cytokine signaling [88]. Dectin-1 recognizes fungal pathogens and, in conjunction with TLR2, promotes production of TNF-α to control fungal pathogenesis [89]. C-type lectin receptors therefore recognize pathogens via their carbohydrate moieties and promote an inflammatory response.

Practical applications for adjuvants

Action

Adjuvants enhance or modulate the immune response in several ways, including formation of an antigen-adjuvant depot, chemoattraction of appropriate immune cells to the site of antigen administration, targeting or delivery to APCs, and direct or indirect immunomodulation [90] (see Chapter 26). Redundancy of PRRs suggests that the host can sense pathogens in many different tissues through a variety of cells and within various cellular compartments. There is evidence that TLRs and NLRs may regulate and/or compensate for each other to prevent overproduction or underproduction of proinflammatory cytokines, respectively. NOD1 and NOD2 agonists synergize with TLR ligands to promote a strong proinflammatory response (reviewed in [58]; [91]. For example, OVA and FK156 prime antigen-specific T-cell and B-cell immunity with a predominant T helper (Th2) polarization profile; however, in the presence of TLR agonists, FK156 can promote increased Th1, Th2, and Th17 responses [92]. The live-attenuated yellow fever vaccine 17D (YF-17D), one of the most successful vaccines available, activates TLR2, 7, 8, and 9 [93], suggesting that the success of at least some of the live vaccines may be due to their ability to activate a number of TLR combinations. Thus, the requirement for multiple agonists to induce potent responses may be a mechanism by which the immune system exerts a stringent "combinatorial security code" whereby at least two microbial products are required to stimulate a strong immune response to pathogen invasion [94].

Safety

Regardless of the mechanism of adjuvanticity, a certain level of inflammation at the injection site is required for recruitment of immune cells, in particular APCs, and generally is considered necessary for vaccines to be effective. A relationship exists between the immune response and tissue reactions induced by adjuvants, with stronger adjuvants often generating more tissue damage.

However, for new adjuvants to become licensed, a balance between safety and adjuvanticity leading to maximal immunogenicity is essential. Although multiple compounds have adjuvant activity under experimental conditions, many of them cause significant tissue damage or other adverse effects following immunization. FCA, a very effective and commonly used adjuvant in experimental animal models, causes significant side effects, including pyrogenicity, leukocytosis, uveitis, and adjuvant arthritis. EMULSIGEN®, an oil-in-water adjuvant licensed for veterinary use, can cause cellulitis and myositis after intramuscular injection when used at 30% (v/v) [95]. Quil-A and ISCOMs can cause an acute hypersensitivity reaction, hemolytic activity, and minor local reactions due to the detergent activity of Quil-A [90], although QS-21, the less toxic purified fraction of Quil-A, is currently used in the recently licensed adjuvant AS02 [96]. Alum may cause side effects in some instances, including erythema, subcutaneous nodules, contact hypersensitivity, and granulomatous inflammation [97]. It is generally accepted that cats immunized with vaccines formulated with alum show a prevalence for the development of sarcomas although whether alum is the direct cause is still a matter of conjecture [98].

The safety and suitability of an adjuvant is also determined by its ability to direct the immune response to be Th1- or Th2-biased, or balanced immunity (see Chapter 23). The tendency of conventional adjuvants such as alum to induce a Th2-type biased immune response may result in failure of protection or even immunopathologic responses following intracellular infections with organisms such as *Leishmania major* [99] and *Schistosoma mansoni* [100], both of which require a Th1-type immune response for control. Formalin-inactivated respiratory syncytial virus (FI-RSV) vaccine given to children in the 1960s [101–103] was not protective and even enhanced clinical disease, sometimes resulting in death, after subsequent exposure to RSV. In this case both the inactivation procedure and the adjuvant likely played a role in the induction of a non-neutralizing Th2-biased response. T-helper type 2-dominant immune responses are also associated with allergy, asthma, and autoimmune disease [104,105]. Thus, safe but effective adjuvants are urgently needed for future vaccines.

Summary

Adjuvants have long been used to improve the immune responses to vaccines. Historically, the choice of substances for use as adjuvants was highly intuitive, a process that resulted in the identification of only a few adjuvants that have proven safe and effective for use in human and animal vaccines. To be efficacious, vaccines must stimulate the development of both innate and adaptive immunity. Therefore, a deeper understanding of the complex and intimate links between innate and adaptive immune responses and the ways in which adjuvants can be used to enhance and refine these responses is required for the efficient development of vaccines. The research summarized in this chapter has done much to help us understand the mechanisms by which adjuvants work. Investigations along these lines will continue to be essential to the process of identifying and developing safer and more effective vaccine adjuvants.

Acknowledgements

The authors' laboratories are funded through grants from the Bill & Melinda Gates Foundation, the Krembil Foundation, Merial Ltd, Genome Canada, the Canadian Institutes for Health Research, the Natural and Engineering Science Council of Canada, Alberta Funding Consortium, Saskatchewan Agriculture Development Fund, Alberta Beef Producers, Beef Cattle Producers Industry Development Fund of British Columbia, and Agriculture and Food Council of Alberta.

References

1 Janeway CA, Jr. Approaching the asymptote? Evolution and revolution in immunology. *Cold Spring Harb Symp Quant Biol* 1989;**54**(Pt 1):1–13.

2 Banchereau J, Briere F, Caux C, *et al.* Immunobiology of dendritic cells. *Annu Rev Immunol* 2000;**18**: 767–811.

3 Adams S, O'Neill DW, Bhardwaj N. Recent advances in dendritic cell biology. *J Clin Immunol* 2005; **25**(3):177–88.

4 Dieu MC, Vanbervliet B, Vicari A, *et al.* Selective recruitment of immature and mature dendritic cells by distinct chemokines expressed in different anatomic sites. *J Exp Med* 1998;**188**(2):373–86.

5 Sallusto F, Schaerli P, Loetscher P, *et al.* Rapid and coordinated switch in chemokine receptor expression during dendritic cell maturation. *Eur J Immunol* 1998;**28**(9):2760–69.

6 Vecchi A, Massimiliano L, Ramponi S, *et al.* Differential responsiveness to constitutive vs. inducible chemokines of immature and mature mouse dendritic cells. *J Leukoc Biol* 1999;**66**(3):489–94.

7 Netea MG, Van der Meer JW, Sutmuller RP, Adema GJ, Kullberg BJ. From the Th1/Th2 paradigm towards a Toll-like receptor/T-helper bias. *Antimicrob Agents Chemother* 2005;**49**(10):3991–6.

8 Murphy KM, Reiner SL. The lineage decisions of helper T cells. *Nat Rev Immunol* 2002;**2**(12):933–44.

9 Steinman RM, Hawiger D, Liu K, *et al.* Dendritic cell function in vivo during the steady state: a role in peripheral tolerance. *Ann N Y Acad Sci* 2003;**987**: 15–25.

10 Bianchi ME. DAMPs, PAMPs and alarmins: all we need to know about danger. *J Leukoc Biol* 2007; **81**(1):1–5.

11 Medzhitov R, Janeway CA. Innate immunity: the virtues of a nonclonal system of recognition. *Cell* 1997;**91**(3):295–8.

12 Takeda K, Kaisho T, Akira S. Toll-like receptors. *Annu Rev Immunol* 2003;**21**: 335–76.

13 Iwasaki A, Medzhitov R. Toll-like receptor control of the adaptive immune responses. *Nat Immunol* 2004;**5**(10):987–95.

14 Martin MU, Wesche H. Summary and comparison of the signaling mechanisms of the Toll/interleukin-1 receptor family. *Biochim Biophys Acta* 2002;**1592**(3):265–80.

15 Bell JK, Mullen GE, Leifer CA, *et al.* Leucine-rich repeats and pathogen recognition in Toll-like receptors. *Trends Immunol* 2003;**24**(10):528–33.

16 Kobe B, Kajava AV. The leucine-rich repeat as a protein recognition motif. *Curr Opin Struct Biol* 2001; **11**(6):725–32.

17 van Duin D, Medzhitov R, Shaw AC. Triggering TLR signaling in vaccination. *Trends Immunol* 2006;**27**(1):49–55.

18 Schjetne KW, Thompson KM, Nilsen N, *et al.* Link between innate and adaptive immunity: Toll-like receptor 2 internalizes antigen for presentation to CD4+ T cells and could be an efficient vaccine target. *J Immunol* 2003;**171**(1):32–6.

19 Means TK, Hayashi F, Smith KD, Aderem A, Luster AD. The Toll-like receptor 5 stimulus bacterial flagellin induces maturation and chemokine production in human dendritic cells. *J Immunol* 2003; **170**(10):5165–75.

20 Roman M, Martin-Orozco E, Goodman JS, *et al.* Immunostimulatory DNA sequences function as T helper-1-promoting adjuvants. *Nat Med* 1997; **3**(8):849–54.

21 Schulz O, Diebold SS, Chen M, *et al.* Toll-like receptor 3 promotes cross-priming to virus-infected cells. *Nature* 2005;**433**(7028):887–92.

22 Heit A, Huster KM, Schmitz F, *et al.* CpG-DNA aided cross-priming by cross-presenting B cells. *J Immunol* 2004;**172**(3):1501–7.

23 Pasare C, Medzhitov R. Toll pathway-dependent blockade of CD4+CD25+ T cell-mediated suppression by dendritic cells. *Science* 2003;**299**(5609): 1033–6.

24 Yang Y, Huang CT, Huang X, Pardoll DM. Persistent Toll-like receptor signals are required for reversal of regulatory T cell-mediated CD8 tolerance. *Nat Immunol* 2004;**5**(5):508–15.

25 Serra P, Amrani A, Yamanouchi J, *et al.* CD40 ligation releases immature dendritic cells from the control of regulatory CD4+CD25+ T cells. *Immunity* 2003;**19**(6):877–89.

26 Peng G, Guo Z, Kiniwa Y, *et al.* Toll-like receptor 8-mediated reversal of CD4+ regulatory T cell function. *Science* 2005;**309**(5739):1380–84.

27 Hertz CJ, Kiertscher SM, Godowski PJ, *et al.* Microbial lipopeptides stimulate dendritic cell maturation via Toll-like receptor 2. *J Immunol* 2001; **166**(4):2444–50.

28 Cella M, Engering A, Pinet V, Pieters J, Lanzavecchia A. Inflammatory stimuli induce accumulation of MHC class II complexes on dendritic cells. *Nature* 1997;**388**(6644):782–7.

29 Alexopoulou L, Thomas V, Schnare M, *et al.* Hyporesponsiveness to vaccination with *Borrelia burgdorferi* OspA in humans and in TLR1- and TLR2-deficient mice. *Nat Med* 2002;**8**(8): 878–84.

30 Yoder A, Wang X, Ma Y, *et al.* Tripalmitoyl-*S*-glyceryl-cysteine-dependent OspA vaccination of toll-like receptor 2-deficient mice results in effective protection from *Borrelia burgdorferi* challenge. *Infect Immun* 2003;**71**(7):3894–900.

31 Latz E, Franko J, Golenbock DT, Schreiber JR. *Haemophilus influenzae* type b-outer membrane protein complex glycoconjugate vaccine induces cytokine production by engaging human toll-like receptor 2 (TLR2) and requires the presence of TLR2 for optimal immunogenicity. *J Immunol* 2004; **172**(4):2431–8.

32 Patel M, Xu D, Kewin P, *et al.* TLR2 agonist ameliorates established allergic airway inflammation by promoting Th1 response and not via regulatory T cells. *J Immunol* 2005;**174**(12):7558–63.

33 Borsutzky S, Kretschmer K, Becker PD, *et al.* The mucosal adjuvant macrophage-activating lipopeptide-2 directly stimulates B lymphocytes via the TLR2 without the need of accessory cells. *J Immunol* 2005;**174**(10):6308–13.

34 Takeuchi O, Kawai T, Muhlradt PF, *et al.* Discrimination of bacterial lipoproteins by Toll-like receptor 6. *Int Immunol* 2001;**13**(7):933–40.

35 Takeuchi O, Sato S, Horiuchi T, *et al.* Role of Toll-like receptor 1 in mediating immune response to microbial lipoproteins. *J Immunol* 2002;**169**(1):10–14.

36 Robinson RA, DeVita VT, Levy HB, *et al.* A phase I-II trial of multiple-dose polyriboinosic-polyribocytidylic acid in patients with leukemia or solid tumors. *J Natl Cancer Inst* 1976;**57**(3):599–602.

37 Asahi-Ozaki Y, Itamura S, Ichinohe T, *et al.* Intranasal administration of adjuvant-combined recombinant influenza virus HA vaccine protects mice from the lethal H5N1 virus infection. *Microbes Infect* 2006;**8**(12–13):2706–14.

38 Masihi KN, Lange W, Brehmer W, Ribi E. Immunobiological activities of nontoxic lipid A: enhancement of nonspecific resistance in combination with trehalose dimycolate against viral infection and adjuvant effects. *Int J Immunopharmacol* 1986; **8**(3):339–45.

39 Cluff CW, Baldridge JR, Stover AG, *et al.* Synthetic toll-like receptor 4 agonists stimulate innate resistance to infectious challenge. *Infect Immun* 2005;**73**(5):3044–52.

40 Evans JT, Cluff CW, Johnson DA, *et al.* Enhancement of antigen-specific immunity via the TLR4 ligands MPL adjuvant and Ribi. *529. Expert Rev Vaccines* 2003;**2**(2):219–29.

41 Hoffman ES, Smith RE, Renaud RC, Jr. From the analyst's couch: TLR-targeted therapeutics. *Nat Rev Drug Discov* 2005;**4**(11):879–80.

42 Ishizaka ST, Hawkins LD. E6020: a synthetic Toll-like receptor 4 agonist as a vaccine adjuvant. *Expert Rev Vaccines* 2007;**6**(5):773–84.

43 Huleatt JW, Nakaar V, Desai P, *et al.* Potent immunogenicity and efficacy of a universal influenza vaccine candidate comprising a recombinant fusion protein linking influenza M2e to the TLR5 ligand flagellin. *Vaccine* 2008;**26**(2):201–14.

44 Hemmi H, Kaisho T, Takeuchi O, *et al.* Small antiviral compounds activate immune cells via the TLR7 MyD88-dependent signaling pathway. *Nat Immunol* 2002;**3**(2):196–200.

45 Diebold SS, Kaisho T, Hemmi H, *et al.* Innate antiviral responses by means of TLR7-mediated recognition of single-stranded RNA. *Science* 2004; **303**(5663):1529–31.

46 Gorden KB, Gorski KS, Gibson SJ, *et al.* Synthetic TLR agonists reveal functional differences between human TLR7 and TLR8. *J Immunol* 2005; **174**(3):1259–68.

47 McInturff JE, Modlin RL, Kim J. The role of toll-like receptors in the pathogenesis and treatment of dermatological disease. *J Invest Dermatol* 2005;**125**(1):1–8.

48 Stockfleth E, Trefzer U, Garcia-Bartels C, *et al.* The use of Toll-like receptor-7 agonist in the treatment of basal cell carcinoma: an overview. *Br J Dermatol* 2003;**149**(Suppl 66):53–6.

49 Lysa B, Tartler U, Wolf R, *et al.* Gene expression in actinic keratoses: pharmacological modulation by imiquimod. *Br J Dermatol* 2004;**151**(6): 1150–59.

50 Wille-Reece U, Flynn BJ, Lore K, *et al.* HIV Gag protein conjugated to a Toll-like receptor 7/8 agonist improves the magnitude and quality of Th1 and CD8$^+$ T cell responses in nonhuman primates. *Proc Natl Acad Sci U S A* 2005;**102**(42):15190–94.

51 Wilson HL, Dar A, Napper SK, *et al.* Immune mechanisms and therapeutic potential of CpG oligodeoxynucleotides. *Int Rev Immunol* 2006;**25** (3–4): 183–213.

52 Pham CT. Neutrophil serine proteases: specific regulators of inflammation. *Nature Rev Immunol* 2006;**6**(7):541–50.

53 Berahovich RD, Miao Z, Wang Y, *et al.* Proteolytic activation of alternative CCR1 ligands in inflammation. *J Immunol* 2005;**174**(11):7341–51.

54 Wittamer V, Bondue B, Guillabert A, *et al.* Neutrophil-mediated maturation of chemerin: a link between innate and adaptive immunity. *J Immunol* 2005;**175**(1):487–93.

55 Brinkmann V, Reichard U, Goosmann C, *et al.* Neutrophil extracellular traps kill bacteria. *Science* 2004;**303**(5663):1532–5.

56 Reeves EP, Lu H, Jacobs HL, *et al.* Killing activity of neutrophils is mediated through activation of proteases by K$^+$ flux. *Nature* 2002;**416**(6878): 291–7.

57 Belaaouaj A, McCarthy R, Baumann M, *et al.* Mice lacking neutrophil elastase reveal impaired host defense against gram negative bacterial sepsis. *Nat Med* 1998;**4**(5):615–18.

58 Franchi L, Warner N, Viani K, Nunez G. Function of Nod-like receptors in microbial recognition and host defense. *Immunol Rev* 2009;**227**(1):106–28.

59 Chamaillard M, Hashimoto M, Horie Y, *et al.* An essential role for NOD1 in host recognition of bacterial peptidoglycan containing diaminopimelic acid. *Nat Immunol* 2003;**4**(7):702–7.

60 Girardin SE, Boneca IG, Viala J, *et al.* Nod2 is a general sensor of peptidoglycan through muramyl dipeptide (MDP) detection. *J Biol Chem* 2003; **278**(11):8869–72.

61 Ellouz F, Adam A, Ciorbaru R, Lederer E. Minimal structural requirements for adjuvant activity of bacterial peptidoglycan derivatives. *Biochem Biophys Res Commun* 1974;**59**(4):1317–25.

62 Geddes K, Magalhaes JG, Girardin SE. Unleashing the therapeutic potential of NOD-like receptors. *Nat Rev Drug Discov* 2009;**8**(6):465–79.

63 Martinon F, Burns K, Tschopp J. The inflammasome: a molecular platform triggering activation of inflammatory caspases and processing of proIL-beta. *Mol Cell* 2002;**10**(2):417–26.

64 Freche B, Reig N, van der Goot F. The role of the inflammasome in cellular responses to toxins and bacterial effectors. *Sem Immunopathol* 2007; **29**(3):249–60.

65 Kanneganti T-D, Lamkanfi M, Kim Y-G, *et al.* Pannexin-1-mediated recognition of bacterial molecules activates the cryopyrin inflammasome independent of Toll-like receptor signaling. *Immunity* 2007;**26**(4):433–43.

66 Amer A, Franchi L, Kanneganti TD, *et al.* Regulation of Legionella phagosome maturation and infection through flagellin and host Ipaf. *J Biol Chem* 2006;**281**(46):35217–23.

67 Franchi L, Amer A, Body-Malapel M, *et al.* Cytosolic flagellin requires Ipaf for activation of caspase-1 and interleukin 1beta in salmonella-infected macrophages. *Nat Immunol* 2006;**7**(6):576–82.

68 Franchi L, Stoolman J, Kanneganti TD, *et al.* Critical role for Ipaf in *Pseudomonas aeruginosa*-induced caspase-1 activation. *Eur J Immunol* 2007; **37**(11):3030–39.

69 Faustin B, Lartigue L, Bruey JM, *et al.* Reconstituted NALP1 inflammasome reveals two-step mechanism of caspase-1 activation. *Mol Cell* 2007;**25**(5): 713–24.

70 Pelegrin P, Surprenant A. Pannexin-1 mediates large pore formation and interleukin-1beta release by the ATP-gated P2X7 receptor. *EMBO J* 2006; **25**(21):5071–82.

71 Martinon F, Petrilli V, Mayor A, Tardivel A, Tschopp J. Gout-associated uric acid crystals activate the NALP3 inflammasome. *Nature* 2006; **440**(7081):237–41.

72 Li P, Allen H, Banerjee S, *et al.* Mice deficient in IL-1 beta-converting enzyme are defective in production of mature IL-1 beta and resistant to endotoxic shock. *Cell* 1995;**80**(3):401–11.

73 Martinon F, Agostini L, Meylan E, Tschopp J. Identification of bacterial muramyl dipeptide as activator of the NALP3/cryopyrin inflammasome. *Curr Biol* 2004;**14**(21):1929–34.

74 Morefield GL, Sokolovska A, Jiang D, *et al.* Role of aluminum-containing adjuvants in antigen internalization by dendritic cells in vitro. *Vaccine* 2005; **23**(13):1588–95.

75 Jordan MB, Mills DM, Kappler J, Marrack P, Cambier JC. Promotion of B cell immune responses via an alum-induced myeloid cell population. *Science* 2004;**304**(5678):1808–10.

76 Kool M, Soullie T, van Nimwegen M, *et al.* Alum adjuvant boosts adaptive immunity by inducing uric acid and activating inflammatory dendritic cells. *J Exp Med* 2008;**205**(4):869–82.

77 Vajdy M, Selby M, Medina-Selby A, *et al.* Hepatitis C virus polyprotein vaccine formulations capable of inducing broad antibody and cellular immune responses. *J Gen Virol* 2006;**87**(Pt 8):2253–62.

78 Franchi L, Nunez G. The Nlrp3 inflammasome is critical for aluminium hydroxide-mediated IL-1beta secretion but dispensable for adjuvant activity. *Eur J Immunol* 2008;**38**(8):2085–9.

79 Li H, Willingham SB, Ting JP, Re F. Inflammasome activation by alum and alum's adjuvant effect are mediated by NLRP3. *J Immunol* 2008;**181**(1): 17–21.

80 Takahashi K, Kawai T, Kumar H, *et al.* Roles of caspase-8 and caspase-10 in innate immune responses to double-stranded RNA. *J Immunol* 2006;**176**(8):4520–4.

81 Balachandran S, Thomas E, Barber GN. A FADD-dependent innate immune mechanism in mammalian cells. *Nature* 2004;**432**(7015):401–5.

82 Garcia MA, Meurs EF, Esteban M. The dsRNA pro-
    tein kinase PKR: virus and cell control. *Biochimie*
    2007;**89**(6–7): 799–811.

83 Braun D, Caramalho I, Demengeot J. IFN-
    alpha/beta enhances BCR-dependent B cell re-
    sponses. *Int Immunol* 2002;**14**(4):411–19.

84 Marrack P, Kappler J, Mitchell T. Type I interfer-
    ons keep activated T cells alive. *J Exp Med* 1999;
    189(3):521–30.

85 Zhang J, Tachado SD, Patel N, *et al.* Negative reg-
    ulatory role of mannose receptors on human alve-
    olar macrophage proinflammatory cytokine release
    in vitro. *J Leukoc Biol* 2005;**78**(3):665–74.

86 Shibata Y, Metzger WJ, Myrvik QN. Chitin particle-
    induced cell-mediated immunity is inhibited by sol-
    uble mannan: mannose receptor-mediated phago-
    cytosis initiates IL-12 production. *J Immunol*
    1997;**159**(5):2462–7.

87 Sturge J, Todd SK, Kogianni G, McCarthy A,
    Isacke CM. Mannose receptor regulation of
    macrophage cell migration. *J Leukoc Biol* 2007;**82**(3):
    585–93.

88 den Dunnen J, Gringhuis S, Geijtenbeek T. In-
    nate signaling by the C-type lectin DC-SIGN dic-
    tates immune responses. *Cancer Immunol Immunother*
    2009;**58**(7):1149–57.

89 Brown GD, Herre J, Williams DL, *et al.* Dectin-1 me-
    diates the biological effects of beta-glucans. *J Exp
    Med* 2003;**197**(9):1119–24.

90 Allison AC, Byars NE. Immunological adjuvants
    and their mode of action. *Biotechnology* 1992;**20**:
    431–49.

91 Tada H, Aiba S, Shibata K, Ohteki T, Takada H. Syn-
    ergistic effect of Nod1 and Nod2 agonists with toll-
    like receptor agonists on human dendritic cells to
    generate interleukin-12 and T helper type 1 cells.
    Infect Immun 2005;**73**(12):7967–76.

92 Fritz JH, Le Bourhis L, Sellge G, *et al.* Nod1-mediated
    innate immune recognition of peptidoglycan con-
    tributes to the onset of adaptive immunity. *Immunity*
    2007;**26**(4):445–59.

93 Querec T, Bennouna S, Alkan S, *et al.* Yellow fever
    vaccine YF-17D activates multiple dendritic cell sub-
    sets via TLR2, 7, 8, and 9 to stimulate polyvalent
    immunity. *J Exp Med* 2006;**203**(2):413–24.

94 Napolitani G, Rinaldi A, Bertoni F, Sallusto F,
    Lanzavecchia A. Selected Toll-like receptor agonist
    combinations synergistically trigger a T helper type

1-polarizing program in dendritic cells. *Nat Immunol*
    2005;**6**(8):769–76.

95 Ioannou XP, Gomis SM, Karvonen B, *et al.* CpG-
    containing oligodeoxynucleotides, in combination
    with conventional adjuvants, enhance the magni-
    tude and change the bias of the immune responses
    to a herpesvirus glycoprotein. *Vaccine* 2002;**21**(1–2):
    127–37.

96 Tritto E, Mosca F, De Gregorio E. Mechanism of ac-
    tion of licensed vaccine adjuvants. *Vaccine* 2009;**27**
    (25–26): 3331–4.

97 Ross JS, Smith NP, White IR. Role of aluminium
    sensitivity in delayed persistent immunisation reac-
    tions. *J Clin Pathol* 1991;**44**(10):876–7.

98 Hendrick MJ, Goldschmidt MH, Shofer FS, Wang
    YY, Somlyo AP. Postvaccinal sarcomas in the
    cat: epidemiology and electron probe microanalyt-
    ical identification of aluminum. *Cancer Res* 1992;
    52(19):5391–4.

99 Heinzel FP, Sadick MD, Mutha SS, Locksley RM.
    Production of interferon gamma, interleukin 2, in-
    terleukin 4, and interleukin 10 by CD4$^+$ lym-
    phocytes in vivo during healing and progressive
    murine leishmaniasis. *Proc Natl Acad Sci U S A* 1991;
    88(16):7011–15.

100 Sher A. Schistosomiasis. Parasitizing the cytokine
    system. *Nature* 1992;**356**(6370):565–6.

101 Chin J, Magoffin RL, Shearer LA, Schieble JH,
    Lennette EH. Field evaluation of a respiratory syn-
    cytial virus vaccine and a trivalent parainfluenza
    virus vaccine in a pediatric population. *Am J Epi-
    demiol* 1969;**89**(4):449–63.

102 Kapikian AZ, Mitchell RH, Chanock RM, Shved-
    off RA, Stewart CE. An epidemiologic study of al-
    tered clinical reactivity to respiratory syncytial (RS)
    virus infection in children previously vaccinated
    with an inactivated RS virus vaccine. *Am J Epidemiol*
    1969;**89**(4):405–21.

103 Kim HW, Canchola JG, Brandt CD, *et al.* Respira-
    tory syncytial virus disease in infants despite prior
    administration of antigenic inactivated vaccine. *Am
    J Epidemiol* 1969;**89**(4):422–34.

104 Kline JN, Waldschmidt TJ, Businga TR, *et al.*
    Modulation of airway inflammation by CpG
    oligodeoxynucleotides in a murine model of
    asthma. *J Immunol* 1998;**160**(6):2555–9.

105 Klinman DM, Barnhart KM, Conover J. CpG motifs
    as immune adjuvants. *Vaccine* 1999;**17**(1):19–25.

CHAPTER 3

Antigen Processing and Presentation by MHC Class I, II, and Nonclassical Molecules

Antony N. Antoniou[1], Izabela Lenart[1], David B. Guiliano[1], & Simon J. Powis[2]

[1]Department of Infection and Immunity/Centre for Rheumatology, University College London, London, UK
[2]School of Medicine, University of St Andrews, Fife, UK

Almost all human nucleated cells express classical major histocompatibility complex (MHC) class I molecules, while MHC class II molecule expression is generally restricted to specialized antigen-presenting cells (APCs), including dendritic cells (DCs), macrophages, B cells, and thymic epithelial cells. MHC class I molecules can sample both the intracellular and extracellular environment for defective and foreign proteins by presenting peptide fragments to immune effector cells. MHC class I-peptide complexes are monitored by cells of both the innate and acquired immune systems, namely natural killer (NK) cells and CD8[+] cytotoxic T lymphocytes (CTL), respectively. MHC class II molecules predominantly sample the extracellular environment and present their peptide cargo to CD4[+] T helper cells, which can modulate both T and B cell responses by providing help in the form of either cytokines or co-stimulatory molecules. Successful vaccination requires the activation of the acquired immune response and must therefore activate both CD4[+] and CD8[+] T cells by providing both their respective ligands and activation signals. A further category of molecules referred to as nonclassical MHC molecules have limited expression patterns, reflecting their specialized and restricted functions with respect to both their antigen presentation function and immune stimulatory capacity.

This chapter will therefore cover how MHC class I, II, and nonclassical molecules can acquire their respective ligands (antigen presentation) and how these ligands are generated (antigen processing).

MHC class I and II structure

Structural composition

Both MHC class I and II molecules share similar structural and functional characteristics; however, distinct differences in both three-dimensional composition and assembly reflect their respective roles in the immune response [1,2].

Classical MHC class I molecules are encoded by the HLA-A, -B, and -C loci and are composed of a trimolecular complex of heavy (H) chain (approximately 43–45 kDa), beta-2-microglobulin (β2m) light chain (approximately 12 kDa), and a peptide between 8 and 10 amino acids long. The MHC class I H chain can be divided into three distinct extracellular domains, plus a transmembrane and cytoplasmic domain. The α1 and α2 domains form two α helices and a series of β pleated sheets, comprising the walls and floor of the peptide-binding groove, respectively. The α3 domain adopts an immunoglobulin (Ig) -like fold, forming noncovalent interactions with β2m. The H chain

Vaccinology: Principles and Practice, First Edition. Edited by W. John W. Morrow, Nadeem A. Sheikh, Clint S. Schmidt and D. Huw Davies.
© 2012 Blackwell Publishing Ltd. Published 2012 by Blackwell Publishing Ltd.

possesses two conserved disulfide bonds within the α2 and α3 domains (Figure 3.1a,b).

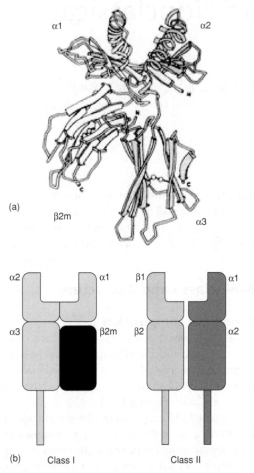

(a)

(b)   Class I   Class II

MHC class II molecules are encoded by the HLA-DR, -DQ, and -DP loci and are comprised of an α (heavy) and β (light) chain, which noncovalently associate with each other, and a peptide of at least 12–14 amino acids in length. The α and β chains are comprised of two extracellular domains, the α1/α2 and β1/β2 domains, with each composed of a transmembrane and cytosolic domain (Figure 3.1b). The α and β chains of MHC class II molecules can pair with other α and β chains of the same class II molecule but of a different haplotype (mixed haplotype) or between different class II molecules (mixed isotype) (Figure 3.2). The α chain possesses a conserved disulfide bond within the α2 domain while the β chain possesses two conserved disulfide bonds within the β1 and β2 domains.

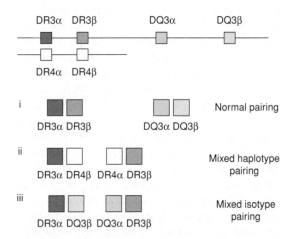

Figure 3.1 MHC class I and II structure. (a) The structure of HLA-A2 represented in ribbons as determined by X-ray crystallography. HLA-A2 consists of a heavy chain subdivided into three domains, the α1, α2, and α3 domains, and a β2m light chain. The H chain possesses four highly conserved cysteine (C) residues within the extracellular domains, forming two structurally important disulfide bonds within the α2 and α3 domains between C101–C164 and C203–C259, respectively. Reprinted by permission of Macmillan Publishers Ltd [1] copyright (1986). (b) MHC class I and II polypeptide organization. MHC class I molecules are composed of a heavy and light (β2m) chain. MHC class II molecules are composed of a heavy (α) and light (β) chain. Reproduced from Bjorkman *et al.* [1] with permission from *Nature*.

Figure 3.2 MHC class II α and β chain pairings. Hypothetical representation of the MHC locus encoding MHC class II molecules, HLA-DR3 and -DQ3 on the maternal chromosome 6 and part of the paternal chromosome 6 encoding the HLA-DR4 subtype. MHC class II molecules can be composed of α and β chains encoded within (i) an MHC allele locus (normal pairing) represented here as a DR3 and DQ3 α/β chain pair; and (ii) MHC class II subtypes to form mixed haplotype pairs, represented here as a DR3α/DR4β and DR4α/DR3β pairs. MHC class II pairings between alleles can give rise to mixed isotype pairs (iii), represented here as DR3α/DQ3β and DQ3α/DR3β pairs.

The peptide-binding grooves

The peptide-binding grooves are structurally different between MHC class I, II, and nonclassical molecules. The MHC class I antigen-binding groove is composed from the single H chain, forming a series of deep pockets at both the amino (N) and carboxy (C) termini, which act as anchors for the peptide. Such a structure leads to stringent quality control for binding. Peptides require specific sequences at both the N and C termini to associate with the B and F pockets of the peptide-binding groove, respectively, thus limiting peptide length to between 8 and 10 residues. However, bulging in the middle of the peptide can occur to accommodate longer peptides (Figure 3.3a,b) [3]. In some cases, molecules such as HLA-B27 can bind the same peptide in different orientations as a result of increased flexibility of the antigen-binding groove [4].

In contrast, both the α and β chains of MHC class II molecules make up the peptide-binding groove, with the α1 and β1 domains both forming α helices and contributing to the β sheets. The MHC class II peptide-binding groove is a more open ended and shallower structure, resulting in peptides of variable and longer length that are not so deeply embedded within the molecule (Figure 3.3c,d). Peptide binding therefore does not display such a stringent requirement for particular peptide sequences in comparison to MHC class I molecules [5].

Nonclassical MHC class I molecules

Nonclassical MHC molecules encoded within the MHC locus include the products of the HLA-E, -F, -G, and -H loci and demonstrate more specialized antigen processing and presentation roles. HLA-H, renamed HFE after it was reported to be mutated in patients with hemochromatosis [6], is involved in iron uptake regulation [7]. HLA-E and -G present a restricted pool of peptides due to structural constraints imposed on the antigen-binding groove [8,9]. Such restrictive peptide presentation probably reflects their specialized functions. For instance, HLA-E and its mouse homologue Qa-1 present peptides derived from MHC class I H chain signal sequences [10,11] and heat shock protein 60 (HSP60)

[12], which are monitored by NK cells. Cellular stress, leading to MHC class I downmodulation and a decrease in signal peptide presentation or the production of HSP60, can lead to NK activation and elimination of the affected cell [12]. The function of HLA-G remains speculative, but its limited expression by trophoblast cells of the placenta suggests it is involved in tolerance and/or protection of the fetus [13].

One of the most intriguing of the nonclassical MHC molecules are the CD1 antigens that are nonpolymorphic and encoded outside the MHC locus [14]. CD1 molecules are divided into two groups based on sequence homology. CD1a, -b, and -c constitute group 1 and CD1d molecules form group II. CD1 molecules combine the structural characteristics of MHC class I molecules, that is, they are composed of an H chain and β2m (CD1d can also be expressed as a free H chain) (Figure 3.3e), but exploit part of the MHC class II pathway by sampling the endocytic environment. CD1 molecules use cytoplasmic YXXZ sequence motifs (where Z is a hydrophobic bulky amino acid) and associate with both MHC class II molecules and invariant (Ii) chain complexes to localize to the endocytic pathway [15,16]. CD1 molecules present lipid-derived structures; for example, the natural self-ligands for CD1d appear to be the most abundant lipid present within the various accessible cellular compartments [17]. In addition, CD1d can present a marine sponge derived lipid, α-galactosylceramide, to innate immune cells known as iNKT cells, a group of T cells expressing an invariant T cell receptor. Structural analysis of CD1d complexed with α-galactosylceramide has revealed that the antigen-binding pockets are complex with very deep grooves [18,19] (Figure 3.3f,g). By activating the innate immune system (see Chapters 2 and 26), CD1 molecules could subsequently enable effective adaptive responses, thus making them attractive vaccine targets.

MHC molecule assembly

Though the ultimate aim is to deliver peptide to MHC molecules, an important element in vaccine

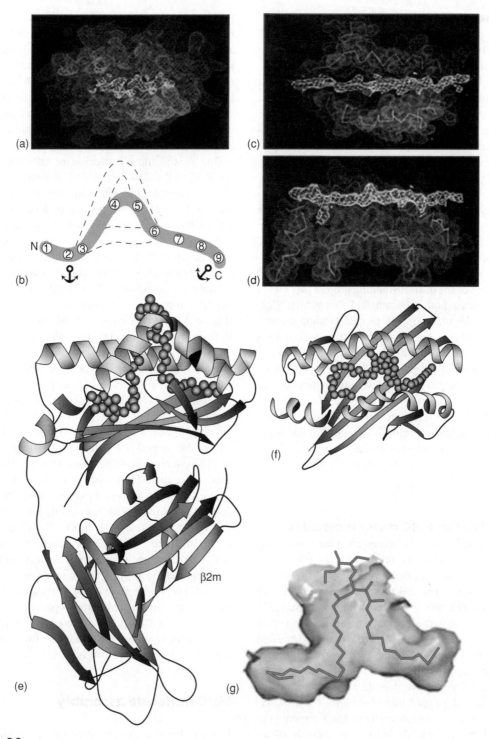

Figure 3.3

design often overlooked is the folding and assembly of MHC molecules, which can vary between MHC molecules, tissues, and cell types. MHC class I, II, and nonclassical MHC molecules begin their folding within the oxidizing environment of the endoplasmic reticulum (ER) via a series of interactions with ER-resident molecules referred to as chaperones. These transient interactions between MHC and chaperone molecules result in appropriate folding of the MHC molecule.

For MHC class I molecules, these folding events can be divided into two stages: (i) an early assembly pathway, governing the folding of the H chain with β2m, and (ii) a latter stage characterized by the formation of the peptide-loading complex (PLC) and the acquisition of optimal peptides [20] (Figure 3.4a). MHC class II and some nonclassical MHC molecules do not associate with their ligands in the ER, but predominantly within vesicles of the endocytic pathway, where their cargo is actually generated. To associate with their peptide ligands, MHC class II molecules need to be directed to the appropriate location. The regulated, endocytic transit of MHC class II molecules is governed by a multifunctional protein known as the invariant (Ii) chain (CD74).

Pre-peptide loading complex stage of MHC class I folding

Newly synthesized MHC class I H chains begin their biosynthesis by associating with the ER-resident chaperone calnexin [21], via a monoglucosylated carbohydrate unit chemically attached to a conserved asparagine residue at position 86 of the H chain [22] (Figure 3.5). Through a proline-rich extended arm-like domain referred to as the P domain, calnexin can recruit the oxidoreductase ERp57, a member of the protein disulfide isomerase (PDI) family of proteins, which reduce, oxidize, or isomerize disulfide bonds and possess two reactive thioredoxin-like CXXC motifs at positions C57–C60 and C405–C408. ERp57 forms several direct conjugates with the MHC class I H chain via transient disulfide bonds [23,24]. Throughout the folding process, misfolded MHC class I molecules

---

Figure 3.3 MHC class I, II, and nonclassical antigen-binding grooves. (a) X-ray crystallography structure of the MHC class I peptide-binding groove of HLA-A2 as observed from the top of the molecule. The high electron dense structure (white) represents bound peptide. Notice that the peptide is enclosed at the N and C termini and is relatively short compared to the MHC class II peptide in (c). The elucidation of the MHC class I structure was a milestone in protein structure determination as it demonstrated the MHC-antigen association. Reproduced from Bjorkman *et al.* [1] with permission from *Nature*. (b) Schematic of MHC class I peptides and how they can occupy the peptide-binding groove [121]. Peptides associate with the binding groove via anchor residues at the N and C termini of the peptides normally located at positions 2 and 8/9, respectively. Peptides can form extreme or shallow bulges. The N and C termini of MHC class I associated peptides interact with the binding groove in distinct ways. The N terminus associates with the groove in a lock and key type mechanism, while interactions with the C terminus lead to conformational changes within the molecule. Peptide interactions with the antigen-binding groove occur via a series of complex hydrogen bonding networks. Reproduced from Parham [121] with permission from *Nature*. (c) X-ray crystallography structure of the MHC class II (HLA-DR1) peptide-binding groove as observed from the top of the molecule. The high electron dense structure (white) represents bound peptide. Notice that the peptide is longer and the ends of the groove are more open at the N and C termini compared to that of MHC class I molecules in (a). Reproduced from Brown *et al.* [2] with permission from *Nature*. (d) MHC class II-peptide complex viewed head on. MHC class II peptides are not buried but sit in a shallower structure when compared to MHC class I associated peptides. Reproduced from Brown *et al.* [2] with permission from *Nature*. (e) Human CD1d structure, as depicted by ribbon structure, composed of a CD1d heavy chain with α-Galcer peptide (beads). (f,g) Human CD1d antigen-binding groove. Notice how the α-Galcer is deeply buried within the CD1d structure. This is better illustrated in (f), a demonstration of α-Galcer in association with the mouse CD1d molecule [18,19]. Reproduced from Koch *et al.* [18] and Zajonc *et al.* [19] with permission from *Nature*.

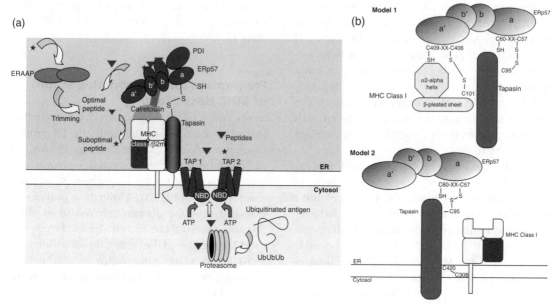

Figure 3.4 The peptide-loading complex. (a) The PLC is composed of partially folded MHC class I molecules, associated with calreticulin and tethered to the TAP heterodimer via the MHC class I specific accessory molecule tapasin, which can form a covalent interaction with the oxidoreductase ERp57. ERp57 can be structurally divided into five distinct domains, the **a** and **a**′ domains, which possess two reactive thioredoxin-like CXXC motifs; the **b** and **b**′ domains, which serve mainly structural roles; and the acidic C terminal region (not shown), which can govern the interactions with ER-resident chaperones. The main function of the PLC is for the optimization of the peptide cargo, which is catalyzed by the activity of tapasin. PDI is also thought to participate in the peptide association by binding peptides

that are transported from the cytosol into the lumen of the ER by the TAP heterodimer. Peptides are generated by the proteolytic degradation of ubiquitinated tagged proteins by the proteasome within the cytoplasm. Also shown is the trimming of peptides by ERAAP to generate optimal peptides. However, how ERAAP activity relates to the PLC or whether ERAAP is part of the PLC remains unresolved. (b) Two proposed models for the PLC. It has been postulated that the H chain can directly bind PDI [37] and/or ERp57 either through the conserved cysteines within the α2 domain [122] (model 1) or by binding to tapasin via cysteine residues within the transmembrane domain of class I H chains [123] (model 2).

can probably be removed at any point and targeted for elimination by a process referred to as ER-associated degradation (ERAD) [25]. This process involves removal of the H chain from the ER into the cytosol, where it is targeted for proteasome-mediated degradation by the addition of ubiquitin (Ub), a small 76 amino acid protein, whose C terminal glycine forms an isopeptide bond with the ε-amino group of lysines (K) or the NH_2 group at the N terminus of proteins. Ubiquitination involves the sequential action of three enzymes, a Ub-activating enzyme (E1), a Ub-conjugating enzyme (E2), and a Ub-ligase (E3) [26].

The peptide-loading complex and export to the cell surface

Once MHC class I H chains associate with β2m, calnexin is displaced and replaced by a soluble ER lectin chaperone, calreticulin [27], which also binds to monoglucosylated N-linked glycans and possesses an extended P domain to recruit ERp57 [28,29]. Partially folded MHC class I molecules, together with calreticulin, associate with the transporter associated with antigen processing (TAP) via a specific multifunctional accessory molecule known as tapasin, which also allows for stable TAP protein expression [27,30] (see Figure 3.4a).

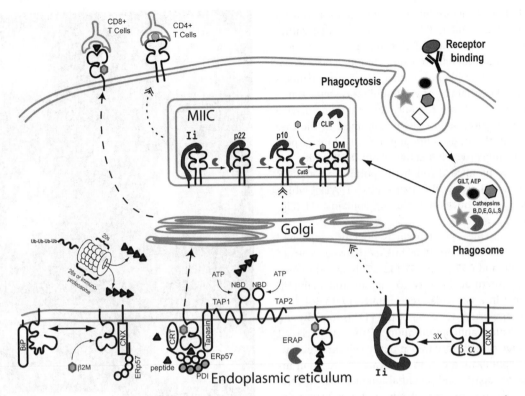

Figure 3.5 MHC class I and II pathways. Newly synthesized MHC class I heavy chains associate with the ER-resident chaperones calnexin (CNX) and immunoglobulin binding protein (BiP). The relationship of the MHC class I heavy chains associated with CNX and BiP is undetermined. CNX can recruit the oxidoreductase ERp57 via a proline-rich P domain. On binding to the light chain β2m, CNX is displaced and replaced by calreticulin (CRT). Together, the partially folded MHC class I molecules are tethered to the transporter associated with antigen processing (TAP) by the MHC class I specific accessory molecule tapasin to form the PLC. Peptides generated by the proteolytic activity of the proteasome, which degrades ubiquitin-tagged proteins, are transported into the ER in an ATP-dependent manner by TAP. MHC class I associated peptides can be N-terminally trimmed by the ER-associated peptidase (ERAP). This stage in the assembly process is represented separately as it remains undetermined whether ERAP trimming occurs before PLC formation or within the PLC. The MHC class I peptide cargo is optimized by the catalytic activity of tapasin, which is disulfide-bonded to ERp57. The oxidoreductase PDI can also be detected within the PLC and is thought to participate in MHC class I disulfide bond formation and peptide loading. Once an appropriate peptide cargo has been attained, MHC class I molecules transit through the Golgi apparatus to the cell surface (block arrow, dashed line) for recognition by cytotoxic CD8$^+$ T cells. MHC class II molecules are synthesized within the ER and associate with CNX. Invariant chain (Ii) then associates with MHC class II molecules forming a "trimer of trimers." Ii chain occludes peptides from the MHC class II peptide-binding groove and targets the MHC class II molecule to the endocytic pathway via the Golgi apparatus (double-headed arrows, dashed line). MHC class II molecules are localized to the MHC class II peptide loading compartment (MIIC). The Ii chain is processed by endocytic proteases into distinct fragments referred to p22 and p10 until the class II associated peptide (CLIP) is generated by cathepsin S. The CLIP peptide is removed and class II peptides are optimized by the activity of HLA-DM. MHC class II peptides are generated from extracellular antigens either by receptor-mediated or phagocytic uptake into the endocytic/phagocytic pathway. MHC class II associated peptides are generated by lysosomal proteases depicted by cathepsins B, D, E, G, L, GILT, and AEP. These proteases are depicted within phagosomes for simplicity of the schematic. On binding peptides, MHC class II molecules transit to the cell surface (double-headed arrow, dotted line) and are recognized by CD4$^+$ T helper cells.

TAP is a heterodimer composed of two subunits, TAP1 and TAP2, which are encoded within the MHC locus. Both TAP subunits are composed of an ER luminal, transmembrane, and cytosolic nucleotide binding domains and are members of the large family of ATP-binding cassette transporters, which are responsible for moving a wide range of substrates across membranes. In the case of TAP, the transmembrane domains form a portal through which peptides transit. Peptides are actively pumped through the portal, into the ER lumen, following the hydrolysis of ATP, which binds to the nucleotide-binding domain [31] (Figures 3.5 and 3.6).

Within the PLC, tapasin is directly conjugated to ERp57 by a disulfide linkage between C95 of tapasin and C57 of ERp57 [32]. This serves to provide structural integrity to tapasin and maintain ERp57 in a particular redox state [17,33,34]. The most important function of the PLC is to allow the acquisition and optimization of the MHC class I peptide cargo before transit to the cell surface. Peptide optimization occurs via a catalytic reaction involving tapasin and potential interactions with the F pocket residues at positions 114 and 116 of the MHC class I H chain [35,36].

PDI, the archetypal member of the PDI family, has also been described to be part of the PLC [37] and has been ascribed a similar function to ERp57, as well as directly binding peptides required for MHC class I loading. How ERp57, PDI, and MHC class I interact within the PLC remains undefined (see Figure 3.4b for proposed models and Figure 3.5).

Calreticulin also plays a key role in allowing MHC class I molecules to acquire an optimal peptide cargo. In the absence of calreticulin, MHC class I molecules are expressed poorly at the cell surface, with a cargo of low-affinity peptides [38]. The precise mechanism of calreticulin activity remains poorly defined, but it could either participate in monitoring peptide-loaded molecules or in actively recruiting and retaining partially folded complexes until optimal peptide loading has been achieved.

The transit and release of MHC class I molecules from the PLC to the cell surface depends on

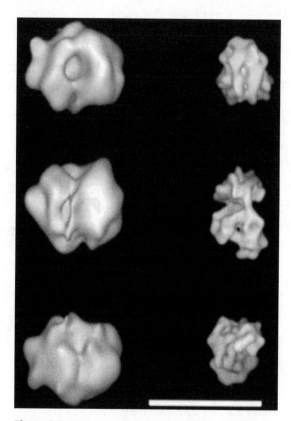

Figure 3.6 TAP structure resolved by single-particle image analysis. The pore-like structure of a detergent-extract immunoaffinity purified TAP particle is shown for three different rotations in the left-hand images [31], whilst a deresolved MHC class I-peptide structure is shown in the right-hand images, with the top panel representing a top view of the peptide-binding groove. Bar = 10 nm. Courtesy of Professor Robert Ford.

both optimal peptide binding and conformational changes within the TAP complex [39] (Figure 3.5). Upon dissociation from TAP, peptide-loaded class I molecules can cluster at ER exit sites, and associate with a putative transport receptor BAP31, a 28 kDa transmembrane protein previously found associated with IgD [40]. These exit sites exclude TAP and tapasin, suggesting that MHC class I ER export is highly regulated and possibly receptor mediated.

The MHC class I cytoplasmic domain can regulate trafficking to and from the cell surface. For instance, HLA-G has a prolonged cell surface half-life, which is due to its truncated cytoplasmic tail domain [41]. Furthermore, endocytosis of cell surface MHC class I molecules requires the cytoplasmic domain and is dependent on a conserved tyrosine (Y) at position 320 [42]. Other trafficking motifs appear to be cell type specific, such as the dihydrophobic leucine/isoleucine (LI) internalization and lysosomal targeting signal located within the HLA-C cytoplasmic domain [43].

MHC class II molecules and the invariant chain

A key difference between MHC class I and II molecule folding within the ER lumen, is that class II molecules associate with the nonpolymorphic Ii chain, a type II transmembrane protein. The Ii chain can exist in several distinct isoforms created by alternative translation initiation and exon splicing (Figure 3.7a). The human Ii chain exists as four different isoforms, p33 (also known as p31), p35, p41, and p45 [44,45], while in the mouse only the p33 and p41 forms have been described, the most common being p33.

MHC class II and Ii chain molecules associate in a trimeric complex consisting of three Ii chain and three MHC class II molecules [46] (Figure 3.7b). An important function of the Ii chain within the ER is to occupy the peptide-binding groove and prevent the possible acquisition of peptides found within the ER, therefore enabling class II molecules to attain peptide in the appropriate endocytic environment [47,48]. Ii chain can direct MHC class II molecules to the correct compartment via a dilysine trafficking motif within its cytoplasmic tail domain [49] (Figure 3.5). Ii chain can control DC motility via interactions with myosin [50], thus coupling Ii chain processing (see below) and antigen presentation to APC motility.

Ii chain must be removed to allow MHC class II molecule peptide loading. Transit through the endocytic pathway exposes the MHC class II/Ii chain complex to proteases that degrade the Ii chain in a stepwise fashion. These same enzymes participate in both the activation of lysosomal proteases and class II peptide generation [51] (Figure 3.5). Thus it is difficult experimentally to dissect the role of proteases in MHC class II antigen presentation.

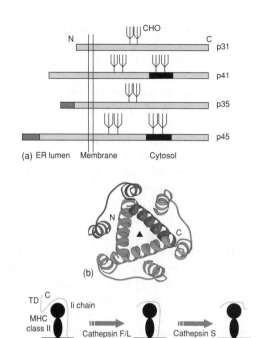

Figure 3.7 Invariant (Ii) chain. (a) The different Ii chain isoforms expressed by human and mouse. The p33 form is 216 amino acids in length and is composed of a 30 amino acid long N-terminal cytoplasmic domain, followed by a 26 amino acid long hydrophobic transmembrane domain and a C-terminal domain of 160 amino acids. Initiation of translation at an alternative upstream AUG codon gives rise to the p35 form, which, as a result, has an additional 16 amino acids at the N terminus. An alternative spliced transcript of an additional exon encodes for p41. The 64 additional residues encode for a cysteine-rich thyroglobulin-like segment, located within the C-terminal luminal region between residues 192 and 193. The p43 form is also generated from the additional exon but includes the N terminal extension. The Ii chain is N-glycosylated (CHO) at positions 114 and 120 in the C-terminal domain. (b) Overhead view of the Ii chain-MHC class II trimer of trimers structure [46]. Reproduced from Jasanoff *et al.* [46] with permission from Nature. (c) Schematic representation of the distinct stages in Ii chain processing. Ii chain trimerizes via the trimerization domain (TD) and associates with three MHC molecules. The initial Ii chain cleavage occurs by an undefined enzymatic activity; however, the generation of the p10/p22 can be governed by cathepsin F in macrophages and cathepsin L in thymic epithelial cells. Cathepsin S is involved in the generation of CLIP.

Ii chain removal from MHC class II molecules occurs in two stages. The first involves the cleavage of Ii chain by the activity of lysosomal proteases and the second involves the displacement of the short fragment that occupies the peptide-binding groove, referred to as the *c*lass II associated *I*i chain *p*eptide (CLIP) (Figure 3.7c).

The removal of Ii chain involves an initial cleavage and the generation of distinct intermediates p22 and p10 before the displacement of CLIP. However, Ii chain degradation remains poorly defined, with the protease initiating the cleavage and the generation of the p22 intermediate remaining unknown. The protease(s) generating the p10 intermediate appears to be cell type specific, involving cathepsin L in thymic epithelium [52] and cathepsin F in macrophages [53], though the latter has yet to be confirmed by gene knockout analysis. Both gene knockout and protease inhibitor studies indicate that cathepsin S can generate the terminal CLIP fragment [54–56] (Figures 3.5 and 3.7c).

The MHC class II peptide loading complex

In order for peptides to associate with MHC class II molecules, the CLIP peptide must be removed. The fact that CLIP removal is a distinct and regulated stage was highlighted by mutant cell lines expressing MHC class II molecules, which associated with Ii chain normally, but were unable to load antigenic peptides [57]. Cell surface MHC class II molecules were found to be predominantly associated with the CLIP peptide [58,59].

Genetic analysis revealed that the defect in these cell lines was attributable to the lack of a molecule referred to as HLA-DM in human or H-2M in mouse. HLA-DM is encoded within the MHC class II locus and is composed of an α and a β chain with similarities to MHC class II molecules [60,61]. HLA-DM does not require peptide for stable expression, can stabilize empty MHC class II molecules, and catalyzes the release of CLIP [62–64]. HLA-DM can catalyze the release of peptides that do not enhance or allow class II molecules to attain appropriate stability [65] and is thought to act by a "compare and exchange" mechanism [66]. This process is known as peptide editing and can be viewed as

the analogous step of MHC class I peptide optimization catalyzed by tapasin [67] (Figure 3.5).

Peptide acquisition and presentation by MHC class II molecules can occur throughout the endocytic pathway. The intersection point between newly synthesized MHC class II molecules and the endocytic location of their peptide acquisition occurs within a distinct cellular compartment known as the MHC class II compartment (MIIC) [68–70].

HLA-DM can associate with HLA-DO, an intracellular MHC class II like αβ heterodimer found in B cells, thymic epithelial cells, and primary DC populations. The precise function of HLA-DO remains undetermined, but it has been suggested to modulate B cell responses by regulating their antigen presentation capacity [71]. Furthermore, HLA-DO can inhibit HLA-DM function at pH levels associated with early endocytic compartments, thus limiting HLA-DM function to the MIIC [72].

Peptide generation

Successful antigen presentation of vaccines will depend on how and where peptides are generated. The cellular localization of MHC class I and II molecules dictates whether peptides are derived endogenously or exogenously, respectively. This division of labor is not always clear cut, especially for MHC class I molecules, which can present peptides from exogenous antigens by a mechanism known as cross-presentation.

Peptide generation in the MHC class I pathway

Proteasome structure and function

MHC class I molecules bind short peptides, generated by the multicatalytic activity of the proteasome in the cytosol (Figure 3.5). The main source of peptides are protein substrates targeted for degradation by ubiquitination, including those generated by mistranslation from standard open reading frames (referred to as defective ribosomal products [DRiPs]) [73], products translated from alternate reading frames via the use of alternative or downstream initiation codons or stop codon read-through [74].

The proteasome is a cylindrical complex found in all eukaryotes, and, depending on the organism, is composed of 13–28 subunits, ranging from 20 to 30 kDa in size. The proteasome is evolutionarily well conserved throughout eukaryotes, yeast, and Archaebacteria, and exists in different forms, the 19S, 20S, 26S, and immunoproteasome.

Proteasome components are categorized as either α- or β-type subunits. The subunits are stacked in four layers around a hollow cylindrical structure [75]. The α subunits make up the two outer rings and are involved in assembly and regulation. The β-type subunits make up the two inner rings and are involved in the generation of proteolytic active sites, which can cleave substrates after acidic, hydrophobic, or basic residues. Together the α and β subunits form the 20S core cylindrical structure. The attachment of the 19S cap (also known as the PA700 regulator) to either end of the 20S structure makes up the 26S form and confers ubiquitin- and ATP- dependent degradative activities of protein substrates [26].

The immunoproteasome

Upon stimulation with IFN-γ, three specific constitutive 20S β subunits, Y/δ, X/MB1, and Z/MC14, can be replaced with the low molecular weight proteins (LMP) -2 and -7, whose genes map between TAP-1 and -2 within the MHC locus and the non-MHC encoded multicatalytic endopeptidase complex-like (MECL) -1 subunit. These latter β subunits, together with the IFN-γ inducible proteasome regulators PA28a and b, which associate with the 20S proteasome, come together and form the immunoproteasome.

The proteasome can generate peptides of varying lengths but with fixed C termini [76]. In the presence of IFN-γ, the cleavage site preference but not the cleavage site itself can change, with chymotrypsin (a measure of cleavage preference of large hydrophobic side chains of phenylalanine, tyrosine, and tryptophan) and trypsin (a measure of cleavage at amino acids lysine and arginine) activities being enhanced. The PA28 regulator appears to be necessary for incorporating the LMP-2, -7, and MECL-1 subunits, with the latter depending on LMP-2 incorporation [77]. However, the bulk

of MHC ligands can be generated in the absence of LMP-2, -7, and MECL-1 [78–80]. These IFN-γ inducible subunits can affect the CD8+ T cell repertoire, MHC class I cell surface expression, and the generation of some peptides. As PA28 can affect all three of these subunits, its absence can lead to altered antigen processing of specific endogenous and viral associated peptides, and leads to MHC class I molecules being loaded with low-affinity peptides [77].

A more complex form of peptide generation has also been attributed to the proteasome. Certain peptides can be generated by ligation of two distal protein sequences [81]. The frequency of such events remains undetermined but may be a further consideration in the hunt for immunogenic peptides and their incorporation into vaccines (see Chapter 9).

Peptide proteolysis

The cytoplasmically located tripeptidyl peptidase II (TPPII) enzyme has been proposed to act in concert with the proteasome by generating MHC class I peptides [82]. TPPII can N-terminally trim peptides 14 amino acids in length or longer, but it remains undetermined whether this proteolytic activity is a main contributor to MHC class I binding ligands [83].

Peptides of varying lengths can be translocated into the ER by TAP. Though their C termini are predominantly fixed and hydrophobic in nature, the N termini can vary, thus requiring further trimming. Several enzymes are thought to generate the appropriate N terminus. The best described is the IFN-γ inducible endoplasmic reticulum associated amino peptidase (ERAAP, also referred to as ERAP1) [84–86]. ERAAP activity is sensitive to N-terminal flanking residues, especially to X-proline bonds, which are resistant to ERAAP cleavage [87]. Other residues located throughout the peptide itself can influence ERAAP activity [88], and MHC class I molecules themselves may contribute to ERAAP activity by regulating the generation of the final peptide [89] (Figure 3.5). In human cell lines, a second aminopeptidase, known as ERAP2, can act in concert with ERAAP [90]. Peptides can be categorized as ERAAP independent,

dependent, or sensitive; that is, those destroyed by ERAAP activity [91]. Thus, the above would suggest that presentation of peptide-based vaccines, such as those proposed to combat HIV, may be sensitive to both surrounding and internal sequences of target peptides.

Peptide generation in the MHC class II pathway

Proteases in the MHC class II pathway

Peptide generation within the endocytic pathway is governed by a number of different enzymes, which must strike a balance between antigen destruction and immunogenic peptide production. Underlying mechanisms of antigen unfolding and peptide generation remain poorly defined. The aspartate endoprotease cathepsin D and a subset of endosomal cysteine proteases, which include cathepsins B, C, H, S, and X (also known as Z), appear to be constitutively expressed in all APCs. Some of these APC-associated cathepsins are not uniformly distributed throughout the endosomal pathway. For instance, cathepsin B is concentrated in early endosomes, while cathepsin S can be found throughout the endocytic pathway, but mainly in MHC class II and HLA-DM-rich compartments [92]. Proteolytic activity can be enhanced or suppressed by pro- and anti-inflammatory cytokines, respectively [93], with certain cytokines altering the peptide presentation capacity of APCs [94].

Cathepsin S has been widely implicated in antigen processing but a direct role in this process is difficult to dissect from its effects on Ii chain processing [95]. However, two proteases, asparaginyl endopeptidase (AEP) and interferon-gamma (γ) inducible lysosomal thiol reductase (GILT), have defined requirements and can control proteolysis of specific antigens. GILT is important in unfolding disulfide bond-containing antigens [96]. AEP cleaves at asparagine residues and was demonstrated to be important in unlocking antigenic peptides from the asparagine-rich antigen, tetanus toxin C fragment [97]. These two examples illustrate the importance of protein sequence in determining antigen processing, but also demonstrate that some antigens can exhibit an apparent bias for

specific proteases. This was further illustrated for the candidate multiple sclerosis associated myelin basic protein autoantigen, whose processing is controlled by cathepsin G, a serine protease released by granulocytes and monocytes and found at the cell surface of B cells [98]. However, most antigens described to date do not depend on single enzymes to generate immunogenic peptides.

Antigen modifications

Exogenous antigen uptake by APCs can occur by phagocytic processes and receptor-mediated uptake. Autophagy, a degradative mechanism used by cells to degrade cytoplasmic proteins and organelles during maintenance of cellular homeostasis, can contribute to MHC class II associated peptides [99]. Antigen proteolysis may differ depending on uptake, protease content, and receptor associations. For instance, receptor-mediated uptake can directly influence the degradation of antigen as the complex of receptor-ligand creates a different protein substrate. This was illustrated for Ig binding of tetanus toxin, which can both enhance and suppress T cell epitope presentation [100].

Post-translational modifications can be detected on both MHC class I and II associated peptides, such as O-linked glycosylation, while phosphorylated peptides can be predominantly found on MHC class I associated peptides [101]. In some instances modifications can affect peptide presentation such as deamidation of asparagines residues to aspartic or iso-aspartic acid. These modifications can affect processing or generate a T-cell response specific to the modified peptide [102]. Modifications can occur during the inflammatory process; for instance, the production of inducible nitric oxide synthase (iNOS) can lead to the release of oxygen reactive species. Nitric oxide and superoxide can form peroxynitrite, which can cause the formation of 3-nitrotyrosine, leading to enhanced peptide presentation [103].

Cross- and criss-cross presentation

The conventional paradigm of MHC class I antigen presentation when applied to peptide generation from endogenous proteins would appear particularly potent against viral- and tumor-derived peptides. This pathway can be exploited by virus-based vaccines (see Chapters 15 and 16) such as those incorporating integrating lentiviral vectors [104]. However, many successful vaccines use attenuated pathogens to elicit an effective protective response. The generation of antibody and CD4+ T helper responses makes biological sense with respect to exogenous antigen presentation by MHC class II molecules. However, to generate an effective CD8+ T-cell response, exogenous antigens must access MHC class I molecules, which occurs via a distinct pathway referred to as cross-presentation [105].

Cross-presentation is restricted to bone marrow derived APCs such as DCs and macrophages. If cross-presentation were a ubiquitous process performed by all MHC class I expressing cells, the immune system would be unable to discriminate between healthy and unhealthy cells. Several routes for cross-presentation have been described, reflecting the cell type, antigen, and route of entry.

An important development in the study of cross-presentation was the description that antigen internalized via phagolysosomes (specialized acidified vesicles) could be presented by MHC class I molecules [106–108]. Phagocytosed antigens can enter the cytosol, possibly via the Sec61 translocation machinery, be degraded by the proteasome, and be transported back into phagosomes via the TAP complex [109]. Most PLC components can be found within the phagolysosome, and peptide-MHC class I complexes can be generated within this compartment [106,107]. Antigens can be internalized via endosomal compartments, transported to the ER, followed by translocation into the cytosol for degradation and subsequent TAP transport [110]. Alternatively, MHC class I molecules can present peptides generated directly within the endocytic pathway [111], which can involve cysteine proteases such as cathepsin S [112]. A "criss-cross" pathway of presentation has been described, whereby peptide from one cell can cross over through gap junctions and be presented by neighboring cells [113]. Though potentially healthy cells would be at risk from immune destruction by this latter pathway, this may act to limit the spread of infection.

Not only do there appear to be multiple cellular pathways governing cross-presentation, but these pathways can be enhanced by innate immune responses to pathogens, such as the production of interferon-α/β during viral infection [114], and can differ between cell types [115]. DCs are not a homogenous population but can be categorized into distinct subsets, of which some seem to be especially efficient at cross-presentation. For instance, CD8α^+, rather than CD8α^-, DCs are more efficient at cross-presenting particulate or soluble antigens [116], but both can cross-present antigen following activation via the Fcγ receptor [117].

Thus antigen processing and presentation pathways are not ubiquitous among APCs, and cell-type targeting in vaccination protocols must be a careful consideration as this can lead to both effective [118] and non-effective immunization [119].

Summary

The expanding knowledge of the mechanics of antigen processing and presentation could well be used as a template for future vaccine design, especially for the generation of recombinant protein- and peptide-based vaccines. One area of intensive research is the development of an effective anti-HIV vaccine. One approach has been to generate vaccines directed against multiple MHC class I peptides. An important recent study demonstrated how each stage in the MHC class I processing and presentation pathway not only affected peptide presentation from HIV, but also determined the hierarchy of peptide generation [120]. From protein sequences, to cell type and cellular location, these parameters will have a bearing on effective peptide presentation. Though many of the key stages in peptide generation have been uncovered, other areas remain poorly understood. For example, it remains undetermined how the kinetics of peptide presentation relate to the overall protein structure and how antigens can be altered during the inflammatory response, which is an important step in recruiting the appropriate immune effector cells.

Acknowledgments

Antony N. Antoniou is supported by an ARC UK Fellowship (15293). Izabela Lenart is supported by an Arthritis Research Campaign (ARC) studentship (17868). David Guiliano is supported by an ARC UK project grant (17222). The authors would like to thank Ms Zofia Prokopowicz for advice and critical evaluation.

References

1 Bjorkman PJ, Saper MA, Samraoui B, et al. Structure of the human class I histocompatibility antigen, HLA-A2. *Nature* 1987;**329**(6139):506–12.

2 Brown JH, Jardetzky TS, Gorga JC, et al. Three-dimensional structure of the human class II histocompatibility antigen HLA-DR1. *Nature* 1993;**364** (6432):33–9.

3 Madden DR, Gorga JC, Strominger JL, Wiley DC. The structure of HLA-B27 reveals nonamer self-peptides bound in an extended conformation. *Nature* 1991;**353**(6342):321–5.

4 Fabian H, Huser H, Narzi D, et al. HLA-B27 subtypes differentially associated with disease exhibit conformational differences in solution. *J Mol Biol* 2008;**376**(3):798–810.

5 Jardetzky TS, Gorga JC, Busch R, et al. Peptide binding to HLA-DR1: a peptide with most residues substituted to alanine retains MHC binding. *EMBO J* 1990;**9**(6):1797–803.

6 Feder JN, Gnirke A, Thomas W, et al. A novel MHC class I-like gene is mutated in patients with hereditary haemochromatosis. *Nat Genet* 1996; **13**(4):399–408.

7 Feder JN, Penny DM, Irrinki A, et al. The hemochromatosis gene product complexes with the transferrin receptor and lowers its affinity for ligand binding. *Proc Natl Acad Sci U S A* 1998;**95**(4):1472–7.

8 O'Callaghan CA, Tormo J, Willcox BE, et al. Structural features impose tight peptide binding specificity in the nonclassical MHC molecule HLA-E. *Mol Cell* 1998;**1**(4):531–41.

9 Clements CS, Kjer-Nielsen L, Kostenko L, et al. Crystal structure of HLA-G: a nonclassical MHC class I molecule expressed at the fetal-maternal interface. *Proc Natl Acad Sci U S A* 2005;**102**(9):3360–65.

10 Braud VM, Allan DS, Wilson D, McMichael AJ. TAP- and tapasin-dependent HLA-E surface expression correlates with the binding of an MHC class I leader peptide. *Curr Biol* 1998;**8**(1):1–10.

11 Aldrich CJ, DeCloux A, Woods AS, et al. Identification of a Tap-dependent leader peptide recognized by alloreactive T cells specific for a class Ib antigen. *Cell* 1994;**79**(4):649–58.

12 Michaelsson J, Teixeira de Matos C, Achour A, et al. A signal peptide derived from hsp60 binds HLA-E and interferes with CD94/NKG2A recognition. *J Exp Med* 2002;**196**(11):1403–14.

13 Shawar SM, Vyas JM, Rodgers JR, Rich RR. Antigen presentation by major histocompatibility complex class I-B molecules. *Annu Rev Immunol* 1994;**12**: 839–80.

14 Porcelli SA, Modlin RL. The CD1 system: antigen-presenting molecules for T cell recognition of lipids and glycolipids. *Annu Rev Immunol* 1999;**17**: 297–329.

15 Kang SJ, Cresswell P. Regulation of intracellular trafficking of human CD1d by association with MHC class II molecules. *EMBO J* 2002;**21**(7):1650–60.

16 Sugita M, Jackman RM, van Donselaar E, et al. Cytoplasmic tail-dependent localization of CD1b antigen-presenting molecules to MIICs. *Science* 1996; **273**(5273):349–52.

17 Im JS, Arora P, Bricard G, et al. Kinetics and cellular site of glycolipid loading control the outcome of natural killer T cell activation. *Immunity* 2009;**30**(6):888–98.

18 Koch M, Stronge VS, Shepherd D, et al. The crystal structure of human CD1d with and without alpha-galactosylceramide. *Nat Immunol* 2005;**6**(8): 819–26.

19 Zajonc DM, Cantu C, 3rd, Mattner J, et al. Structure and function of a potent agonist for the semi-invariant natural killer T cell receptor. *Nat Immunol* 2005;**6**(8):810–18.

20 Antoniou AN, Powis SJ, Elliott T. Assembly and export of MHC class I peptide ligands. *Curr Opin Immunol* 2003;**15**(1):75–81.

21 Degen E, Cohen-Doyle MF, Williams DB. Efficient dissociation of the p88 chaperone from major histocompatibility complex class I molecules requires both beta 2- microglobulin and peptide. *J Exp Med* 1992;**175**(6):1653–61.

22 Zhang Q, Tector M, Salter RD. Calnexin recognizes carbohydrate and protein determinants of class I major histocompatibility complex molecules. *J Biol Chem* 1995;**270**(8):3944–8.

23 Antoniou AN, Santos SG, Campbell EC, et al. ERp57 interacts with conserved cysteine residues in the

MHC class I peptide-binding groove. *FEBS Lett* 2007; **581**(10):1988–92.

24 Antoniou AN, Ford S, Alphey M, *et al.* The oxidoreductase ERp57 efficiently reduces partially folded in preference to fully folded MHC class I molecules. *EMBO J* 2002;**21**(11):2655–63.

25 Hughes EA, Hammond C, Cresswell P. Misfolded major histocompatibility complex class I heavy chains are translocated into the cytoplasm and degraded by the proteasome. *Proc Natl Acad Sci U S A* 1997;**94**(5):1896–901.

26 Hershko A, Ciechanover A. The ubiquitin system. *Annu Rev Biochem* 1998;**67**: 425–79.

27 Sadasivan B, Lehner PJ, Ortmann B, Spies T, Cresswell P. Roles for calreticulin and a novel glycoprotein, tapasin, in the interaction of MHC class I molecules with TAP. *Immunity* 1996;**5**(2):103–14.

28 Frickel EM, Riek R, Jelesarov I, *et al.* TROSY-NMR reveals interaction between ERp57 and the tip of the calreticulin P-domain. *Proc Natl Acad Sci U S A* 2002;**99**(4):1954–9.

29 Oliver JD, Roderick HL, Llewellyn DH, High S. ERp57 functions as a subunit of specific complexes formed with the ER lectins calreticulin and calnexin. *Mol Biol Cell* 1999;**10**(8):2573–82.

30 Ortmann B, Copeman J, Lehner PJ, *et al.* A critical role for tapasin in the assembly and function of multimeric MHC class I-TAP complexes. *Science* 1997;**277**(5330):1306–9.

31 Velarde G, Ford RC, Rosenberg MF, Powis SJ. Three-dimensional structure of transporter associated with antigen processing (TAP) obtained by single particle image analysis. *J Biol Chem* 2001;**276**(49):46054–63.

32 Dick TP, Bangia N, Peaper DR, Cresswell P. Disulfide bond isomerization and the assembly of MHC class I-peptide complexes. *Immunity* 2002;**16**(1):87–98.

33 Peaper DR, Cresswell P. The redox activity of ERp57 is not essential for its functions in MHC class I peptide loading. *Proc Natl Acad Sci U S A* 2008; **105**(30):10477–82.

34 Peaper DR, Wearsch PA, Cresswell P. Tapasin and ERp57 form a stable disulfide-linked dimer within the MHC class I peptide-loading complex. *EMBO J* 2005;**24**(20):3613–23.

35 Williams AP, Peh CA, Purcell AW, McCluskey J, Elliott T. Optimization of the MHC class I peptide cargo is dependent on tapasin. *Immunity* 2002; **16**(4):509–20.

36 Chen M, Bouvier M. Analysis of interactions in a tapasin/class I complex provides a mechanism for peptide selection. *EMBO J* 2007;**26**(6):1681–90.

37 Park B, Lee S, Kim E, *et al.* Redox regulation facilitates optimal peptide selection by MHC class I during antigen processing. *Cell* 2006;**127**(2):369–82.

38 Gao B, Adhikari R, Howarth M, *et al.* Assembly and antigen-presenting function of MHC class I molecules in cells lacking the ER chaperone calreticulin. *Immunity* 2002;**16**(1):99–109.

39 Knittler MR, Alberts P, Deverson EV, Howard JC. Nucleotide binding by TAP mediates association with peptide and release of assembled MHC class I molecules. *Curr Biol* 1999;**9**(18):999–1008.

40 Adachi T, Schamel WW, Kim KM, *et al.* The specificity of association of the IgD molecule with the accessory proteins BAP31/BAP29 lies in the IgD transmembrane sequence. *EMBO J* 1996;**15**(7):1534–41.

41 Park B, Lee S, Kim E, *et al.* The truncated cytoplasmic tail of HLA-G serves a quality-control function in post-ER compartments. *Immunity* 2001;**15**(2): 213–24.

42 Santos SG, Antoniou AN, Sampaio P, Powis SJ, Arosa FA. Lack of tyrosine 320 impairs spontaneous endocytosis and enhances release of HLA-B27 molecules. *J Immunol* 2006;**176**(5):2942–9.

43 Schaefer MR, Williams M, Kulpa DA, *et al.* A novel trafficking signal within the HLA-C cytoplasmic tail allows regulated expression upon differentiation of macrophages. *J Immunol* 2008;**180**(12):7804–17.

44 Strubin M, Berte C, Mach B. Alternative splicing and alternative initiation of translation explain the four forms of the Ia antigen-associated invariant chain. *EMBO J* 1986;**5**(13):3483–8.

45 O'Sullivan DM, Noonan D, Quaranta V. Four Ia invariant chain forms derive from a single gene by alternate splicing and alternate initiation of transcription/translation. *J Exp Med* 1987;**166**(2):444–60.

46 Jasanoff A, Wagner G, Wiley DC. Structure of a trimeric domain of the MHC class II-associated chaperonin and targeting protein Ii. *EMBO J* 1998; **17**(23):6812–18.

47 Busch R, Cloutier I, Sekaly RP, Hammerling GJ. Invariant chain protects class II histocompatibility antigens from binding intact polypeptides in the endoplasmic reticulum. *EMBO J* 1996;**15**(2):418–28.

48 Bijlmakers MJ, Benaroch P, Ploegh HL. Assembly of HLA DR1 molecules translated in vitro: binding of peptide in the endoplasmic reticulum precludes association with invariant chain. *EMBO J* 1994;**13**(11):2699–707.

49 Bakke O, Dobberstein B. MHC class II-associated invariant chain contains a sorting signal for endosomal compartments. *Cell* 1990;**63**(4):707–16.

50 Faure-Andre G, Vargas P, Yuseff MI, *et al.* Regulation of dendritic cell migration by CD74, the MHC class II-associated invariant chain. *Science* 2008; **322**(5908):1705–10.

51 Jensen PE. Recent advances in antigen processing and presentation. *Nat Immunol* 2007;**8**(10):1041–8.

52 Nakagawa T, Roth W, Wong P, *et al.* Cathepsin L: critical role in Ii degradation and CD4 T cell selection in the thymus. *Science* 1998;**280**(5362):450–53.

53 Shi GP, Bryant RA, Riese R, *et al.* Role for cathepsin F in invariant chain processing and major histocompatibility complex class II peptide loading by macrophages. *J Exp Med* 2000;**191**(7):1177–86.

54 Riese RJ, Wolf PR, Bromme D, *et al.* Essential role for cathepsin S in MHC class II-associated invariant chain processing and peptide loading. *Immunity* 1996;**4**(4):357–66.

55 Shi GP, Villadangos JA, Dranoff G, *et al.* Cathepsin S required for normal MHC class II peptide loading and germinal center development. *Immunity* 1999;**10**(2):197–206.

56 Nakagawa TY, Brissette WH, Lira PD, *et al.* Impaired invariant chain degradation and antigen presentation and diminished collagen-induced arthritis in cathepsin S null mice. *Immunity* 1999;**10**(2):207–17.

57 Fling SP, Arp B, Pious D. HLA-DMA and -DMB genes are both required for MHC class II/peptide complex formation in antigen-presenting cells. *Nature* 1994;**368**(6471):554–8.

58 Mellins E, Kempin S, Smith L, Monji T, Pious D. A gene required for class II-restricted antigen presentation maps to the major histocompatibility complex. *J Exp Med* 1991;**174**(6):1607–15.

59 Sette A, Ceman S, Kubo RT, *et al.* Invariant chain peptides in most HLA-DR molecules of an antigen-processing mutant. *Science* 1992;**258**(5089):1801–4.

60 Fremont DH, Crawford F, Marrack P, Hendrickson WA, Kappler J. Crystal structure of mouse H2-M. *Immunity* 1998;**9**(3):385–93.

61 Mosyak L, Zaller DM, Wiley DC. The structure of HLA-DM, the peptide exchange catalyst that loads antigen onto class II MHC molecules during antigen presentation. *Immunity* 1998;**9**(3):377–83.

62 Denzin LK, Cresswell P. HLA-DM induces CLIP dissociation from MHC class II alpha beta dimers and facilitates peptide loading. *Cell* 1995;**82**(1):155–65.

63 Sloan VS, Cameron P, Porter G, *et al.* Mediation by HLA-DM of dissociation of peptides from HLA-DR. *Nature* 1995;**375**(6534):802–6.

64 Sherman MA, Weber DA, Jensen PE. DM enhances peptide binding to class II MHC by release of invariant chain-derived peptide. *Immunity* 1995;**3**(2):197–205.

65 Weber DA, Evavold BD, Jensen PE. Enhanced dissociation of HLA-DR-bound peptides in the presence of HLA-DM. *Science* 1996;**274**(5287):618–20.

66 Ferrante A, Anderson MW, Klug CS, Gorski J. HLA-DM mediates epitope selection by a "compare-exchange" mechanism when a potential peptide pool is available. *PLoS One* 2008;**3**(11):e3722.

67 Sadegh-Nasseri S, Chen M, Narayan K, Bouvier M. The convergent roles of tapasin and HLA-DM in antigen presentation. *Trends Immunol* 2008;**29**(3): 141–7.

68 West MA, Lucocq JM, Watts C. Antigen processing and class II MHC peptide-loading compartments in human B-lymphoblastoid cells. *Nature* 1994; **369**(6476):147–51.

69 Tulp A, Verwoerd D, Dobberstein B, Ploegh HL, Pieters J. Isolation and characterization of the intracellular MHC class II compartment [see comments]. *Nature* 1994;**369**(6476):120–26.

70 Qiu Y, Xu X, Wandinger-Ness A, Dalke DP, Pierce SK. Separation of subcellular compartments containing distinct functional forms of MHC class II. *J Cell Biol* 1994;**125**(3):595–605.

71 Glazier KS, Hake SB, Tobin HM, *et al.* Germinal center B cells regulate their capability to present antigen by modulation of HLA-DO. *J Exp Med* 2002; **195**(8):1063–9.

72 van Ham M, van Lith M, Lillemeier B, *et al.* Modulation of the major histocompatibility complex class II-associated peptide repertoire by human histocompatibility leukocyte antigen (HLA)-DO. *J Exp Med* 2000;**191**(7):1127–36.

73 Schubert U, Anton LC, Gibbs J, *et al.* Rapid degradation of a large fraction of newly synthesized proteins by proteasomes. *Nature* 2000;**404**(6779):770–74.

74 Zook MB, Howard MT, Sinnathamby G, Atkins JF, Eisenlohr LC. Epitopes derived by incidental translational frameshifting give rise to a protective CTL response. *J Immunol* 2006;**176**(11):6928–34.

75 Baumeister W, Walz J, Zuhl F, Seemuller E. The proteasome: paradigm of a self-compartmentalizing protease. *Cell* 1998;**92**(3):367–80.

76 Craiu A, Akopian T, Goldberg A, Rock KL. Two distinct proteolytic processes in the generation of a major histocompatibility complex class I-presented peptide. *Proc Natl Acad Sci U S A* 1997;**94**(20):10850–55.

77 Preckel T, Fung-Leung WP, Cai Z, *et al.* Impaired immunoproteasome assembly and immune responses in PA28$^{-/-}$ mice. *Science* 1999;**286**(5447):2162–5.

78 Van Kaer L, Ashton-Rickardt PG, Eichelberger M, *et al.* Altered peptidase and viral-specific T cell response in LMP2 mutant mice. *Immunity* 1994;**1**(7): 533–41.

79 Fehling HJ, Swat W, Laplace C, *et al.* MHC class I expression in mice lacking the proteasome subunit LMP-7. *Science* 1994;**265**(5176):1234–7.

80 Basler M, Moebius J, Elenich L, Groettrup M, Monaco JJ. An altered T cell repertoire in MECL-1-deficient mice. *J Immunol* 2006;**176**(11):6665–72.

81 Vigneron N, Stroobant V, Chapiro J, *et al.* An antigenic peptide produced by peptide splicing in the proteasome. *Science* 2004;**304**(5670):587–90.

82 Reits E, Neijssen J, Herberts C, *et al.* A major role for TPPII in trimming proteasomal degradation products for MHC class I antigen presentation. *Immunity* 2004;**20**(4):495–506.

83 York IA, Bhutani N, Zendzian S, Goldberg AL, Rock KL. Tripeptidyl peptidase II is the major peptidase needed to trim long antigenic precursors, but is not required for most MHC class I antigen presentation. *J Immunol* 2006;**177**(3):1434–43.

84 York IA, Chang SC, Saric T, et al. The ER aminopeptidase ERAP1 enhances or limits antigen presentation by trimming epitopes to 8–9 residues. *Nat Immunol* 2002;**3**(12):1177–84.

85 Saric T, Chang SC, Hattori A, *et al.* An IFN-gamma-induced aminopeptidase in the ER, ERAP1, trims precursors to MHC class I-presented peptides. *Nat Immunol* 2002;**3**(12):1169–76.

86 Serwold T, Gonzalez F, Kim J, Jacob R, Shastri N. ERAAP customizes peptides for MHC class I molecules in the endoplasmic reticulum. *Nature* 2002;**419**(6906):480–83.

87 Serwold T, Gaw S, Shastri N. ER aminopeptidases generate a unique pool of peptides for MHC class I molecules. *Nat Immunol* 2001;**2**(7):644–51.

88 Chang SC, Momburg F, Bhutani N, Goldberg AL. The ER aminopeptidase, ERAP1, trims precursors to lengths of MHC class I peptides by a "molecular ruler" mechanism. *Proc Natl Acad Sci U S A* 2005; **102**(47):17107–12.

89 Kanaseki T, Blanchard N, Hammer GE, Gonzalez F, Shastri N. ERAAP synergizes with MHC class I molecules to make the final cut in the antigenic peptide precursors in the endoplasmic reticulum. *Immunity* 2006;**25**(5):795–806.

90 Saveanu L, Carroll O, Lindo V, *et al.* Concerted peptide trimming by human ERAP1 and ERAP2 aminopeptidase complexes in the endoplasmic reticulum. *Nat Immunol* 2005;**6**(7):689–97.

91 Hammer GE, Kanaseki T, Shastri N. The final touches make perfect the peptide-MHC class I repertoire. *Immunity* 2007;**26**(4):397–406.

92 Lautwein A, Kraus M, Reich M, *et al.* Human B lymphoblastoid cells contain distinct patterns of cathepsin activity in endocytic compartments and regulate MHC class II transport in a cathepsin S-independent manner. *J Leukoc Biol* 2004;**75**(5):844–55.

93 Fiebiger E, Meraner P, Weber E, *et al.* Cytokines regulate proteolysis in major histocompatibility complex class II-dependent antigen presentation by dendritic cells. *J Exp Med* 2001;**193**: 881–92.

94 Drakesmith H, O'Neil D, Schneider SC, *et al.* In vivo priming of T cells against cryptic determinants by dendritic cells exposed to interleukin 6 and native antigen. *Proc Natl Acad Sci U S A* 1998; **95**(25):14903–8.

95 Hsieh CS, deRoos P, Honey K, Beers C, Rudensky AY. A role for cathepsin L and cathepsin S in peptide generation for MHC class II presentation. *J Immunol* 2002;**168**(6):2618–25.

96 Maric M, Arunachalam B, Phan UT, *et al.* Defective antigen processing in GILT-free mice. *Science* 2001;**294**(5545):1361–5.

97 Antoniou AN, Blackwood SL, Mazzeo D, Watts C. Control of antigen presentation by a single protease cleavage site. *Immunity* 2000;**12**(4):391–8.

98 Burster T, Beck A, Tolosa E, *et al.* Cathepsin G, and not the asparagine-specific endoprotease, controls the processing of myelin basic protein in lysosomes from human B lymphocytes. *J Immunol* 2004;**172**(9):5495–503.

99 Schmid D, Pypaert M, Munz C. Antigen-loading compartments for major histocompatibility complex class II molecules continuously receive input from autophagosomes. *Immunity* 2007;**26**(1):79–92.

100 Simitsek PD, Campbell DG, Lanzavecchia A, Fairweather N, Watts C. Modulation of antigen processing by bound antibodies can boost or suppress class II major histocompatibility complex presentation of different T cell determinants. *J Exp Med* 1995; **181**(6):1957–63.

101 Engelhard VH, Altrich-Vanlith M, Ostankovitch M, Zarling AL. Post-translational modifications of naturally processed MHC-binding epitopes. *Curr Opin Immunol* 2006;**18**(1):92–7.

102 McAdam SN, Fleckenstein B, Rasmussen IB, *et al.* T cell recognition of the dominant I-A(k)-restricted hen egg lysozyme epitope: critical role for asparagine deamidation. *J Exp Med* 2001;**193**(11): 1239–46.

103 Birnboim HC, Lemay AM, Lam DK, Goldstein R, Webb JR. MHC class II-restricted peptides containing the inflammation-associated marker 3-nitrotyrosine evade central tolerance and elicit a robust cell-mediated immune response. *J Immunol* 2003;**171**(2): 528–32.

104 Breckpot K, Emeagi PU, Thielemans K. Lentiviral vectors for anti-tumor immunotherapy. *Curr Gene Ther* 2008;**8**(6):438–48.

105 Rock KL, Shen L. Cross-presentation: underlying mechanisms and role in immune surveillance. *Immunol Rev* 2005;**207**: 166–83.

106 Gagnon E, Duclos S, Rondeau C, *et al.* Endoplasmic reticulum-mediated phagocytosis is a mechanism of entry into macrophages. *Cell* 2002;**110**(1):119–31.

107 Guermonprez P, Saveanu L, Kleijmeer M, *et al.* ER-phagosome fusion defines an MHC class I cross-presentation compartment in dendritic cells. *Nature* 2003;**425**(6956):397–402.

108 Houde M, Bertholet S, Gagnon E, *et al.* Phagosomes are competent organelles for antigen cross-presentation. *Nature* 2003;**425**(6956):402–6.

109 Wiertz EJ, Tortorella D, Bogyo M, *et al.* Sec61-mediated transfer of a membrane protein from the endoplasmic reticulum to the proteasome for destruction [see comments]. *Nature* 1996;**384**(6608): 432–8.

110 Ackerman AL, Kyritsis C, Tampe R, Cresswell P. Access of soluble antigens to the endoplasmic reticulum can explain cross-presentation by dendritic cells. *Nat Immunol* 2005;**6**(1):107–13.

111 Di Pucchio T, Chatterjee B, Smed-Sorensen A, *et al.* Direct proteasome-independent cross-presentation of viral antigen by plasmacytoid dendritic cells on major histocompatibility complex class I. *Nat Immunol* 2008;**9**(5):551–7.

112 Shen L, Sigal LJ, Boes M, Rock KL. Important role of cathepsin S in generating peptides for TAP-independent MHC class I crosspresentation in vivo. *Immunity* 2004;**21**(2):155–65.

113 Neijssen J, Herberts C, Drijfhout JW, *et al.* Cross-presentation by intercellular peptide transfer through gap junctions. *Nature* 2005;**434**(7029): 83–8.

114 Le Bon A, Etchart N, Rossmann C, *et al.* Cross-priming of CD8+ T cells stimulated by virus-induced type I interferon. *Nat Immunol* 2003;**4**(10):1009–15.

115 Dudziak D, Kamphorst AO, Heidkamp GF, *et al.* Differential antigen processing by dendritic cell subsets in vivo. *Science* 2007;**315**(5808):107–11.

116 den Haan JM, Lehar SM, Bevan MJ. CD8(+) but not CD8(-) dendritic cells cross-prime cytotoxic T cells in vivo. *J Exp Med* 2000;**192**(12):1685–96.

117 den Haan JM, Bevan MJ. Constitutive versus activation-dependent cross-presentation of immune complexes by CD8(+) and CD8(-) dendritic cells in vivo. *J Exp Med* 2002;**196**(6):817–27.

118 Lopes L, Dewannieux M, Gileadi U, *et al.* Immunization with a lentivector that targets tumor antigen expression to dendritic cells induces potent CD8+ and CD4+ T-cell responses. *J Virol* 2008;**82**(1):86–95.

119 Follenzi A, Battaglia M, Lombardo A, *et al.* Targeting lentiviral vector expression to hepatocytes limits transgene-specific immune response and establishes long-term expression of human antihemophilic factor IX in mice. *Blood* 2004;**103**(10):3700–709.

120 Tenzer S, Wee E, Burgevin A, *et al.* Antigen processing influences HIV-specific cytotoxic T lymphocyte immunodominance. *Nat Immunol* 2009; **10**(6):636–46.

121 Parham P. Immunology. Deconstructing the MHC. *Nature* 1992;**360**(6402):300–301.

122 Santos SG, Campbell EC, Lynch S, *et al.* MHC class I-ERp57-tapasin interactions within the peptide-loading complex. *J Biol Chem* 2007;**282**: 17587–93.

123 Chambers JE, Jessop CE, Bulleid NJ. Formation of a major histocompatibility complex class I tapasin disulfide indicates a change in spatial organization of the peptide-loading complex during assembly. *J Biol Chem* 2008;**283**(4):862–9.

CHAPTER 4

Understanding the Mucosal Immune System for Better Mucosal Vaccine Design

Janine Bilsborough & Joanne L. Viney
Inflammation Research, Amgen, Thousand Oaks, CA, USA

Introduction

Mucosal surfaces of the respiratory, gastrointestinal, and urogenital tracts constitute an immense surface area that is exposed to a diverse array of antigenic material including both harmful and innocuous environmental substances. Pathogens such as virus, parasites, or bacteria, and for the intestine, beneficial commensal microorganisms and essential dietary proteins can be present at mucosal surfaces. As a consequence to this overwhelming antigenic insult, the mucosal immune system has developed sophisticated immunoregulatory mechanisms to prevent damaging inflammatory responses to harmless antigens. In essence these mechanisms translate to the phenomenon referred to as mucosal tolerance, where delivery of antigen via the mucosal route is poorly immunogenic and can often induce long-lasting systemic antigen-specific hyporesponsiveness [1].

Although essential for the maintenance of healthy mucosal tissues, mucosal tolerance is an obvious impediment to the development of effective mucosal vaccines. To overcome the poor immunogenicity associated with mucosal vaccines many groups have turned to the development of mucosal adjuvants, including bacterial toxins and Toll-like receptor (TLR) ligands or unique delivery systems such as live microbial vectors ([2];

see Chapter 14 for more details). These modifications, however, may carry certain risks such as unwanted immunoresponsiveness to innocuous antigens, resulting in allergies such as celiac disease or asthma, or the possible risk of reversion of modified live vectors to a pathogenic state. Thus a better understanding of the regulatory mechanisms of the mucosal immune system may facilitate the development of more effective and safe mucosal vaccines. To this end, we present an overview of the immunobiology of the mucosal immune system and highlight some of the recent efforts to manipulate this biology for effective mucosal vaccine design.

Anatomy of the mucosal immune system

The common basic architecture of all mucosal sites includes an epithelial barrier that borders mucosal tissues and provides both protection from the external environment and support for the functional integrity of the underlying tissues; the mucosal-associated lymphoreticular tissue (MALT), which is dispersed throughout the tissue beneath the layer of epithelial cells and represents the primary inductive sites for mucosal immunity; the highly organized secondary lymphoid tissues, which serve

---

Vaccinology: Principles and Practice, First Edition. Edited by W. John W. Morrow, Nadeem A. Sheikh, Clint S. Schmidt and D. Huw Davies.
© 2012 Blackwell Publishing Ltd. Published 2012 by Blackwell Publishing Ltd.

to centralize the immune response and protect mucosal tissues from repeated antigenic insult; and the lamina propria, a thin layer of loose connective tissue that lies beneath the epithelium and constitutes the effector site for mucosal immune responsiveness (Figure 4.1). Within this anatomy of the mucosal immune system, various players interact to provide an appropriately balanced response to the plethora of antigens that may be encountered at mucosal surfaces.

Players of the mucosal immune system

Mucosal epithelium

Epithelial cells (ECs) that border the mucosal surfaces serve as the first line of defense for the mucosal immune system. These specialized cells are polarized both physically and functionally. The apical surface (the luminal facing side) of ECs is protected by a glycocalyx coating covered in mucus, while their basolateral side (the side facing the underlying mucosal tissues) is in close contact with mucosal leukocytes. The glycocalyx and mucus coating on the apical surface of ECs comprises glycoproteins, proteoglycans, enzymes, and immunolglobulin (Ig) (primarily of the IgA isotype) and provides host defense, by limiting accessibility of microbes and particulate antigens to EC as well as forming a matrix for antimicrobial peptides [3] and support for nutrient adsorption from the lumen [4].

Far from being a passive barrier to antigens, ECs are acknowledged as active participants in maintaining intestinal homeostasis and directing immune responsiveness to antigen in the face of constant antigen exposure. Under normal, non-inflammatory conditions, ECs are not recognized as professional antigen-presenting cells (APC) due to the absence of the traditional co-stimulatory molecules. However, ECs express both major histocompatability complex (MHC) class I and II antigens on their basolateral side and can uptake, process, and present mostly soluble luminal antigens to antigen-specific lymphocytes within the mucosae (reviewed [5]; see Chapter 3 for more

details). Larger particulate antigens are generally prevented access to ECs by the glycocalyx/mucus coating and will gain entry to the mucosal immune system via specialized ECs known as M cells, which will be described in more detail later in this chapter. ECs can, however, sample particulate luminal bacterial antigens by recycling IgG complex bound to the neonatal Fc receptor (FcRn) and deliver these antigens to professional dendritic cells (DCs) in the underlying lamina propria [6]. Moreover, ECs can support antigen uptake by M cells through secreted IgA. IgA produced in the lamina propria is exported from the basolateral side of epithelium to the intestinal lumen via EC receptor-specific transcytosis through the polymeric immunoglobulin receptor (pIgR) [7]. The pIgR is then cleaved to release soluble IgA (SIgA) with an attached remnant of the pIgR that protects SIgA from the action of proteases in the mucus. This model of SIgA secretion is generally accepted as the means by which both IgA and IgM are exported to the lumen [8]. Thus, ECs are both perfectly positioned and adequately equipped to direct antigen-specific immune responses to luminal antigens.

Within the EC layer, intraepithelial lymphocytes (IEL) are present. In the intestine, these T lymphocytes consist mostly of two populations: traditional CD4$\alpha\beta$ or CD8$\alpha\beta$ T cells expressing the $\alpha\beta$ T cell receptor (TCR), and unconventional IEL cells that express the CD8$\alpha\alpha$ homodimer that express either the $\alpha\beta$ or $\gamma\delta$ TCR (reviewed in [9]). Unconventional IELs are hypothesized to maintain homeostasis and epithelial repair (reviewed in [10]). Traditional CD4$\alpha\beta$ and CD8$\alpha\beta$ T cells can also be found in the lamina propria in close association with EC basolateral projections (reviewed [11]). Similarly, T cells in the lung can be found in close association with squamous type I and cuboidal type II ECs that line the alveolar surface. Unique to the lung, however, is the fact that T cells can be present in the lumen of the airways, closely associated with ECs, but essentially outside the body [12].

Since presentation of antigen to lymphocytes in the absence of co-stimulatory molecules induces tolerance (reviewed [13]), ECs are thought

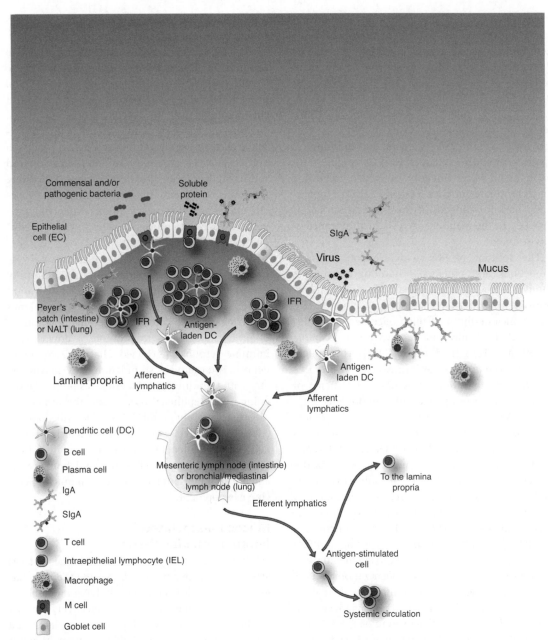

Figure 4.1 Players in the mucosal immune system. The common basic architecture of all mucosal sites includes an epithelial barrier with a mucus coating, the mucosal-associated lymphoreticular tissue (MALT) dispersed throughout the mucosal tissue, for example Peyer's patch (PP) in the small intestine or nasal-associated lymphoreticular tissue (NALT) in the lung with the associated interfollicular region (IFR);

highly organized secondary lymphoid tissue to promote lymphocyte activation and redistribution to appropriate tissues, for example mesenteric lymph node (MLN) in the intestine or bronchial lymph node (BLN) in the lung; and the lamina propria, where effector cells migrate, ready to initiate memory immune responses. Soluble IgA (SIgA) is a hallmark of mucosal immunity and is exported from the lamina propria to the lumen through epithelial cells.

to be a major contributor in driving mucosal hyporesponsiveness. Indeed, recent studies of transgenic mice over-expressing a self-antigen in ECs demonstrated a role for ECs in the development of Foxp3+ T regulatory cells [14]. ECs also express novel class I molecules, including CD1d, which, when ligated, cause IL10 secretion and can counteract the inflammatory effects of IFNγ on barrier function [15]. This dampening of immune responses in mucosal tissues by ECs is important to maintain tissue integrity. However, mounting an appropriate immune response against potentially harmful antigens at the mucosal surface is also key to the maintenance of a healthy mucosal environment.

The aptitude of ECs to differentiate between innocuous and potentially harmful antigens is thought to be, at least in part, due to their expression of pattern recognition receptors (PRR), which include the nucleotide oligomerization domain (NOD) family; protease-activated receptors (PAR); and TLRs (reviewed in [16]). This collection of receptors provides a means by which ECs can respond to various structural components of microorganisms or to enzymatic components of allergens. While nonpathogenic commensal microorganisms also express ligands recognized by PRRs [17], it is hypothesized that ECs can differentiate these from pathogenic microorganisms via the presence of virulence factors, including toxins, invasins, and other adherence factors associated with invasive pathogens. Such pathogen-associated virulence factors contribute to EC attachment, invasion, and replication, thus triggering a PRR-mediated inflammatory response to aid in pathogen clearance [18]. Interestingly, polarization of PRR expression on ECs appears to influence the subsequent response to PRR signaling. In polarized ECs, basolateral but not apical activation of TLR3, TLR5, and TLR9 induced IL8 secretion [19], suggesting that stimulation of TLR at the luminal side of ECs, the side most likely to encounter antigens, was less likely to induce an immune response and perhaps more tolerant of PRR stimulation than the basolateral side, which may indicate pathogen entry into mucosal tissues and a requirement for an immediate immune response.

In addition to PRR-mediated pathogen recognition, polarized compartmentalization of antigen processing by ECs is suggested to be important to the functional outcome of antigen presentation to T cells [20]. This hypothesis proposes that apical and basolateral antigen-processing pathways affect the immunogenicity of antigens. It is proposed that "pathogenic epitopes" within an antigen that normally elicit no significant response when processed apically may be unmasked by internalization and trafficking from the basolateral surface. Processing from the basolateral side would more likely occur under pathological conditions when the antigen gains access to mucosal tissues through "leaky" epithelial tight junctions [20].

One potential mechanism by which mucosal vaccine adjuvants can help induce mucosal immunity is through stimulation of EC PRRs. This activation could result in production of EC-derived cytokines and chemokines to attract and induce maturation of professional APCs to promote a downstream immune response [21] (see Chapter 2 for more details). Alternatively, stimulation of EC may interfere with tight junction integrity, resulting in loosening of the epithelial barrier and the promotion of antigen presentation by ECs as described above. Although the precise mechanism by which mucosal adjuvants can affect ECs directly is unclear, ECs are a key factor for controlling mucosal homeostasis and are an important consideration in mucosal vaccine development.

Mucosal-associated lymphoreticular tissue

While the single layer of ECs at mucosal surfaces acts as a protective barrier to exclude the vast majority of antigens from the underlying mucosal tissue, mucosal inductive sites, collectively known as the mucosal-associated lymphoreticular tissue (MALT), stand as sentinels below the epithelium to quickly mount appropriate immune responses against those antigens that either evade exclusion or are permitted entry (Figure 4.1). The MALT sites do not possess afferent lymphatics, making them distinct from the highly organized structures of the mucosal draining lymph nodes (mDLN). Consequently, the MALT samples antigens directly from the lumen whereas the mDLN generally obtain antigen in the context of immune cells from the draining lymphatics.

The MALT sites are subclassified according to organ and tissue. The tonsils and adenoids compose the nasopharyngeal-associated lymphoreticular tissue (NALT) of the upper airway, and the bronchial-associated lymphoid tissue (BALT) is associated with the airway branches. The gut-associated lymphoreticular tissues (GALT) include the Peyer's patches (PP), which reside in the small intestine, isolated lymphoid follicles (ILF), which are present in both the small and large intestine, and the appendix. The lymphoid tissues of the urogenital tract are more loosely defined and lack organized lymphoid follicles analogous to the PP and it is perhaps this lack of PP that renders vaginal mucosal immune responses unimpressive (reviewed in [22]).

The PP of the gastrointestinal tract has been the most commonly studied MALT. Structurally, PPs are aggregates of B cell rich follicles interspersed with T cell rich interfollicular regions (IFR) capped off or separated from the lumen by a layer of specialized follicle-associated epithelium (FAE) containing a unique population of cells known as M cells (Figure 4.1). M cells are a common feature of the inductive sites of the mucosal immune system and are present in both the gastrointestinal and respiratory tracts [23,24]. Interaction of ECs with lymphocytes *in vitro* can induce the differentiation of M-like cells, highlighting the close relationship between M cell differentiation and EC/lymphocyte interaction (reviewed in [25]). M cells form tight junctions with ECs but lack surface microvilli and have a microfold surface, hence the name. The basolateral membrane of M cells is invaginated to form pockets that harbor B and T cells and occasional DCs (reviewed in [26]). This proximal association supports one of the major functions of M cells: uptake and transport of particulate antigens from the gut lumen to the underlying mucosal immune system. In M cells, unlike most epithelial cells, transepithelial vesicular transport is the major pathway for endocytosed material with little to no material directed to lysosomes and therefore no antigen processing (reviewed in [27]). M cells are also a major site of luminal SIgA uptake, though

the surrounding FAE do not secrete poly IgA (due to lack of pIgR expression), luminal SIgA from ECs adheres selectively to the apical membrane of M cells. SIgA-antigen complexes are transported into the intraepithelial pocket to generate mucosal immune responses. Although M cells are important in sampling luminal antigens for the generation of local immune responses, many microorganisms, including bacteria, parasites, and viruses, can utilize M cells to actively cross the intestinal epithelial barrier to cause infection. Thus the association of M cells with the underlying organized lymphoid structure of the PP and the affiliated DC, B cells, T cells, and macrophages is important to maintain host defense against potential pathogens.

DCs, as professional APCs, are critical for priming naïve T cells and driving the immune responses for mucosal-specific immunity or tolerance at inductive sites. M cells are a major source of antigen uptake for DCs in PPs, though lamina propria DCs are reported to sample luminal antigens via extension of transepithelial dendrites [28,29]. In general, however, antigen acquisition in the PP is thought to be more efficient than antigen acquisition in the lamina propria since prodigious uptake of fluorescent bacteria by PP-derived DCs compared to those from the lamina propria has been demonstrated [30]. DC antigen uptake and activation in the PP results in migration of DCs to the T cell IFR where T cell activation can occur [31]. Antigen-laden DCs can also migrate to the distant mesenteric lymph nodes (MLN) but appear restricted from entering systemic sites such as the spleen, a process thought to limit dissemination of potentially harmful microorganisms [30]. Continuous antigen acquisition by DCs in mucosal tissues and subsequent trafficking to distant lymph nodes monitors the antigenic environment and maintains mucosal tolerance, and occurs even in the absence of inflammation [32].

T cell encounter with antigen-bearing DCs in the mucosal inductive sites can result in multiple outcomes depending on the form of antigen and the "state" or "flavor" of the APC. Particulate antigens such as bacteria, virus, material from dead or dying cells, and immune complexes are thought to be more immunogenic compared to soluble material. Delivery of soluble proteins such as ovalbumin

(OVA) either orally or to the lungs via intranasal or aerosol administration induces antigen-specific systemic T cell tolerance, either through T cell deletion, anergy, or through the differentiation of regulatory T cells (reviewed in [33,34]). Moreover, the diverse array and precise location of DC subsets present in PP, MLN, and intestinal lamina propria may have significance to the outcome of immune responses within mucosal tissues (reviewed [18,35]). Like ECs, mucosal DCs also express PRR but appear either refractory to TLR-ligand engagement [36] or are hard-wired to respond to antigen in a manner that promotes antigen-specific tolerance [37–39]. Under healthy conditions, therefore, the apparent default nature of mucosal DC is tolerance, which restricts the effectiveness of mucosal vaccines.

Studies have shown, however, that mucosal DC can be modulated by proinflammatory cytokines to enhance oral immunization [40]. Furthermore, comparative analysis of different mucosal vaccine adjuvants has shown that adjuvant delivery can induce a rapid increase in the number of DCs within the FAE, a major site of antigen entry. This marked increase in DC chemotaxis is consistent with the hypothesis that stimulation of ECs by adjuvant components such as endotoxins and TLR agonists can result in release of chemokines to attract DCs to the site of antigen for uptake and maturation [41]. At later time points following adjuvant delivery, DCs move to the T cell areas of the PP to presumably promote T cell activation [42]. It is also possible that adjuvant components such as cholera toxin (CT) and *Escherichia coli* heat labile toxin (LT) can directly activate DCs after being transcytosed by M cells [43]. Clearly, a complex network of cytokine, chemokine, and cell-tissue interactions can control DC activation and migration within mucosal inductive sites to influence the outcome of mucosal immune responses (reviewed in [18]).

Macrophages are also abundantly present in mucosal tissues, including the bronchoalveolar spaces of the lung, and differ from DCs primarily in their decreased efficiency as APCs. Though less efficient at inducing T cell activation, macrophages are more efficient at capturing and killing microbes [44]. These differences highlight the general idea

that macrophages are specialized for clearance of microbes and cellular debris, rather than induction of adaptive immune responses. Macrophages in the intestine also appear to be less proinflammatory than circulating monocytes, showing suppressed responses to cytokines and TLR ligands, constitutive IL10 production, and the capacity to induce regulatory T cells (reviewed in [45]). Similarly, analysis of lung alveolar and interstitial macrophages suggests they promote an immunosuppressive environment in the lung (reviewed in [46]). Thus macrophages may be a major contributor in the modulation of mucosal immune responses.

The most predominate cell type in the PP is the IgA+ B cell. The production of SIgA and its presence in the mucocilliary blanket of the mucosae is perhaps the most distinguishing feature of mucosal immunity. The primary means by which SIgA is exported to the lumen is through EC transcytosis. In the lung, however, SIgA can also transudate from the serum into the bronchial secretions. In humans, IgA consists of two subclasses, IgA1 (predominantly found in serum, nasal tissue, and upper digestive tract) and IgA2 (predominantly found in the colon) [47]. Although IgA is the most predominant isotype in respiratory secretions, IgG may play an important role in the protection of the lower respiratory tract against viral infection and is the predominant isotype in alveoli secretions (reviewed in [46]). In the genital tract, IgG is efficiently transported from the circulation into genital tract secretion as well, and there is generally more IgG than IgA [48]. IgA is produced following activation and class switch recombination (CSR) by B cells. Early studies in rabbits have shown that IgA CSR takes place mainly in PP [49] while recent evidence, though more controversial, suggests IgA CSR can take place in the lamina propria, outside mucosal inductive sites (reviewed in [50–53]).

Although T cell help is required for the production of high-affinity IgA antibody, recent studies have suggested that mucosal-derived DCs alone are sufficient for the induction of low-affinity IgA by B cells, primarily through retinoic acid (RA) and IL6 production [54]. Exposure of B cells to RA also induces the upregulation of the mucosal tissue homing receptors CCR9 and α4β7, thus ensuring activated B cells return to the site of antigen for antibody production and antigen clearance [54]. The vast majority of IgA produced by DC-stimulated B cells in the gut is directed against commensal microorganisms, primarily through capture and presentation of commensal bacteria by mucosal DCs [30]. Decreasing commensal microorganism content in the gut can decrease IgA concentration, while IgA deficiency results in increased bacterial load [30]. Interestingly, IgA can also be produced against bacterial toxins and, unlike IgA production against commensal bacteria, anti-toxin IgA requires T cell help, presumably to raise the affinity of the IgA response [55]. It therefore appears that high-affinity IgA is important for the exclusion of toxins and pathogenic microorganisms from mucosal tissues, whereas low-affinity IgA might be important in limiting binding of commensal bacteria to epithelial cells.

SIgA responses appear to be the most important defensive molecule for protection against infections, though protective IgG responses have also been demonstrated and highlight the value of generating both mucosal SIgA responses and systemic IgG with vaccination. In the lung, for example, SIgA has been shown to be more important in the upper respiratory tract for protection against Influenza virus, whereas IgG is important for protection in the lower lung [56]. However, it should be noted that IgG, unlike SIgA, is sensitive to the proteolytic activity of luminal enzymes and will have a limited sustainability against antigen challenge. Moreover, non-neutralizing SIgA can prevent infection of mucosal epithelial cells through immune exclusion (SigA-mediated cross-linking and entrapment in the mucus) and blocking transcytosis [57]. Thus, generation of SIgA responses will be key for effective long-lived mucosal immune responses against pathogens. It is generally accepted that mucosal vaccination is required to generate mucosal SIgA production (reviewed in [58]).

Mucosal draining lymph nodes

Whereas the MALT acquires antigens directly from the lumen, mDLN are distant from mucosal surfaces and acquire antigens, and immune cells, from peripheral mucosal tissues via afferent lymphatics (Figure 4.1). The mDLN for mucosal organs consist of the cervical and bronchial/mediastinal lymph nodes for the upper and lower airway, respectively; the mesenteric lymph nodes (MLN) for the gastrointestinal tract; and the iliac lymph nodes for the urogenital tract. The mDLN are sites in which mucosal-derived DCs (from both PP and lamina propria) and blood-derived DCs merge and where systemic T and B cell immune responses can be initiated. In mucosal tissues, the phenomenon of antigen-specific tolerance is paramount to the maintenance of healthy tissues, and in the gut, MLNs have been identified as the site where oral tolerance is thought to occur. Oral tolerance cannot be induced in mice lacking MLN [59] and remains intact when PP are absent [60]. Moreover, studies have demonstrated that intact afferent lymph circulation of antigen-laden DCs to the MLNs is required for oral tolerance induction [61]. In addition to its central role in tolerance, the MLN also appears critical for preventing commensal organisms from gaining access to the systemic immune system [30].

Since MLNs are central to mucosal tolerance, they provide a platform in which to study the mechanism involved in the switch from tolerance to immunity, particularly in the context of vaccine strategies. Early studies in rats have demonstrated that DCs continually migrate to the MLNs via the afferent lymph. Under steady state conditions, a population of these migrating DCs, characterized by low expression of CD172a, was shown to carry fragments of apoptotic ECs and has been implicated in the maintenance of self-tolerance [62]. Conversely, a second population of DCs, expressing high levels of CD172a, was thought to be more potent as APCs [63]. Recent investigation into the effect of the oral adjuvant *E. coli* heat labile enterotoxin on DC migration in the MLN has shown that although this mucosal adjuvant boosts immune responses to orally delivered antigen, it does not do so by increasing DC migration. Rather, delivery of antigen with adjuvant results in increased antigen loading by DCs, increased DC activation status, and redistribution of CD172a high DC into the central T cell zones within the MLN, all of which result in an amplified antigen-specific T cell response [64].

In contrast to these studies, similar experiments using the structurally analogous mucosal adjuvant, cholera toxin (CT), did induce an increase in DC numbers migrating to the MLN, as well as inducing highly immunostimulatory DCs, similar to LT [21]. These data suggest that a significant mechanism by which adjuvants can improve immune responses to oral antigens is to induce robust lymphocyte priming through increased DC activity in the MLN.

Lamina propria

Once priming, activation, and imprinting have occurred in the draining lymph nodes, effector immune cells migrate to mucosal effector sites [54, 65]. Since the vast majority of T cells present in the lamina propria, including the unique population of IELs, are of the effector/memory phenotype (reviewed in [66]), it is largely accepted that the lamina propria is primarily a site for effector immune responses. Residing within the lamina propria is a variety of innate and adaptive immune cells, including T cells, B cells, IgA-producing plasma cells, regulatory T cells, invariant T cells, natural killer cells, $\gamma\delta$ T cells, mast cells, macrophages, and DCs. The lung parenchyma is somewhat analogous to the intestinal lamina propria in that it is composed of loosely organized connective tissue containing immune cells of both the innate and adaptive immune systems. However, only in the respiratory tract can cells be found outside the body, in the bronchoalveolar space.

The lamina propria of the intestine also contains structures known as isolated lymphoid follicles (ILF), which develop in response to gut flora and represent an alternative site for IgA production (reviewed in [67]). ILFs are composed of a single B cell follicle surrounded by DC and IL7R$^+$ c-kit$^+$ cells that can be found closely associated with the epithelium. There are relatively few T cells and no distinct T cell zones. The IL7R$^+$ c-kit$^+$ cells present in ILF, known as lymphoid tissue inducer (LTi) cells, are believed to be of hematopoietic origin, express CD45 and CD4 but not CD3, and can differentiate into APC, NK cells, and follicular cells, but not T or B cells [68]. LTi are important for the generation of secondary lymphoid organs like PP (reviewed in [67]) but also appear central to

ILF formation. ILF formation requires interaction between LTi cells and stromal organizer cells, and is hypothesized to occur following a series of events, including intestinal bacteria activation of lamina propria DCs and production of cytokines and chemokines, that enhances the interaction between LTi and stromal organizer cells. This leads to upregulation of adhesion molecules and chemokines that recruit B cells to the gut. Within the ILFs, B cells are either activated directly or by local DCs to induce preferential IgA class switching and differentiation to IgA-producing plasma cells [69]. This mechanism is proposed to restrict stimulation of the immune system by bacteria, thus avoiding damaging inflammatory responses.

Mucosal adjuvants such as CT can increase DC numbers in the subepithelial mucosa, thereby increasing antigen acquisition and potential presentation to B cells for T-independent antibody production (see Chapter 23 for more detail). Moreover, direct targeting of vaccine antigens to mucosal ECs could also induce chemotaxis of DCs to epithelial cells for antigen uptake. Defining the balance between rapid mobilization of immune cells and limiting local inflammation in the lamina propria will be important for the development of safe and effective vaccines.

Mucosal vaccines: current strategies and ongoing challenges

Due to the phenomenon of oral tolerance and other factors intrinsic to the mucosal environment such as acidic pH and proteolytic enzymes, mucosal vaccine development faces significant challenges. Nevertheless, biologists have sought to improve vaccine strategies through, for example: encapsulation of vaccine antigens, delivery of antigens with mucosal adjuvants, conjugation of antigens to ligands of EC receptors for targeted antigen uptake, and/or the use of live attenuated microbial vectors (see Chapters 12 and 22 for more details).

Antigen encapsulation provides a means to deliver large amounts of antigen in encapsulated form to protect it from degradation. In addition, some antigen encapsulation modalities contain intrinsic adjuvant properties. Biodegradable particles such as microspheres, liposomes, immunostimulating complex (ISCOMS), proteosomes, and calcium phosphate nanoparticles (CaP) represent just a few encapsulation technologies [70]. Plant-based vaccines, including tobacco, tomato, potato, lettuce, spinach, banana, corn, rice, and algae, also provide a means to encapsulate antigen and provide a stable vehicle for vaccine delivery. A number of these vaccine candidates have entered early human clinical trials and have shown induction of immune responses when taken orally [71]. However, there are still numerous hurdles to overcome in order for plant-based vaccines to be successful. These nonreplicating vaccines are limited by the dose of antigen they can deliver for effective immunity. Moreover, environmental concerns about crop transgene escape may produce a hurdle for adequate production [72].

Other targeting vaccine strategies that utilize cell-specific receptors to facilitate antigen absorption and uptake by ECs and M cells are also under investigation. Specifically, integrins, PRRs such as TLRs, lectins, specific carbohydrate residues, or microbial vectors can be used to target M cells ([73]; see Chapter 26 for more detail). Microbial vectors, bacterial or viral vehicles that encode defined genetic material from a pathogen to which immunity is desired, take advantage of the natural route of infection to generate improved immune responses. Live attenuated microbial vaccines are thought to provide better protection compared to killed or subunit vaccines but are plagued by the threat of reversion to a pathogenic phenotype. Thus commensal microorganisms such as *Lactobacillus* spp. are favored as noninvasive vectors. Nevertheless, a number of attenuated pathogens such as *Salmonella*, *Shigella*, and *Listeria*, to name a few, have been explored as potential vaccine vectors [2]. Common viral vectors for vaccine development include adenovirus, herpes virus, measles virus, and poxviruses, though pre-existing immunity to some of these vectors have hampered vaccine efficacy [74].

Mucosal vaccines for human use

According to the World Health Organization (WHO), mucosally transmitted diseases such as lower respiratory tract infections, diarrheal diseases, and HIV/AIDS were in the top six causes of death worldwide in 2008 and in the top three for lower-income countries, representing 1.05, 0.76, and 0.72 million deaths per year in this group, respectively (www.who.int/mediacentre/factsheets/fs310_2008.pdf). The potential for these highly infectious diseases to turn pandemic is significant, highlighting the need for effective vaccines that can be administered rapidly and with little need for training, particularly in developing countries.

Unfortunately, current approved vaccines against influenza, for example, include mostly parenteral administration, which requires administration by trained personnel. Furthermore, although parenteral administration of influenza vaccines can reduce severity of infection and induce serum immunoglobulin, it does not inhibit infection nor elicit significant SIgA, and provides little or no cross-protection against other viral strains [75]. In contrast, intranasal administration of the influenza vaccine in humans can provide protection against heterologous viruses [76], presumably because SIgA are more cross-reactive compared to IgG. But intranasal vaccination often does not induce adequate serum immunoglobulin, which is also thought to be important. These data indicate that a combination of intranasal and parenteral delivery may work best [77]. Live attenuated vaccines for influenza have been shown to be efficacious [78], but there are safety concerns for some age groups. Inactivated or killed vaccines are considered safer, more affordable, and easier to distribute in lower economic countries but may not be as immunogenic as live vaccines. Inactivated influenza vaccines are classified based on whether they contain whole virus particles, partially disrupted virus ("split" vaccines), or purified envelope proteins ("subunit" vaccines). Adjuvants have been used to enhance the immunogenicity of subunit vaccines, though LT has been associated with adverse clinical side effects such as facial paralysis (Bell's palsy) [79]. New clinically safe adjuvants are under investigation (reviewed in [80]); however, recent studies of a whole inactivated virus have shown efficacy without the use of adjuvants [81], supporting the view that particulate antigens may be more immunogenic to the mucosal immune system as they promote targeting to local M cells and DCs. Both a parenterally administered inactivated vaccine and an intranasal spray live attenuated vaccine (FluMist®) are currently approved for commercial use.

Human trials for parenterally delivered HIV vaccines have yet to show efficacy and it is speculated that this is partly due to the lack of SIgA production and mucosal immunity following parenteral administration (reviewed in [82]). In addition, there is evidence to suggest that the HIV replicates in the gut even when no systemic viral RNA is detectible [83], suggesting mucosal immunity may be paramount to virus eradication. Although systemic immunization has shown the ability to generate mucosal cytotoxic C lymphocyte (CTL) responses, studies in animals suggest that mucosal immunization is more effective at clearing virus from the major site of replication in the gastrointestinal tract [84]. Different routes for mucosal immunization have been investigated for HIV. In mice, intranasal vaccination showed superiority over vaginal, gastric, or rectal routes for induction of mucosal antibody responses [85]. Studies in nonhuman primates demonstrated that intranasal immunization can induce SIgA responses at other mucosal sites as well [86]. Comparison of vaccination routes in humans using a cholera vaccine suggests that although intravaginal vaccination can induce local immune responses, intranasal vaccination was able to induce SIgA at other mucosal sites, consistent with the animal studies (reviewed in [58]). Intravaginal vaccination in humans may also be hampered by hormonal effects (reviewed in [87]). In addition to the route of vaccine administration, consideration of existing mucosal infections in target populations, particularly in developing countries, needs to be taken into account and will likely complicate our understanding of the effectiveness of mucosal HIV vaccines [88]. No vaccine against HIV is commercially available at this time.

Diarrheal diseases caused by pathogens including *Vibrio cholerae* (cholera), Salmonella spp (particularly *S. typhi*), Shigella spp, Campylobacter spp, *Escherichia coli* strains (Enterotoxigenic *E. coli* [ETEC]) and rotavirus are transmitted by the fecal-oral route. Mucosal vaccines are currently available for: cholera (either an oral live attenuated [CVD 103-HgR] or killed oral vaccine [Dukoral™], both of which have been shown to be safe, immunogenic, and efficacious; reviewed in [2]), *S. typhi* (either an oral live-attenuated [Ty2la] or parenteral inactive vaccine [Vi], both of which have been shown to be safe and efficacious in preventing typhoid fever [89]), and rotavirus (two oral live attenuated vaccines, Rotarix™ and RotaTeq™, both of which have been shown to be efficacious, inducing SIgA and cell-mediated immunity [90]). Vaccines are being developed for ETEC, *Shigella*, and *Campylobacter* but no vaccine is commercially available for these agents as yet. Despite the availability of safe and efficacious vaccines for the treatment of high-burden diarrheal diseases, such as typhoid fever and cholera, vaccination compliance remains low. Reasons include bias against vaccination, accessibility, and cost, particularly in lower economic countries. Of note, there is also concern for lack of efficacy of mucosal vaccines in developing countries due to existing infections or chronic environmental enteropathy (CEE) and nutritional deficiencies [91]. Efforts to decrease mucosal vaccine costs while increasing efficacy and accessibility will be important in curbing the pandemic potential of these diseases.

Final word

There is considerable interest in utilizing nonparenteral routes for vaccine delivery as oral or nasal delivery of vaccines offers a method to overcome the inconveniences and problems of vaccine injections and could potentially augment the effectiveness of vaccination against mucosal pathogens. Oral tolerance and other factors of the mucosal environment can present significant hurdles to the efficacy of oral vaccination. However, a firm understanding of the mechanisms employed by the mucosal immune system in dealing with mucosal antigens is continuing to give rise to unique strategies to overcome these challenges and allow for development of effective and accessible mucosal vaccines for the future.

References

1 Faria AM, Weiner HL. Oral tolerance. *Immunol Rev* 2005;**206**: 232–59.

2 Mestecky J, Nguyen H, Czerkinsky C, Kiyono H. Oral immunization: an update. *Curr Opin Gastroenterol* 2008;**24**(6):713–19.

3 Linden SK, Sutton P, Karlsson NG, Korolik V, McGuckin MA. Mucins in the mucosal barrier to infection. *Mucosal Immunol* 2008;**1**(3):183–97.

4 Bugaut M. Occurrence, absorption and metabolism of short chain fatty acids in the digestive tract of mammals. *Comp Biochem Physiol B* 1987;**86**(3):439–72.

5 Dahan S, Roth-Walter F, Arnaboldi P, Agarwal S, Mayer L. Epithelia: lymphocyte interactions in the gut. *Immunol Rev.* 2007 Feb;**215**: 243–53.

6 Yoshida M, Claypool SM, Wagner JS, *et al.* Human neonatal Fc receptor mediates transport of IgG into luminal secretions for delivery of antigens to mucosal dendritic cells. *Immunity* 2004;**20**(6):769–83.

7 Mostov KE, Verges M, Altschuler Y. Membrane traffic in polarized epithelial cells. *Curr Opin Cell Biol* 2000;**12**(4):483–90.

8 Brandtzaeg P. Transport models for secretory IgA and secretory IgM. *Clin Exp Immunol* 1981;**44**(2):221–32.

9 Guy-Grand D, Vassalli P. Gut intraepithelial lymphocyte development. *Curr Opin Immunol* 2002;**14**(2): 255–9.

10 Havran WL, Jameson JM, Witherden DA. Epithelial cells and their neighbors. III. Interactions between intraepithelial lymphocytes and neighboring epithelial cells. *Am J Physiol Gastrointest Liver Physiol* 2005;**289**(4):G627–30.

11 Hershberg RM, Mayer LF. Antigen processing and presentation by intestinal epithelial cells – polarity and complexity. *Immunol Today* 2000;**21**(3):123–8.

12 Eghtesad M, Jackson HE, Cunningham AC. Primary human alveolar epithelial cells can elicit the transendothelial migration of CD14$^+$ monocytes and CD3$^+$ lymphocytes. *Immunology* 2001;**102**(2):157–64.

13 McAdam AJ, Schweitzer AN, Sharpe AH. The role of B7 co-stimulation in activation and differentiation of CD4$^+$ and CD8$^+$ T cells. *Immunol Rev* 1998;**165**: 231–47.

14 Westendorf AM, Fleissner D, Groebe L, *et al.* CD4$^+$Foxp3$^+$ regulatory T cell expansion induced by antigen-driven interaction with intestinal epithelial cells independent of local dendritic cells. *Gut* 2009; **58**(2):211–19.

15 Colgan SP, Hershberg RM, Furuta GT, Blumberg RS. Ligation of intestinal epithelial CD1d induces bioactive IL-10: critical role of the cytoplasmic tail in autocrine signaling. *Proc Natl Acad Sci U S A* 1999 **23;96**(24):13938–43.

16 Vroling AB, Fokkens WJ, van Drunen CM. How epithelial cells detect danger: aiding the immune response. *Allergy* 2008;**63**(9):1110–23.

17 Rakoff-Nahoum S, Medzhitov R. Innate immune recognition of the indigenous microbial flora. *Mucosal Immunol* 2008;**1**(Suppl 1):S10–14.

18 Iwasaki A. Mucosal dendritic cells. *Annu Rev Immunol* 2007;**25**: 381–418.

19 Lee J, Gonzales-Navajas JM, Raz E. The "polarizing-tolerizing" mechanism of intestinal epithelium: its relevance to colonic homeostasis. *Semin Immunopathol* 2008;**30**(1):3–9.

20 Hershberg RM. The epithelial cell cytoskeleton and intracellular trafficking. V. Polarized compartmentalization of antigen processing and Toll-like receptor signaling in intestinal epithelial cells. *Am J Physiol Gastrointest Liver Physiol* 2002;**283**(4):G833–9.

21 Anjuere F, Luci C, Lebens M, *et al.* In vivo adjuvant-induced mobilization and maturation of gut dendritic cells after oral administration of cholera toxin. *J Immunol* 2004 **15;173**(8):5103–11.

22 Mestecky J, Moldoveanu Z, Russell MW. Immunologic uniqueness of the genital tract: challenge for vaccine development. *Am J Reprod Immunol* 2005;**53**(5):208–14.

23 Fujihashi K, Dohi T, Rennert PD, *et al.* Peyer's patches are required for oral tolerance to proteins. *Proc Natl Acad Sci U S A* 2001 **13;98**(6):3310–15.

24 Teitelbaum R, Schubert W, Gunther L, *et al.* The M cell as a portal of entry to the lung for the bacterial pathogen *Mycobacterium tuberculosis*. *Immunity* 1999;**10**(6):641–50.

25 Mach J, Hshieh T, Hsieh D, Grubbs N, Chervonsky A. Development of intestinal M cells. *Immunol Rev* 2005;**206**: 177–89.

26 Neutra MR, Mantis NJ, Kraehenbuhl JP. Collaboration of epithelial cells with organized mucosal lymphoid tissues. *Nat Immunol* 2001;**2**(11):1004–9.

27 Kraehenbuhl JP, Neutra MR. Epithelial M cells: differentiation and function. *Annu Rev Cell Dev Biol* 2000;**16**: 301–32.

28 Niess JH, Brand S, Gu X, *et al.* CX3CR1-mediated dendritic cell access to the intestinal lumen and bacterial clearance. *Science* 2005;**307**(5707):254–8.

29 Rescigno M, Urbano M, Valzasina B, *et al.* Dendritic cells express tight junction proteins and penetrate gut epithelial monolayers to sample bacteria. *Nat Immunol* 2001;**2**(4):361–7.

30 Macpherson AJ, Harris NL. Interactions between commensal intestinal bacteria and the immune system. *Nat Rev Immunol* 2004;**4**(6):478–85.

31 Iwasaki A, Kelsall BL. Localization of distinct Peyer's patch dendritic cell subsets and their recruitment by chemokines macrophage inflammatory protein (MIP)-3alpha, MIP-3beta, and secondary lymphoid organ chemokine. *J Exp Med* 2000;**191**(8):1381–94.

32 Liu LM, MacPherson GG. Antigen acquisition by dendritic cells: intestinal dendritic cells acquire antigen administered orally and can prime naive T cells in vivo. *J Exp Med* 1993;**177**(5):1299–307.

33 Akbari O, DeKruyff RH, Umetsu DT. Pulmonary dendritic cells producing IL-10 mediate tolerance induced by respiratory exposure to antigen. *Nat Immunol* 2001;**2**(8):725–31.

34 Mowat AM. Anatomical basis of tolerance and immunity to intestinal antigens. *Nat Rev Immunol* 2003;**3**(4):331–41.

35 Coombes JL, Powrie F. Dendritic cells in intestinal immune regulation. *Nat Rev Immunol* 2008;**8**(6): 435–46.

36 Monteleone I, Platt AM, Jaensson E, Agace WW, Mowat AM. IL-10-dependent partial refractoriness to Toll-like receptor stimulation modulates gut mucosal dendritic cell function. *Eur J Immunol* 2008; **38**(6):1533–47.

37 Bilsborough J, George TC, Norment A, Viney JL. Mucosal CD8alpha$^+$ DC, with a plasmacytoid phenotype, induce differentiation and support function of T cells with regulatory properties. *Immunology* 2003; **108**(4):481–92.

38 Coombes JL, Siddiqui KR, Arancibia-Carcamo CV, *et al.* A functionally specialized population of mucosal CD103$^+$ DCs induces Foxp3$^+$ regulatory T cells via a TGF-beta and retinoic acid-dependent mechanism. *J Exp Med* 2007;**204**(8):1757–64.

39 Iwasaki A, Kelsall BL. Freshly isolated Peyer's patch, but not spleen, dendritic cells produce interleukin 10 and induce the differentiation of T helper type 2 cells. *J Exp Med.* 1999 Jul 19;**190**(2):229–39.

40 Williamson E, Westrich GM, Viney JL. Modulating dendritic cells to optimize mucosal immunization protocols. *J Immunol* 1999;**163**(7):3668–75.

41 Anosova NG, Chabot S, Shreedhar V, *et al.* Cholera toxin, *E. coli* heat-labile toxin, and non-toxic derivatives induce dendritic cell migration into the follicle-associated epithelium of Peyer's patches. *Mucosal Immunol* 2008;**1**(1):59–67.

42 Shreedhar VK, Kelsall BL, Neutra MR. Cholera toxin induces migration of dendritic cells from the subep-

ithelial dome region to T- and B-cell areas of Peyer's patches. *Infect Immun* 2003;**71**(1):504–9.

43 Frey A, Giannasca KT, Weltzin R, *et al.* Role of the glycocalyx in regulating access of microparticles to apical plasma membranes of intestinal epithelial cells: implications for microbial attachment and oral vaccine targeting. *J Exp Med* 1996;**184**(3):1045–59.

44 Nagl M, Kacani L, Mullauer B, *et al.* Phagocytosis and killing of bacteria by professional phagocytes and dendritic cells. *Clin Diagn Lab Immunol* 2002; **9**(6):1165–8.

45 Kelsall B. Recent progress in understanding the phenotype and function of intestinal dendritic cells and macrophages. *Mucosal Immunol* 2008;**1**(6):460–49.

46 Macaubas C, DeKruyff RH, Umetsu DT. Respiratory tolerance in the protection against asthma. *Curr Drug Targets Inflamm Allergy* 2003;**2**(2):175–86.

47 Brandtzaeg P, Johansen FE. Mucosal B cells: phenotypic characteristics, transcriptional regulation, and homing properties. *Immunol Rev* 2005;**206**: 32–63.

48 Moldoveanu Z, Huang WQ, Kulhavy R, Pate MS, Mestecky J. Human male genital tract secretions: both mucosal and systemic immune compartments contribute to the humoral immunity. *J Immunol* 2005;**175**(6):4127–36.

49 Craig SW, Cebra JJ. Peyer's patches: an enriched source of precursors for IgA-producing immunocytes in the rabbit. 1971. *J Immunol* 2008;**180**(3):1295–307.

50 Barone F, Patel P, Sanderson J, Spencer J. Gut-associated lymphoid tissue contains the molecular machinery to support T-cell-dependent and T-cell-independent class switch recombination. *Mucosal Immunol* 2009;**2**(6):495–503.

51 Cerutti A. The regulation of IgA class switching. *Nat Rev Immunol* 2008;**8**(6):421–34.

52 Macpherson AJ, McCoy KD, Johansen FE, Brandtzaeg P. The immune geography of IgA induction and function. *Mucosal Immunol* 2008;**1**(1):11–22.

53 Suzuki K, Fagarasan S. Diverse regulatory pathways for IgA synthesis in the gut. *Mucosal Immunol* 2009;**2**(6):468–71.

54 Mora JR, Iwata M, Eksteen B, *et al.* Generation of gut-homing IgA-secreting B cells by intestinal dendritic cells. *Science* 2006;**314**(5802):1157–60.

55 Hornquist CE, Ekman L, Grdic KD, Schon K, Lycke NY. Paradoxical IgA immunity in CD4-deficient mice. Lack of cholera toxin-specific protective immunity despite normal gut mucosal IgA differentiation. *J Immunol* 1995;**155**(6):2877–87.

56 Renegar KB, Small PA, Jr, Boykins LG, Wright PF. Role of IgA versus IgG in the control of influenza

viral infection in the murine respiratory tract. *J Immunol* 2004;**173**(3):1978–86.

57 Brandtzaeg P. Induction of secretory immunity and memory at mucosal surfaces. *Vaccine* 2007;**25**(30): 5467–84

58 Neutra MR, Kozlowski PA. Mucosal vaccines: the promise and the challenge. *Nat Rev Immunol* 2006; **6**(2):148–58.

59 Spahn TW, Weiner HL, Rennert PD, *et al.* Mesenteric lymph nodes are critical for the induction of high-dose oral tolerance in the absence of Peyer's patches. *Eur J Immunol* 2002;**32**(4):1109–13.

60 Kraus TA, Brimnes J, Muong C, *et al.* Induction of mucosal tolerance in Peyer's patch-deficient, ligated small bowel loops. *J Clin Invest* 2005;**115**(8): 2234–43.

61 Worbs T, Bode U, Yan S, *et al.* Oral tolerance originates in the intestinal immune system and relies on antigen carriage by dendritic cells. *J Exp Med* 2006;**203**(3):519–27.

62 Huang FP, Platt N, Wykes M, *et al.* A discrete subpopulation of dendritic cells transports apoptotic intestinal epithelial cells to T cell areas of mesenteric lymph nodes. *J Exp Med* 2000;**191**(3):435–44.

63 Liu L, Zhang M, Jenkins C, MacPherson GG. Dendritic cell heterogeneity in vivo: two functionally different dendritic cell populations in rat intestinal lymph can be distinguished by CD4 expression. *J Immunol* 1998;**161**(3):1146–55.

64 Milling SW, Yrlid U, Jenkins C, *et al.* Regulation of intestinal immunity: effects of the oral adjuvant *Escherichia coli* heat-labile enterotoxin on migrating dendritic cells. *Eur J Immunol* 2007;**37**(1):87–99.

65 Mora JR, Bono MR, Manjunath N, *et al.* Selective imprinting of gut-homing T cells by Peyer's patch dendritic cells. *Nature* 2003;**424**(6944):88–93.

66 Lefrancois L, Puddington L. Intestinal and pulmonary mucosal T cells: local heroes fight to maintain the status quo. *Annu Rev Immunol* 2006;**24**: 681–704.

67 Finke D. Induction of intestinal lymphoid tissue formation by intrinsic and extrinsic signals. *Semin Immunopathol* 2009;**31**(2):151–69.

68 Mebius RE, Rennert P, Weissman IL. Developing lymph nodes collect CD4$^+$CD3$^-$ LTbeta$^+$ cells that can differentiate to APC, NK cells, and follicular cells but not T or B cells. *Immunity* 1997;**7**(4):493–504.

69 Tsuji M, Suzuki K, Kitamura H, *et al.* Requirement for lymphoid tissue-inducer cells in isolated follicle formation and T cell-independent immunoglobulin A generation in the gut. *Immunity* 2008**15**;29(2): 261–71.

70 Peek LJ, Middaugh CR, Berkland C. Nanotechnology in vaccine delivery. *Adv Drug Deliv Rev* 2008;**60**(8): 915–28.

71 Streatfield SJ. Mucosal immunization using recombinant plant-based oral vaccines. *Methods* 2006;**38**(2): 150–57.

72 Rybicki EP. Plant-produced vaccines: promise and reality. *Drug Discov Today* 2009;**14**(1–2): 16–24.

73 Brayden DJ, Jepson MA, Baird AW. Intestinal Peyer's patch M cells and oral vaccine targeting. *Drug Discov Today* 2005;**10**(17):1145–57.

74 Robert-Guroff M. Replicating and non-replicating viral vectors for vaccine development. *Curr Opin Biotechnol* 2007;**18**(6):546–56.

75 Muszkat M, Yehuda AB, Schein MH, *et al.* Local and systemic immune response in community-dwelling elderly after intranasal or intramuscular immunization with inactivated influenza vaccine. *J Med Virol* 2000;**61**(1):100–106.

76 Belshe RB, Gruber WC, Mendelman PM, *et al.* Efficacy of vaccination with live attenuated, cold-adapted, trivalent, intranasal influenza virus vaccine against a variant (A/Sydney) not contained in the vaccine. *J Pediatr* 2000;**136**(2):168–75.

77 Keitel WA, Cate TR, Nino D, *et al.* Immunization against influenza: comparison of various topical and parenteral regimens containing inactivated and/or live attenuated vaccines in healthy adults. *J Infect Dis* 2001;**183**(2):329–32.

78 Belshe RB, Ambrose CS, Yi T. Safety and efficacy of live attenuated influenza vaccine in children 2–7 years of age. *Vaccine* 2008;**26**(Suppl 4):D10–16.

79 Mutsch M, Zhou W, Rhodes P, *et al.* Use of the inactivated intranasal influenza vaccine and the risk of Bell's palsy in Switzerland. *N Engl J Med* 2004;**350**(9):896–903.

80 Hasegawa H, Ichinohe T, Ainai A, Tamura S, Kurata T. Development of mucosal adjuvants for intranasal vaccine for H5N1 influenza viruses. *Ther Clin Risk Manag* 2009;**5**(1):125–32.

81 Greenbaum E, Engelhard D, Levy R, *et al.* Mucosal (SIgA) and serum (IgG) immunologic responses in young adults following intranasal administration of one or two doses of inactivated, trivalent anti-influenza vaccine. *Vaccine* 2004;**22**(20):2566–77.

82 Demberg T, Robert-Guroff M. Mucosal immunity and protection against HIV/SIV infection: strategies and challenges for vaccine design. *Int Rev Immunol* 2009;**28**(1):20–48.

83 Veazey RS, DeMaria M, Chalifoux LV, *et al.* Gastrointestinal tract as a major site of CD4$^+$ T cell

depletion and viral replication in SIV infection. *Science* 1998;**280**(5362):427–31.

84 Belyakov IM, Hel Z, Kelsall B, *et al.* Mucosal AIDS vaccine reduces disease and viral load in gut reservoir and blood after mucosal infection of macaques. *Nat Med* 2001;**7**(12):1320–26.

85 Staats HF, Montgomery SP, Palker TJ. Intranasal immunization is superior to vaginal, gastric, or rectal immunization for the induction of systemic and mucosal anti-HIV antibody responses. *AIDS Res Hum Retroviruses* 1997;**13**(11):945–52.

86 Imaoka K, Miller CJ, Kubota M, *et al.* Nasal immunization of nonhuman primates with simian immunodeficiency virus p55gag and cholera toxin adjuvant induces Th1/Th2 help for virus-specific immune responses in reproductive tissues. *J Immunol* 1998;**161**(11):5952–8.

87 Mestecky J. Humoral immune responses to the human immunodeficiency virus type-1 (HIV-1) in the genital tract compared to other mucosal sites. *J Reprod Immunol* 2007;**73**(1):86–97.

88 Pala P, Gomez-Roman VR, Gilmour J, Kaleebu P. An African perspective on mucosal immunity and HIV-1. *Mucosal Immunol* 2009;**2**(4):300–14.

89 Fraser A, Paul M, Goldberg E, Acosta CJ, Leibovici L. Typhoid fever vaccines: systematic review and meta-analysis of randomised controlled trials. *Vaccine* 2007;**25**(45):7848–57.

90 Ward RL. Rotavirus vaccines: how they work or don't work. *Expert Rev Mol Med* 2008;**10**(10):e5.

91 Czerkinsky C, Holmgren J. Enteric vaccines for the developing world: a challenge for mucosal immunology. *Mucosal Immunol* 2009;**2**(4):284–7.

CHAPTER 5

Immunologic Memory: T Cells in Humans

Maria Candela Iglesias, Victor Appay, & Arnaud Moris

INSERM UMR S 945, Infections and Immunity, Avenir Group, Université Pierre et Marie Curie (UPMC), Sorbonne Universités, and Hôpital Pitié-Salpêtrière, Paris, France

Introduction

Neuroscientists define memory as the ability to store and recall observations and sensations, so that one is able to remember information and to recognize people and places over time. Our immunity is said to have a memory for most invading agents (e.g., bacteria, toxins, and viruses) because a second encounter with the same agent prompts a swifter and more vigorous immune response than the primary invasion. This memory, which can last for decades, is the basis for immunization or vaccination, aimed at rendering an individual immune to a particular agent.

Immunologic memory is a property of the adaptive immunity (as opposed to innate immunity), system, which consists of two principal arms: the cellular response and the humoral response, mediated by T cells and antibody-producing B cells, respectively (see Chapter 6). Although related and sharing common features, these two responses represent distinct and complex systems. This chapter concentrates on immunologic memory within the T-cell arm of immunity in humans. Initial descriptions portrayed memory T lymphocytes as cells that subsist in the absence of antigenic stimulation and have the capacity to expand rapidly upon secondary challenge. In recent years, we have learnt that the memory population consists of multiple subsets with specialized functions. Moreover, numerous factors have been shown to influence the generation and maintenance of T-cell memory responses. Here, we discuss this knowledge and its implication for the induction of effective T-cell immunity using vaccines.

Generation of memory T cells

Different types of memory T cells in humans

Originally, memory T cells were divided into two main lineages: the CD4[+] helper T cells, which assist in both cellular and humoral immunity through the secretion of various cytokines, and the CD8[+] killer T cells, which eliminate cells expressing foreign antigens (Ag). However, in recent years, detailed characterizations of these cells have led to a complex classification of an increasing number of CD4[+] or CD8[+] memory T-cell subpopulations, distinguished by their phenotype, functional profile, and potential role in the immune response.

CD8[+] T-cell subsets

The CD8[+] T-cell population can be divided into different subsets based on their phenotype; that is, the expression of diverse cell-surface receptors. The most commonly used markers are CD45RA (or CD45RO), CCR7, CD27, and CD28, the expression of which enables the distinction between subsets referred to as central memory, and early, intermediate, or late effector memory cells (Figure 5.1a).

Vaccinology: Principles and Practice, First Edition. Edited by W. John W. Morrow, Nadeem A. Sheikh, Clint S. Schmidt and D. Huw Davies.
© 2012 Blackwell Publishing Ltd. Published 2012 by Blackwell Publishing Ltd.

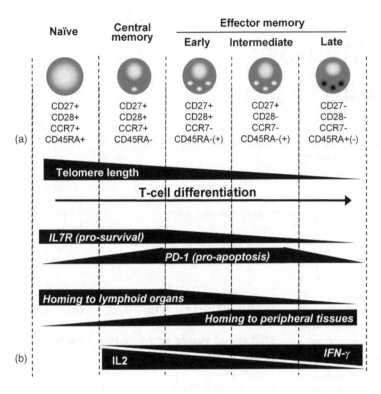

Figure 5.1 Subsets of memory CD8+ T cells. (a) Distinct subsets of CD8+ T cells can be identified according to the expression of the cell-surface molecules CD45RA, CCR7, CD27, and CD28 and placed along a pathway of differentiation on the basis of the average length of their telomeres. (b) These subsets present distinct cell-surface receptors or intracellular molecules, which confer upon them distinct properties like survival capacity, homing potential, or functional potential.

Measurements of telomere lengths (which provide information on the replicative history of the cells and therefore their biological age) in these subsets suggest that they can be positioned along a putative pathway of differentiation or post-thymic development. Of note, the expression of a large number of cell-surface molecules overlaps or is associated with this CD8+ T-cell classification (reviewed in [1]). For instance, central memory CD8+ T cells express high levels of molecules like IL7R and CD62L and low levels of PD-1 and CX3CR1, in contrast to more differentiated CD8+ T cells. These receptors and molecules are often involved in key cellular functions, including T-cell activation (e.g., CD45RA or CD45RO), co-stimulation (e.g., CD27 and CD28), regulation and apoptosis (e.g., PD-1), homeostatic maintenance and survival (e.g., IL7R), as well as migration (e.g., CCR7 and CX3CR1) or adhesion (e.g., CD11a and CD62L). Moreover, these subsets differ with regard to their effector functions, reflected by the expression of various intracellular molecules. For instance, granzyme K production is a trait of CCR7$^-$CD27$^+$CD28$^+$CD8$^+$ T cells, whereas granzyme B production is predominant in CCR7$^-$CD27$^-$CD28$^-$CD8$^+$ T cells. Distinct CD8$^+$ T-cell subsets have also been reported to have different capacity to produce cytokines like IL2 or IFN-γ [2]. The differential expression of surface receptors and intracellular molecules implies different requirements for stimulation and survival, different homing potential (e.g., to lymphoid organs or to peripheral tissues), and immediate effector functions, so that distinct memory T-cell subsets display specific sets of attributes (Figure 5.1b). The precise role of the distinct differentiated CD8$^+$ T-cell subsets in the immune response remains to be characterized.

CD4+ T-cell subsets

Although the dissection of T-lymphocyte subsets based on their phenotype (as described above) has mainly concerned CD8$^+$ T cells, it can also

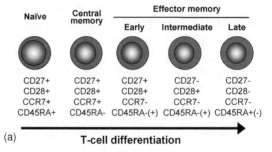

(a)

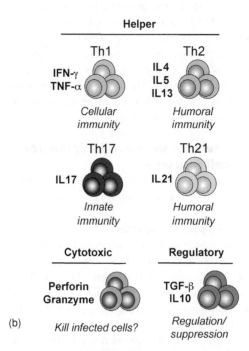

(b)

Figure 5.2 Subsets of memory CD4+ T cells. (a) The CD4+ T-cell population can be separated into subsets with distinct phenotype and placed along a pathway of differentiation, in the same way as for CD8+ T cells. (b) Independently, several CD4+ T cell subsets with distinct functional profile and various roles in the immune response have been characterized.

be applied to CD4+ T cells. Different CD4+ T-cell subsets (like central and effector memory cells) can be identified and placed along a similar pathway of differentiation based on their telomere length (Figure 5.2a). However, the distinction between CD4+ T-cell subpopulations has been commonly based on their functional/cytokine secretion profile, rather

than their phenotype (Figure 5.2b). Initial works distinguished Th1 and Th2 CD4+ T cells. Th1 CD4+ T cells are characterized by secretion of IFN-γ and TNF-α, and are necessary for the establishment of cellular responses (by maximizing the killing efficacy of macrophages and the proliferation of CD8+ T cells). Instead, Th2 CD4+ T cells secrete cytokines like IL4, IL5, IL6, IL10, or IL13 and contribute to the humoral response (by stimulating B-cell proliferation, inducing B-cell antibody class switching, and increasing neutralizing antibody production). In recent years, two additional major subsets have emerged. The first (referred to as Th17 cells) is characterized by IL17 secretion, and is involved in the recruitment, activation, and migration of neutrophils. The second is characterized by IL21 secretion (referred to as Th21 or follicular Th cells), and is necessary for mounting effective humoral responses (e.g., germinal center formation and generation of high-affinity antibodies) [3]. A number of studies have also shown that the expression of certain chemokine receptors on CD4+ T cells is associated with specific Th profiles (reviewed in [4]). CCR5 and CXCR3 expression discriminates CD4+ T cells with a Th1 cytokine profile, while CCR3 and CCR4 expression identifies CD4+ T cells with a Th2 cytokine profile. The expression of CCR6 and CCR4, or CXCR5 has been reported to characterize Th17 or Th21 cells, respectively. These associations provide a link between CD4+ T-cell function and migratory potential, although this remains complex. For instance, expression of CCR6 and CXCR3 identifies a heterogeneous population composed of Th1 cells and cells producing both IFN-γ and IL17. In addition to helper CD4+ T-cell subsets, the existence of CD4+ T cells with apparent cytotoxic properties (i.e., harboring cytolytic granules containing perforin and granzymes, and able to kill target cells) has also been reported by several investigators (including [5]). They appear to be highly differentiated CD4+ memory cells; however, their physiological role remains unclear. Last, regulatory T cells represent another major subtype of CD4+ T cells, which are identified using Foxp3, CD25 expression, and lack of IL7R expression. These cells play key roles in modulating and deactivating immune responses, and establishing tolerance. Although it is still not clear if they can really be considered as memory cells *per se* (e.g., their Ag specificity has not been reported to date), recent studies reported the distinction between naïve and standard regulatory T cells, suggesting that primed or memory regulatory T cells may be defined (reviewed in [6]). Though the role of the different CD4$^+$ T-cell subsets is roughly defined, it is still necessary to reconcile Th profiling and phenotypic distinction of CD4$^+$ T cells.

Different pathogens and distinct T-cell responses

Distinct profiles of T-cell responses are established when generating memory or maintaining latency to different pathogens. For instance, Ag-specific CD8$^+$ T cells display unique profiles depending on their viral specificity: cells are predominantly CCR7$^+$CD27$^+$CD28$^+$, CCR7$^-$CD27$^+$CD28$^+$, CCR7$^-$CD27$^+$CD28$^-$, or CCR7$^-$CD27$^-$CD28$^-$ during latent infection with hepatitis C virus (HCV), Epstein-Barr virus (EBV), HIV, or cytomegalovirus (CMV), respectively [7]. Following the clearance of an acute viral infection such as influenza or respiratory syncytial virus (RSV), virus-specific CD8$^+$ T cells appear predominantly CCR7$^+$CD27$^+$CD28$^+$ [8,9]. Of note, CD4$^+$ T cells specific for these viruses also present very similar phenotypic distributions. The reasons for the associations between viruses and T-cell phenotype profiles remain unclear; however, the type and level of stimulation, which differ between distinct infection settings, are likely to have a role in dictating these profiles. Indeed, the Ag load and recurrence, co-stimulation, and cytokine environment have been shown to influence the phenotype of T cells [10,11].

Beyond T-cell phenotype, interesting associations between the functional attributes of CD4$^+$ or CD8$^+$ T cells and different pathogens have also been described. In line with their phenotype, Influenza- or EBV-specific CD8$^+$ T cells express high levels of granzyme K but not B, whereas CMV-specific T cells express abundantly granzyme B, but little K [12]. Of particular interest, CD4$^+$ T cells that lack CD28 expression and display cytolytic potential [13] are associated with CMV infection [14]. In healthy adults, CD4$^+$ T cells specific

for *Staphylococcus aureus*, *Candida albicans*, tetanus toxoid or streptococcal kinase were found primarily in the Th17 subset, whereas CD4$^+$ T cells specific for pathogens like HIV, adenovirus, CMV, EBV, influenza virus, or *Mycobacterium tuberculosis* (MTB) were present in the Th1 subset [15,16]. Most likely, these distinct T-cell profiles reflect differential immune requirements to control different pathogens. Pathogens differ in tropism, replication kinetics, and other biological properties (e.g., immune evasion mechanisms). The immune system has adapted to these specific traits by mounting specialized T-cell responses. This introduces the concept of pathogen-specific T-cell memory profile, which is obviously central in the context of vaccination. A vaccine should induce memory responses adapted to a given pathogen in order to protect against that specific infection.

Parameters influencing the induction of a T-cell response

The generation, differentiation, and maintenance of memory T cells rely on multiple parameters.

Type of Ag-presenting cells

T-cell priming is controlled by dendritic cells (DC). DCs are a family of professional antigen-presenting cells (APC) present in low numbers in virtually all organs. DCs have unique capacities to process and present pathogen-derived Ag to T cells, which distinguishes them from other APC such as B cells and macrophages. DCs are engaged in functional cross-talks with naïve T cells, leading to their activation, proliferation, and differentiation into memory cells. These immunostimulatory properties depend on the type of DC and their maturation status.

DCs are divided into several subsets based on their hematopoietic origins, the expression of cell-surface markers, and their localization in the body. Two major DC subpopulations have been identified: CD11c^{high} myeloid (myDC, expressing CD1b/CD1c, CD16, or BDCA3) and CD11c^{low} plasmacytoid DC (pDC, expressing CD123, BDCA2, and BDCA4) [17]. pDC are important mediators of antiviral immunity: they process and present Ag to T cells, and secrete large amounts of IFN-α during viral infection [18]. However, their role in the induction and regulation of T-cell activation is a matter of debate. In contrast, the function of myDC in directing T-cell immunity is well documented. In the skin, at least three different myDC subsets have been characterized: epidermal Langerhans cells (LC) (that express Langerin or CD207) and CD14$^+$ or CD14$^-$CD207$^-$CD1a$^+$ dermal interstitial DC (intDC) [17]. These distinct skin DC subpopulations present functional specialization; for example, CD14$^+$ intDC and LC preferentially activate humoral and cellular immunity, respectively [19]. However, assigning one particular function to one DC subset might be over-simplistic. Coordinated exchanges between DC subsets most likely occur throughout the course of an immune response [20].

A primary location of DCs is the mucosa; that is, the portal of pathogen entry where DCs sense the presence of pathogen-associated molecular patterns (PAMP) and can initiate antimicrobial defenses. To this end, DCs express an array of pathogen recognition receptors (PRR) that have diverse cellular localizations, structures, and ligands. C-type lectins (e.g., Dectin-1, DC-SIGN) and Toll-like receptors (TLR) are transmembrane proteins that interact with glycoproteins or specific molecular structures such as bacterial deoxycytidyl-deoxyguanosin (CpG), respectively. NOD-like receptors (NLR) and RIG-like receptors (RLR) are cytosolic proteins that bind bacterial peptidoglycans and viral RNA/DNA, respectively (reviewed in [21]). PRR engagement triggers cytokine/chemokine secretion, migration to lymph nodes, and functional maturation of DCs. Immature DCs (imDC) are devoted to scanning the environment for antigenic material. ImDC engulf pathogen-derived Ag through receptor-dependent (lectins or FcR) or -independent mechanisms (macropinocytosis) but are relatively inefficient at processing and presenting Ag. In contrast, mature DCs (mDC) reduce their capacity to uptake Ag and acquire the capacity to present Ag to pathogen-specific T cells. The role of mDC is not limited to presenting Ag via MHC molecules; mDC provide also the signals required by T cells to become protective effector T cells and determine their differentiation profile (such as Th1 or Th2).

Antigen processing and presentation pathways

Two distinct pathways of Ag presentation involving MHC class I and II molecules are used for the activation of Ag-specific CD8$^+$ and CD4$^+$ T cells, respectively. MHC-I and -II complexes use similar peptide-binding domains to present antigenic peptides to T-cell receptors (TCR). The origin, processing pathways, and length of the peptides distinguish MHC-I and MHC-II complexes (see Chapter 3).

Peptides presented by MHC-II molecules originate from protein that gained access to endosomal compartments. Peptide proteolysis is mediated by endosomal proteases whose function is regulated by acidic pH. MHC-II molecules are composed of an α and a β chain. Newly formed MHC-II $\alpha\beta$ heterodimers are stabilized by invariant chain Ii and accumulate in late endositic compartments. Antigenic peptides are then loaded on these immature MHC-II heterodimers in a process that requires a peptide exchange tightly regulated by the chaperone HLA-DM. It is generally assumed that MHC-II binding peptides originate solely from exogenous sources (protein or pathogen) taken up by membrane engulfment (e.g., macropinocitosis or phagocytosis). However, accumulating evidence suggests that cytosolic or nuclear proteins also represent a source of Ag, provided that the precursor peptide gains access to endosomal compartments [22].

To a large extent, MHC-I molecules present peptides that originate from endogenous proteins. Nascent MHC molecules acquire the antigenic peptide during their initial assembly in the endoplasmic reticulum (ER). Peptide precursors are generated from the catabolism of endogenous proteins by the proteasomes and other proteases. Peptides are then translocated into the ER by TAP (transporters associated with antigen processing) pumps, where they undergo a final trimming by aminopeptidases and bind MHC-I molecules. In addition, in a process called cross-presentation, MHC molecules display peptides coming from engulfed material such as apoptotic cells or virus [23,24]. This process involves the uptake of antigenic material into specialized compartments equipped with the classical

MHC-I presentation machinery [25] or delivery of the viral Ag to the cytosol [26].

TLR signaling and antigen processing/presentation

The function of PRR in cytokine and chemokine secretion has been extensively studied (see Chapter 26). More recently, it has been proposed that PRR signaling also regulates Ag uptake, DC migration, and Ag processing/presentation. TLRs are expressed either at the cell surface (e.g., TLR2, TLR4, TLR6) or inside late endosomal compartments (e.g., TLR3, TLR7, TLR9). Depending on their cellular localization, TLRs control phagosome formation and maturation. TLR signaling within the Ag-loaded phagosome might facilitate the fusion with lysosome or access to MHC-II loading compartments [27]. PRR also induce the expression of antiviral factors, such as the DNA editing enzyme APOBEC3G, that contribute to the generation of MHC-I epitopes and thus enhance CTL activation [28]. PRR, including lectins and TLRs, are implicated in MHC-I cross-presentation (see, for instance, [24,29]). In addition, TLR signaling triggers a remodeling of the intravesicular compartments, leading to the recruitment at the cell surface of peptide-MHC complexes and of co-stimulatory molecules required for optimal T-cell activation. Overall, PRR, such as TLR, determine the nature of the signals delivered to T cells and thus, T-cell activation, clonal expansion, and T-cell differentiation.

Strength of T-cell receptor stimulation

The strength of the signal received by the TCR during priming depends on several complementary parameters: density of Ag presented by MHC molecules on the APC, duration of the TCR-peptide:MHC interaction, the presence and engagement of co-stimulatory molecules, and the affinity of the TCR for its cognate peptide:MHC complex. Ag density (or quantity) and duration of T-cell priming dictate not only the level of initial cell proliferation (burst size), but also the size and quality of the resulting memory pool (reviewed in [30]). As for TCR-peptide:MHC affinity, it has been shown that while low-affinity interactions are sufficient

for T-cell activation, higher affinity interactions are needed for sustained T-cell expansion, resulting in larger memory T cell pools [31]. Meanwhile, co-stimulation not only lowers the activation threshold of T cells [32] but also improves T-cell differentiation [33] (see Chapter 25).

Frequency of precursors

The frequency of naïve T-cell precursors can vary widely between populations with different MHC-Ag specificities. In mice, precursor frequency can correlate with the magnitude of the primary T-cell response and memory cell immunodominance patterns [34,35]. Moreover, it can affect the differentiation kinetics of memory T cells. Indeed, experiments in mice have shown that higher precursor frequencies permit a more rapid transition of T cells to a central memory phenotype [36,37]. Precursor frequency is thus emerging as another variable that can shape T-cell memory.

Maintenance/homeostasis of memory T cells

The maintenance of memory T cell pools is critical to provide life-long immunity to the desired pathogen or cancer. Decades ago, it was assumed that Ag persistence was required to preserve effective memory T cells. However, it appears now that preservation of memory cells could be independent of TCR signaling (for review see [38]). Memory T-cell maintenance is regulated by a combination of IL7 and IL15, which primarily support cell viability and basal homeostatic proliferation, respectively. Signaling through IL7 receptors induces the expression of anti-apoptotic factors such as bcl-2 in T cells [39,40]. Interestingly, the first observation that persistence of memory T cells required cytokine secretions came from studies on TLR ligands like poly I:C and lipopolysaccharide (LPS) [41,42]. These molecules are able to induce the secretion of type I IFN, which in turn triggers the synthesis of IL15 by a variety of cell types, including APCs [43]. IL15 receptor is composed of CD122 (IL15Rb) and CD132 (γc), which are expressed by memory CD8$^+$ and CD4$^+$ T cells.

In conclusion, multiple parameters determine the fate of T cells and their differentiation into diverse memory T cells (Figure 5.3): on the APC

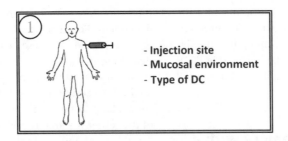

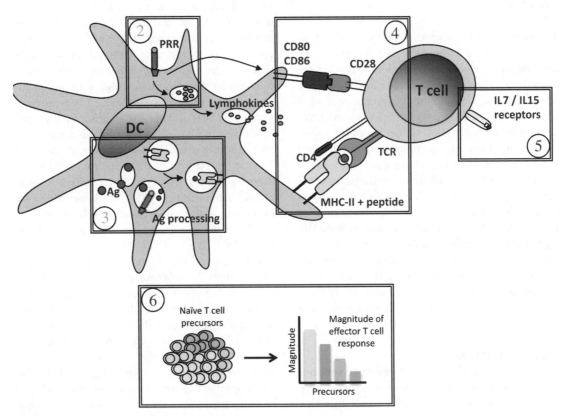

Figure 5.3 Parameters influencing the induction of a T-cell response. The intimate contacts established between T cells and DCs during the initial activation of antigen-specific T cells will determine the generation and differentiation of memory T cells. The site of injection, hence the type of DC encountered, and the diversity of PRR expressed by the DC will be fundamental (1). PRR-induction influences lymphokine secretion and the upregulation of co-stimulatory molecules (2), as well as phagosome maturation, antigen processing, and presentation by MHC molecules (3). Overall, the strength of the signal delivered by DC, meaning the resultant of multiple engagements including TCR-MHC and co-stimulatory molecules (such as CD28/CD80 or CD86), will impact on T cell differentiation (4). To that regard, the antigen sensitivity of the T cell *per se* probably plays a major role. Notably, the precursor frequency of the antigen-specific T cells (5) and the expression of IL15/IL7 receptors (6) may also influence the establishment and maintenance of memory responses.

side, the type of DC (subset, localization) and the signal received for maturation (type of PRR engaged) influence the nature and strength of the signals delivered to T cells; on the T cell side, TCR signaling and the precursor frequency shape T-cell memory.

Induction of T-cell memory with a vaccine

The most successful vaccines developed to date protect against acute rather than chronic infections, and induce predominantly humoral immune responses, in particular neutralizing antibodies. For these vaccines, a certain titer of specific antibodies has been defined as a surrogate marker – or correlate – of protection. Recent studies have also shown that cellular immunity may play a role in licensed vaccines, for instance in protecting against hepatitis A virus (HAV), MTB, influenza, varicella, and typhoid fever [44–48]. Developing vaccines against pathogens that cause chronic infections, such as HIV, HCV, MTB, or *Plasmodium falciparum* (malaria) represents a particular challenge. Elimination of these pathogens is likely to require the induction of strong T cell-immunity, since (i) neutralizing antibodies do not seem to confer protection, due to a high variability of pathogen outer components, and (ii) infected cells must be destroyed.

Major obstacles

The development of successful T-cell based vaccines has been hampered by three major obstacles: (i) the lack of reliable correlates of protection in humans; (ii) the choice of a good immunogen to induce T-cell responses; and (iii) the diversity of the host, particularly in terms of HLA polymorphism.

Defining the correlates of protection

Correlates of protection refer to an immunologic variable that can be measured in vaccinated/naturally-immunized individuals and is predictive of protection against a given pathogen. It differs from immunogenicity – that is, the capacity of a vaccine to induce an immune response – which is not necessarily protective. Correlates of

protection are vaccine- and infection/pathogen-dependent. For major epidemics like HIV, malaria, and tuberculosis, these correlates are still ill defined [49].

Which characteristics of T-cell responses generated by a vaccine may correlate with protection? By analogy to humoral responses, the magnitude of the response – that is, the number of Ag-specific T cells – may be a critical parameter. This can be assessed using tetramers (which enable the detection of T cells specific for a certain HLA-epitope combination) or by measuring their capacity to secrete soluble factors (e.g., IFN-γ) upon stimulation with the cognate Ag (either by ELISPOT or by intracellular fluorescent staining). However, it has been shown that not all Ag-specific T cells are functional, and that attempts to measure their magnitude might not be enough to ascertain protection [50]. Another candidate for correlate of protection may be the breadth of the response – that is, the diversity of antigens targeted by T cells. The initial assumption is that the broader the better. However, in the case of HIV infection, some infected individuals seem to control the virus using narrow Ag diversity [51].

The quality of the response rather than its magnitude might be determinant for protection. The quality is defined as the capacity of T cells to elicit a wide variety of effector functions: proliferation in response to Ag or induction of proliferation of other cells, cytokine and chemokine secretion, expression of antiviral factors, and the capacity to lyse target cells. It remains a challenge to determine which specific effector functions correlate with protection against a particular infection. T cells capable of eliciting several effector functions simultaneously (referred to as polyfunctional) may be better at controlling infections. Indeed, the "polyfunctionality" of Ag-specific T cells correlates with improved control of HIV replication in humans [52,53] and with predicted protection against *Leishmania major* in mouse [54]. These polyfunctional T cells are not only better because they can perform multiple tasks, but also, apparently, because they are better at each particular function; for example, a polyfunctional T cell secretes more IFN-γ than a monofunctional one [54,55]. However, in a particular infectious setting, more polyfunctionality is not necessary better; the best "quality" might be a specific balance of different effector functions.

Another qualitative aspect that may correlate with protection is Ag sensitivity (or avidity) of T cells; that is, the efficiency to recognize its cognate Ag at a given Ag density. T cells with high Ag sensitivity recognize Ag presented by MHC molecules at lower densities and are more efficient at controlling or clearing infected or transformed cells (reviewed in [56]). The efficacy of high-avidity T cells can be attributed to several – probably complementary – mechanisms: they recognize and kill infected cells earlier and faster (cells are eliminated before new viral progeny are made); their effector functions are triggered more readily and more efficiently (e.g., cells are more polyfunctional) [57,58]. High-avidity T cells could thus be better at controlling infection or deleting tumor cells than low-avidity counterparts. However, they may also be more sensitive to deletion by apoptosis in the presence of high densities of Ag [59].

A key parameter for protection is also the location of the T cells. Induction of good quality T cells with a vaccine in blood or lymph nodes but not at mucosal surfaces or other compartments that represent entry or replication sites for pathogens (e.g., vaginal or rectal tract for sexually transmitted diseases; respiratory tract for MTB; liver for *Plasmodium falciparum*) may lack protective efficacy. These potential correlates of protection (quantitative: magnitude, breadth; and qualitative: polyfunctionality, Ag sensitivity, location) may even be interdependent (Figure 5.4). A major challenge for immunologists is to define reliable correlate(s) of protection to guide rational vaccine design.

Choice of immunogen

Whole proteins, peptides, and inactivated or attenuated whole pathogens are not equivalent sources of Ag, and can result in distinct T-cell responses. Upon infection with a pathogen, the host generates a panel of T cells against several, but not every possible, epitopes, a phenomenon termed immunodominance. Immunodominant epitopes presented in the natural course of an infection might not be optimal for inducing protective immunity, particu-

larly in chronic infections. This may be related to several factors. First, immunodominant Ag may be derived from proteins that support high sequence variability, thus facilitating the generation of CTL escape mutations. In HIV infection, CTL targeting the conserved HIV Gag protein have been associated with lower viral loads, while CTL targeting the variable HIV Env protein are associated with higher viral loads [60]. Naturally processed epitopes may induce a lower magnitude and/or low-quality T-cell response. Finally, the kinetics of epitope expression might have a direct impact on the induction of protective T-cell responses. Targeting proteins that are present or expressed early during infection might dampen pathogen spread. In HIV infection, the HIV Gag protein is carried into the cell by the infecting virions, and this protein can be processed and presented without *de novo* synthesis [24,26], making it a good candidate for targeting. In the case of malaria infection, targeting proteins from the early pre-erythrocitic stage might be a promising vaccination strategy [61].

Another major hurdle in the choice of the immunogen is the sequence variability of a given pathogen. Some pathogens, such as HIV, HCV, dengue virus, or *Plasmodium*, mutate rapidly and/or differ largely from one geographic region to another. Hence, the antigen to be included in a vaccine should be adapted to the particular region of the globe where the vaccine will be eventually applied. Alternatively, the vaccine might target the most conserved proteins, for which evolution and sequence diversity are limited and thus mutations might come at a great fitness cost. Another possibility would be to design mosaic vaccines that include consensus, ancestral sequences, or variants of the same protein [62].

Overcoming host diversity

Ideally, a vaccine should provide protection to all individuals, regardless of age, ethnicity (genetics), co-infections, or immunodeficiencies. However, even highly effective vaccines such as the one against smallpox can generate severe adverse effects in some individuals [63], while immunodeficient and elderly patients do not respond as well to influenza [64] and possibly other vaccines.

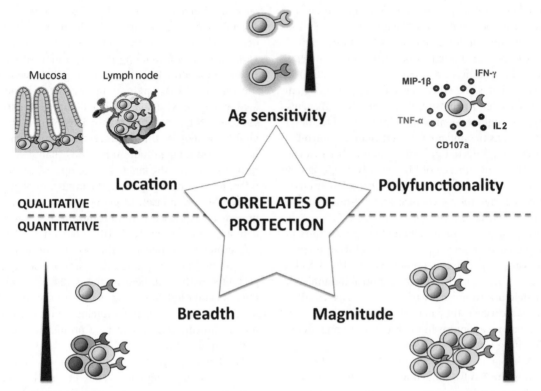

Figure 5.4 Correlates of immune protection. To date, several potential correlates of immune protection have been evaluated in different infectious settings. Quantitative parameters that may correlate with protection in some settings include the magnitude – that is, the number of antigen-specific T cells – and the breadth of the T-cell response – that is, the diversity of antigens against which the T-cell response is directed. Qualitative parameters that have more recently been studied as possible correlates of protection include polyfunctionality, the capacity of an antigen-specific T cell to elicit different effector functions simultaneously (secreting several cytokines and/or chemokines such as IL2, IFN-γ, TNF-α or MIP-1β, degranulating, as measured by CD107a mobilization); antigen sensitivity, the efficiency with which a given T cell recognizes an antigen at a specific antigen density; and the location or compartmentalization of the induced T-cell response, which in some settings may require to be mucosal as well as in blood and lymph nodes.

With age, the capacity of the immune system declines, resulting in an increased incidence and/or severity of many infectious diseases (e.g., influenza, pneumonia, meningitis, sepsis, varicella zoster virus, severe acute respiratory syndrome) and a higher prevalence of cancers in the elderly. The T-cell compartment is particularly affected during the process of aging: the thymus naturally atrophies, a process termed "thymic involution" [65]. Progressive decay of the thymus results in a decreased production of T cells and lower numbers of naïve T cells. Restricted T-cell repertoire and accumulation of highly differentiated memory T cells are also characteristics of older individuals [66]. Thus, the immune system of the elderly likely recognizes a narrower range of Ag, which may affect the effectiveness of vaccination.

Host genetics, and particularly HLA polymorphism, have been shown to be vitally important in the control of some chronic infections. Specific HLA class I molecules are consistently associated with progression to AIDS: while HLA-B27 and -B57 are predominant in individuals who control HIV, HLA-B35 has been associated with a more rapid disease progression (reviewed in [51]). Particular HLA alleles have also been shown to contribute to HCV clearance and chronicity (reviewed in [67]). HLA-B35 has been associated with lower risk of malaria complications. HLA diversity probably plays a role in driving pathogen evolution at the population level, and the frequency of the protective allele in the population can also alter the infection spread (reviewed in [51]). Ideally, T-cell vaccines must overcome these HLA-based differences and provide protective responses in all populations. The choice of the immunogen will be crucial. Conserved proteins that are targeted by a wide array of different HLA molecules might be good candidates.

Manipulating the immune response with a vaccine

A number of parameters can be manipulated in order to influence the attributes of vaccine-induced T cells.

The antigen: quality and quantity

Concerning the "quality" of the Ag, as we have seen, immunodominant epitopes generated in the course of an infection might not be the best for inducing protective T-cell responses. However, immunodominant and subdominant epitopes can be improved in order to obtain better responses. This "epitope enhancement" can be achieved in various ways: (i) by changing the anchor residues of the epitope to improve its binding to the MHC class I molecule; (ii) by altering the MHC-peptide complexes to increase their affinity to the TCR; or (iii) by altering the epitope to obtain a more broadly cross-reactive T-cell response that recognizes more strains of the pathogen (reviewed in [68]). As for the quantity of the Ag, T cells require a minimal quantitative threshold of Ag to react and the Ag must last a certain minimum time to trigger an immune response (reviewed in [30]). During the expansion phase, the Ag quantity might directly impact the size of the effector populations; that is, the number of pathogen-specific T cells (reviewed in [69]). However, the exact quantity of Ag required

for the activation of T-cell response is still a matter of debate. Some studies showed that a higher quantity of Ag increases the number of activated T cells and improves their quality [70,71]. In contrast, studies focusing on Ag sensitivity suggest that lower Ag concentrations may lead to the induction of T cells with higher Ag sensitivity [54,72] which, as we have seen, may correlate with protection. The risk of using low levels of Ag that may selectively induce higher avidity CTLs is to go below the threshold needed to induce a response. However, recent studies have shown that augmenting co-stimulation or adding cytokines such as IL15 can compensate for low Ag levels and induce high-avidity T cells [73]. The careful manipulation of the Ag (its quality as well as its quantity) to ensure optimal T-cell responses will most likely determine vaccine efficacy.

Antigen-delivery systems

Ag delivery systems, or vectors, that induce endogenous expression of the Ag within cells tend to be more immunogenic than peptides or proteins [74] (see Part 5 of this book for novel Ag-delivery systems). Ag can be delivered using DNA or virus-derived vectors. T cell-based vaccines are currently being developed using adenoviruses (AdV), poxviruses, alphaviruses, lentiviruses, retroviruses, and measles virus. Viral vectors can be divided into replicating and nonreplicating systems, and several viruses have been engineered to enter both categories (e.g., adenoviruses, alphaviruses). The type of vaccine/vector delivery system will determine the level and kinetics of Ag exposure. Short-lived nonreplicating vaccines provide Ag for a shorter time period (until the transfected/transduced cell dies or is destroyed). On the other hand, replicating vaccines provide Ag for a longer time and the quantity of Ag delivered may *in fine* be higher. Viral vectors can infect cells, such as DCs, and tissues of interest but also provide a natural adjuvant effect, leading to cytokine and chemokine secretions. Thus, vectors, replicating and nonreplicating alike, differ not only in the quantity of Ag-specific T cells they induce, but also in their quality. For example, comparing nonreplicating anti-HIV vaccines, it has been shown that AdV-5 vectors induce stronger and more polyfunctional CTL responses than poxvirus vectors [75]. Interestingly, two of the most effective vaccines known to date, against yellow fever and smallpox, can replicate in the host and induce numerous long-lived vaccine-specific CTL responses quickly after immunization [76,77]. However, vaccination with live viral vectors might cause adverse reactions, particularly in immunosuppressed individuals or the elderly [78].

Regimen: doses and prime-boosts

Many classical vaccines require several immunizations to provide complete protection. The same is probably true for T-cell vaccines, unless a highly immunogenic Ag is chosen. Repeated boosts might not only increment the quantity of Ag-specific T cells and maintain the memory T-cell pool, but also provide a mechanism for skewing the population of memory T cells toward higher affinity T-cell clones [79]. However, this strategy could backfire if too many immunizations exhaust the higher affinity T cells through repeated stimulation that pushes the cells to replicative senescence [80]. Prime-boost immunization strategies can be homologous – using the same Ag-vector combination on all immunizations – or heterologous, using the same Ag, but provided by a different vector in the prime and the boost(s). While homologous prime-boosts work well for antibody-induced vaccines, heterologous prime-boost strategies seem to induce higher numbers and better quality of Ag-specific T cells than homologous prime-boost strategies (reviewed in [81]). Heterologous prime-boosts can circumvent vector-specific immunity that may have developed with the first immunization and might dampen vaccine-specific T-cell response. These strategies are often used to augment the immunogenicity of nonreplicating vaccines. However, using replicating vectors for prime-boost in mice, a recent study achieved outstanding results, not only on the frequency, but also on the phenotype (mostly effector memory cells) and location (enriched in nonlymphoid tissues) of T-cell responses [82]. Prime-boost strategies can also be used to induce high-sensitivity T-cell clones: for instance, priming with DNA provides low levels of Ag and could in-

duce highly sensitive T cells, which could be expanded with a heterologous boost. There is now a large variety of Ag-delivery systems available that might be combined to induce optimal T-cell responses in terms of protection and durability.

Route of immunization

The route of immunization can regulate the recruitment of T cells at the site of infection, a critical factor for protection. Attracting CTL at the portal of pathogen entry such as mucosal surfaces might participate in clearance and/or containment of infections. Ideally, vaccination at a single point should induce humoral and cellular responses not only systemically but also at the periphery, for example mucosal surfaces. Research in mice and monkeys showed that mucosal immunization (e.g., intranasal, intrarectal, intravaginal) might be more prone to induce potent mucosal T-cell responses than systemic immunization (e.g., intramuscularly or subcutaneous administration) [83,84]. Transcutaneous immunization, considered a systemic route of immunization, seems to be the exception to this rule [85]. Note that mucosal immunization can also induce systemic responses, probably through migration of mucosal DCs to lymph nodes and spleen [86], and generates responses at all other mucosal surfaces [87]. However, even within the mucosal compartment, distinct routes of vaccination may influence the outcome of Ag-specific CD8+ T cells. Thus, while nasal immunization has been shown to protect against vaginal challenges in a simian immunodeficiency virus (SIV) model [88], optimal protection of the gastrointestinal tract, the rectum, and the female genital tract might still require oral, rectal, or vaginal vaccines. Nasal immunization, on the other hand, seems particularly promising for effective protection against respiratory pathogens such as MTB [89]. The route of immunization can also influence the nature of vaccine-induced T cells, probably due to the presence of distinct Ag-presenting cells at different sites. For instance, in some animal studies, mucosal immunizations induced T cells with higher Ag sensitivities compared to subcutaneous immunization [90,91]. The route of vaccination is therefore critical to recruit highly sensitive and protective T-cell responses at the site of pathogen entry.

Adjuvants

As discussed previously, in contrast to recombinant subunit vaccines, attenuated viral vectors possess natural adjuvant effects. Hence, by analogy with viruses, viral vectors induce different qualities of T-cell and antibody responses, due to their diverse tropism and/or interplay with the innate immunity [7,77,92]. Thus, vaccine design strongly relies on our knowledge of the interactions between these vaccine vectors and the immune system. However, with few exceptions, such as modified vaccinia Ankara (MVA) [93,94] and yellow fever (YF) [77,92], little is known on the biology of the different vectors in humans. On the other hand, recombinant proteins or subunits of pathogens lack immunostimulatory properties and require the development of new adjuvants (see Chapters 23 and 26). Aluminum salts (alum) is currently the major adjuvant approved for human use and is successfully used for vaccination, for example tetanus, diphteria-tetanus-pertussis (DTP). Alum induces inflammation and recruitment of APC, Ag uptake, DC maturation, and T-cell differentiation. It is very effective in inducing antibody responses. However, it is a poor stimulator of CTLs. The discovery of PRR opened new avenues for the development of safe and effective adjuvants. TLR ligands are incorporated in newly licensed adjuvants for humans [95]. Since pDC and myDC show mutually exclusive expression profiles of some TLRs [96], TLR ligands might be used to target specific DC populations, thus enhancing a desired immune response. In addition, inducing DC maturation through distinct PRR/TLR pathways might influence T-cell differentiation and memory responses [97]. Other PRR ligands, such as NLR ligands, are also good adjuvant candidates [98].

In conclusion, there is still much to learn on ways to exploit different combinations of Ag, Ag-delivery systems, adjuvants, regimen, and route of immunization in order to create a T-cell vaccine that could confer durable protection to desired pathogens.

Examples of vaccine-induced memory T-cell responses

In recent years, a number of vaccine strategies have been used in humans and nonhuman primates to assess the quality of memory T-cell responses.

Vaccinia virus immunization, which provides lifelong protection against smallpox, has been reported to induce vaccinia virus-specific CD8$^+$ T cells, which are highly polyfunctional [99]. In another study, IFN-γ-producing effector memory CD4$^+$ T cells could be observed in vaccinees 13–25 years after their last vaccinia immunization, and proliferative responses remained detectable up to 45 years after priming [100].

Recombinant poxvirus (NYVAC or MVA) is also used to induce HIV- or MTB-specific T cells. In healthy volunteers, a DNA prime/NYVAC boost vaccine regimen was shown to induce robust (detected in 90% of vaccinees), polyfunctional, and durable (present in 70% of vaccinees after 1.5 years) HIV-specific CD4$^+$ and CD8$^+$ T-cell responses [101]. Immunization with *Mycobacterium bovis* Bacille Calmette-Guérin (BCG) or MVA expressing 85A (MTB Ag) also induced long-lasting MTB-specific effector memory CD4$^+$ memory T cells presenting polyfunctional profiles and robust proliferative capacities following antigenic stimulation [102]. Interestingly, vaccination with live attenuated flavivirus such as YF induces effector memory YF-specific T-cell responses with polyfunctional properties [92,103].

In rhesus macaques, based on the observation that herpes viruses naturally induce life-long effector memory T-cell responses, a recombinant rhesus cytomegalovirus (RhCMV) has been recently tested. RhCMV vectors expressing SIV proteins persistently infected macaques, and primed and maintained robust polyfunctional SIV-specific CD4$^+$ and CD8$^+$ effector memory T cells. Upon repeated low-dose intrarectal challenge, vaccinated animals showed increased resistance to SIVmac239 infection, including four macaques that controlled rectal mucosal infection without progressive systemic dissemination [104].

In the field of cancer, efforts to develop T-cell based vaccines have mainly concentrated on immunization with peptides, derived from tumor-associated Ag, in combination with adjuvants. For instance, the induction of potent $CD8^+$ T-cell responses was achieved after vaccination with the melanoma Ag A (Melan-A or MART-1) and CpG oligodeoxynucleotides (ODNs), which trigger TLR9, resulting in DC maturation and enhanced co-stimulation. The frequency of Melan-A–specific T cells reached over 3% of circulating $CD8^+$ T cells, which was 10 times higher than the frequency in donors treated without CpG. This T cell population consisted primarily of effector memory cells, which in part secreted IFN-γ and expressed granzyme B and perforin *ex vivo* [105]. As an alternative, APC expressing various co-stimulatory molecules (i.e., B7-1, LFA-3, and ICAM-1) were shown *in vitro* to promote activation and expansion of human carcinoembryonic Ag (CEA) -specific memory $CD8^+$ T cells producing multiple cytokines [106]. Altogether, vaccine trials in the field of cancer highlight the central role of co-stimulation in inducing T-cell responses.

Concluding remarks

Vaccine design remains rather empirical because our knowledge of the immunologic memory is still incomplete. We know that the nature and the strength of the signal delivered to T cells upon priming will determine the activation, proliferation, and differentiation into protective memory T-cell subsets. However, multiple parameters influence this key process, including the type of DC, adjuvant (used to provoke inflammation and DC maturation], the quality/quantity of Ag presentation and co-stimulation, the cytokinic environment, and the Ag sensitivity of the T cells. The pathogen and its portal of entry provide another level of complexity. For different pathogens a local (mucosal) or systemic immunity might be preferred. Rational vaccine design will require defining the ins and outs of these different steps and parameters. Hopefully, mimicking, with viral or bacterial vectors, the natural immunostimulatory properties of attenuated pathogens may offer a way out. The recent discovery of PRR (see Chapter 26) and the development of sensitive techniques to measure T-cell efficacy (see Chapter 28) offer new avenues for vaccine development.

Acknowledgments

We would like to thank the members of the INSERM UMR S 945 and our collaborators for challenging scientific discussions. We would also like to thank scientists around the world for their amazing contributions in the field of T-cell immunity. We apologize to those that we could not quote due to size constraints.

References

1 Appay V, van Lier RA, Sallusto F, *et al.* Phenotype and function of human T lymphocyte subsets: consensus and issues. *Cytometry A* 2008;**73**:975–83.

2 Hamann D, Baars PA, Rep MH, *et al.* Phenotypic and functional separation of memory and effector human CD8+ T cells. *J Exp Med* 1997;**186**:1407–18.

3 Fazilleau N, Mark L, McHeyzer-Williams LJ, *et al.* Follicular helper T cells: lineage and location. *Immunity* 2009;**30**:324–35.

4 Sallusto F, Lanzavecchia A. Heterogeneity of $CD4^+$ memory T cells: functional modules for tailored immunity. *Eur J Immunol* 2009;**39**:2076–82.

5 Appay V, Papagno L, Spina CA, *et al.* Dynamics of T cell responses in HIV infection. *J Immunol* 2002;**168**:3660–66.

6 Sakaguchi S, Miyara M, Costantino CM, *et al.* $FOXP3^+$ regulatory T cells in the human immune system. *Nat Rev Immunol* 2010;**10**:490–500.

7 Appay V, Dunbar PR, Callan M, *et al.* Memory $CD8^+$ T cells vary in differentiation phenotype in different persistent virus infections. *Nat Med* 2002;**8**:379–85.

8 He XS, Mahmood K, Maecker HT, *et al.* Analysis of the frequencies and of the memory T cell phenotypes of human $CD8^+$ T cells specific for influenza A viruses. *J Infect Dis* 2003;**187**:1075–84.

9 Tussey LG, Nair US, Bachinsky M, *et al.* Antigen burden is major determinant of human immunodeficiency virus-specific $CD8^+$ T cell maturation state: potential implications for therapeutic immunization. *J Infect Dis* 2003;**187**:364–74.

10 Gamadia LE, van Leeuwen EM, Remmerswaal EB, *et al.* The size and phenotype of virus-specific T cell populations is determined by repetitive antigenic

stimulation and environmental cytokines. *J Immunol* 2004;**172**:6107–14.

11 Papagno L, Spina CA, Marchant A, *et al.* Immune activation and CD8(+) T-Cell differentiation towards senescence in HIV-1 infection. *PLoS Biol* 2004;**2**:E20.

12 Harari A, Enders FB, Cellerai C, *et al.* Distinct profiles of cytotoxic granules in memory CD8 T cells correlate with function, differentiation stage, and antigen exposure. *J Virol* 2009;**83**:2862–71.

13 Appay V, Zaunders JJ, Papagno L, *et al.* Characterization of CD4(+) CTLs ex vivo. *J Immunol* 2002;**168**:5954–8.

14 van Leeuwen EM, Remmerswaal EB, Vossen MT, *et al.* Emergence of a CD4$^+$CD28$^-$ granzyme B$^+$, cytomegalovirus-specific T cell subset after recovery of primary cytomegalovirus infection. *J Immunol* 2004;**173**:1834–41.

15 Acosta-Rodriguez EV, Rivino L, Geginat J, *et al.* Surface phenotype and antigenic specificity of human interleukin 17-producing T helper memory cells. *Nat Immunol* 2007;**8**:639–46.

16 Brenchley JM, Paiardini M, Knox KS, *et al.* Differential Th17 CD4 T-cell depletion in pathogenic and nonpathogenic lentiviral infections. *Blood* 2008;**112**:2826–35.

17 Shortman K, Naik SH. Steady-state and inflammatory dendritic-cell development. *Nat Rev Immunol* 2007;**7**:19–30.

18 Villadangos JA, Young L. Antigen-presentation properties of plasmacytoid dendritic cells. *Immunity* 2008;**29**:352–61.

19 Klechevsky E, Morita R, Liu M, *et al.* Functional specializations of human epidermal Langerhans cells and CD14$^+$ dermal dendritic cells. *Immunity* 2008;**29**:497–510.

20 de Heusch M, Blocklet D, Egrise D, *et al.* Bidirectional MHC molecule exchange between migratory and resident dendritic cells. *J Leukoc Biol* 2007;**82**:861–8.

21 Kawai T, Akira S. The roles of TLRs, RLRs and NLRs in pathogen recognition. *Int Immunol* 2009;**21**:317–37.

22 Crotzer VL, Blum JS. Autophagy and its role in MHC-mediated antigen presentation. *J Immunol* 2009;**182**:3335–41.

23 Albert ML, Sauter B, Bhardwaj N. Dendritic cells acquire antigen from apoptotic cells and induce class I-restricted CTLs. *Nature* 1998;**392**:86–9.

24 Moris A, Nobile C, Buseyne F, *et al.* DC-SIGN promotes exogenous MHC-I-restricted HIV-1 antigen presentation. *Blood* 2004;**103**:2648–54.

25 Saveanu L, Carroll O, Weimershaus M, *et al.* IRAP identifies an endosomal compartment required for MHC class I cross-presentation. *Science* 2009;**325**:213–17.

26 Buseyne F, Le Gall S, Boccaccio C, *et al.* MHC-I-restricted presentation of HIV-1 virion antigens without viral replication. *Nat Med* 2001;**7**:344–9.

27 Blander JM, Medzhitov R. Toll-dependent selection of microbial antigens for presentation by dendritic cells. *Nature* 2006;**440**:808–12.

28 Casartelli N, Guivel-Benhassine F, Bouziat R, *et al.* The antiviral factor APOBEC3G improves CTL recognition of cultured HIV-infected T cells. *J Exp Med* 2010;**207**:39–49.

29 Sancho D, Joffre OP, Keller AM, *et al.* Identification of a dendritic cell receptor that couples sensing of necrosis to immunity. *Nature* 2009;**458**:899–903.

30 Bushar ND, Farber DL. Recalling the year in memory T cells. *Ann N Y Acad Sci* 2008;**1143**:212–25.

31 Zehn D, Lee SY, Bevan MJ. Complete but curtailed T-cell response to very low-affinity antigen. *Nature* 2009;**458**:211–14.

32 Viola A, Lanzavecchia A. T cell activation determined by T cell receptor number and tunable thresholds. *Science* 1996;**273**:104–6.

33 Fuse S, Zhang W, Usherwood EJ. Control of memory CD8$^+$ T cell differentiation by CD80/CD86-CD28 costimulation and restoration by IL-2 during the recall response. *J Immunol* 2008;**180**:1148–57.

34 Moon JJ, Chu HH, Pepper M, *et al.* Naive CD4(+) T cell frequency varies for different epitopes and predicts repertoire diversity and response magnitude. *Immunity* 2007;**27**:203–13.

35 Obar JJ, Khanna KM, Lefrancois L. Endogenous naive CD8$^+$ T cell precursor frequency regulates primary and memory responses to infection. *Immunity* 2008;**28**:859–69.

36 Hataye J, Moon JJ, Khoruts A, *et al.* Naive and memory CD4$^+$ T cell survival controlled by clonal abundance. *Science* 2006;**312**:114–16.

37 Marzo AL, Klonowski KD, Le Bon A, *et al.* Initial T cell frequency dictates memory CD8$^+$ T cell lineage commitment. *Nat Immunol* 2005;**6**:793–9.

38 Surh CD, Sprent J. Homeostasis of naive and memory T cells. *Immunity* 2008;**29**:848–62.

39 Carrio R, Rolle CE, Malek TR. Non-redundant role for IL-7R signaling for the survival of CD8$^+$ memory T cells. *Eur J Immunol* 2007;**37**:3078–88.

40 Osborne LC, Dhanji S, Snow JW, *et al.* Impaired CD8 T cell memory and CD4 T cell primary

responses in IL-7R alpha mutant mice. *J Exp Med* 2007;**204**:619–31.

41 Tough DF, Borrow P, Sprent J. Induction of by-stander T cell proliferation by viruses and type I interferon in vivo. *Science* 1996;**272**:1947–50.

42 Tough DF, Sun S, Sprent J. T cell stimulation in vivo by lipopolysaccharide (LPS). *J Exp Med* 1997;**185**:2089–94.

43 Zhang X, Sun S, Hwang I, *et al.* Potent and selective stimulation of memory-phenotype CD8$^+$ T cells in vivo by IL-15. *Immunity* 1998;**8**:591–9.

44 Arvin A. Aging, immunity, and the varicella-zoster virus. *N Engl J Med* 2005;**352**:2266–7.

45 Lazarevic V, Flynn J. CD8$^+$ T cells in tuberculosis. *Am J Respir Crit Care Med* 2002;**166**:1116–21.

46 Salerno-Goncalves R, Pasetti MF, Sztein MB. Characterization of CD8(+) effector T cell responses in volunteers immunized with *Salmonella enterica* serovar Typhi strain Ty21a typhoid vaccine. *J Immunol* 2002;**169**:2196–203.

47 Schmidtke P, Habermehl P, Knuf M, *et al.* Cell mediated and antibody immune response to inactivated hepatitis A vaccine. *Vaccine* 2005;**23**:5127–32.

48 Thomas PG, Keating R, Hulse-Post DJ, *et al.* Cell-mediated protection in influenza infection. *Emerg Infect Dis* 2006;**12**:48–54.

49 Seder RA, Darrah PA, Roederer M. T-cell quality in memory and protection: implications for vaccine design. *Nat Rev Immunol* 2008;**8**:247–58.

50 Gea-Banacloche JC, Migueles SA, Martino L, *et al.* Maintenance of large numbers of virus-specific CD8$^+$ T cells in HIV-infected progressors and long-term nonprogressors. *J Immunol* 2000;**165**:1082–92.

51 Goulder PJ, Watkins DI. Impact of MHC class I diversity on immune control of immunodeficiency virus replication. *Nat Rev Immunol* 2008;**8**:619–30.

52 Almeida JR, Price DA, Papagno L, *et al.* Superior control of HIV-1 replication by CD8$^+$ T cells is reflected by their avidity, polyfunctionality, and clonal turnover. *J Exp Med* 2007;**204**:2473–85.

53 Betts MR, Nason MC, West SM, *et al.* HIV nonprogressors preferentially maintain highly functional HIV-specific CD8$^+$ T cells. *Blood* 2006;**107**:4781–9.

54 Darrah PA, Patel DT, De Luca PM, et al. Multifunctional TH1 cells define a correlate of vaccine-mediated protection against *Leishmania major*. *Nat Med* 2007;**13**:843–50.

55 Kannanganat S, Ibegbu C, Chennareddi L, *et al.* Multiple-cytokine-producing antiviral CD4 T cells are functionally superior to single-cytokine-producing cells. *J Virol* 2007;**81**:8468–76.

56 Appay V, Douek DC, Price DA. CD8$^+$ T cell efficacy in vaccination and disease. *Nat Med* 2008;**14**:623–8.

57 Almeida JR, Sauce D, Price DA, *et al.* Antigen sensitivity is a major determinant of CD8$^+$ T-cell polyfunctionality and HIV-suppressive activity. *Blood* 2009;**113**:6351–60.

58 Derby M, Alexander-Miller M, Tse R, *et al.* High-avidity CTL exploit two complementary mechanisms to provide better protection against viral infection than low-avidity CTL. *J Immunol* 2001;**166**:1690–97.

59 Alexander-Miller MA, Derby MA, Sarin A, *et al.* Supraoptimal peptide-major histocompatibility complex causes a decrease in bc1-2 levels and allows tumor necrosis factor alpha receptor II-mediated apoptosis of cytotoxic T lymphocytes. *J Exp Med* 1998;**188**:1391–9.

60 Kiepiela P, Ngumbela K, Thobakgale C, *et al.* CD8$^+$ T-cell responses to different HIV proteins have discordant associations with viral load. *Nat Med* 2007;**13**:46–53.

61 Alonso PL, Sacarlal J, Aponte JJ, *et al.* Efficacy of the RTS,S/AS02A vaccine against *Plasmodium falciparum* infection and disease in young African children: randomised controlled trial. *Lancet* 2004;**364**:1411–20.

62 Nickle DC, Rolland M, Jensen MA, *et al.* Coping with viral diversity in HIV vaccine design. *PLoS Comput Biol* 2007;**3**:e75.

63 Poland GA, Grabenstein JD, Neff JM. The US smallpox vaccination program: a review of a large modern era smallpox vaccination implementation program. *Vaccine* 2005;**23**:2078–81.

64 Kamps BS, Hoffmann C, Preiser W (Eds). *Influenza Report.* Flying Publisher, 2006. Available at www.influenzareport.com/influenzareport.pdf. Accessed January 2012.

65 Lynch HE, Goldberg GL, Chidgey A, *et al.* Thymic involution and immune reconstitution. *Trends Immunol* 2009;**30**:366–73.

66 Weng NP, Akbar AN, Goronzy J. CD28(-) T cells: their role in the age-associated decline of immune function. *Trends Immunol* 2009;**30**:306–12.

67 Isaguliants MG, Ozeretskovskaya NN. Host background factors contributing to hepatitis C virus clearance. *Curr Pharm Biotechnol* 2003;**4**:185–93.

68 Berzofsky JA, Ahlers JD, Belyakov IM. Strategies for designing and optimizing new generation vaccines. *Nat Rev Immunol* 2001;**1**:209–19.

69 Lanzavecchia A, Sallusto F. Antigen decoding by T lymphocytes: from synapses to fate determination. *Nat Immunol* 2001;**2**:487–92.

70 La Gruta NL, Turner SJ, Doherty PC. Hierarchies in cytokine expression profiles for acute and resolving influenza virus-specific CD8[+] T cell responses: correlation of cytokine profile and TCR avidity. *J Immunol* 2004;**172**:5553–60.

71 Valitutti S, Muller S, Dessing M, *et al.* Different responses are elicited in cytotoxic T lymphocytes by different levels of T cell receptor occupancy. *J Exp Med* 1996;**183**:1917–21.

72 Alexander-Miller MA, Leggatt GR, Berzofsky JA. Selective expansion of high- or low-avidity cytotoxic T lymphocytes and efficacy for adoptive immunotherapy. *Proc Natl Acad Sci U S A* 1996;**93**: 4102–7.

73 Oh S, Hodge JW, Ahlers JD, *et al.* Selective induction of high avidity CTL by altering the balance of signals from APC. *J Immunol* 2003;**170**:2523–30.

74 Sedlik C, Dadaglio G, Saron MF, *et al.* In vivo induction of a high-avidity, high-frequency cytotoxic T-lymphocyte response is associated with antiviral protective immunity. *J Virol* 2000;**74**: 5769–75.

75 Sun Y, Santra S, Schmitz JE, *et al.* Magnitude and quality of vaccine-elicited T-cell responses in the control of immunodeficiency virus replication in rhesus monkeys. *J Virol* 2008;**82**:8812–19.

76 Demkowicz WE, Jr, Littaua RA, Wang J, *et al.* Human cytotoxic T-cell memory: long-lived responses to vaccinia virus. *J Virol* 1996;**70**:2627–31.

77 Querec TD, Akondy RS, Lee EK, *et al.* Systems biology approach predicts immunogenicity of the yellow fever vaccine in humans. *Nat Immunol* 2009;**10**:116–25.

78 Kretzschmar M, Wallinga J, Teunis P, *et al.* Frequency of adverse events after vaccination with different vaccinia strains. *PLoS Med* 2006;**3**:e272.

79 Busch DH, Pamer EG. T cell affinity maturation by selective expansion during infection. *J Exp Med* 1999;**189**:701–10.

80 Narayan S, Choyce A, Fernando GJ, *et al.* Secondary immunisation with high-dose heterologous peptide leads to CD8 T cell populations with reduced functional avidity. *Eur J Immunol* 2007;**37**:406–15.

81 Woodland DL. Jump-starting the immune system: prime-boosting comes of age. *Trends Immunol* 2004;**25**:98–104.

82 Masopust D, Ha SJ, Vezys V, *et al.* Stimulation history dictates memory CD8 T cell phenotype: implications for prime-boost vaccination. *J Immunol* 2006;**177**:831–9.

83 Egan MA, Chong SY, Rose NF, *et al.* Immunogenicity of attenuated vesicular stomatitis virus vectors expressing HIV type 1 Env and SIV Gag proteins: comparison of intranasal and intramuscular vaccination routes. *AIDS Res Hum Retroviruses* 2004;**20**:989–1004.

84 Qimron U, Paul L, Bar-Haim E, *et al.* Nonreplicating mucosal and systemic vaccines: quantitative and qualitative differences in the Ag-specific CD8(+) T cell population in different tissues. *Vaccine* 2004;**22**:1390–94.

85 Belyakov IM, Hammond SA, Ahlers JD, *et al.* Transcutaneous immunization induces mucosal CTLs and protective immunity by migration of primed skin dendritic cells. *J Clin Invest* 2004;**113**:998–1007.

86 Iwasaki A, Kelsall BL. Unique functions of CD11b+, CD8 alpha+, and double-negative Peyer's patch dendritic cells. *J Immunol* 2001;**166**:4884–90.

87 Mestecky J. The common mucosal immune system and current strategies for induction of immune responses in external secretions. *J Clin Immunol* 1987;**7**:265–76.

88 Enose Y, Ui M, Miyake A, *et al.* Protection by intranasal immunization of a nef-deleted, nonpathogenic SHIV against intravaginal challenge with a heterologous pathogenic SHIV. *Virology* 2002;**298**:306–16.

89 Kallenius G, Pawlowski A, Brandtzaeg P, *et al.* Should a new tuberculosis vaccine be administered intranasally? *Tuberculosis (Edinb)* 2007;**87**:257–66.

90 Belyakov IM, Isakov D, Zhu Q, *et al.* A novel functional CTL avidity/activity compartmentalization to the site of mucosal immunization contributes to protection of macaques against simian/human immunodeficiency viral depletion of mucosal CD4[+] T cells. *J Immunol* 2007;**178**:7211–21.

91 Ranasinghe C, Turner SJ, McArthur C, *et al.* Mucosal HIV-1 pox virus prime-boost immunization induces high-avidity CD8+ T cells with regime-dependent cytokine/granzyme B profiles. *J Immunol* 2007;**178**:2370–9.

92 Gaucher D, Therrien R, Kettaf N, *et al.* Yellow fever vaccine induces integrated multilineage and polyfunctional immune responses. *J Exp Med* 2008;**205**:3119–31.

93 Brandler S, Lepelley A, Desdouits M, *et al.* Preclinical studies of a modified vaccinia virus Ankara-based HIV candidate vaccine: antigen presentation and antiviral effect. *J Virol* 2010;**84**:5314–28.

94 Delaloye J, Roger T, Steiner-Tardivel QG, *et al.* Innate immune sensing of modified vaccinia virus Ankara (MVA) is mediated by TLR2-TLR6, MDA-5 and the NALP3 inflammasome. *PLoS Pathog* 2009;**5**:e1000480.

95 Harandi AM, Davies G, Olesen OF. Vaccine adjuvants: scientific challenges and strategic initiatives. *Expert Rev Vaccines* 2009;**8**:293–8.

96 Kadowaki N, Ho S, Antonenko S, *et al.* Subsets of human dendritic cell precursors express different toll-like receptors and respond to different microbial antigens. *J Exp Med* 2001;**194**:863–9.

97 Fritz JH, Le Bourhis L, Sellge G, *et al.* Nod1-mediated innate immune recognition of peptidoglycan contributes to the onset of adaptive immunity. *Immunity* 2007;**26**:445–59.

98 Geddes K, Magalhaes JG, Girardin SE. Unleashing the therapeutic potential of NOD-like receptors. *Nat Rev Drug Discov* 2009;**8**:465–79.

99 Precopio ML, Betts MR, Parrino J, *et al.* Immunization with vaccinia virus induces polyfunctional and phenotypically distinctive CD8(+) T cell responses. *J Exp Med* 2007;**204**:1405–16.

100 Combadiere B, Boissonnas A, Carcelain G, *et al.* Distinct time effects of vaccination on long-term proliferative and IFN-gamma-producing T cell memory to smallpox in humans. *J Exp Med* 2004;**199**:1585–93.

101 Harari A, Bart PA, Stohr W, *et al.* An HIV-1 clade C DNA prime, NYVAC boost vaccine regimen induces reliable, polyfunctional, and long-lasting T cell responses. *J Exp Med* 2008;**205**:63–77.

102 Beveridge NE, Price DA, Casazza JP, *et al.* Immunisation with BCG and recombinant MVA85A induces long-lasting, polyfunctional *Mycobacterium tuberculosis*-specific CD4+ memory T lymphocyte populations. *Eur J Immunol* 2007;**37**:3089–100.

103 Miller JD, van der Most RG, Akondy RS, *et al.* Human effector and memory CD8+ T cell responses to smallpox and yellow fever vaccines. *Immunity* 2008;**28**:710–22.

104 Hansen SG, Vieville C, Whizin N, *et al.* Effector memory T cell responses are associated with protection of rhesus monkeys from mucosal simian immunodeficiency virus challenge. *Nat Med* 2009;**15**:293–9.

105 Speiser DE, Lienard D, Rufer N, *et al.* Rapid and strong human CD8+ T cell responses to vaccination with peptide, IFA, and CpG oligodeoxynucleotide 7909. *J Clin Invest* 2005;**115**:739–46.

106 Yang S, Tsang KY, Schlom J. Induction of higher-avidity human CTLs by vector-mediated enhanced costimulation of antigen-presenting cells. *Clin Cancer Res* 2005;**11**:603–15.

CHAPTER 6

Immunologic Memory: B Cells

F. Eun-Hyung Lee[1] & Iñaki Sanz[2]

[1]Division of Pulmonary and Critical Care Medicine, and [2]Division of Allergy, Immunology, and Rheumatology, University of Rochester Medical Center, Rochester, NY, USA

Introduction

The objective of any immunization is to provide protective immunity from disease, and resistance to disease or reducing severity with microbial challenge is the only true marker of vaccine efficacy. These studies are often difficult to perform in human subjects, and so vaccine efficacy is often measured epidemiologically with reduction in disease from natural infection or by correlates of protection by immune measurements. Traditionally, *in vitro* serum neutralizing antibody titers have been used as immune measures. The cells responsible for this "serologic memory" are the long-lived plasma cells and memory B cells that make up the "memory B-cell response." Understanding the cellular component of the humoral response is under extensive investigation. However, it is noteworthy that despite more than 200 years since the introduction of Edward Jenner's smallpox vaccine in 1798 [1] and the availability of over 20 different human vaccines, the mechanisms of how long-lived immune protection is produced and preserved for decades are not entirely known.

Human evaluation of B-cell vaccine responses

Historically, immune correlates of vaccinology have been based on the B-cell memory response to guarantee immediate protection from dangerous pathogens. Two compartments constitute this B-cell memory response: (i) the long-lived plasma cells that are responsible for the sustained levels of protective antibodies, and (ii) the memory B cells, which are the precursors of the plasma cell compartment. We will outline the current understanding of B-cell vaccinology in the context of these two compartments.

Vaccine immune responses are primed in secondary lymphoid structures such as lymph nodes, and the long-lived plasma cells are found in the bone marrow. These compartments are difficult to sample routinely in human subjects. Thus, the blood containing the protective antibodies has been used routinely as an immune surrogate for vaccine efficacy. Interestingly, the blood also contains memory B cells, and for a transient time after vaccine priming, circulating vaccine-specific antibody-secreting cells (ASCs) can be found. Characterizing the memory B cells and ASCs in the blood responsible for the memory B-cell responses during immunization is an active area of research and can lead to important immune biomarkers in the evaluation of novel vaccines. In this chapter, we will define some of the important questions in the field of vaccinology: how long-lived antibodies may be generated and maintained; whether the role of memory B cells is important in protection and assays to measure this compartment; as well as understanding the heterogeneity of the ASCs at the time of

Vaccinology: Principles and Practice, First Edition. Edited by W. John W. Morrow, Nadeem A. Sheikh, Clint S. Schmidt and D. Huw Davies.
© 2012 Blackwell Publishing Ltd. Published 2012 by Blackwell Publishing Ltd.

priming that may prognosticate long-lived humoral protection.

Variability in antibody maintenance is dependent on the type of vaccine

With administration of potent live attenuated vaccines, there is the initial rise of serum antibodies within two weeks and rapid decay to a new long-lived or sustained steady state level that can last for years [2,3] (Figure 6.1). Depending on the vaccine, the magnitude of the initial antibody rise can be highly variable, as can the steady state half-lives. For many live viral infections such as measles, mumps, and varicella viruses or live attenuated vaccines such as vaccinia for smallpox, antibody levels can be maintained for over 50 years to a lifetime [3]. With protein-toxoid based vaccines, such as tetanus and diphtheria, antibody titers decrease with half-lives at 11–19 years [3]. With pro-

tein vaccines such as acellular pertussis or hepatitis B, antibody levels can wane even more rapidly, within 3–5 years [4–6]. Lastly, pure polysaccharide vaccines generate no sustained levels after the initial rise, suggesting that these vaccines do not trigger generation of long-lived plasma cells, presumably due to the inability of this type of polysaccharide alone (or of the responding B cells) to recruit T-cell help [7]. Clearly, the variability in duration of the antibody levels suggests that how the immune system is primed with different vaccine strategies determines plasma cell survival long-term and antibody maintenance.

Primary B-cell immune response

B cells are generated in the bone marrow with estimates of less than 10% released into circulation as transitional and naïve B cells [8]. Upon antigen encounter, naïve or antigen-inexperienced B cells

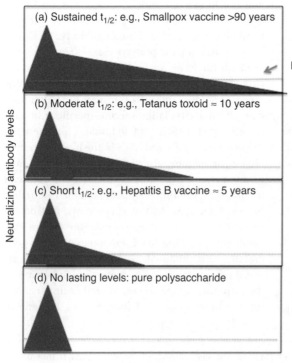

(a) Sustained $t_{1/2}$: e.g., Smallpox vaccine >90 years

Protective titer

(b) Moderate $t_{1/2}$: e.g., Tetanus toxoid ≈ 10 years

(c) Short $t_{1/2}$: e.g., Hepatitis B vaccine ≈ 5 years

(d) No lasting levels: pure polysaccharide

Neutralizing antibody levels

Time (years)

Figure 6.1 Variability of long-lived antibody levels after the initial rise in serum antibody levels with different immunizations. Dotted line represents the protective titers. (a) Represents kinetics of antibody titers with live attenuated vaccines. (b) Kinetics of antibody titers with tetanus toxoid vaccine. (c) Kinetics of antibody levels with recombinant protein vaccines. (d) No sustained antibody levels with pure polysaccharide vaccines.

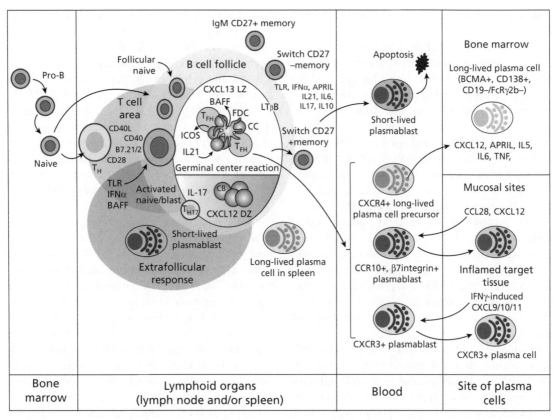

Figure 6.2 B-cell development and differentiation from the pro-B cell bone marrow stage to long-lived plasma cells resident in the bone marrow, mucosal sites, and target tissues. With vaccination, naïve B cells are activated and undergo proliferation through B cell-CD4 T cell (Th) interactions via CD40L-CD40 and B7.1/2 co-stimulation in the early phases, and with GC formation in the late phases via stimulation with ICOS and IL21. GC formation is dependent on the LTβR and its structure and survival is influenced by chemokines CXCL12, CXCL13, and survival factors BAFF. IL17 can also influence output of GC B cells. From the GC reactions, heterogeneous populations of memory B cells arise that include IgM CD27+, conventional isotype-switched CD27+ memory, and isotype-switched CD27− memory, and a heterogeneous ASC population of CD19+ short-lived plasmablasts and long-lived precursors is released into the blood. CXCR4+ ASC are likely to be long-lived plasma cell precursors homing to the bone marrow sites where CXCL12, APRIL, IL5, IL6, and TNF are found. CCR10+, β7+ ASCs are presumed to migrate to mucosal sites and CXCR3+ ASCs to inflamed tissue sites. Phenotypic long-lived plasma cells can also be found in the human spleen.

take up antigen through the B-cell receptor (BCR), interact with activated CD4 T cells, and can adopt two different fates: (i) migration into the follicle, where they proliferate, differentiate, and establish germinal centers to establish memory B cells and long-lived plasma cell precursors, or (ii) movement to the extrafollicular area followed by proliferation and differentiation into short-lived plasma cells [9,10] (see Figure 6.2). Cognate B cell/T cell inter-

actions form through CD40-CD40L [11] and co-stimulatory molecules CD28-B7. These activated naïve B cells within the follicles or B cell centroblasts proliferate massively in the dark zones and exit the cell cycle. Follicular dendritic cells (FDCs) also play a major role as a depot of vaccine antigens and are situated in the light zones. The B cells then move to the light zones and are now called centrocytes; here they differentiate into memory B cells and ASCs, which may be the precursors of long-lived plasma cells [9].

It has been found that the CD40L-CD40 B cell/T cell interactions are required in the germinal center (GC) formation for isotype switching [12] and somatic hypermutation [13,14] to take place, a process by which the B-cell receptor mutates to eventually produce antibodies with increased affinity to the antigens. These GC reactions are fully formed within 4 days after the cognate T cell/B cell interactions and can last for 14–28 days [15,16]. During a primary immune response as early as day 7, ASCs that secrete high-affinity antibodies due to somatic mutation in the antibody variable region genes can be found [17–19]. Those ASCs generated from extrafollicular areas become short-lived plasmablasts with lower affinity and fewer mutations [10,15,20,21]. These ASCs are released into the blood and are often called "plasmablasts" since they have many features of both activated B cells and plasma cells.

In addition to ASCs, memory B-cell clones with increased mutations also arise from the GC [17,22]. Memory B-cell clones are also generated and typically peak in the blood at one month and wane over 90% within a year [23]. Unlike plasma cells, which secrete antibodies years after the vaccine, memory B cells require days for new antibodies to be formed upon re-encountering the pathogen.

Secondary B-cell immune responses

Memory B cells can persist for long periods and are the basis of the enhanced secondary humoral responses. They have lower thresholds of activation than naïve cells [24] and are characterized by more rapid B-cell activation, proliferation, and differentiation to high-affinity ASCs as early as day 4, instead of day 7 as with a primary immune response [25,26]. The timing of the peak of the ASC response after secondary influenza immunization can occur as early as day 5 and as late as day 8 [27]. Major differences between memory and naïve B-cell activation are the stimulation requirements. Distinct from naïve B cells, memory B cells may not require

cognate antigens or the presence of antigen-BCR interactions for activation. Some studies show that memory B cells can differentiate into ASCs in response to bystander or noncognate T-cell help via CD40L and cytokines [24,28]. In addition, memory B cells express Toll-like receptor 2 (TLR2), TLR6, TLR7, TLR9, and TLR10; and when triggered by TLR agonists such as CpG (TLR9 agonists) or R848 (TLR7/8 agonists) in the absence of antigen, memory B cells undergo proliferation and differentiation into ASCs [29,30]. These lower thresholds of activation may be mechanisms for quicker responses.

The kinetics of ASCs in secondary immunization is several days faster than with primary responses, and peak antibody titers occur 1–5 days faster than ASCs [19,27]. Moreover, high-affinity class-switched antibodies are generated more rapidly than in a primary immune response. The magnitude of the ASC frequencies or the rise in the antibody titers can be higher [19] but may depend on the level of pre-existing antibodies from the primary immunization. This ability to generate high-affinity antibodies more rapidly in a secondary immune response is the crux of vaccine responses as the replication of invading pathogen competes with the host response to eradicate it.

Factors important for long-lived plasma cell generation

Although not entirely known, several major elements during the initial priming event of an immune response appear important for the generation of long-lived memory B cells and long-lived antibody responses. Clearly, germinal center formation, requiring both T- and B-cell interactions, cytokines, and the ability of ASCs to migrate and relocate to appropriate survival niches, have all been shown to be critical for long-lived plasma cell formation.

Classically, cytokines such as IL-4, IFN-γ, and TGF-β have been shown to be essential for isotype switching of B cells [31]. Cytokines such as IL-10 have a modest role in isotype switching and Ig secretion [32,33], and IL-6 has also been shown to play a role in Ig secretion [34,35]. Most interestingly of late, IL21 has emerged as a key cytokine for establishing, maintaining, and regulating the antibody responses [36–38]. IL-21 produced by follicular helper T cells (Tfh) has been shown to be a potent inducer of BLIMP-1, a major transcription factor for plasma cell differentiation [39]. Tfh are a CXCR5+CD4+ T-cell subset that resides in the secondary lymphoid structures and are critical in antibody production [40]. In humans, IL-21 plays a key role in generation of ASC, memory B cells, and class switching through STAT3 signaling [41]. Although patients with STAT3 mutations have normal total immunoglobulin levels, they have difficulty developing high-affinity antibodies to many new pathogens [41]. Also, Th17 cells (CD4 T cells producing IL17) may in fact produce higher levels of IL21 [42–44]. Lastly, IL21 may have a role not only in the generation of short-lived plasmablasts but in that of the more valuable long-lived plasma cells as well [41].

After a primary immune response, ASCs are eventually released into the circulation as early as day 7, peak in the blood circulation on day 10, and disappear by day 28, as demonstrated with rabies vaccination [19]. ASCs found in the blood after an immune response can be quite heterogeneous. Early studies from the 1960s described plasma cell half-lives of days to weeks since they were detected during a transient period [45–50]. Despite the 21-day half-life of human serum IgG, kinetics of the antibody levels suggested survival of the plasma cells with much longer half-lives, lasting many years. Eventually, elegant mouse studies demonstrated survival of bone marrow resident plasma cells for over a year [23]. Reconciliation of these data led to the conclusion that ASCs are quite heterogeneous, with both short-lived plasmablasts and long-lived plasma cells generated during a primary vaccine response [21].

The B-cell survival factors BAFF (BLyS, TNFSF13b) and APRIL (for "a proliferation-inducing ligand") are members of the tumor necrosis factor (TNF) family and also play a role in ASC survival [51]. While BAFF prolongs B-cell survival, APRIL, through the receptor BCMA (B cell maturation antigen), induces B-cell proliferation and class switching as well as survival [52,53] and is particularly important for survival of plasmablasts [54,55]. It is possible that increased levels of APRIL during priming may prolong survival of plasma cells, and at present, APRIL has been shown to be a promising survival factor for short-lived ASCs. But it is not clear if it is required for survival of long-lived plasma cells [52].

Location of the final plasma cell residence also plays a role in longevity. It was found that the circulating ASCs removed *ex vivo* would eventually die within a few days and that bone marrow stroma promoted survival, suggesting the importance of essential survival factors from bone marrow privileged sites [56–58]. In humans, between days 14 and 28, ASCs effectively disappear from the blood and migrate to secondary lymphoid organs, primarily the bone marrow, where it is thought they establish niches and become long-lived plasma cells [59]. Chemokine receptors such as CXCR4 are important in migration to the bone marrow, and it is possible that CXCR4+ ASCs may eventually become long-lived plasma cells. Many of these short-lived plasmablasts without this migratory potential are believed to undergo apoptosis, which reflects the initial decay of the antibody levels. At present, it is still unclear if ASCs generated during an immune response are homogenous, and further differentiation is dependent on the migratory site, or if the circulating ASCs are predestined heterogeneous populations with short- and long-lived fates. Evidence seems to point to the latter.

Heterogeneity of the circulating newly formed ASCs

After vaccination peak vaccine-specific ASC frequencies correlate with the peak rises in the ASC [59a]. However, understanding the ASC subsets reveals valuable information about the intensity of the vaccine priming that is occurring at the lymph nodes. Days after immunization, it is known that upwards of 90% of plasmablasts found in the blood can be specific for the vaccine [19,26,60]. Therefore, phenotyping all ASC can still be quite useful since it mirrors the vaccine-specific cells. As an example, identifying vaccine-specific memory B cells and circulating ASC subsets with bone marrow migratory potential may reflect a robust GC response. Thus, the circulating ASCs are likely to be important immune biomarkers for vaccine evaluation.

Currently, the ASCs can be divided into subsets based on markers of proliferation, homing, survival, and apoptosis. Homing markers can reveal information about the future location of vaccine-specific ASCs. For example, markers of inflammation such as IFN-gamma and TNF-alpha may recruit ASC that are positive for CXCR3 to inflamed target tissues [61]. In addition, migration to other body sites such as the gastrointestinal and respiratory tract may be critical for mucosal vaccines. It has been proposed that ASC that express CCR10 and beta7 integrins may preferentially be recruited to mucosal sites [62]. These cells as well as the CXCR3$^+$ ASCs are likely to become plasma cells resident in target tissues. Lastly, CXCR4 is an important homing receptor for CXCL12, which is secreted by bone marrow stromal cells and is expressed on a subset of ASCs [61] that migrate to the specialized niches in the bone marrow. Quite possibly, this marker may identify long-lived plasma cell precursors.

Specific receptors for B-cell survival factors may also reveal important ASC subsets. BCMA is one of the two receptors for APRIL, which is an important survival factor for plasmablasts [52,54,55], and mouse models demonstrate that BCMA is essential for survival of long-lived plasma cells [55]. Thus, a small population of circulating ASCs expressing cell-surface BCMA may have a survival advantage over the others.

Another mechanism important for maintenance of long-lived plasma cells may be linked with the level of antibody-antigen complexes. The FcRγIIb is a potent inhibitory receptor that induces suppression of B cells and apoptosis of plasma cells [63]. It is through immune complexes that crosslinking FcRγIIb induces apoptosis of both short-lived plasmablasts and bone marrow resident plasma cells in mice. Therefore, higher levels of antigen-antibody complexes eliminate excess plasma cells, which

makes for an ideal homeostatic system to maintain antibody titers. Some suggest that by this mechanism, plasmablasts and plasma cells during immune priming may selectively be deleted to decrease the number of long-lived plasma cells for which survival niches are limited. Therefore, circulating ASCs with this receptor would readily undergo apoptosis, and ASCs without this receptor would survive to migrate to privileged sites. This mechanism may also be important for the homeostasis of long-lived plasma cells since bone marrow plasma cell tumors (myelomas) with this receptor also undergo apoptosis [63]. Again quite promising at present, it is unclear if normal human bone marrow resident plasma cells contain this receptor and are regulated by this mechanism.

Models of long-lived plasma cells maintenance

Long-lived protective serum antibodies are sustained by long-lived plasma cells. How these long-lived plasma cells are generated is not entirely known. Historically, live infections with greater immune intensity can generate life-long antibody levels [3,64] as compared to waning antibody levels with protein immunizations [3]. Three major models are proposed. The first model suggests that long-lived plasma cells acquire longevity by migrating to special niches in bone marrow sites where space is limited to acquire survival factors [65]. They are long-lived, radio-resistant, nonproliferating, and constitutively secrete antibodies [23]. With each infection or vaccination, old plasma cells are released and replaced by newly formed plasma cells, resulting in the slow sustained decay. The second model states that long-lived plasma cells are constantly being replenished by the memory B-cell compartment in a non-antigen-specific fashion through TLRs with each infectious or vaccine stimulation [66]. Unlike naïve B cells, memory B cells express TLRs, which when triggered by TLR agonists undergo proliferation and differentiation into ASCs in the absence of cognate antigen [29,30]. In this model, the memory B-cell compartment would be closely linked to the long-lived antibody levels, which has been difficult to prove. Finally, yet a more complex third model proposes that a depot of antigen through basophils is required to maintain long-lived antibody production [67].

Whether the relationship between memory B cells and long-lived plasma cells is dependent or independent has tremendous implications for vaccine biology. If indeed these compartments are independent of one another, measurements of memory B cells after vaccination would not be needed to predict long-lived antibody protection. Several studies have demonstrated this independent relationship between antibody levels and memory B-cell frequencies [2,3,68]. Others argue a link between these two compartments. Studies with conjugate pneumococcal vaccine show a link between quantitative antibody titers at 28 days and the memory B-cell frequencies [29,69]. This concept supports the second model of long-term antibody maintenance, where memory B cells are tightly linked to replenishing the long-lived plasma cell compartment. Unfortunately, long-term measurements of the memory B cells were not obtained in this study, and the correlative relationship between these two compartments could just reflect the intensity of immune priming and not necessarily a true link between long-lived memory B cells and long-lived plasma cells. Therefore, the importance of memory B cells for antibody maintenance needs further study.

Heterogeneity of human memory B-cell subsets

Memory B cells themselves in the absence of protective antibody may have a limited role in prevention and a more substantial role in decreasing morbidity of disease. The reason for this limitation is that memory B cells still require time (days) to proliferate and differentiate into effector ASCs that secrete high-affinity antibodies. These kinetics may explain the limited protection against rapidly replicating blood-borne bacterial infections afforded by pre-existing memory B cells [70], whereas for viral infections, memory B cells may be able to play a significant protective role since symptoms can de-

velop several days after inoculation, as illustrated by the timing of new antibody production in human challenge studies with influenza and respiratory syncytial virus [71,72].

It should be noted, however, that our knowledge of B-cell memory, its heterogeneity, and protective functions is quite poorly developed in both humans and animal models. Indeed, as recently discussed by others [73], our understanding of memory B-cell populations is hampered by preconceived notions based on a strict definition of memory cells expressing isotype-switched, somatically mutated antibodies and generated through a T cell-dependent GC reaction. Yet, the heterogeneity of B-cell memory responses, while poorly understood, is likely to be substantial [74–81]. In addition to conventional IgG memory to T cell-dependent (TD) protein antigens, mouse IgM memory to T cell-independent type 2 (TI-2) antigens can be provided by B1b cells [82–84]. Recent evidence indicates that, in the mouse, TI-2 antigens can also induce IgG memory responses mediated by B2 cells with a phenotype different from both follicular and marginal zone (MZ) B cells [85].

Substantial heterogeneity is also apparent among human memory B cells. In fact, while their functional heterogeneity is less well understood, several phenotypic subsets have been recognized and facilitated by the higher abundance of human memory cells and the usefulness of CD27 as a marker of human B-cell memory [86]. Of significant interest, less than half of all human CD27$^+$ memory B cells have undergone isotype switch, while the rest express surface IgM. Whether IgM memory cells represent a homogeneous subset remains controversial but several reports and our own experience indicate that the vast majority of IgM memory cells also express at least low levels of surface IgD [77–79,87]. IgM/IgD memory cells, which may develop through GC-independent pathways, have been proposed to represent the human functional equivalents of B1 and MZ B cells and to mediate protection against infections with encapsulated organisms [77–79,87]. Significant controversy, however, still exists regarding the concept that IgM/IgD memory cells may represent a re-circulating subset of MZ B cells.

Current schemes of classification of human memory B-cell populations

Flow cytometric analysis of human B cells has thus far relied on the expression of four major surface markers: CD19, IgD, CD38, and CD27 [87,88]. With this four-color approach, two major classification schemes can be produced depending on the relative expression of either IgD and CD38 or IgD and CD27. Thus IgD/CD38 staining provides the so-called Bm1-Bm5 classification [89] and can be used to identify multiple subsets in the human tonsil, including virgin naïve cells (Bm1: IgD$^+$CD38$^-$); activated naïve cells (Bm2: IgD$^+$CD38$^+$); pre-GC cells (Bm2′; IgD$^+$CD38^{++}); GC cells (Bm3-centroblasts and Bm4-centrocytes; both are IgD$^-$CD38^{++}); and memory cells (Bm5: IgD$^-$CD38$^{+/-}$). Bm5 memory cells that express levels of CD38 ranging from moderately positive to negative have been further divided into early Bm5 (CD38$^+$) and late Bm5 (CD38$^-$) [90]. In the peripheral blood the Bm1-Bm5 classification recognizes similar subsets with the exception of GC cells. While this classification has been quite useful and represents an almost mandatory point of reference in the field, it also suffers from significant limitations, including the inclusion of unswitched CD27$^+$ cells within the naïve subset and the inability to recognize heterogeneity within the Bm5 memory compartment.

The IgD/CD27 classification builds on the notion of CD27 as a universal marker of human memory B cells to distinguish between memory cells (CD27$^+$) and naïve B cells (CD27$^-$IgD$^+$). In turn, CD27$^+$ memory cells can be divided into IgD$^+$ (usually together with IgM) and IgD$^-$, with the latter subset usually labeled as isotype switched (predominantly IgG$^+$ or IgA$^+$). An obvious drawback of this classification is its inability to recognize memory cells that lack expression of CD27. However, recent studies have identified a novel human memory B-cell subset as defined by isotype-switched CD19$^+$CD27$^-$IgD$^-$ population [88]. Originally reported in tonsils, and thereby labeled as tissue-based memory, this population has also been reported as significantly expanded in the peripheral blood lymphocytes (PBL) of patients with active systemic lupus erythematosis (SLE) [91,92] and in patients with chronic infections, including HIV [93]

and malaria. Interestingly, in the infectious situations (as in tonsils), these cells are characterized by increased expression of the inhibitory FcRL4, a property not shared by their SLE counterpart. Based on the expression of this and other inhibitory receptors, their decreased expression of CD21 (presumably due to chronic antigenic stimulation) as well as poor *in vitro* proliferation and decreased differentiation into ASC, tissue-based memory cells (also described by others as atypical memory) have been proposed to represent exhausted memory cells. Moreover, the finding that at least in chronic HIV infection these cells appear to be enriched for virus-specific responses has led to the suggestion that a shift of memory cells into this compartment may contribute to poor viral clearance and disease progression. In all, the compartment in which the vaccine-specific memory B cell resides may be quite critical for both swift antibody generation and other effector functions such as antigen presentation or cytokine responses upon re-encounter of the pathogen. It is therefore apparent that there is significant phenotypic and functional heterogeneity among human memory B cells, and that this diversity bears significant implications for our understanding of vaccine responses and our ability to measure them and to devise immunization strategies that optimize the generation and survival of antigen-specific memory B cells within the most beneficial compartment.

Measuring memory B-cell responses to vaccines

Most assays to interrogate the memory B-cell repertoire after a vaccine response for the most part require *in vitro* differentiation of B cells for a final read-out of antibody production. Methods include measuring frequencies of vaccine-specific ASC by ELISPOT after *in vitro* proliferation of peripheral blood mononuclear cells (PBMC) [94, 95]. This method has routinely been used to measure antigen-specific memory B-cell frequencies after many vaccines, including influenza [96, 97], tetanus, pneumococcal [98], and rabies [69]. However, this method makes several assumptions and requires "universal" differentiation of ASC. Bias of memory B-cell populations that differentiate into ASCs and not other functions may be favored. Furthermore, using "universal" differentiation conditions to differentiate all B-cell isotypes is extremely difficult but essential to reflect the true memory B-cell frequencies. Lastly, caution should be used in enumerating the frequencies during the days when spontaneous ASCs (generated *in vivo*) are in circulation because they may falsely increase the memory B-cell numbers. Other methods include generation of monoclonal antibody from single memory B-cells or ASCs [99,100]. Although quite informative for one particular memory B cell clone, the technique is cumbersome, labor intensive, and cannot adequately sample the entire repertoire. Other newly described methods, such as Cellspot™ [101–103], "immunospot array assay on a chip" (ISAAC) [104], and introduction of Bcl-6 and Bcl-xL genes into memory B cells for the generation of monoclonal antibodies [105], all have similar limitations. For each of these memory B-cell assays, using crude B-cell populations without proper fractionation could lead to over-representation of one subset under any given set of conditions.

It is likely that the routine measurements of vaccine-specific memory B cells may not identify all subsets equally. Tracking memory B cells with labeled antigens (such as tetanus and influenza) can be done but has proven to be technically challenging [106–108] and is not routinely measured after vaccination. However, greater insights are likely to be gained by identifying antigen-specific B cells with direct labeling because it eliminates the need for *in vitro* differentiation that may under-represent novel B-cell functions.

Antibody maintenance is dependent on the age of the host

The magnitude of the initial surge of antibody and long-term antibody maintenance is less in young children as compared to adults with primary immunization. It is well established that young children are susceptible to severe infections with polysaccharide-encapsulated bacteria such as

Streptococcus pneumoniae, Hemophilus influenza type b (Hib), and *Neisseria meningitidis* due to the "immaturity" of the immune system [109]. Thus, development of polysaccharide vaccines is targeted for this young population. Yet antibody levels after three doses of MenC (a vaccine for *N. meningitidis*) during infancy do not persist. At one year of age, only 50% of the infants are protected and the numbers fall to 12% in the fourth year of life [110]. Also, with Hib vaccines, a rapid decline of antibody titers leading to waning of protection is well documented in young children [111]. In direct comparison of young adults with infants after a primary immunization with the same conjugated pneumococcal vaccine, young adults had better memory B-cell responses and a longer duration of sustained antibody levels [112]. Amazingly, as little as a few months can matter such that, during infancy, antibody persistence is better when the first dose of the vaccine is given after 12 months of age [112].

These findings may be due to the differential intensity of the vaccine priming and immaturity of the GC reaction in children as well as decreased survival factors from specialized niches in the infant bone marrow. A recent mouse study compared neonatal to adult bone marrow stroma and found that the neonatal stroma had decreased levels of APRIL, an important survival factor for ASCs [113]. At present, it is not known if supplementing with APRIL can improve vaccine efficacy. Thus, age plays a significant role in the ability to generate long-lived immunity, and so dissecting of these mechanisms can lead to better strategies to improve infant vaccine efficacy.

Location of memory B cells and plasma cells may play a role in protection

Mucosal vaccines can sometimes be more effective in protection than intramuscular vaccines. As an example, cold-adapted live attenuated influenza vaccine (LAIV) has better efficacy compared to inactivated influenza vaccine in children [114]. Reductions of influenza attack rates with LAIV range from 35% to 53% as compared to the intramuscular vaccine [114–116]. The mechanism of this increased protection may be multifactorial, including both T-cell and B-cell compartments. Yet, one major speculation is that with mucosal vaccines, the location of long-lived humoral immunity matters. Since influenza virus causes disease in the upper and lower respiratory tract, priming intranasally at the target tissue site appears logical. With LAIV, few systemic antibodies are generated, and nasal IgA levels correlate with protection [117–119]. Thus, IgA secreted from long-lived plasma cells in the respiratory tract provide better immediate and localized protection compared to systemic antibodies to influenza virus. Therefore, understanding mechanisms of how long-lived tissue-resident plasma cells are generated, migrate, and survive in target tissue sites is fundamental for mucosal vaccine protection.

Biomarkers of long-lived humoral immunity during vaccine priming

The goal for any novel vaccine is protective antibody maintenance due to long-lived plasma cells. At present, whether the long-lived plasma cell compartment is dependent or independent of the memory B-cell compartment is yet to be determined. Furthermore, the memory B-cell subset best suited for a protective vaccine response will also require further elucidation. With the development of new vaccines, only the tincture of time will tell if they are long lasting. Therefore, distinguishing immune biomarkers of vaccines with history of long-lived immunity compared to short-lived responses will be important to identify novel biomarkers of long-lived immunity. Clearly, the quality and quantity of the antibody at the peak of the vaccine response are currently the only major immune surrogates of protection. However, careful interrogation and analysis of the ASC repertoire and memory B-cell subsets in the blood with accurate immune measurements are likely to lead to novel immune surrogates during vaccine priming. Hopefully, these new biomarkers will better prognosticate effective long-lived humoral protection.

In conclusion, historically serologic correlates of vaccine efficacy have been useful but ignore the complexity of the human memory B-cell responses to vaccines. Using modern tools to dissect the cellular underpinnings of the human circulating ASC and memory B-cell biology will clearly advance the immunology of immunizations. By studying the heterogeneity and complexity of ASC and memory B-cell subsets, new vaccine-specific immune surrogates or biomarkers will be discovered, which will be effective in evaluating new vaccine strategies.

References

1 Jenner E. *An Inquiry into the Cause and Effects of the Variolae Vaccineae, a Disease Discovered in Some of the Western Counties of England, Particularly Gloucestershire, and Known by the Name of the Cow Pox.* London, Printed by Samson Low, 1798.

2 Crotty S, Felgner P, Davies H, *et al.* Long-term B cell memory in humans after smallpox vaccination. *J Immunol* 2003;**171**:4969–73.

3 Amanna IJ, Carlson NE, Slifka MK. Duration of humoral immunity to common viral and vaccine antigens. *N Engl J Med* 2007;**357**:1903–15.

4 Edwards KM, Talbot TR. The challenges of pertussis outbreaks in healthcare facilities: is there a light at the end of the tunnel? *Infect Control Hosp Epidemiol* 2006;**27**:537–40.

5 Edwards K, Freeman DM. Adolescent and adult pertussis: disease burden and prevention. *Curr Opin Pediatr* 2006;**18**:77–80.

6 West DJ, Calandra GB. Vaccine induced immunologic memory for hepatitis B surface antigen: implications for policy on booster vaccination. *Vaccine* 1996;**14**:1019–27.

7 Kelly DF, Snape MD, Clutterbuck EA, *et al.* CRM197-conjugated serogroup C meningococcal capsular polysaccharide, but not the native polysaccharide, induces persistent antigen-specific memory B cells. *Blood* 2006;**108**:2642–7.

8 Crowley JE, Scholz JL, Quinn WJ, 3rd, *et al.* Homeostatic control of B lymphocyte subsets. *Immunol Res* 2008;**42**:75–83.

9 Allen CD, Okada T, Cyster JG. Germinal-center organization and cellular dynamics. *Immunity* 2007;**27**:190–202.

10 Toellner KM, Gulbranson-Judge A, Taylor DR, Sze DM, MacLennan IC. Immunoglobulin switch transcript production in vivo related to the site and time of antigen-specific B cell activation. *J Exp Med* 1996;**183**:2303–12.

11 MacLennan IC. Germinal centers. *Annu Rev Immunol* 1994;**12**:117–39.

12 Foy TM, Laman JD, Ledbetter JA, *et al.* gp39-CD40 interactions are essential for germinal center formation and the development of B cell memory. *J Exp Med* 1994;**180**:157–63.

13 Clarke SH, Huppi K, Ruezinsky D, *et al.* Inter- and intraclonal diversity in the antibody response to influenza hemagglutinin. *J Exp Med* 1985;**161**:687–704.

14 Berek C, Berger A, Apel M. Maturation of the immune response in germinal centers. *Cell* 1991;**67**:1121–9.

15 Liu YJ, Zhang J, Lane PJ, Chan EY, MacLennan IC. Sites of specific B cell activation in primary and secondary responses to T cell-dependent and T cell-independent antigens. *Eur J Immunol* 1991;**21**:2951–62.

16 Hanna MG, Jr. An autoradiographic study of the germinal center in spleen white pulp during early intervals of the immune response. *Lab Invest* 1964;**13**:95–104.

17 Tarlinton DM, Smith KG. Dissecting affinity maturation: a model explaining selection of antibody-forming cells and memory B cells in the germinal centre. *Immunol Today* 2000;**21**:436–41.

18 Ueki Y, Goldfarb IS, Harindranath N, *et al.* Clonal analysis of a human antibody response. Quantitation of precursors of antibody-producing cells and generation and characterization of monoclonal IgM, IgG, and IgA to rabies virus. *J Exp Med* 1990;**171**:19–34.

19 Blanchard-Rohner G, Pulickal AS, Jol-van der Zijde CM, Snape MD, Pollard AJ. Appearance of peripheral blood plasma cells and memory B cells in a primary and secondary immune response in humans. *Blood* 2009;**114**:4998–5002.

20 Jacob J, Kelsoe G. In situ studies of the primary immune response to (4-hydroxy-3-nitrophenyl)acetyl. II. A common clonal origin for periarteriolar lymphoid sheath-associated foci and germinal centers. *J Exp Med* 1992;**176**:679–87.

21 Ho F, Lortan JE, MacLennan IC, Khan M. Distinct short-lived and long-lived antibody-producing cell populations. *Eur J Immunol* 1986;**16**:1297–1301.

22 Blink EJ, Light A, Kallies A, *et al.* Early appearance of germinal center-derived memory B cells and plasma cells in blood after primary immunization. *J Exp Med* 2005;**201**:545–54.

23 Slifka MK, Antia R, Whitmire JK, Ahmed R. Humoral immunity due to long-lived plasma cells. *Immunity* 1998;**8**:363–72.

24 Tangye SG, Avery DT, Deenick EK, Hodgkin PD. Intrinsic differences in the proliferation of naive and memory human B cells as a mechanism for enhanced secondary immune responses. *J Immunol* 2003;**170**:686–94.

25 Kelly DF, Snape MD, Perrett KP, *et al.* Plasma and memory B-cell kinetics in infants following a primary schedule of CRM 197-conjugated serogroup C meningococcal polysaccharide vaccine. *Immunology* 2009;**127**:134–43.

26 Cox RJ, Brokstad KA, Zuckerman MA, *et al.* An early humoral immune response in peripheral blood following parenteral inactivated influenza vaccination. *Vaccine* 1994;**12**:993–99.

27 Halliley JL, Kyu S, Kobie JJ, *et al.* Peak frequencies of circulating human influenza-specific antibody secreting cells correlate with serum antibody response after immunization. *Vaccine* 2010;**28**:3582–87.

28 Lanzavecchia A, Parodi B, Celada F. Activation of human B lymphocytes: frequency of antigen-specific B cells triggered by alloreactive or by antigen-specific T cell clones. *Eur J Immunol* 1983;**13**:733–8.

29 Bernasconi NL, Traggiai E, Lanzavecchia A. Maintenance of serological memory by polyclonal activation of human memory B cells. *Science* 2002;**298**:2199–202.

30 Bernasconi NL, Onai N, Lanzavecchia A. A role for Toll-like receptors in acquired immunity: up-regulation of TLR9 by BCR triggering in naive B cells and constitutive expression in memory B cells. *Blood* 2003;**101**:4500–504.

31 Stavnezer J. Immunoglobulin class switching. *Curr Opin Immunol* 1996;**8**:199–205.

32 Rousset F, Garcia E, Defrance T, *et al.* Interleukin 10 is a potent growth and differentiation factor for activated human B lymphocytes. *Proc Natl Acad Sci U S A* 1992;**89**:1890–93.

33 Briere F, Servet-Delprat C, Bridon JM, Saint-Remy JM, Banchereau J. Human interleukin 10 induces naive surface immunoglobulin D+ (sIgD+) B cells to secrete IgG1 and IgG3. *J Exp Med* 1994;**179**:757–62.

34 Ellyard JI, Avery DT, Phan TG, *et al.* Antigen-selected, immunoglobulin-secreting cells persist in human spleen and bone marrow. *Blood* 2004;**103**:3805–12.

35 Good KL, Bryant VL, Tangye SG. Kinetics of human B cell behavior and amplification of proliferative responses following stimulation with IL-21. *J Immunol* 2006;**177**:5236–47.

36 Ozaki K, Spolski R, Feng CG, *et al.* A critical role for IL-21 in regulating immunoglobulin production. *Science* 2002;**298**:1630–34.

37 Pene J, Gauchat JF, Lecart S, *et al.* IL-21 is a switch factor for the production of IgG1 and IgG3 by human B cells. *J Immunol* 2004;**172**:5154–7.

38 Bryant VL, Ma CS, Avery DT, *et al.* Cytokine-mediated regulation of human B cell differentiation into Ig-secreting cells: predominant role of IL-21 produced by CXCR5+ T follicular helper cells. *J Immunol* 2007;**179**:8180–90.

39 Ozaki K, Spolski R, Ettinger R, *et al.* Regulation of B cell differentiation and plasma cell generation by IL-21, a novel inducer of Blimp-1 and Bcl-6. *J Immunol* 2004;**173**:5361–71.

40 McHeyzer-Williams LJ, Pelletier N, Mark L, Fazilleau N, McHeyzer-Williams MG. Follicular helper T cells as cognate regulators of B cell immunity. *Curr Opin Immunol* 2009;**21**:266–73.

41 Avery DT, Deenick EK, Ma CS, *et al.* B cell-intrinsic signaling through IL-21 receptor and STAT3 is required for establishing long-lived antibody responses in humans. *J Exp Med* 2010;**207**:155–71.

42 Korn T, Bettelli E, Gao W, *et al.* IL-21 initiates an alternative pathway to induce proinflammatory T(H)17 cells. *Nature* 2007;**448**:484–7.

43 Nurieva R, Yang XO, Martinez G, *et al.* Essential autocrine regulation by IL-21 in the generation of inflammatory T cells. *Nature* 2007;**448**:480–83.

44 Zhou L, Ivanov, II, Spolski R, *et al.* IL-6 programs T(H)-17 cell differentiation by promoting sequential engagement of the IL-21 and IL-23 pathways. Nat Immunol 2007;**8**:967–74.

45 Slifka MK, Ahmed R. Long-lived plasma cells: a mechanism for maintaining persistent antibody production. *Curr Opin Immunol* 1998;**10**:252–8.

46 Cooper EH. Production of lymphocytes and plasma cells in the rat following immunization with human serum albumin. *Immunology* 1961;**4**:219–31.

47 Schooley JC. Autoradiographic observations of plasma cell formation. *J Immunol* 1961;**86**:331–7.

48 Nossal GJ, Makela O. Kinetic studies on the incidence of cells appearing to form two antibodies. *J Immunol* 1962;**88**:604–12.

49 Makela O, Nossal GJ. Autoradiographic studies on the immune response. II. DNA synthesis amongst

50 Nossal GJ, Makela O. Autoradiographic studies on the immune response. I. The kinetics of plasma cell proliferation. *J Exp Med* 1962;**115**:209–30.

51 Moore PA, Belvedere O, Orr A, *et al.* BLyS: member of the tumor necrosis factor family and B lymphocyte stimulator. *Science* 1999;**285**:260–63.

52 Avery DT, Kalled SL, Ellyard JI, *et al.* BAFF selectively enhances the survival of plasmablasts generated from human memory B cells. *J Clin Invest* 2003;**112**:286–97.

53 Litinskiy MB, Nardelli B, Hilbert DM, *et al.* DCs induce CD40-independent immunoglobulin class switching through BLyS and APRIL. *Nat Immunol* 2002;**3**:822–9.

54 Benson MJ, Dillon SR, Castigli E, *et al.* The dependence of plasma cells and independence of memory B cells on BAFF and APRIL. *J Immunol* 2008;**180**:3655–9.

55 O'Connor BP, Raman VS, Erickson LD, *et al.* BCMA is essential for the survival of long-lived bone marrow plasma cells. *J Exp Med* 2004;**199**:91–8.

56 Cassese G, Arce S, Hauser AE, *et al.* Plasma cell survival is mediated by synergistic effects of cytokines and adhesion-dependent signals. *J Immunol* 2003;**171**:1684–90.

57 Hauser AE, Muehlinghaus G, Manz RA, *et al.* Long-lived plasma cells in immunity and inflammation. *Ann N Y Acad Sci* 2003;**987**:266–9.

58 Nossal GJ, Szenberg A, Ada GL, Austin CM. Single cell studies on 19s antibody production. *J Exp Med* 1964;**119**:485–502.

59 Tokoyoda K, Egawa T, Sugiyama T, Choi BI, Nagasawa T. Cellular niches controlling B lymphocyte behavior within bone marrow during development. *Immunity* 2004;**20**:707–18.

59a Halliley JL, Kyu S, Kobie JJ, *et al.* Peak frequencies of circulating human influenza-specific antibody secreting cells correlate with serum antibody response after immunization. *Vaccine* 2010;**28**:3582–7.

60 Moldoveanu Z, Clements ML, Prince SJ, Murphy BR, Mestecky J. Human immune responses to influenza virus vaccines administered by systemic or mucosal routes. *Vaccine* 1995;**13**:1006–12.

61 Odendahl M, Mei H, Hoyer BF, *et al.* Generation of migratory antigen-specific plasma blasts and mobilization of resident plasma cells in a secondary immune response. Blood 2005;**105**:1614–21.

single antibody-producing cells. *J Exp Med* 1962;**115**:231–44.

62 Mei HE, Yoshida T, Sime W, *et al.* Blood-borne human plasma cells in steady-state are derived from mucosal immune responses. Blood 2008;**113**(11): 2461–9.

63 Xiang Z, Cutler AJ, Brownlie RJ, *et al.* FcgammaRIIb controls bone marrow plasma cell persistence and apoptosis. *Nat Immunol* 2007;**8**(4):419–29.

64 Yu X, Tsibane T, McGraw PA, *et al.* Neutralizing antibodies derived from the B cells of 1918 influenza pandemic survivors. *Nature* 2008;**455**:532–6.

65 Radbruch A, Muehlinghaus G, Luger EO, *et al.* Competence and competition: the challenge of becoming a long-lived plasma cell. *Nat Rev Immunol* 2006;**6**:741–50.

66 Lanzavecchia A, Bernasconi N, Traggiai E, *et al.* Understanding and making use of human memory B cells. *Immunol Rev* 2006;**211**:303–9.

67 Denzel A, Maus UA, Rodriguez Gomez M, *et al.* Basophils enhance immunological memory responses. *Nat Immunol* 2008;**9**:733–42.

68 Leyendeckers H, Odendahl M, Lohndorf A, *et al.* Correlation analysis between frequencies of circulating antigen-specific IgG-bearing memory B cells and serum titers of antigen-specific IgG. *Eur J Immunol* 1999;**29**:1406–17.

69 Blanchard Rohner G, Snape MD, Kelly DF, *et al.* The magnitude of the antibody and memory B cell responses during priming with a protein-polysaccharide conjugate vaccine in human infants is associated with the persistence of antibody and the intensity of booster response. *J Immunol* 2008; **180**:2165–73.

70 Pollard AJ, Perrett KP, Beverley PC. Maintaining protection against invasive bacteria with protein-polysaccharide conjugate vaccines. *Nat Rev Immunol* 2009;**9**:213–20.

71 Lee FE, Walsh EE, Falsey AR, Betts RF, Treanor JJ. Experimental infection of humans with A2 respiratory syncytial virus. *Antiviral Res* 2004;**63**:191–6.

72 Hayden FG, Treanor JJ, Fritz RS, *et al.* Use of the oral neuraminidase inhibitor oseltamivir in experimental human influenza: randomized controlled trials for prevention and treatment. *JAMA* 1999;**282**:1240–46.

73 Anderson SM, Hannum LG, Shlomchik MJ. Memory B cell survival and function in the absence of secreted antibody and immune complexes on follicular dendritic cells. *J Immunol* 2006;**176**:4515–19.

74 Weller S, Faili A, Garcia C, *et al.* CD40-CD40L independent Ig gene hypermutation suggests a second B cell diversification pathway in humans. *Proc Natl Acad Sci U S A* 2001;**98**:1166–70.

75 Toyama H, Okada S, Hatano M, *et al.* Memory B cells without somatic hypermutation are generated from Bcl6-deficient B cells. *Immunity* 2002;**17**:329–39.

76 Harada Y, Muramatsu M, Shibata T, Honjo T, Kuroda K. Unmutated immunoglobulin M can protect mice from death by influenza virus infection. *J Exp Med* 2003;**197**; 1779–85.

77 Kruetzmann S, Rosado MM, Weber H, *et al.* Human immunoglobulin M memory B cells controlling *Streptococcus pneumoniae* infections are generated in the spleen. *J Exp Med* 2003;**197**:939–45.

78 Shi Y, Agematsu K, Ochs HD, Sugane K. Functional analysis of human memory B-cell subpopulations: IgD$^+$CD27$^+$ B cells are crucial in secondary immune response by producing high affinity IgM. *Clin Immunol* 2003;**108**:128–37.

79 Weller S, Braun MC, Tan BK, *et al.* Human blood IgM "memory" B cells are circulating splenic marginal zone B cells harboring a pre-diversified immunoglobulin repertoire. *Blood* 2004;**104**(12): 3647–54.

80 Ma CS, Pittaluga S, Avery DT, *et al.* Selective generation of functional somatically mutated IgM$^+$CD27$^+$, but not Ig isotype-switched, memory B cells in X-linked lymphoproliferative disease. *J Clin Invest* 2006;**116**:322–33.

81 Anderson SM, Tomayko MM, Ahuja A, Haberman AM, Shlomchik MJ. New markers for murine memory B cells that define mutated and unmutated subsets. *J Exp Med* 2007;**204**(9):2103–14.

82 Alugupalli KR, Leong JM, Woodland RT, *et al.* B1b lymphocytes confer T cell-independent long-lasting immunity. *Immunity* 2004;**21**:379–90.

83 Haas KM, Poe JC, Steeber DA, Tedder TF. B-1a and B-1b cells exhibit distinct developmental requirements and have unique functional roles in innate and adaptive immunity to S. pneumoniae. *Immunity* 2005;**23**:7–18.

84 Hsu M-C, Toellner K-M, Vinuesa CG, MacLennan ICM. B cell clones that sustain long-term plasmablast growth in T-independent extrafollicular antibody responses. *PNAS* 2006;**103**:5905–10.

85 Obukhanych TV, Nussenzweig MC. T-independent type II immune responses generate memory B cells. *J Exp Med* 2006;**203**:305–10.

86 Klein U, Rajewsky K, Kuppers R. Human immunoglobulin (Ig)M$^+$IgD$^+$ peripheral blood B cells expressing the CD27 cell surface antigen carry somatically mutated variable region genes: CD27 as a general marker for somatically mutated (memory) B cells. *J Exp Med* 1998;**188**:1679–89.

87 Carsetti R, Rosado MM, Wardmann H. Peripheral development of B cells in mouse and man. *Immunol Rev* 2004;**197**:179–91.

88 Wei C, Anolik J, Cappione A, *et al.* A new population of cells lacking expression of CD27 represents a notable component of the B cell memory compartment in systemic lupus erythematosus. *J Immunol* 2007;**178**:6624–33.

89 Pascual V, Liu YJ, Magalski A, *et al.* Analysis of somatic mutation in five B cell subsets of human tonsil. *J Exp Med* 1994;**180**:329–39.

90 Bohnhorst J, Bjorgan MB, Thoen JE, Natvig JB, Thompson KM. Bm1-bm5 classification of peripheral blood B cells reveals circulating germinal center founder cells in healthy individuals and disturbance in the B cell subpopulations in patients with primary Sjogren's syndrome. *J Immunol* 2001;**167**: 3610–18.

91 Jacobi AM, Reiter K, Mackay M, *et al.* Activated memory B cell subsets correlate with disease activity in systemic lupus erythematosus: delineation by expression of CD27, IgD, and CD95. *Arthritis Rheum* 2008;**58**:1762–73.

92 Jenks SA, Sanz I. Altered B cell receptor signaling in human systemic lupus erythematosus. *Autoimmun Rev* 2009;**8**:209–13.

93 Moir S, Ho J, Malaspina A, *et al.* Evidence for HIV-associated B cell exhaustion in a dysfunctional memory B cell compartment in HIV-infected viremic individuals. *J Exp Med* 2008;**205**:1797–1805.

94 Crotty S, Aubert RD, Glidewell J, Ahmed R. Tracking human antigen-specific memory B cells: a sensitive and generalized ELISPOT system. *J Immunol Methods* 2004;**286**:111–22.

95 Czerkinsky CC, Nilsson LA, Nygren H, Ouchterlony O, Tarkowski A. A solid-phase enzyme-linked immunospot (ELISPOT) assay for enumeration of specific antibody-secreting cells. *J Immunol Methods* 1983;**65**:109–21.

96 Sasaki S, He XS, Holmes TH, *et al.* Influence of prior influenza vaccination on antibody and B-cell responses. *PLoS One* 2008;**3**:e2975.

97 Sasaki S, Jaimes MC, Holmes TH, *et al.* Comparison of the influenza virus-specific effector and memory B-cell responses to immunization of children and adults with live attenuated or inactivated influenza virus vaccines. *J Virol* 2007;**81**:215–28.

98 Clutterbuck EA, Oh S, Hamaluba M, *et al.* Serotype-specific and age-dependent generation of pneumococcal polysaccharide-specific memory B-cell and antibody responses to immunization with a pneumococcal conjugate vaccine. *Clin Vaccine Immunol* 2008;**15**:182–93.

99 Tiller T, Meffre E, Yurasov S, *et al.* Efficient generation of monoclonal antibodies from single human B cells by single cell RT-PCR and expression vector cloning. *J Immunol Methods* 2008;**329**:112–24.

100 Wrammert J, Smith K, Miller J, *et al.* Rapid cloning of high-affinity human monoclonal antibodies against influenza virus. *Nature* 2008;**453**:667–71.

101 Harriman WD, Collarini EJ, Sperinde GV, *et al.* Antibody discovery via multiplexed single cell characterization. *J Immunol Methods* 2009;**341**:135–45.

102 Harriman WD, Collarini EJ, Cromer RG, *et al.* Multiplexed Elispot assay. *J Immunol Methods* 2009; **341**:127–34.

103 Collarini EJ, Lee FE, Foord O, *et al.* Potent high-affinity antibodies for treatment and prophylaxis of respiratory syncytial virus derived from B cells of infected patients. *J Immunol* 2009;**183**:6338–45.

104 Jin A, Ozawa T, Tajiri K, *et al.* A rapid and efficient single-cell manipulation method for screening antigen-specific antibody-secreting cells from human peripheral blood. *Nat Med* 2009;**15**:1088–92.

105 Kwakkenbos MJ, Diehl SA, Yasuda E, *et al.* Generation of stable monoclonal antibody-producing B cell receptor-positive human memory B cells by genetic programming. *Nat Med* 2010;**16**:123–8.

106 Townsend SE, Goodnow CC, Cornall RJ. Single epitope multiple staining to detect ultralow frequency B cells. *J Immunol Methods* 2001;**249**:137–46.

107 Amanna IJ, Slifka MK. Quantitation of rare memory B cell populations by two independent and complementary approaches. *J Immunol Methods* 2006;**317**:175–85.

108 Doucett VP, Gerhard W, Owler K, *et al.* Enumeration and characterization of virus-specific B cells by multicolor flow cytometry. *J Immunol Methods* 2005;**303**:40–52.

109 MacLennan J, Obaro S, Deeks J, *et al.* Immunologic memory 5 years after meningococcal A/C conjugate vaccination in infancy. *J Infect Dis* 2001;**183**:97–104.

110 Snape MD, Pollard AJ. Meningococcal polysaccharide-protein conjugate vaccines. *Lancet Infect Dis* 2005;**5**:21–30.

111 McVernon J, Johnson PD, Pollard AJ, Slack MP, Moxon ER. Immunologic memory in Haemophilus influenzae type b conjugate vaccine failure. *Arch Dis Child* 2003;**88**:379–83.

112 Snape MD, Kelly DF, Lewis S, *et al.* Seroprotection against serogroup C meningococcal disease in

adolescents in the United Kingdom: observational study. *BMJ* 2008;**336**:1487–91.

113 Belnoue E, Pihlgren M, McGaha TL, *et al.* APRIL is critical for plasmablast survival in the bone marrow and poorly expressed by early-life bone marrow stromal cells. *Blood* 2008;**111**:2755–64.

114 Belshe RB, Edwards KM, Vesikari T, *et al.* Live attenuated versus inactivated influenza vaccine in infants and young children. *N Engl J Med* 2007;**356**: 685–96.

115 Ashkenazi S, Vertruyen A, Aristegui J, *et al.* Superior relative efficacy of live attenuated influenza vaccine compared with inactivated influenza vaccine in young children with recurrent respiratory tract infections. *Pediatr Infect Dis J* 2006;**25**:870–79.

116 Fleming DM, Crovari P, Wahn U, *et al.* Comparison of the efficacy and safety of live attenuated cold-adapted influenza vaccine, trivalent, with triva-

lent inactivated influenza virus vaccine in children and adolescents with asthma. *Pediatr Infect Dis J* 2006;**25**:860–69.

117 Belshe RB, Mendelman PM, Treanor J, *et al.* The efficacy of live attenuated, cold-adapted, trivalent, intranasal influenzavirus vaccine in children. *N Engl J Med* 1998;**338**:1405–12.

118 Treanor JJ, Kotloff K, Betts RF, *et al.* Evaluation of trivalent, live, cold-adapted (CAIV-T) and inactivated (TIV) influenza vaccines in prevention of virus infection and illness following challenge of adults with wild-type influenza A (H1N1), A (H3N2), and B viruses. *Vaccine* 1999;**18**: 899–906.

119 Nichol KL, Mendelman PM, Mallon KP, *et al.* Effectiveness of live, attenuated intranasal influenza virus vaccine in healthy, working adults: a randomized controlled trial. *JAMA* 1999;**282**:137–44.

CHAPTER 7

Utility of Mouse Models in Vaccine Design and Development

Catharine M. Bosio[1], Megan MacLeod[2]*, Philippa Marrack[2], & Ross M. Kedl[3]

[1]Rocky Mountain Laboratories, National Institute of Allergy and Infectious Diseases, National Institutes of Health, Hamilton, MT, USA
[2]Integrated Department of Immunology, Howard Hughes Medical Institute, National Jewish Health, Denver, CO, USA
[3]Department of Immunology, University of Colorado Denver, Denver, CO, USA
*Present address

Why the Mouse?

The adjective murine applies to any members, including rats and mice, of a fairly large family of rodents. As far as use in the laboratory is concerned, the most used are members of the genus *Rattus* and, even more dominantly, the species *Mus musculus*. Despite the common usage in the early 20th century of the brown rat or even the guinea pig, a favorite subject for experimentation because of its need for vitamin C, *Mus musculus* became the preferred small mammal in many areas of scientific experimentation. The dominant use of *Mus*, like that of *E. coli*, seems to have occurred because of a combination of convenience, circumstances, luck, and suitability.

It is somewhat amusing to think that our use of the mouse as the dominant animal model for immunologic studies was due in no small part to an inner ear defect in the Japanese waltzing mouse [1]. These mice had been bred for years by mouse fanciers from the East for their curious tendency to, when excited, scramble around the cage in a random fashion until exhausted. This tendency is caused by a single recessive gene that causes an inner ear defect, leading to the curious behavior. In the process of maintaining this behavior through many generations of breeding, the mouse fanciers

had unwittingly, but significantly, reduced the genetic heterogeneity of the species. This reduced heterogeneity made the growth of a tumor derived from a Japanese waltzing mouse far more reproducible [2]. Utilizing this model and knowledge in the early 1900s, investigators such as Clarence Little, Carl Jensen, Leo Loeb, and E.E. Tyzzer began mating mice for many generations, creating inbred strains of mice with known susceptibility to various diseases [1]. These studies led to the theory of the genetic control of tumor susceptibility, and, ultimately, to the use of mice to study what would eventually become the field of immunology. Of course we now know these inbred stains had the added advantage that they responded identically to various forms of test, not just immunologic, allowing reproducible experimentation by biologists around the world.

Why mouse models for vaccine development

Any animal model used for vaccine development must first and foremost be conducive to the study of the basic immune principles underlying potent innate and adaptive immunity. Practically speaking, this means that there must be a variety of molecular

Vaccinology: Principles and Practice, First Edition. Edited by W. John W. Morrow, Nadeem A. Sheikh, Clint S. Schmidt and D. Huw Davies.
© 2012 Blackwell Publishing Ltd. Published 2012 by Blackwell Publishing Ltd.

and cellular tools available for the manipulation of the host, and the host must bear enough similarity to the human to make the comparison valid. The mouse is generally well suited on both counts. First, while the physiology of the mouse differs from that of humans in many respects (e.g., the reproductive cycle, the structure of the lungs, etc.), as luck would have it, the immune systems of *M. musculus* and *H. sapiens* are quite similar. Indeed, years of research have established that most of the molecules found to be important in mouse immunity typically have an ortholog in the human, possessing similar, if not identical, function. A good example is CD40L, an Ig superfamily member expressed on activated T cells. Genetic mutations that eliminate CD40L function in humans lead to hyper- syndrome (HIM) [3–6], a disease in which patients suffer from defects in memory B-cell development, Ig class switching, and T-cell activation. CD40-deficient mice show the same adaptive immune defects [7,8].

Second, crucial to the dominance of the mouse as an animal model has been the development of tools for production of monoclonal antibodies, which can be produced relatively easily in mice and other rodents, and, of course, the capacity to manipulate mice genetically, introducing and removing genes at will. Whole catalogs of mouse-specific reagents

tailored to immune response analysis are available, as well as numerous strains of mice genetically modified to augment or eliminate hundreds of immune-specific signaling pathways/mechanisms.

While the field of Immunology at large has obviously benefited from these tools and mouse strains, such reagents have been particularly invaluable to our understanding of the actions of vaccines. The reason vaccination is the most successful medical intervention in human history is based on the simple principle of immune memory; the ability of the immune system to remember previous pathogen encounters and respond more vigorously to a second challenge years, or even decades, later (Figure 7.1) [9]. The cell types responsible for this immune memory are of course T and B cells. Thus our understanding of the capacity of these cells to form immune memory, and, by extension, our understanding of the principles underlying the efficacy of vaccines, has grown in direct proportion to the development of molecular tools and reagents necessary for the analysis of T and B cell responses.

Indeed, the past 10 years have seen a dramatic expansion in the number of reagents and methods able to qualitatively and quantitatively measure T- and B-cell responses in both mouse and human. These include adoptive transfer models

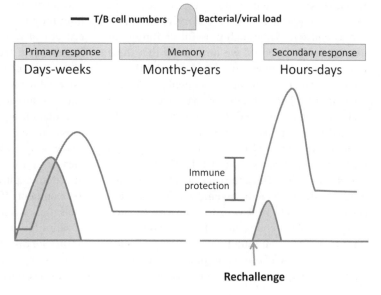

Figure 7.1 Infectious challenge and the development of immune memory. Survival of a primary encounter with an infectious agent produces robust T- and B-cell responses that lead to the elimination of the infection from the host. Immune memory can persist for years, if not decades. Secondary exposure to the infection produces a secondary immune response that is (i) more rapid and (ii) of greater magnitude than the primary response, resulting in a more efficacious clearance of the infection. Vaccination strategies hope to produce the protective capacity of the secondary response without primary encounter with the infectious agent.

utilizing transgenic T and/or B cells; class I [10] and class II [11] major histocompatibility complex (MHC) tetramers, used to identify antigen-specific T cells; and intracellular cytokine staining (ICCS) [12] or ELISPOT [13,14], used to measure the functions of antigen-specific lymphocytes. In many cases these sophisticated reagents and methods are available only for mouse and human, thus cementing the role of the mouse as the primary animal model for vaccine development. While we will go into no further detail in describing these mice, reagents, methods, and tools, their impact on the use of mouse models, and indeed on immunology as a whole, bears emphasis.

That said, while many transgenic and knockout mouse models are useful in the early stages of preclinical development, there are no real surrogates or substitutes for the kind of models described below, which examine the capacity of vaccination to motivate an endogenous response in a wild-type (WT) host to form protective immunity. An excellent example of this is the use of T-cell receptor (TCR) transgenic T-cell adoptive transfer models to track the activation and expansion of antigen-specific T cells in response to vaccination. These models usually involve the transfer of a small number of congenically marked TCR transgenic T cells into a WT recipient. The recipient is then immunized and the activity of the transferred cells monitored by the use of the congenic marker using either flow cytometry or immunohistochemistry. While highly useful and informative for many purposes, we now know that these models are confounded to some extent by the artificial elevation in precursor frequency following T-cell transfer [15–17]. Further, we have observed that the proliferation and differentiation of T cells isolated from a transgenic host is significantly accelerated as compared to the normal endogenous repertoire of antigen-specific T cells ([18] and unpublished results). Thus, the capacity [15–17] to induce transferred TCR transgenic T-cell expansion does not correlate well with the capacity to elicit a similarly robust endogenous T-cell response that leads to protective immunity. Collectively the data show that any use of transgenic or knockout mouse models during preclinical vaccine development requires subsequent confirmation in the kinds of models discussed below in order to validate the capacity of the vaccination to produce protective immune memory from an endogenous T- and B-cell repertoire.

Experimental mouse models of human pathogens

The various infectious models used for assessing immune protection have actually supported two purposes in the history of vaccine development: monitoring immune development and measuring immune protection. The infectious challenges that can be cleared from the host in the absence of prior vaccination have been instrumental in advancing our understanding of the basic immune principles that facilitate potent, protective immune memory. The immune responses resulting from challenge with these agents have been held as gold standards for the generation of optimal cellular and/or humoral immunity against which we can compare the immunity generated by our vaccine method/formulation of interest. Studies from these models systems (such as LCMV or HSV-1) have contributed substantially toward our understanding of basic principles of T-cell and B-cell immunity [19,20].

Ultimately, however, vaccination is about immune-mediated protection. While in the modern era of tetramers and ICCS we have become increasingly focused on the quantitative measurement of various immune parameters, the essential parameter that must be satisfied is that of immune protection: does one's vaccine method or formulation actually protect the host from future infectious encounters? This is assessed by either challenging with a lethal dose of the agent or by measuring the infectious titer at the point of peak infectious replication in a naïve host. Prior to the development of more sophisticated immunologic tools, this was the only way to quantify the degree of immunity generated from a given vaccination. Ironically, this classic parameter of immune protection is sometimes lost in the shuffle amidst today's rapidly advancing technology.

In the following sections, we will discuss examples of clinically and/or experimentally relevant viral and bacterial infections that are used for the purposes of vaccine development and analysis. A general point of mention for almost all mouse infectious model systems is the importance of strain selection. As described above, various inbred strains of mice have been generated over the past century, usually for the purposes of being used in a specific infectious or tumor model system. Extensive study has revealed different strains as being sensitive or resistant to specific infectious challenges [21]. As a general rule, C57BL/6 (B6) mice skew their immune responses toward the Th1 end of the spectrum and, as a result, tend to be the most resistant to mouse-adapted viral or bacterial challenges. In contrast, Balb/C mice skew their immune responses toward the Th2 end of the spectrum, leading to the host either succumbing to the viral or bacterial challenge or establishing chronic infection. Of course these rules are reversed when using paracytic models, such as *Heligmosomoides polygyrus*, which require the establishment of a robust Th2 response for infectious control. Therefore, a single infectious agent can serve as either a model of acute or chronic infection depending on the strain used. For the most part B6 is the strain of choice for immunologists simply because the majority of available reagents for T- and B-cell analysis are specific for the B6 haplotype (H-2^b), and the majority of genetically modified mice are now created on, or backcrossed to, the B6 background.

Vaccinia

Vaccinia virus (VV) is responsible for the only documented eradication of an infectious agent (smallpox) from the globe as a result of human intervention [22,23]. Given our general familiarity with the virus and its impact on human history, it is surprising to note that the origins of this particular virus are clouded in obscurity. Edward Jenner initially used the cowpox virus in his famous vaccination of the 8-year-old boy James Phipps against smallpox. However, as the practice caught on in the early 1800s, practitioners used poxviruses isolated from a variety of hosts, including sheep, goats, horses, and even buffalo [24]. At some point, one particular strain emerged as preferred for performing vaccinations, thereafter referred to as the vaccinia strain. Curiously, though most assume the name of the virus indicates its origins as a cowpox virus (*Vacca* is Latin for cow), sequencing has shown that our modern day VV is more closely related to horsepox than either cowpox or the variola virus against which it is so protective [25].

The capacity of vaccinia to promote long-term immunity is probably unparalleled in the infectious world, eliciting T- and B-cell immunity that has been shown to last 5–6 decades and beyond [26–28]. The potency of this immune memory does not come without some cost, however; the adverse event rate to VV immunization in humans is considerably higher than for other live vaccines [22,29]. However, this potency has been attractive enough to lure modern day researchers into producing less virulent strains of VV [30] to be used as vectors in a host of vaccine strategies against recalcitrant infectious and tumor agents [31,32].

All of these features have made VV virus an easy choice for use in mouse models of vaccination, both in terms of studying the normal mouse immune response to VV to establish the phenotype of a "gold standard" vaccine-elicited immune memory, as well as use in quantifying the protective capacity of other experimental vaccination strategies. In the mouse, the primary site of VV replication is the ovary, although some replication does occur in cells in the lymphoid organs and other tissues [33]. Though this fact is generally well known, the corollary that VV displays a dramatically different course of replication in male versus female mice is much less well publicized. Thus, the use of VV virus to quantitate protective immunity should usually be limited to the use of female mice, at least for systemic challenge models.

At high doses, VV can be lethal, and so the simplest protective model is high-dose systemic challenge followed by monitoring for survival. However, sublethal infections (which are cleared from the host and result in long-term T- and B-cell immunity) can also be utilized followed by the assessment of viral titers in the ovary at the peak time point of viral replication, usually between days 4 and 6 after viral challenge (Figure 7.2). The

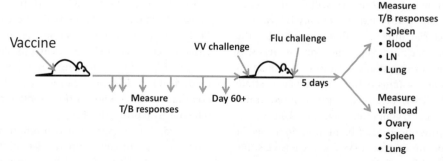

Figure 7.2 Schematic of VV and influenza viral challenge mouse models. Mice are vaccinated through various routes of administration depending on the desired tissue site of immune protection. Primary T- and B-cell responses can be measured in the blood/spleen to assess the peak of the response as well as the level of persisting immune memory. The mice are challenged with the viral agent of choice 1–3 months later and the secondary T- and B-cell responses, as well as viral load, are measured, each in their respective tissues, 3–5 days after challenge.

advantage of using this method is that it provides a more sensitive quantitation of immune protection compared to the use of a lethal challenge. As peak viral load in the host can reach 10^7 infectious particles, or plaque forming units (pfu), this provides the experimenter with a 7 log scale with which to measure protection with one's vaccine strategy [34,35]. Indeed, this marks a useful aspect of less lethal animal models; while a "digital" live versus dead read-out of the lethal challenge models is often seen as more clinically relevant, an "analog" read-out of protection is often more sensitive and can be much more informative with regard to understanding immune mechanisms responsible for protective immunity. To this point, because the peak of a secondary T-cell response in the mouse is usually around day 5 after secondary challenge [35], the use of nonlethal virus challenge allows the simultaneous analysis of viral titers as well as memory T-cell responses (Figure 7.2). Well-described outer coat proteins and recently described dominant epitopes for both CD4 and CD8+ T-cell responses from a number of mouse strains [36, 37] provide a rich source of target antigens against which to generate T- and/or B-cell immunity and subsequently determine protection. In addition, recombinant strains of vaccinia have been made expressing antigens derived from other pathogens [30–32]. These are particularly useful as they allow the assessment of protective immunity against antigens derived from pathogens for which there are no reproducible mouse models. Finally, VV provides an additional advantage with the opportunity to test tissue-specific protective immunity using multiple routes of viral challenge. While most utilize a systemic viral challenge (i.p. or i.v.), topical [38] and even mucosal challenge [39,40] models are well established. Given the capacity of immune memory for tissue-specific homing [41] and its importance in immune protection, these alternative methods of challenge facilitate the assessment of vaccine strategies that promote barrier-specific (gut, skin) protective immune memory. As the vast majority of infectious agents (including HIV, TB, and the family of neglected tropical diseases [42]) gain access to the host via the mucosa and/or skin, there is a need to accurately measure immune protection in these barriers. Given the flexibility and reproducibility of the mouse response to VV infections, this model will undoubtedly be a critical tool in vaccine development directed against a wide range of pathogens.

Influenza

As described above, smallpox was considered eradicated in 1980 [22,23]. Although it retains importance as a potential biological weapon, its eminent threat to the worldwide population is significantly diminished. In contrast, influenza (paramyxovirus) is a human pathogen that continues to pose a serious danger to global human health. Though it is not a natural pathogen for the mouse, it does productively infect the mouse respiratory epithelium, induces similar pathology in the lung as that observed in humans, and can be productively cleared by the immune response [43,44]. Both T- and B-cell response are easily identified in the mouse and numerous CD4$^+$ and CD8$^+$ T-cell epitopes have been identified for a number of mouse MHC haplotypes [43]. Thus, the mouse has become an important surrogate for studying influenza-specific immunity.

There are three strains of influenza virus, A, B, and C. However, influenza A and B are responsible for the majority of human infections [44]. Influenza A is the most variable subtype as a result of two separate processes: genetic drift and genetic shift. Genetic drift results from mutations that occur during viral replication. This predominantly affects the two major surface proteins, hemagglutinin (HA) and neuraminidase (NA), which are the main targets of neutralizing antibodies, and by altering the sequences of HA and NA, the virus can evade pre-existing antibody-mediated (humoral) immunity [45]. Genetic shift occurs when two viruses simultaneously infect the same host, allowing the viral gene segments that code for HA and NA in each virus to mix. Since influenza A can infect many animals, including pigs and birds, it is thought that novel virus strains also arise from genetic shift [44]. The shifting variation of influenza is one of the cornerstones of its virulence and consequentially has been the central topic for development of novel effective influenza vaccines.

The consequence of this variation on immune-mediated protection is one area in which the mouse model has been highly useful [46]. While specific antibody can provide sterile immunity, it cannot detect or clear a different viral subtype [45]. Some protection is seen, however, in mice first infected with one viral subtype and then challenged with a distinct virus, a phenomenon known as heterosubtypic immunity [47,48]. This protection is mediated by CD4 and CD8 T cells that are more likely to recognize conserved epitopes within the virus, for example in the internal viral proteins such as the nucleoprotein; non-neutralizing antibody and B cells

that respond to nucleoprotein may also contribute to heterosubtypic immunity [47–51]. Numerous studies have demonstrated that viral or vaccine-generated cytotoxic CD8 T cells specific for an epitope in the nucleoprotein can reduce influenza infection [48,52–55]. This has led to much interest in the development of universal influenza vaccines that would prime protective memory CD8 T cells specific for nonvariable epitopes in the virus [45, 46,56]. While heterosubtypic immunity has clearly been observed in mouse models, there is little direct evidence for it in humans [57,58]. However, cross-reactive CD4 and CD8 T cells that recognize novel viral subtypes can be identified in humans, suggesting that these cells may offer some protection to pandemic strains [59–64].

The course of infection has been intricately mapped in the mouse, and the signals and molecules required for protective immune responses are fairly well defined [43,65]. The use of intranasal viral challenge offers the opportunity to measure the ensuing response at the natural peripheral site of infection, the lung, and in the draining mediastinal lymph node where the adaptive immune response is initiated. The dose of virus can be altered to allow the mice to develop a mild infection that they completely recover from within 10–12 days or a large dose can be given to measure protection from a lethal challenge (Figure 7.2) [66]. In this model, morbidity resulting from wasting and weight loss can be monitored daily to track progression of the disease. The extent of disease can also be determined by measuring viral titers in the lung early after infection (day 1–4), and recovery correlates with the influx of influenza-specific cytotoxic CD8 T cells into the lungs [66].

Although the mouse provides a useful model for influenza infection, ferrets are often used to test the efficacy of new vaccines [67]. This is because ferrets can be naturally infected with human isolates, infection in ferrets closely resembles that in humans, and vaccine-generated protection in ferrets is a better predictor of successful protection in humans. However, the numerous tools to study the immune response in mice still make them an attractive model to test theories and new vaccine strategies before moving to a larger animal model.

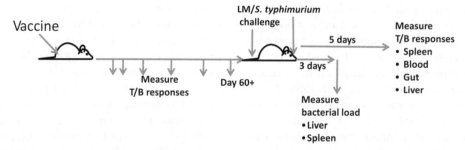

Figure 7.3 Schematic of bacterial challenge mouse models. As in Figure 7.2, mice are vaccinated through various routes of administration depending on the desired tissue site of immune protection. Primary T- and B-cell responses can be measured in the blood/spleen to assess the peak of the response as well as the level of persisting immune memory. The mice are challenged with the bacterial agent of choice 1–3 months later and the secondary T- and B-cell responses, as well as bacterial load, are measured, each in their respective tissues, 3–5 days after challenge.

Listeria monocytogenes

Similar to viral models, there are numerous mouse models of bacterial infection one might choose from. We will focus our discussion here on two bacterial models, *Listeria monocytogenes* (LM) and *Salmonella enterica* serovar *typhimurium*, (hereafter referred to as simply *S. typhimurium*). LM is a Gram-positive, facultative intracellular pathogen, and its use as a mouse model of bacterial infection for use in immunologic studies came as a result of initial studies by George Mackaness in the early 1960s [68,69]. Similar to VV, the importance of LM as a human pathogen is relatively minimal [70]. Rather, its use as an animal model is based on the fact that it is an accessible, granulomatous-inducing infection that requires the participation of cellular responses for immunologic protection. Thus, while the viral models are useful in examining the generation of neutralizing antibodies, LM is an excellent model for examining the protective capacity of vaccine-elicited T cell responses. The cellular response to LM has also achieved "gold standard" status, and much effort has been put into the mechanisms by which LM can generate particularly robust CD8+ T-cell immune memory [71]. One reason for such potent CD8+ T-cell responses is the fact that the primary cell types for LM replication are antigen-presenting cells (APCs) such as DCs and macrophages [72–74]. For nonattenuated strains, bacterial load following a primary challenge in resistant mouse strains such as B6 peaks around day 3–4 after challenge (Figure 7.3). The T-cell response to this primary LM challenge becomes detectable by day 4 and peaks on day 7–8, at which point the bacteria is eliminated [71,72].

As with VV, LM demonstrates multiple uses for the purposes of vaccine development and design. First, as mentioned above, it is often used as a reference point for the generation of potent cellular immune memory against which one can compare an experimental vaccine method or formulation. Second, given its potency for eliciting cellular memory, numerous modified LM strains have been produced and significant effort is currently being directed at their use as vaccine vectors [75,76]. Finally, the ability to measure bacterial load provides a similar analog readout of immune protection as the sublethal VV challenge model (Figure 7.1). With the traditional challenge dose of 2×10^5 colony forming units (cfu), peak bacterial loads in the spleens or livers (both primary sites of bacterial replication) of resistant mouse strains easily reach 10^7–10^9 cfu. Given that the limit of detection of the bacterial plating methods used to assay bacterial load is approximately 10^2, this again provides 5–7 logs of bacterial growth in which to assess the magnitude of immune protection (Figure 7.1).

Salmonella typhimurium

As mentioned above, LM's usefulness as an animal model is not based on its clinical importance. In contrast, *S. typhimurium* is considered an effective model for a significant human pathogen, *Salmonella typhi* (*S. typhi*). While *S. typhi* does not cause typhoid in mice, *S. typhimurium* does cause disease with a progression and tissue involvement similar to that seen in humans infected with *S. typhi* [77]. Thus a significant strength of the model is its relevance to human disease. Further, numerous antigenic epitopes on the H-2^{d,b,k} haplotyopes have been identified within the past 10 years, facilitating the study of both the natural T-cell response to bacterial challenge as well as the protective capacity of vaccine elicited *S. typhimurium*-specific T-cell responses [78]. While CD4$^+$ T-cell responses are critical for resistance to primary *S. typhimurium* challenge [79–81], B cells, CD4$^+$, and CD8$^+$ T cells are all required for immune-mediated protection from secondary challenge [82–85]. Thus, *S. typhimurium* is useful for determining whether an experimental vaccine can generate cellular and/or humoral immunity. Similar to LM, bacterial load is measured in multiple organs 2–4 days after oral challenge with *S. typhimurium* (Figure 7.3) [86]. Lethal, sublethal, and attenuated vaccine strain challenge models are all available for quantitating protective immunity against enteric bacterial challenge [87]. For all the reasons described above regarding the relationship between anatomical location and protective immunity, *S. typhimurium*, being an enteric bacteria, provides the opportunity to examine vaccination and protection within the intestinal mucosa. Indeed, as with LM, the potency with which *S. typhimurium* can elicit long-lasting mucosal immunity is being leveraged in the development and use of attenuated recombinant vaccine strains [87].

While enough similarity between *S. typhi* in humans and *S. typhimurium* in mice exists to warrant the use of the mouse model in early vaccine-related studies, the model does depart from the human disease in some significant ways. Differences in physiologic response (mice become hypothermic rather than hyperthermic, and do not experience diarrhea) and critical virulence factors for disease are limitations of the mouse model as it applies to humans [77,88], as for all models described above. There are, however, a number of mouse models of human disease that have increasing similarity to the human pathology, course of disease, disease

severity, or combinations of any of these. In the following section we will discuss some of these models and their potential for use in vaccine design and development.

Mice as models for lethal human pathogens

As described above, the utilization of mice for discovery of basic mechanisms by which the immune system develops and maintains immunity directed against antigens and attenuated pathogens represented an important step forward in the field of infectious disease immunology. Equally important has been the development of mouse models for diseases mediated by microorganisms that routinely cause severe and/or lethal infections in humans. Ideally, a mouse model of human disease would encompass four primary features: (i) the virulent strain isolated from humans also infects mice; (ii) the infectious dose is similar to that found in humans; (ii) the course of the infection is approximately the same as observed in humans; and (iv) the pathogenesis in mice is similar to that found in humans following the same route of infection. However, fulfillment of each of these criteria in the mouse model is exceedingly rare. This does not mean that rodent models are not useful. Rather, one must be aware of the limitations embodied by each model before developing firm conclusions based on data obtained from that model. Discussed below are several examples of mouse models of disease mediated by highly virulent microorganisms, and the disadvantages and advantages of each model.

Tularemia

Perhaps one of the best, yet underutilized, models of human disease is the mouse model of tularemia. Tularemia is the disease following infection with virulent strains of the Gram-negative bacterium *Francisella tularensis* subspecies *tularensis*. There are four different subspecies of *F. tularensis*, three of which can infect and kill mice. With respect to human pathogens, *F. tularensis* is a fairly new emergent virulent organism. This bacterium was first described at the turn of the 20th century as a "plague-like illness" among California ground squirrels [89]. Within two years it was demonstrated that *F. tularensis* was the causative agent of what is now known as tularemia in humans [90]. Although this bacterium can infect via nearly every imaginable route, the ease and deadly nature of transmission of *F. tularensis* by aerosol made it dangerous as both a natural pathogen and potential biological weapon [91].

F. tularensis is capable of causing lethal disease following inhalation with as few as 10–15 cfu in mice and humans, suggesting that both of these species are equally susceptible to pneumonic tularemia [92–94]. Following inhalation, *F. tularensis* replicates quickly in the lung, with as many as 10^4 organisms present in the pulmonary compartment within 24 hours of infection [95,96]. Despite this rapid replication, *F. tularensis* fails to induce any significant inflammatory response in the lung, in mice or humans, for the first several days after infection [95,97,98]. The failure of *F. tularensis* to induce proinflammatory responses following inoculation into the lung is likely the result of a deficiency in a number of innate immune-related signals and/or functions [99]. Following phagocytosis by host cells, *F. tularensis* evades detection by the host cell by actively inhibiting recognition of unrelated microbial molecules in mouse and human target cells and the lungs during early stages of disease [95,98,100]. Suppression of cytokine and chemokine production by virulent *F. tularensis* not only minimizes local inflammatory responses but inhibits the recruitment of other immune effector cells such as monocytes, granulocytes, natural killer cells, and T cells [95] (Anderson and Bosio, unpublished data). Thus, the profound effect virulent *F. tularensis* has on the innate immune system also negatively impacts development and implementation of adaptive immune responses.

Unfortunately, to date the majority of published work concerning requirements for effective adaptive immunity directed against *F. tularensis* has utilized attenuated and vaccine strains of this family of bacteria. Although this data is important in establishing a baseline for defense against *F. tularensis* infections, attenuated and vaccine strains behave differently in the pulmonary compartment of mice [101]. Thus, extrapolation of findings obtained with these less virulent isolates cannot necessarily be applied to infections with fully virulent strains of *F. tularensis*. Due to these differences among strains of *F. tularensis*, we will restrict our discussion of adaptive immunity to tularemia to infections mediated by virulent strains of the bacteria.

Some of the earliest therapeutic trials consisted of passive transfer of hyperimmune serum obtained from horses [102]. Other studies demonstrated that hyperimmune serum could also be used to protect hosts prior to infection, although this protection was tightly correlated with the dose of serum delivered, the species of the host, and the challenge dose used (as reviewed in [103]). Similar experiments performed in the mouse model have been less successful. The inability of serum to protect mice against *F. tularensis* was attributed to increased susceptibility of these animals to *F. tularensis* infection compared to humans. However, recent studies in our and other's laboratories have shown that passive transfer of immune serum can protect up to 80% of mice from infections with virulent *F. tularensis* infections (Anderson and Bosio, unpublished data; Norgard and Huntley, personal communication). Thus, in mice, like humans, presence of antibody specific for *F. tularensis* plays a critical role in protection against tularemia.

Unsurprisingly, as *F. tularensis* is a facultative intracellular pathogen, cellular immunity also plays an important role in protection against infection. Using the mouse model, it has been shown that both CD4$^+$ and CD8$^+$ T cells are equally capable of mediating protection against virulent *F. tularensis* [104]. Though this remains to be conclusively determined in humans, recent reports have shown that both humans and mice develop strong CD4$^+$ T cell responses against the Francisella lipoprotein antigen Tul4 following either a natural infection or vaccination [105–108].

Mouse models have been developed for a wide variety of diseases. However, there is typically little information that allows for direct comparison of immunity to infection between mice and humans, and thus validation of the model. Disease mediated by *F. tularensis* is an outstanding exception to this scenario. Despite the relatively low numbers of humans infected each year there is a wealth of information from older studies. Importantly, these early experiments and observations in humans support the use of the mouse model of tularemia. Given the strong similarities between the mouse and human manifestation of disease, the mouse model of tularemia may also serve as an important model for testing other, more broadly applicable, immunologic tenants.

Ebola

Ebola virus (EBOV) emerged as a serious human pathogen in the mid-1970s following the infamous outbreak in Yambuku and Kinshasa [109,110]. Following this outbreak, EBOV joined Marburg virus (MARV) in this unique family of Filoviridae. Over the next 20 years, scientists and clinicians struggled to understand the pathogenesis and mechanisms of virulence of this virus. Obviously, a small-animal model had the potential to greatly advance our understanding of the interaction of EBOV with mammalian immune systems. However, the greatest obstacle in development of a mouse model of EBOV infection was that clinical strains of the virus were not infectious in adult immunocompetent mice [111].

Following serial passage of the EBOV Zaire strain in inbred C57Bl/6 and Balb/c as well as outbred ICR (CD-1) mice, Bray and colleagues were successful in generating a mouse-adapted virus that caused uniformly lethal disease following intraperitoneal (i.p.) injection with approximately 1 virion [112]. However, unlike what is believed to occur in humans, injection of up to 100 pfu of virus intradermally (i.d.), subcutaneously (s.c.), or intramuscularly (i.m.) was not lethal in mice. Further, mice exposed to virus via these parenteral routes were completely protected from subsequent i.p. challenge [112]. The route-dependent virulence in mice has not been resolved, but must be considered when directly comparing data gained from rodents to that obtained in nonhuman primates and humans.

Despite these drawbacks, the mouse model has proven to be an important tool for both understanding basic mechanisms of pathogenesis and

screening novel vaccines and therapeutics [113, 114]. Initial studies in the mouse model showed that eVLP could successfully protect against EBOV infection in mice [114]. Later, it was shown that this same eVLP vaccine could also protect nonhuman primates against EBOV infection [115]. Therefore, despite the strange observation that virulence of mouse-adapted EBOV in the murine model is dependent upon the route of inoculation, the reproducibility of results obtained in mice in far more stringent models (e.g., primary human cells and nonhuman primates) suggests that mice serve as a reasonable tool by which to dissect immunity against filoviruses.

Tuberculosis

Unlike tularemia and EBOV infections, disease caused by *Mycobacterium tuberculosis*, tuberculosis (TB), affects large numbers of individuals worldwide. To date, approximately 9 million individuals are newly infected with the bacterium and 2 million people die of TB-related disease each year [116]. *M. tuberculosis* was recognized as the causative agent of TB in 1882 by Robert Koch. Soon after, efforts were made to develop an effective vaccine against this serious, debilitating disease. Initially, investigators tried immunization with fully virulent strains of *M. bovis*. The results of these vaccine trials were disastrous, since *M. bovis* is as virulent in humans as *M. tuberculosis*.

Despite this failure, efforts to develop a safe vaccine continued. While working at the Institute Pasteur de Lille and later at the Paris Pasteur Institute, Drs Albert Calmette and Camille Guérin found that growth of virulent *M. bovis* on glycerin-bile-potato medium attenuated the bacterium. Following repeated passage of virulent *M. bovis* on this medium, the two scientists isolated a strain that no longer caused disease in animals and could protect against challenge with virulent *Mycobacterium* [117]. Within a short two years the new vaccine, dubbed Bacille Calmette-Guérin (BCG), was first used in humans. However, even at this early time, variation in protective immunity engendered by BCG was apparent. Thus, scientists set out to design a new model by which to study the development of adaptive immunity to TB following vaccination with BCG.

Although initial animal studies were conducted in rabbits and guinea pigs, the value of the mouse as an affordable, easily manipulated animal drove investigators to begin exploring these mammals as tools for TB research. Some of the earliest studies evaluated the virulence of *M. tuberculosis* in mice following intravenous inoculation [118]. These studies established that the mouse was indeed susceptible to *M. tuberculosis* infection. However, it took 15 years before a model for reliable aerosol infections with *M. tuberculosis* in mice was established [119]. Here Dr Middlebrook described a machine that could routinely infect nearly 100 mice at once with a low-dose aerosol. Given that this route is the natural means of exposure in humans, the ability to routinely infect mice following exposure to *M. tuberculosis* containing aerosols was a major leap forward in utilizing mice for understanding both manipulation of the host immune response in naïve animals and development of adaptive immunity.

Following Middlebrook's description of the mouse model of pulmonary TB, there have been significant advances in our understanding of the requirements for immunity to TB following aerosol infection. Initially, studies directed at identifying the nature of immunity required for protection against TB utilized cells obtained from mice vaccinated with BCG. The ability of these cells to mediate immunity against virulent *M. tuberculosis* was demonstrated by protection of naïve mice from *M. tuberculosis* following adoptive transfer of T cells harvested from mice vaccinated with BCG [120]. Furthermore, it was discovered that nonviable BCG bacteria were not capable of engendering protective immunity against infection with virulent *M. tuberculosis* [121]. This important observation using the mouse model of TB led to the understanding that proteins secreted by *M. tuberculosis* were highly immunogenic and represented key targets of the cellular immune response responsible for protecting the host against infection [122–124].

Since then the mouse model has continued to contribute to the process of TB vaccine development, examining various TB-specific antigens incorporated into various vaccine methodologies [125,126], in some cases leading to the initiation of phase I clinical trials in humans. Thus, despite the inability of mice to generate pulmonary lesions that are pathologically similar to those observed in humans, these animals represent an important and viable tool for understanding and examining the requirements for generation of memory immune responses directed against *M. tuberculosis*.

Concluding remarks

The mouse models we have described above are incredibly useful, highly malleable models that have been and will continue to be invaluable for the purposes of vaccine design and development. We have attempted to discuss both strengths and weaknesses of each model system as it applies not only to the process of vaccine development, but also to the degree to which the model accurately represents the human disease. It must be remembered, however, that these are only models, which at best can only represent the human condition and cannot replace larger animal models or clinical studies. As such, it should come as no surprise when data generated in nonhuman primates, or human cells or subjects, does not completely recapitulate what is found in the mouse. Furthermore, it should probably be stressed that this incomplete representation of the human condition will be maintained outside of future technological developments: new technology will never be able to fully bridge the gap between the results obtained in mouse models and that experienced in human disease. Rather, any future advances will simply solidify the role of mouse models in their capacity to reveal and manipulate immune mechanisms that have potential in mediating protection against infectious processes.

References

1 Klein J. *Biology of the Mouse Histocompatibility-2 Complex: Principles of immunogenetics Applied to a Single System*. Springer, New York, 1975.

2 Loeb L. Uber Entstehung eines Sarkoms nach Transplantation eines Adenocarcinoma einer japanischen Maus. *Z Krebsforsch* 1908;**7**:80–110.

3 Allen RC, Armitage RJ, Conley ME, *et al.* CD40 ligand gene defects responsible for X-linked hyper-IgM syndrome. *Science* 1993;**259**:990–93.

4 Aruffo A, Farrington M, Hollenbaugh D, *et al.* The CD40 ligand, gp39, is defective in activated T cells from patients with X-linked hyper-IgM syndrome. *Cell* 1993;**72**:291–300.

5 DiSanto JP, Bonnefoy JY, Gauchat JF, Fischer A, de Saint Basile G. CD40 ligand mutations in x-linked immunodeficiency with hyper-IgM. *Nature* 1993;**361**:541–3.

6 Korthauer U, Graf D, Mages HW, *et al.* Defective expression of T-cell CD40 ligand causes X-linked immunodeficiency with hyper-IgM. *Nature* 1993;**361**:539–41.

7 Quezada SA, Jarvinen LZ, Lind EF, Noelle RJ. CD40/CD154 interactions at the interface of tolerance and immunity. *Annu Rev Immunol* 2004;**22**:307–28.

8 Renshaw BR, Fanslow WC, 3rd, Armitage RJ, *et al.* Humoral immune responses in CD40 ligand-deficient mice. *J Exp Med* 1994;**180**:1889–1900.

9 Marrack P, McKee AS, Munks MW. Towards an understanding of the adjuvant action of aluminium. *Nat Rev Immunol* 2009;**9**:287–293.

10 Altman JD, Davis MM. MHC-peptide tetramers to visualize antigen-specific T cells. *Curr Protoc Immunol* 2003;Chapter **17**:Unit 17.3.

11 Crawford F, Kozono H, White J, Marrack P, Kappler J. Detection of antigen-specific T cells with multivalent soluble class II MHC covalent peptide complexes. *Immunity* 1998;**8**:675–82.

12 Sander B, Andersson J, Andersson U. Assessment of cytokines by immunofluorescence and the paraformaldehyde-saponin procedure. *Immunol Rev* 1991;**119**:65–93.

13 Taguchi T, McGhee JR, Coffman RL, *et al.* Analysis of Th1 and Th2 cells in murine gut-associated tissues. Frequencies of CD4+ and CD8+ T cells that secrete IFN-gamma and IL-5. *J Immunol* 1990;**145**:68–77.

14 Taguchi T, McGhee JR, Coffman RL, *et al.* Detection of individual mouse splenic T cells producing IFN-gamma and IL-5 using the enzyme-linked immunospot (ELISPOT) assay. *J Immunol Methods* 1990;**128**:65–73.

15 Badovinac VP, Haring JS, Harty JT. Initial T cell receptor transgenic cell precursor frequency dictates critical aspects of the CD8(+) T cell response to infection. *Immunity* 2007;**26**:827–41.

16 Hataye J, Moon JJ, Khoruts A, Reilly C, Jenkins MK. Naive and memory CD4+ T cell survival controlled by clonal abundance. *Science* 2006;**312**:114–16.

17 Marzo AL, Klonowski KD, Le Bon A, *et al.* Initial T cell frequency dictates memory CD8+ T cell lineage commitment. *Nat Immunol* 2005;**6**:793–99.

18 Haluszczak C, Akue AD, Hamilton SE, *et al.* The antigen-specific CD8+ T cell repertoire in unimmunized mice includes memory phenotype cells bearing markers of homeostatic expansion. *J Exp Med* 2009;**206**(2):435–48.

19 Heath WR, Carbone FR. Cross-presentation, dendritic cells, tolerance and immunity. *Annu Rev Immunol* 2001;**19**:47–64.

20 Murali-Krishna K, Altman JD, Suresh M, *et al.* In vivo dynamics of anti-viral CD8 T cell responses to different epitopes. An evaluation of bystander activation in primary and secondary responses to viral infection. *Adv Exp Med Biol* 1998;**452**:123–42.

21 Kelso A, Troutt AB, Maraskovsky E, *et al.* Heterogeneity in lymphokine profiles of CD4+ and CD8+ T cells and clones activated in vivo and in vitro. *Immunol Rev* 1991;**123**:85–114.

22 Rotz LD, Dotson DA, Damon IK, Becher JA. Vaccinia (smallpox) vaccine: recommendations of the Advisory Committee on Immunization Practices (ACIP). *MMWR Recomm Rep* 2001;**50**:1–25; quiz CE21–7.

23 Wehrle, PF A reality in our time – certification of the global eradication of smallpox. *J Infect Dis* 1980;**142**:636–8.

24 Fenner F, Henderson DA, Arita I, Jezek Z, Ladnyi ID. *Smallpox and its Eradication*. World Health Organization, Geneva, 1988, 1460 pp.

25 Tulman ER, Delhon G, Afonso CL, *et al.* Genome of horsepox virus. *J Virol* 2006;**80**:9244–58.

26 Amanna IJ, Slifka MK, Crotty S. Immunity and immunological memory following smallpox vaccination. *Immunol Rev* 2006;**211**:320–37.

27 Crotty S, Felgner P, Davies H, *et al.* Long-term B cell memory in humans after smallpox vaccination. *J Immunol* 2003;**171**:4969–73.

28 Miller JD, RG van der Most, Akondy RS, *et al.* Human effector and memory CD8+ T cell responses to smallpox and yellow fever vaccines. *Immunity* 2008;**28**:710–22.

29 Kretzschmar M, Wallinga J, Teunis P, Xing S, Mikolajczyk R. Frequency of adverse events after vaccination with different vaccinia strains. *PLoS Med* 2006;**3**:e272.

30 Jacobs BL, Langland JO, Kibler KV, *et al.* Vaccinia virus vaccines: past, present and future. *Antiviral Res* 2009;**84**:1–13.

31 Gomez CE, Najera JL, Krupa M, Esteban M. The poxvirus vectors MVA and NYVAC as gene delivery systems for vaccination against infectious diseases and cancer. *Curr Gene Ther* 2008;**8**:97–120.

32 Kirn DH, Thorne SH. Targeted and armed oncolytic poxviruses: a novel multi-mechanistic therapeutic class for cancer. *Nature Rev* 2009;**9**:64–71.

33 Buller RM, Palumbo GJ. Poxvirus pathogenesis. *Microbiol Rev* 1991;**55**:80–122.

34 Kedl RM, Rees WA, Hildeman DA, *et al.* T cells compete for access to antigen-bearing antigen-presenting cells. *J Exp Med* 2000;**192**:1105–14.

35 Sanchez PJ, McWilliams JA, Haluszczak C, Yagita H, Kedl RM. Combined TLR/CD40 stimulation mediates potent cellular immunity by regulating dendritic cell expression of CD70 in vivo. *J Immunol* 2007;**178**:1564–72.

36 Sette A, Moutaftsi M, Moyron-Quiroz J, *et al.* Selective CD4$^+$ T cell help for antibody responses to a large viral pathogen: deterministic linkage of specificities. *Immunity* 2008;**28**:847–58.

37 Tscharke DC, Karupiah G, Zhou J, *et al.* Identification of poxvirus CD8$^+$ T cell determinants to enable rational design and characterization of smallpox vaccines. *J Exp Med* 2005;**201**:95–104.

38 Howell MD, Gallo RL, Boguniewicz M, *et al.* Cytokine milieu of atopic dermatitis skin subverts the innate immune response to vaccinia virus. *Immunity* 2006;**24**:341–8.

39 Belyakov IM, Moss B, Strober W, Berzofsky JA. Mucosal vaccination overcomes the barrier to recombinant vaccinia immunization caused by preexisting poxvirus immunity. *Proc Natl Acad Sci U S A* 1999;**96**:4512–17.

40 Belyakov IM, Wyatt LS, Ahlers JD, *et al.* Induction of a mucosal cytotoxic T-lymphocyte response by intrarectal immunization with a replication-deficient recombinant vaccinia virus expressing human immunodeficiency virus 89.6 envelope protein. *J Virol* 1998;**72**:8264–72.

41 Denucci CC, Mitchell JS, Shimizu Y. Integrin function in T-cell homing to lymphoid and nonlymphoid sites: getting there and staying there. *Crit Rev Immunol* 2009;**29**:87–109.

42 Liese B, Rosenberg M, Schratz A. Programmes, partnerships, and governance for elimination and control of neglected tropical diseases. *Lancet* **375**:67–76.

43 Doherty PC, Turner SJ, Webby RG, Thomas PG. Influenza and the challenge for immunology. *Nat Immunol* 2006;**7**:449–55.

44 Webster RG, Bean WJ, Gorman OT, Chambers TM, Kawaoka Y. Evolution and ecology of influenza A viruses. *Microbiol Rev* 1992;**56**:152–79.

45 Ellebedy AH, Webby RJ. Influenza vaccines. *Vaccine* 2009;**27**(Suppl 4):D65–8.

46 Thomas PG, Keating R, Hulse-Post DJ, Doherty PC. Cell-mediated protection in influenza infection. *Emerg Infect Dis* 2006;**12**:48–54.

47 Liang S, Mozdzanowska K, Palladino G, Gerhard W. Heterosubtypic immunity to influenza type A virus in mice. Effector mechanisms and their longevity. *J Immunol* 1994;**152**:1653–61.

48 Yewdell JW, Bennink JR, Smith GL, Moss B. Influenza A virus nucleoprotein is a major target antigen for cross-reactive anti-influenza A virus cytotoxic T lymphocytes. *Proc Natl Acad Sci U S A* 1985;**82**:1785–9.

49 Carragher DM, Kaminski DA, Moquin A, Hartson L, Randall TD. A novel role for non-neutralizing antibodies against nucleoprotein in facilitating resistance to influenza virus. *J Immunol* 2008;**181**:4168–76.

50 Rangel-Moreno J, Carragher DM, Misra RS, *et al.* B cells promote resistance to heterosubtypic strains of influenza via multiple mechanisms. *J Immunol* 2008;**180**:454–63.

51 Rimmelzwaan GF, Fouchier RA, Osterhaus AD. Influenza virus-specific cytotoxic T lymphocytes: a correlate of protection and a basis for vaccine development. *Curr Opin Biotechnol* 2007;**18**:529–36.

52 Crowe SR, Miller SC, Woodland DL. Identification of protective and non-protective T cell epitopes in influenza. *Vaccine* 2006;**24**:452–6.

53 Epstein SL, Kong WP, Misplon JA, *et al.* Protection against multiple influenza A subtypes by vaccination with highly conserved nucleoprotein. *Vaccine* 2005;**23**:5404–10.

54 Tite JP, Hughes-Jenkins C, O'Callaghan D, *et al.* Antiviral immunity induced by recombinant nucleoprotein of influenza A virus. II. Protection from influenza infection and mechanism of protection. *Immunology* 1990;**71**:202–7.

55 Topham DJ, Tripp RA, Doherty PC. CD8$^+$ T cells clear influenza virus by perforin or Fas-dependent processes. *J Immunol* 1997;**159**:5197–200.

56 Rimmelzwaan GF, McElhaney JE. Correlates of protection: novel generations of influenza vaccines. *Vaccine* 2008;**26**(Suppl 4):D41–4.

57 Epstein SL. Prior H1N1 influenza infection and susceptibility of Cleveland Family Study participants during the H2N2 pandemic of 1957: an experiment of nature. *J Infect Dis* 2006;**193**:49–53.

58 McMichael AJ, Gotch FM, Noble GR, Beare PA. Cytotoxic T-cell immunity to influenza. *N Engl J Med* 1983;**309**:13–17.

59 Alexander J, Bilsel P, del Guercio MF, *et al.* Universal influenza DNA vaccine encoding conserved CD4$^+$ T cell epitopes protects against lethal viral challenge in HLA-DR transgenic mice. *Vaccine* **28**:664–72.

60 Greenbaum JA, Kotturi MF, Kim Y, *et al.* Pre-existing immunity against swine-origin H1N1 influenza viruses in the general human population. *Proc Natl Acad Sci U S A* 2009;**106**:20365–70.

61 Kreijtz JH, de Mutsert G, van Baalen CA, *et al.* Cross-recognition of avian H5N1 influenza virus by human cytotoxic T-lymphocyte populations directed to human influenza A virus. *J Virol* 2008;**82**:5161–6.

62 Lee LY, Ha do LA, Simmons C, *et al.* Memory T cells established by seasonal human influenza A infection cross-react with avian influenza A (H5N1) in healthy individuals. *J Clin Invest* 2008;**118**:3478–90.

63 Richards KA, Chaves FA, Sant AJ. Infection of HLA-DR1 transgenic mice with a human isolate of influenza a virus (H1N1) primes a diverse CD4 T-cell repertoire that includes CD4 T cells with heterosubtypic cross-reactivity to avian (H5N1) influenza virus. *J Virol* 2009;**83**:6566–77.

64 Wang M, Lamberth K, Harndahl M, *et al.* CTL epitopes for influenza A including the H5N1 bird flu; genome-, pathogen-, and HLA-wide screening. *Vaccine* 2007;**25**:2823–31.

65 Kohlmeier JE, Woodland DL. Immunity to respiratory viruses. *Annu Rev Immunol* 2009;**27**:61–82.

66 Cottey R, Rowe CA, Bender BS. Influenza virus. *Curr Protoc Immunol* 2003;Chapter **19**:Unit 19.12.

67 van der Laan JW, Herberts C, Lambkin-Williams R, *et al.* Animal models in influenza vaccine testing. *Expert Rev Vaccines* 2008;**7**:783–93.

68 Mackaness GB. Cellular resistance to infection. *J Exp Med* 1962;**116**:381–406.

69 Mackaness GB. The immunological basis of acquired cellular resistance. *J Exp Med* 1964;**120**:105–20.

70 Lorber B. Listeriosis. *Clin Infect Dis* 1997;**24**:1–9; quiz 10–11.

71 Zenewicz LA, Shen H. Innate and adaptive immune responses to *Listeria monocytogenes*: a short overview. *Microbes Infect* 2007;**9**:1208–15.

72 Pamer EG. Immune responses to *Listeria monocytogenes*. *Nat Rev Immunol* 2004;**4**:812–23.

73 Pron B, Boumaila C, Jaubert F, *et al.* Dendritic cells are early cellular targets of *Listeria monocytogenes* after intestinal delivery and are involved in bacterial spread in the host. *Cell Microbiol* 2001;**3**:331–40.

74 Vazquez-Boland JA, Kuhn M, Berche P, *et al.* Listeria pathogenesis and molecular virulence determinants. *Clin Microbiol Rev* 2001;**14**:584–640.

75 Bruhn KW, Craft N, Miller JF. Listeria as a vaccine vector. *Microbes Infect* 2007;**9**:1226–35.

76 Schoen C, Loeffler DI, Frentzen A, *et al.* Listeria monocytogenes as novel carrier system for the development of live vaccines. *Int J Med Microbiol* 2008;**298**:45–58.

77 Santos RL, Zhang S, Tsolis RM, *et al.* Animal models of salmonella infections: enteritis versus typhoid fever. *Microbes Infect* 2001;**3**:1335–44.

78 Moon JJ, McSorley SJ. Tracking the dynamics of salmonella specific T cell responses. *Curr Top Microbiol Immunol* 2009;**334**:179–98.

79 Hess J, Ladel C, Miko D, Kaufmann SH. *Salmonella typhimurium* aroA-infection in gene-targeted immunodeficient mice: major role of CD4$^+$ TCR-alpha beta cells and IFN-gamma in bacterial clearance independent of intracellular location. *J Immunol* 1996;**156**:3321–6.

80 Sinha K, Mastroeni P, Harrison J, de Hormaeche RD, Hormaeche CE. *Salmonella typhimurium* aroA, htrA, and aroD htrA mutants cause progressive infections in athymic (nu/nu) BALB/c mice. *Infect Immun* 1997;**65**:1566–9.

81 Weintraub BC, Eckmann L, Okamoto S, *et al.* Role of alphabeta and gammadelta T cells in the host response to salmonella infection as demonstrated in T-cell-receptor-deficient mice of defined Ity genotypes. *Infect Immun* 1997;**65**:2306–12.

82 Lo WF, Ong H, Metcalf ES, Soloski MJ. T cell responses to Gram-negative intracellular bacterial pathogens: a role for CD8$^+$ T cells in immunity to salmonella infection and the involvement of MHC class Ib molecules. *J Immunol* 1999;**162**:5398–406.

83 Mastroeni P, Simmons C, Fowler R, Hormaeche CE, Dougan G. Igh-6(-/-) (B-cell-deficient) mice fail to mount solid acquired resistance to oral challenge with virulent *Salmonella enterica* serovar *typhimurium* and show impaired Th1 T-cell responses to salmonella antigens. *Infect Immun* 2000;**68**:46–53.

84 McSorley SJ, Jenkins MK. Antibody is required for protection against virulent but not attenuated *Salmonella enterica* serovar *typhimurium*. *Infect Immun* 2000;**68**:3344–8.

85 Mittrucker HW, Raupach B, Kohler A, Kaufmann SH. Role of B lymphocytes in protective immunity against *Salmonella typhimurium* infection. *J Immunol* 2000;**164**:1648–52.

86 McSorley SJ, Cookson BT, Jenkins MK. Characterization of CD4$^+$ T cell responses during natural infection with *Salmonella typhimurium*. *J Immunol* 2000;**164**:986–93.

87 Cheminay C, Hensel M. Rational design of salmonella recombinant vaccines. *Int J Med Microbiol* 2008;**298**:87–98.

88 Pasetti MF, Levine MM, Sztein MB. Animal models paving the way for clinical trials of attenuated *Salmonella enterica* serovar typhi live oral vaccines and live vectors. *Vaccine* 2003;**21**:401–18.

89 McCoy GW, Chapin CW. *Bacterium tularense* the cause of a plague-like disease of rodents. *J Infect Dis* 1912;**10**:17–23.

90 Wherry WB, Lamb BH. Infection of man with *Bacterium tularense*. *J Infect Dis* 1914;**15**:331–40.

91 Dennis DT, Inglesby TV, Henderson DA, *et al.* Tularemia as a biological weapon: medical and public health management. *JAMA* 2001;**285**: 2763–73.

92 Conlan JW, Chen W, Shen H, Webb A, KuoLee R. Experimental tularemia in mice challenged by aerosol or intradermally with virulent strains of *Francisella tularensis*: bacteriologic and histopathologic studies. *Microb Pathog* 2003;**34**:239–48.

93 Eigelsbach HT, Downs CM. Prophylactic effectiveness of live and killed tularemia vaccines. I. Production of vaccine and evaluation in the white mouse and guinea pig. *J Immunol* 1961;**87**:415–25.

94 Saslaw S, Eigelsbach HT, Prior JA, Wilson HE, Carhart S. Tularemia vaccine study. II. Respiratory challenge. *Arch Intern Med* 1961;**107**:702–14.

95 Bosio CM, Bielefeldt-Ohmann H, Belisle JT. Active suppression of the pulmonary immune response by *Francisella tularensis* Schu4. *J Immunol* 2007;**178**:4538–47.

96 Chen W, KuoLee R, Shen H, Conlan JW. Susceptibility of immunodeficient mice to aerosol and systemic infection with virulent strains of *Francisella tularensis*. *Microb Pathog* 2004;**36**:311–18.

97 Andersson H, Hartmanova B, Kuolee R, *et al.* Transcriptional profiling of host responses in mouse lungs following aerosol infection with type A *Francisella tularensis*. *J Med Microbiol* 2006;**55**:263–71.

98 Telepnev M, Golovliov I, Grundstrom T, Tarnvik A, Sjostedt A. *Francisella tularensis* inhibits Toll-like receptor-mediated activation of intracellular signalling and secretion of TNF-alpha and IL-1 from murine macrophages. *Cell Microbiol* 2003;**5**:41–51.

99 Chase JC, Bosio CM. The presence of CD14 overcomes evasion of innate immune responses by virulent *Francisella tularensis* in human dendritic cells in vitro and pulmonary cells in vivo. *Infect Immun* 2010;**78**:154–67.

100 Chase JC, Celli J, Bosio CM. Direct and indirect impairment of human dendritic cell function by virulent *Francisella tularensis* Schu S4. *Infect Immun* 2009;**77**:180–95.

101 Hall JD, Woolard MD, Gunn BM, *et al.* Infected-host-cell repertoire and cellular response in the lung following inhalation of *Francisella tularensis* Schu S4, LVS, or U112. *Infect Immun* 2008;**76**:5843–52.

102 Foshay L. A comparative study of the treatment of tularemia with immune serum, hyperimmune serum and streptomycin. *Am J Med* 1946;**1**:180–88.

103 Foshay L. Tularemia. *Annu Rev Microbiol* 1950; **4**:313–30.

104 Wayne Conlan J, Shen H, Kuolee R, Zhao X, Chen W. Aerosol-, but not intradermal-immunization with the live vaccine strain of *Francisella tularensis* protects mice against subsequent aerosol challenge with a highly virulent type A strain of the pathogen by an alphabeta T cell- and interferon gamma-dependent mechanism. *Vaccine* 2005;**23**: 2477–85.

105 Golovliov I, Ericsson M, Sandstrom G, Tarnvik A, Sjostedt A. Identification of proteins of *Francisella tularensis* induced during growth in macrophages and cloning of the gene encoding a prominently induced 23-kilodalton protein. *Infect Immun* 1997;**65**:2183–9.

106 Sjostedt A, Eriksson M, Sandstrom G, Tarnvik A. Various membrane proteins of *Francisella tularensis* induce interferon-gamma production in both CD4$^+$ and CD8$^+$ T cells of primed humans. *Immunology* 1992;**76**:584–92.

107 Sjostedt A, Sandstrom G, Tarnvik A. Several membrane polypeptides of the live vaccine strain *Francisella tularensis* LVS stimulate T cells from naturally infected individuals. *J Clin Microbiol* 1990;**28**:43–8.

108 Valentino MD, Hensley LL, Skrombolas D, *et al.* Identification of a dominant CD4 T cell epitope in the membrane lipoprotein Tul4 from *Francisella tularensis* LVS. *Mol Immunol* 2009;**46**:1830–38.

109 Ebola haemorrhagic fever in Zaire, 1976. *Bull World Health Organ* 1978;**56**(2):271–93.

110 Ebola haemorrhagic fever in Sudan, 1976. Report of a WHO/International Study Team. *Bull World Health Organ* 1978;**56**(2):247–70.

111 van der Groen G, Jacob W, Pattyn SR. Ebola virus virulence for newborn mice. *J Med Virol* 1979; **4**:239–40.

112 Bray M, Davis K, Geisbert T, Schmaljohn C, Huggins J. A mouse model for evaluation of prophylaxis and therapy of Ebola hemorrhagic fever. *J Infect Dis* 1999;**179**(Suppl 1):S248–58.

113 Fuller CL, Ruthel G, Warfield KL, *et al.* NKp30-dependent cytolysis of filovirus-infected human dendritic cells. *Cell Microbiol* 2007;**9**:962–76.

114 Warfield KL, Perkins JG, Swenson DL, *et al.* Role of natural killer cells in innate protection against lethal Ebola virus infection. *J Exp Med* 2004;**200**:169–79.

115 Warfield KL, Swenson DL, Olinger GG, *et al.* Ebola virus-like particle-based vaccine protects nonhuman primates against lethal Ebola virus challenge. *J Infect Dis* 2007;**196**(Suppl 2):S430–37.

116 CDC. *A Global Perspective on Tuberculosis*. CDC Fact Sheet – TB. CDC, Atlanta, GA, 2009.

117 Calmette A. *Ann Inst Pasteur* 1928;**42**:1–34.

118 Schwabacher H, Wilson G. Vaccination of mice against tuberculosis with killed cultures and living BCG. *Tubercle* 1937;**18**:492–8.

119 Middlebrook G. An apparatus for airborne infection of mice. *Proc Soc Exp Biol Med* 1952;**80**:105–10.

120 Orme IM, Collins FM. Adoptive protection of the *Mycobacterium tuberculosis*-infected lung. Dissociation between cells that passively transfer protective immunity and those that transfer delayed-type hypersensitivity to tuberculin. *Cell Immunol* 1984;**84**:113–20.

121 Orme IM. Induction of nonspecific acquired resistance and delayed-type hypersensitivity, but not specific acquired resistance in mice inoculated with killed mycobacterial vaccines. *Infect Immun* 1988;**56**:3310–12.

122 Andersen P. The T cell response to secreted antigens of *Mycobacterium tuberculosis*. *Immunobiology* 1994;**191**:537–47.

123 Andersen P, Askgaard D, Gottschau A, *et al.* Identification of immunodominant antigens during infection with *Mycobacterium tuberculosis*. *Scand J Immunol* 1992;**36**:823–31.

124 Andersen P, Askgaard D, Ljungqvist L, Bennedsen J, Heron I. Proteins released from *Mycobacterium tuberculosis* during growth. *Infect Immun* 1991; **59**:1905–10.

125 Olsen I, Tryland M, Wiker HG, Reitan LJ. AhpC, AhpD, and a secreted 14-kilodalton antigen from *Mycobacterium avium* subsp. *paratuberculosis distinguish* between paratuberculosis and bovine tuberculosis in an enzyme-linked immunosorbent assay. *Clin Diagn Lab Immunol* 2001;**8**:797–801.

126 Skeiky YA, Alderson MR, Ovendale PJ, *et al.* Differential immune responses and protective efficacy induced by components of a tuberculosis polyprotein vaccine, Mtb72F, delivered as naked DNA or recombinant protein. *J Immunol* 2004;**172**:7618–28.

CHAPTER 8

Utility of Nonhuman Primate Models for Vaccines

Preston A. Marx, Jr[1] & Alexander F. Voevodin[2]

[1]Tulane National Primate Research Center, Tulane University, Covington, LA, USA
[2]Vir&Gen, Toronto, ON, Canada

Introduction

The principal utility of nonhuman primates (NHPs) as vaccine models lies in their obvious close relationship to human beings. The common chimpanzee, *Pan troglodytes*, is widely appreciated as the closest living NHP relative of human beings. However, there are other considerations in addition to relatedness, especially availability and cost. Therefore, the use of more distantly related monkey species such as the macaques and African green monkeys is much more common than chimpanzees. This chapter focuses on AIDS vaccine research, but many of the principles described here will apply to other types of vaccines.

NHPs commonly used for all types of vaccines are members of the great ape and monkey families shown in Table 8.1. Rhesus macaques (*Macaca mulatta*) are a commonly used species; however, it is not widely appreciated that all rhesus are not the same and individual subspecies and even breeds may respond differently to infectious agents.

The macaque AIDS models began with the description of a fatal immunodeficiency syndrome associated with lymphoma, reported in 1971 from the California National Primate Research Center (NPRC) [1]. This outbreak led to a series of events that resulted in the discovery of simian immunodeficiency viruses (SIVs) in macaques (SIVmac),

which are the most commonly used SIVs for AIDS animal model research. The discoveries were both serendipitous and unintended. SIVmac emerged as an unintended consequence of animal model research on kuru [2,3]; SIVB670, a virus that emerged in the early 1980s, resulted from the unintended consequences of animal model research on leprosy [4,5]. There exists a law for unintended consequences, which states, "the purposeful actions of people and especially of governments always have effects that are unintended" [6]. This law applies to economics and government, but also to medical research. It was not until AIDS was reported in human beings in 1981 [7] that veterinarians and research scientists at primate centers recognized the macaque immunosuppressive diseases as AIDS.

SIVs have their natural origins in healthy African monkeys and apes and the infection is mostly silent in the naturally infected African host species [5, 8–10]. The virus was unintentionally transmitted and serially passaged to Asian species, rhesus monkeys (rh), and cynomolgus macaques. The SIV infections manifested clinically as typical AIDS [5, 11,12]. The combination of the close genetic relationship between SIV and HIV-2 [8] and the induction of AIDS in commonly available laboratory NHP species led to the development of SIV infection in macaques (SIVmac) as the model most widely

Vaccinology: Principles and Practice, First Edition. Edited by W. John W. Morrow, Nadeem A. Sheikh, Clint S. Schmidt and D. Huw Davies.
© 2012 Blackwell Publishing Ltd. Published 2012 by Blackwell Publishing Ltd.

Table 8.1 Nonhuman primate species and subspecies commonly used in vaccine research.

Species/subspecies[a]	Common name	Geographical distribution (free living)
Macaca mulatta	**Rhesus monkey**	Afghanistan, India to China, north Thailand
M. mulatta mulatta	Indian rhesus monkey	East Afghanistan, Bangladesh, Bhutan, north peninsular India, Nepal, north Pakistan
M. mulatta lasiota	West Chinese rhesus monkey	China (southeast Qinghai, west Sichuan, northeast Yunnan)
Macaca fascicularis	**Cynomolgus macaque or crab-eating macaque**	Indonesia, Philippines, India
M. fascicularis philippinensis	Philippine long-tailed macaque	Philippines (Balabac, Culion, Leyte, Luzon, northeast Mindanao, Mindoro, Palawan, Samar)
Macaca nemistrina	**Pig-tailed macaque**	Burma to Malay peninsula and Sumatra
Chlorocebus aethiops	**African green monkey**	Africa (multiple countries) (natural)
Chlorocebus aethiops sabeus	Sabeus monkey	Caribbean (introduced), Senegal to Ghana
Chlorocebus aethiops pygerytrus	Vervet monkey	Ethiopia, Somalia, Kenya, Tanzania, Zambia, Zimbabwe, Republic of South Africa
Pan troglydytes	**Common chimpanzee**	
P. troglodytes verus	West African chimpanzee	Senegal to Ghana
P. troglodytes troglodytes	Central African Chimpanzee	Cameroon south to Gabon, east to Congo and west Central African Republic, south Burundi
P. troglodytes schweinfurthi	East African chimpanzee	West Uganda, west Tanzania, north Democratic Republic of Congo, east Central African Republic

[a]Species names are in bold.

used for AIDS research, including vaccine research. The number of publications on different aspects of this NHP model of AIDS exceeds 5000 and increases every day. This chapter will describe the major findings in vaccine research using the SIV-macaque model, undoubtedly the model of choice in the context of AIDS vaccine development.

Notably, several important discoveries were made in the SIVmac model before they were found in human AIDS. For example, early immunopathogenesis of SIV was characterized in SIV-infected rh [13,14] before the same studies were done in humans [15]. Proof that AIDS was a disease of the mucosal immune system was also done first in SIV-infected rh [16,17], showing a sharp decline in mucosal CD4$^+$ cells in acute infection.

There has been much discussion in the literature about the value of AIDS animal models [18,19].

The viewpoint as to what constitutes a "perfect" AIDS model is a matter of opinion. The ideal model for AIDS and for any other infectious disease is the induction of the human disease in a common laboratory animal with a virus isolated from human tissue. These conditions are not rigorously met by any of the AIDS animal models. The most common AIDS virus is HIV-1 and it does not reproducibly infect or cause AIDS in any available laboratory animal species, although many species were tested in vitro and in vivo [20–22]. HIV-1 readily infects chimpanzees although AIDS is a relatively rare outcome, but chimpanzees are hardly a common laboratory animal [23–25]. There are reports of HIV-1 infection in pig-tailed macaques (*M. nemestrina*) and HIV-2 infection in baboons (*Papio* spp.) and cynomolgus macaques (*M. fascicularis*). HIV-1 infection in pig-tailed macaques has been of limited

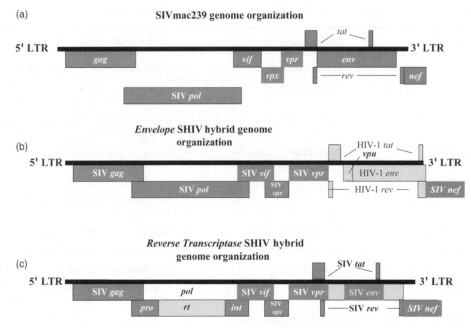

Figure 8.1 Genomic organization of simian immunodeficiency virus (SIV) and simian-human immunodeficiency virus (SHIV). The genome organization for (a) SIVmac239, (b) SHIV containing HIV-1 env, and (c) HIV-1 reverse transcriptase. The SIV genes are dark gray and the HIV-1 genes are light gray.

value due to the transient nature of the HIV-1 infection [26]. Infection of baboons and cynomolgus macaques with HIV-2 has not been widely used because of the transient nature of infection [27–29], although the cynomolgus model does show persistent infections and AIDS in some cases. SIVmac in macaques represents an animal model compromise in a sense that SIVmac is related to HIV-2, the less prevalent of the two human AIDS viruses. Nevertheless, the ability of SIVmac to readily induce a disease that closely mimics human AIDS in rhesus monkeys, and the fact that rh are a well-characterized and common laboratory animal provides the justification for using this most appropriate model of human AIDS.

SIVs and SIV/HIV hybrid viruses (SHIV) used for vaccine studies

SIVs and SIV-derived viruses commonly used in AIDS animal model research belong to the following three groups: SIVmac, SIVB670, and simian-human immunodeficiency viruses (SHIVs). The lat-

ter are hybrid viruses derived from SIV and HIV-1 genes. Figure 8.1 shows the representative genomic maps of these viruses. Table 8.2 provides a list of the commonly used SIV and SHIV strains and their characteristics with regard to pathogenesis and sensitivity to neutralizing antibody. All SIVs in Table 8.2 are derived from sooty mangabeys. Interestingly, although nine separate phylogenetic lineages of SIV are known in sooty mangabeys, the vast majority of AIDS animal model research is performed using strains belonging to only two of these lineages, the SIVmac lineage 8 and the SIVB670/H5 lineage 1 [30].

SIVmac group: SIVmac251, SIVmac239, and vaccine challenge viruses

The SIVmac group strains are the most used for modeling AIDS. The SIVmac group originated from a monkey in the sooty mangabey colony held at the California NPRC [30,31] in the 1970s. At that time the California colony was used by Carleton

Table 8.2 SIVs and SHIVs used in nonhuman primate model of AIDS vaccine research.

SIVs commonly used	Major co-receptors *in vitro*[a]/*in vivo*	In vivo pathogenesis[b] in rh	Remarks
SIVmac group	CCR5, BONZO/CCR5 [191]		
SIVmac251 [12]	CCR5, BONZO/CCR5	Medium pathogenic swarm	Four serial passages
SIVmac251 TCLA [119]	CCR5, BONZO/CCR5	Not tested *in vivo*	T-cell line adapted neutralization sensitive
SIVmac251 CX-1 [92]	CCR5, BONZO/CCR5	Pathogenic swarm	Moderately neutralization sensitive
SIVmac239 [31]	ND	Highly pathogenic swarm	Seven serial passages
SIVmac239 (clone) [192]	CCR5, BONZO/CCR5	Highly pathogenic molecular clone[c]	Seven serial passages, neutralization resistant
SIVmac142 [31]	ND	Less commonly used	
SIVmne [37]	CCR5, BONZO/CCR5	Least pathogenic of SIVmac group	
SIVmac32H [38]	CCR5, BONZO/CCR5	Pathogenic molecular clone derived from SIVmac251	
SIVB670 group	CCR5, BONZO/CCR5		
SIVB670 [5]	CCR5, BONZO/CCR5	Pathogenic swarm	Neutralization resistant
SIVE660 [43]	CCR5, BONZO/CCR5	Pathogenic swarm	Moderately sensitive to neutralization
SHIV group [53]			Clade/HIV-1 donor strain
SHIV vpu[−] [54]	CXCR4/CXCR4		B/HXBc2
SHIV89.6P [61]	CCR5[+], CXCR4/CXCR4	Pathogenic	B/89.6
SHIVKu-1, KU-2 [59]	CXCR4/CXCR4	Pathogenic	B/HXBc2
SHIV162p3/4 [57]	CCR5/CCR5	Transient infection in most rh	B/162p
SHIV-SF33A [57]	CXCR4/CXCR4	Moderately pathogenic	B/SF33
SHIV DH12 [56]	CCR5,CXCR4/CxCR4	Pathogenic	B/DH12
RT-SHIV [77]	CCR5/CCR5 (same as SIVmac239)	Moderately pathogenic	B/HXBc2
SHIV1157i [70]	CCR5/CCR5	Transient infection or moderately pathogenic	C/{1157i}
RT-SHIVrti/3mP [80]	CXCR4	Transient infection	B/{NL432}

[a]SIV and SHIV are promiscuous *in vitro*. Co-receptors used *in vitro* may or may not be the major co-receptors *in vivo* BOB (gpr15) and BONZO (STRL33).
[b]Relative pathogenesis defined as time to AIDS and plasma virus load. Highly pathogenic strains induce AIDS in shortest time with higher virus loads compared to moderately pathogenic strains [64,192].
[c]This clone is also used for SIV vaccine vectors.
[d]Passaged in rh.

Gajdusek's group to develop an animal model of kuru disease [24,32,33]. In the course of their experiments, tissues from kuru-inoculated sooty mangabeys were passaged from sooty mangabeys to rhesus monkeys to develop the model in a more commonly available monkey species. This passage was responsible for an outbreak of B-cell lymphomas in outdoor rhesus colonies at the California NPRC [1,3,34].

Apparently healthy animals from the outbreak-affected colonies at the California NPRC were sent to the New England NPRC where several additional serial passages, monkey to monkey, were performed. The highly pathogenic SIVmac viruses SIVmac251 and SIVmac239 [35] are derived from passages 4 and 7, respectively [31]. Soon after human AIDS was first described [7], the epizootic of fatal immunosuppressive disease in rhesus macaques was recognized at both primate centers as a simian counterpart to human AIDS [36]. SIVmne, a less pathogenic member of the SIVmac group, surfaced in pig-tailed macaques (*M. nemestrina*) [37] from a colony at the Washington NPRC. SIVmne also has its origin in the rhesus monkey colony at California NPRC unintentionally "contaminated" with sooty mangabey SIV [31,37]. SIVmne is less pathogenic compared to SIVmac239 because SIVmne was not serially passaged to the same extent as SIVmac239 [31]. An additional virus derived from SIVmac is SIV32H [38], which is a re-isolated strain of SIVmac251 (Table 8.2).

Sequence data of SIVmac142 shows this virus to be closely related to SIVmac239 and SIVmac251. It was derived from the same series of animal passages at the New England Primate Center that generated all SIVmac isolates [31]. SIVmac142 is not widely used because the molecular clone was less pathogenic, and in a vaccine-related experiment, SIVmac142 infection did not protect monkeys from superinfection with pathogenic SIVmac251 [39,40].

SIVB670/H4/H9 group and vaccine challenge viruses

The SIVB670/H4/H9 group was derived from three sooty mangabeys in the colony at the Tulane NPRC.

Again, the discovery was the untended consequence of a completely different set of experiments. The research group at this center had developed a leprosy model using the sooty mangabey colony, in which a naturally occurring case of leprosy had been identified [41,42]. As in the kuru experiments at the California NPRC [2], the Tulane group passaged affected tissues from sooty mangabeys to rhesus monkeys with the goal of further developing the model in a more common laboratory NHP species [4]. After a period of time immunosuppression was seen in some of the rhesus macaques and the disease was later characterized as SIV-induced AIDS [5,10]. SIVB670 [10], SIVE660 [43,44], an uncloned isolate that is pathogenic and moderately susceptible to neutralizing antibody [44–46], and SIVpbj [47,48], all belonging to the SIVsmm lineage 1, have their origin in this outbreak. SIVE660 is emerging as a more appropriate vaccine challenge virus due to its moderate sensitivity to neutralizing antibody. A pathogenic molecular clone of lineage 1 SIV, E543-3, is also available [44]. SIVpbj induces a particularly virulent and frequently fatal infection in pig-tailed macaques that is characterized by extensive lymphoid hyperplasia of T-cell zones in the gut-associated lymphoid tissue [49]. It is not widely used for vaccines, since the disease it induces is different from AIDS. The names B670, E660, pbj, and E543-3 are derived from the monkey numbers. B670 was one of the rhesus monkeys in the original leprosy serial passage group.

The SIVB670 strain was originated derived from sooty mangabey SM-022. This monkey was followed for clinical signs and was shown to be free of AIDS. The same observation was also made at the Yerkes NPRC in their sooty mangabey colony [50]. These studies were the first to associate SIV with sooty mangabeys that were free of disease and led to the theory that SIV was not pathogenic in its natural host. This theory holds largely true, with only a few exceptions [51,52].

SIV H4 virus was derived from SM-038, a sooty mangabey in the Tulane NPRC colony. SIV H4 was passaged in rhesus monkeys and was the first SIV sequenced that could be directly traced to a sooty mangabey [8]. This seminal paper showed that SIVsm was the most likely source of HIV-2. This hypothesis was proven by further studies in sooty mangabeys in West Africa [9]. Molecular clones are available for constructing vaccines for which SIVE660 is the homologous challenge virus [44].

SHIV group

The concept of simian-human hybrid viruses, the SHIVs, was first reported by Shibata *et al.* in 1991 [53] and followed by Li *et al.* [54]. The early SHIVs included clade B HIV-1 *env, tat,* and *rev* genes. The HIV-1 genes of this virus were from the CXCR4 HIV-1 strain HXBc2 and HIV-1 (NL432) and the rest of the genome was from the pathogenic molecular clone of SIVmac239 (Figure 8.1) [54,55]. Because this SHIV lacked the HIV-1 *vpu* gene, it was named SHIVvpu$^-$. The virus was non-pathogenic [55]. Subsequently many more SHIVs have been made and the major ones are summarized in Table 8.2. SHIVs produced after vpu$^-$ SHIV had a functional *vpu* and were initially designated SHIVvpu$^+$. Since SHIVvpu$^-$ were no longer used the early distinctions of vpu$^-$ and vpu$^+$ were dropped. The next generation of SHIVs (SHIV89.6p, SHIVDH12, KU-SHIVs, SHIV-SF33A) were dual CCR5/CXCR4 tropic *in vitro*, but, importantly, behaved like CXCR4 tropic *in vivo* [56–61]. The need for a pure CCR5 tropic SHIV was met by SHIV162, which is CCR5 tropic both *in vitro* and *in vivo* [56,62]. SHIV162 was passaged up to four times to increase pathogenicity for rhesus monkeys [63]. SHIV162/passage 3 and passage 4 (SHIV162p3/p4) are commonly used; however, the passaged SHIV162 viruses are not as pathogenic as other CXCR4 tropic SHIVs and some infected rhesus monkeys naturally suppress the infection [64].

HIV-1 strains are divided into phylogenetic clades, A, B, C, etc. All SHIVs described above are clade B SHIVs. Clade B viruses are common in the USA and Europe; other clades are more prevalent in other geographical areas [65]. For example clade C HIV-1s are very common in India and some parts of Africa, whereas clade E HIV-1s are common in some parts of Asia. SHIVs containing clade C and clade E HIV-1 *env*, instead of clade B *env*, were developed to provide a model to assess vaccines in-

tended for the regions where clade C and clade E viruses predominate [66–70].

Attempts have continued to expand the HIV-1 genes that could be used in SHIV macaque models. SHIVs containing the reverse transcriptase (RT) coding region of HIV-1 were made. These viruses are used for *in vivo* testing of RT inhibitor vaccines and microbicides that are restricted to blocking HIV-1 RT activity, such as non-nucleoside RT inhibitors (NNRTI) [71–79].

The most "humanized" SHIV produced thus far is SHIVrti/3rnP, which combines an env-SHIV with an RT-SHIV and also includes the *int* region of *pol* [80]. Only the *gag, prt* (*pro*), *vif* are of SIV origin. After being serially passaged in rhesus monkeys this virus is capable of transient replication in rh of Chinese origin. Rhesus monkeys of Indian origin are more permissive for replication of SIVmac239 and its derivatives [81,82]. It may be that Indian-origin rh would confer better *in vivo* replication for SHIV-rti/3rnP. However, proof of this is lacking.

HIV infection of chimpanzees

The only animal species routinely susceptible to HIV-1 infection is the common chimpanzee (*Pan troglodytes*). Two subspecies have been used, *P. t. troglodytes* and *P. t. schweinfurthi* (Table 8.1). The two explanations for this unique susceptibility are: (i) chimpanzees are the nearest human relatives in the animal kingdom, and (ii) chimpanzees are the natural host of HIV-1 ancestral viruses, therefore HIV-1 infection is a natural or near natural infection. Both explanations are probably correct. Chimpanzees inoculated by HIV-1 either by intravenous or mucosal routes become persistently infected [83–85]. However HIV-1 infected chimpanzees develop only transient lymphadenopathy and immunosuppression [23] and then maintain their immunocompetence and mount cellular immune responses to HIV-1 antigens [86]. AIDS develops only rarely in this model [87]. HIV-1 subtype B infected chimpanzees can be superinfected with HIV-1 subtype E [88]. Moreover, recombination between the two subtypes was observed [89]. Chimpanzees are now used much less frequently for AIDS research compared to the early days of the epidemic. High cost is frequently cited, but the fact that the vast majority of chimpanzees do not develop persistent immunosuppression and AIDS is also a major factor.

HIV-1 infection of pig-tailed macaques

Experimental transmission of HIV-1 to pig-tailed macaques has been reported [90,91]. HIV-1 infection in this species induces cell-mediated immune responses. However, the infection was not persistent [26]. For this reason the model, which initially appeared as promising, is not in common use.

Challenge routes of infection for testing vaccine efficacy

There are four entry points for HIV transmission: (i) mucosal surfaces, (ii) blood stream, (iii) placenta, and (iv) through skin, either by injection or through a break in the skin. Mucosal transmission is further divided into genital, oral, and rectal. NHP models have been developed for each of the four routes of transmission.

The simplest and most commonly used transmission mode is intravenous (IV) injection. This route of infection is the most efficient and requires the least amount of infectious virus [93] because blood presents no barrier to infection, unlike mucous membranes, which provide an epithelial barrier to virus penetration.

Vaginal transmission is frequently used, especially in vaccine experiments in which the vaccine is being tested for efficacy in preventing sexual transmission. Typically, 1–4 mL of titrated SIV or SHIV is placed atraumatically into the vaginal vault [92]. The volume of the macaque vagina is approximately 4 cc. Atraumatic exposure is used to model the natural penetration of the virus through the intact mucosa. Chimpanzees can also be infected with HIV-1 by this route [84]. Vaginal infection requires a higher dose of virus compared to IV inoculation, as much as a 100- to 1000-fold increase in the dose compared to the IV route [92]. Susceptibility to vaginal transmission can be increased by pretreat-

ing macaques with progesterone or progestins such as Depo-Provera [93,94]. The correlate of increased transmission is the thinning of the vaginal epithelium [93,95,96]. Estrogen thickens the vaginal epithelium and renders macaques more resistant to infection [96]. Progesterone, an estrogen antagonist, causes the epithelium to thin and therefore increases susceptibility. In addition to the thinning of the mucosa, progestins are reported to be immunosuppressive in macaque AIDS models and may contribute to disease progression or breaking vaccine protection [97,98]. Other factors in the vagina may also play a role, such as vaginal pH and thickening of mucous.

The intact rectal mucosa is also susceptible to infection and this model is widely used for vaccine efficacy studies [99,100]. The clinical outcome of infection is the same by any of the infection routes. The foreskin and urethra of the macaque penis are also susceptible tissues [92,101].

Oral transmission of HIV to infants by breast milk is an important route of transmission in humans [102,103]. This route can be used in vaccine experiments and has been effectively modeled in SIVB670 infected lactating females, in which 10 of 14 transmitted SIV to their infants in 1 year. Four infants remained SIV-negative despite their mothers' progressing to AIDS [104–106].

SIVB670 transplacental transmission has been demonstrated in dams inoculated at mid-gestation [107]. However, in another study, infants delivered by caesarian section were SIV-negative [108].

AIDS vaccine models

The greatest challenge for AIDS vaccine development using NHP models is the successful testing of a candidate vaccine that is both safe and effective against a relevant immunosuppressive primate lentivirus. The key word is "relevant" since protection in NHPs can be achieved against tissue culture-adapted HIVs and SHIVs that are neutralization sensitive.

The search for an AIDS vaccine using NHP models began with simple killed-virus vaccines and now encompasses numerous sophisticated replicating/single-cycle vectors, DNA vaccines, and others. The number of publications reporting specifically on AIDS vaccines in NHP models is over 1000. There is no single source covering the entire field of AIDS vaccine design and testing. The major issues of vaccine design, correlates of protection, escape from vaccine-induced immunity, and vaccine safety are dealt with in a series of reviews [109–112]. Representative vaccine approaches in the NHP models are covered here. This chapter serves mainly as a starting point for understanding how to use this model for vaccine testing and what has been done.

The gold standard for vaccines is prophylaxis of infection, often called "sterilizing immunity." Protection from disease is also a criterion for judging vaccine candidates, if sterilizing immunity is not achieved. Classically, protective immunity is achieved through priming with the vaccine, followed by one or more boosts with the same vaccine or a different formulation that carries the same antigens of interest. Table 8.3 is a list of the major types of vaccines that have been tested in the SIV and SHIV macaque model.

Killed-virus vaccines

In the late 1980s reports were published in high-profile journals that reported protection claiming sterilizing immunity against SIV using immunization with simple killed-virus vaccines [113–115]. Protection was achieved using a low-dose challenge of SIV grown in human cells and inactivated with formalin or nonionic detergent. Another study was unable to show protection using a relatively high challenge dose [116]. It was later shown that the protection by the killed-virus vaccines was due to "anti-human" antibodies [117,118]. This was a major setback in the progress toward an effective AIDS vaccine. The anti-human antibodies were induced by human-cell antigens that coated SIV when virions budded from the cultured human cells in which vaccine virus was grown. These anti-human antibodies were able to neutralize the challenge virus. The necessary control consisting of cellular antigens from the cells used to grow the vaccine virus was omitted in earlier studies. When killed-virus SIV vaccines were prepared using the virus

grown in macaque cells, no protection was found [118]. Killed-virus vaccines induced antibodies that were largely ineffective in neutralizing SIV and HIV [119].

After the failure with killed vaccines in the NHP model, the criterion for efficacy was ratcheted down from complete protection provided by sterilizing immunity to delay of disease and lower virus loads in immunized groups compared to control groups.

Subunit protein vaccines

Soluble HIV and SIV envelope glycoproteins are effective in inducing antibody in chimpanzee and macaque models. Using the HIV-1 chimpanzee model, protection was shown with a soluble gp120-based vaccine. However the challenge in these experiments was done with a tissue culture adapted strain of HIV-1 that was highly susceptible to neutralizing antibody [120]. In humans the situation is quite different – most of the HIV-1s transmitted between persons are relatively resistant to neutralizing antibody [121,122]. A similar vaccine (HIV-1 gp120) was tested in humans and failed to elicit neutralizing antibody and protection.

After these failures, emphasis shifted to vaccines that were capable of inducing cell-mediated immunity (CMI). These include recombinant DNA plasmids encoding SIV and HIV proteins and live virus vectors. DNA plasmids that express SIV proteins *in vivo* are effective in inducing CMI. They are taken up by cells and carry out intracellular expression of the encoded antigens. Antigen-presenting cells process these antigens for induction of cell-mediated immunity [123], resulting in the induction of CD8+ cytotoxic T cells. DNA plasmids have also been used to co-express cytokines, such as IL2, IL12, IL15, and others [124–127], which serve as adjuvants to boost immune responses against viral antigens. These plasmids have been used in the SIVmac model to show enhanced CMI responses and amelioration of plasma virus load [124–126,128].

Replication-competent vaccines

Vaccines based on replication-competent viruses are hybrid viruses containing SIV or HIV genes

Table 8.3 Major types of vaccines tested in nonhuman primate models.

Vaccine type/NHP model	Prime/boost	Adjuvant	Challenge	Protection	Ab/CMI[a]
Killed whole virus/rhesus [114,115]	Killed whole virus/same vaccine	MDP, alum, ICF	SIVmac, SIVB670	Y[b]	+/ND[c]
Soluble antigen/chimpanzee [183]	HIV env/same vaccine	Alum	HIV-1	Y[d]	+/ND
HIV protein cocktail/chimpanzee [184]	HIV virion proteins, peptide/same vaccine	SAF-1	HIV-ILai virus followed by infected Cpz cells	Y[e]	+/ND
Attenuated live SIVmac[f]/rhesus [170,177]	None	None	Various SIVmac strains	Y[f]	+/+
Nonpathogenic HIV-2 SBL-6669/cynomolgus [29,185]	Virus alone or with canary pox HIV-2 env, gag, pol	None	SIVsm	Y	+/+
DNA/rhesus [124,128,142,186]	DNA/DNA or MVA	Cytokine[g]/Bivucaine	SIVmac251	Y[e]	+/+
Attenuated SHIV/rhesus [179]	SHIV/none	None	SIVmac239	Y	+/+
VLP/rhesus [187]	VLP/Semliki Forest virus vector	None or alum	SHIV4	Y[e]	+/+
Fowl pox virus (FPV)/rhesus [188]	DNA/FPV	Lipofectamine or DOTAP	SHIV162p3	Y[e]	+/+
Modified vaccinia Ankara (MVA)/rhesus [189]	MVA/DNA plasmid	None	SHIV89.6p	Y[e]	+/+
Vesicular stomatitis virus (VSV)/rhesus [137]	VSV/VSV[h] (different serotype from prime)	None	SHIV89.6p	Y[e]	+/+

Canary pox vector/chimpanzee [190]	Canary pox/canary pox	None	HIV-1 IIIB infected cells/HIV IIIB virus	N	+/−
Adenovirus vector/rhesus [134,142]	Adeno/soluble viral protein or DNA prime/adeno/SIV proteins	IL12–IL15[g]		Y[e]	+/+
Semliki Forest virus/cynomolgus [138]	Same vaccine	None	SHIV4	Y[e]	+/+
Replicon Venezuelan equine encephalitis virus/rhesus [151]	VEE replicon/same vaccine	None	SIVsmE660	Y[e]	+/+
Bacterial vectors					
Salmonella/rhesus [164]	Salmonella/same vaccine or p27	None/polyphosphazene for p27	SHIV89.6P	N	+/+
Bacille Calmette-Guérin (BCG)/rhesus [160]	BCG/p11c peptide	None/lipid A liposome and alum	SIVmne	N	Weak/+

[a] Antibody/cell-mediated immunity. +/+, antibody-induced/CMI-induced.

[b] Protection due to anticellular antibody induced by vaccine prepared in human cell lines.

[c] No data.

[d] Protection was from a neutralization sensitive laboratory-adapted challenge virus. Primary HIV-1 strains (not adapted to tissue culture) are neutralization resistant.

[e] Virus load reduced, no protection from transmission of virus.

[f] Attenuation of SIVs by deletions in accessory genes, deletion in nef, or multiply deleted viruses in vpr, vpx, and other regions. Viruses tested in newborn rhesus were pathogenic [169].

[g] Cytokine expression by vector, for example IL2, IL15.

[h] Boosting with different VSV serotypes so boosting vector not neutralized by antibody induced by priming vector.

and are viable as candidate AIDS vaccines if the vector viruses that these vaccines are based upon (i) have low pathogenic potential, (ii) are not common in humans, (iii) have the capability to express HIV and SIV genes *in vivo*, and (iv) induce both antibody and cell-mediated immunity. Replicating vectors are often superior for inducing CMI. DNA viruses commonly used as vaccine vectors are vaccinia [129,130] and its derivative, modified vaccinia Ankara (MVA) [131], fowl pox [132], and adenovirus [133–135]. RNA virus vectors include vesicular stomatitis virus (VSV) [136,137], Semliki Forest virus, and simian foamy viruses (SFV), among others [138–141]. The vaccines based on the replicating viral vectors have shown at least limited promise in either SIVmac or SHIV models. Typically, these vaccines are used in various combinations in a framework of "prime and boost" strategy. For example, VSV vectors containing an HIV-1 *env* gene and the SIVmac *gag* gene were used to prime rhesus monkeys against a SHIV challenge (Table 8.3). The boost vaccine contained the same lentivirus genes but the VSV vector encoded a surface protein from a VSV serotype different from the priming vector [136]. Thus, the replication of boost vaccine is not suppressed by the VSV neutralizing antibodies elicited by the priming vaccine. A variation on this approach is to prime with VSV and boost with MVA-based vaccines. This approach has the advantage of boosting with a completely unrelated virus [136].

Replicating adenovirus-SIV and -HIV vaccines have also shown promise in both the SIV and SHIV systems [132,135,139,142–147]. Studies in chimpanzees showed that replicating adenovirus vectors were superior to nonreplicating vectors in inducing HIV immune responses. Immunization with replicating adenovirus type 5 vector containing SIVmac *env/rev/gag* and/or *nef* genes and boosted with soluble gp120 was capable of suppressing SIVmac251 plasma virus loads compared to empty vector controls [134]. Further studies showed that antibody-dependent cell cytotoxicity and antibody-dependent cell-mediated viral inhibition correlated with lower plasma virus loads in rh immunized with adenovirus-SIV hybrid vectors. This model is one of the few to

show an immune correlate of vaccine efficacy [144,145].

Single-cycle vaccine vectors

Single-cycle vectors are vaccines that carry out only a single round of replication, as the name implies [148–150]. The vectors contain the SIV or HIV genes encoding the antigens of interest. The vector viruses contain partial gene deletions that do not allow for complete rounds of replication. Essential missing functions may be provided by proteins from other viruses. For example, one such vector was created by mutating 27 codons in multiple genes of SIVsm251. Envelope functions were provided with the G protein from VSV [150]. The end result is a vaccine candidate that provides all of the viral proteins for priming and boosting the immune system without the risk of disease. It remains to be determined if this approach is potent enough for an effective HIV vaccine.

Replicons

Replicons are DNA or RNA self-replicating vectors encoding a viral replicase that confers the capacity to replicate *in vitro* and *in vivo*. RNA replicons derived from RNA viruses have been engineered to express SIV/HIV proteins for testing as candidate vaccines in NHP models. The capacity to produce particles released by replicon "infected" cells is accomplished through the use of a helper gene [151] or encoded within the replicon itself [152]. Replication of the vector amplifies antigen expression, activates the innate immune system, and induces strong immune responses. Replicons developed for AIDS vaccine testing in NHPs were derived from Venezuelan equine encephalitis virus [151,153], Semliki Forest virus [152], poliovirus [154], Kunjin virus [153], and Sindbis virus [154]. Thus far, these systems have not been widely used for efficacy testing. One vector tested, the Kunjin vector, did not induce SIV immunity in pig-tailed macaques and no protection was observed from SIVmac251 challenge [155].

Bacteria-based vaccines

Bacterial expression systems have been used as live vectors for AIDS vaccine models in macaques.

Expression is adequate for induction of both CMI and antibody; however, antigens will not be glycosylated, which may impair immune responses. The attenuated tuberculosis bacillus, Bacille Calmette-Guérin (BCG), has been used as a candidate vaccine vector in macaques [157–160]. In one study, intradermally inoculated BCG expressing SIV Gag protein and after boosting with the Mamu A01-specific Gag peptide epitope p11c induced CMI in rh but no protection against SIVmne was achieved [160,161].

Expression systems based on salmonella are another example of a bacterial vector in use in AIDS [162–166]. SIV-specific immunity is induced using salmonella-based vaccine, but the protection is not achieved even when relatively "easy" challenge with SHIV89.6P is used [166]. Other bacteria have been used as vaccine vectors, including live attenuated *Listeria monocytogenes*, which induced CMI and humoral responses against Gag [167].

Attenuated live virus vaccines

The attenuated live SIVmac-based vaccines have shown remarkable success in protection of macaques against highly pathogenic SIVmac strains. Unfortunately, after early successes, it was shown that attenuated SIVs were capable of inducing AIDS. Thus, attenuated SIV vaccines have not met, as yet, the minimum criteria of being both safe and effective.

Attenuated SIVs are obtained by deleting genes that are non-essential for replication but reduce pathogenicity. These gene-deleted SIVs replicate *in vitro* and *in vivo*, but their capacity to establish persistent infections and cause disease is reduced compared to wild type virus. Using a pathogenic molecular clone of SIVmac239, the *nef* gene was deleted and shown to be non-essential for transient *in vivo* replication [168,169]. This virus was named SIVmac239Δnef to indicate the deleted gene. This nomenclature has been adopted by the field. SIVmac239Δnef infection of adult rh macaques induced lower virus loads compared to the wild type SIVmac239 clone [169]. Rh macaques inoculated with SIVmac239Δnef survived 3 years without evidence of infection or disease, providing preliminary safety data. These results spurred the development of a *nef*-deleted SIV as a can-didate for an attenuated AIDS vaccine. For the immunization study, adult rh macaques were inoculated with SIVmac239Δnef. The infection was suppressed and was undetectable for more than 2 years. When challenged with pathogenic SIVmac239 or SIVmac251, vaccinated animals did not have detectable virus in blood, achieving the "sterilizing immunity," the "Holy Grail" of vaccinology [170]. Unfortunately, this most promising of vaccine approaches was shown to be unsafe in neonatal rhesus monkeys [171] and, eventually, AIDS was shown in SIVmacΔnef-infected adults as well [172,173]. Multiply deleted SIVmac239 mutants, lacking *nef*, *vpr*, and upstream sequences in U3, protected against pathogenic SIVmac251 [174] but were also pathogenic [172]. Other combinations of gene deletions were either too weak to induce protection or were pathogenic [175]. Deletion of the V1-V2 region of SIVmac239 molecular clone also attenuated SIVmac239. Protection against pathogenic wild type SIVmac239 challenge was observed [176]. Importantly, protection was achieved in the face of low antibody and cell-mediated immunity, suggesting that protection was due to other mechanisms [177]. Nevertheless, proof of the correlates of protection from attenuated SIVs has remained elusive.

The negative impact of experiments showing attenuated SIV vaccines to be unsafe cannot be overestimated. Protection was remarkably strong, and all vaccines that followed have been judged in comparison to live attenuated SIV vaccines. The gold standard of protection was established but not equaled by subsequent vaccines. Finally, the correlates of protection by attenuated SIVs have not been found. Should they be discovered, it may be possible to engineer a safe and effective vaccine based on the promising results obtained by gene-deleted SIVs.

Another approach to attenuated primate lentiviruses as vaccines is the use of low-pathogenic SHIVs as an attenuated vaccine. The nonpathogenic form of SHIV89.6 has been used in this regard and provided protection against pathogenic SIVmac. Recent results show that replication of SIVmac in vaginal tissue was limited by immunization [178]. This model has also been used to explore the correlates of protection provided by attenuated primate lentiviruses [178–182].

Acknowledgments

The authors thank Laura Altman for manuscript preparation. This work was supported by R01 AI076067, R01 AI045510, R01 AI045510, and P51-RR000164.

References

1 Stowell RE, Smith EK, España C, Nelson VG. Outbreak of malignant lymphoma in rhesus monkeys. *Lab Invest* 1971;**25**(5):476–9.

2 Apetrei C, Lerche NW, Pandrea I, *et al.* Kuru experiments triggered the emergence of pathogenic SIVmac. *AIDS* 2006;**20**:317–21.

3 Gajdusek DC, Gibbs CJ, Jr. Transmission of kuru from man to rhesus monkey (*Macaca mulatta*) 8 and one-half years after inoculation. *Nature* 1972;**240**:351.

4 Wolf RH, Gormus BJ, Martin LN, *et al.* Experimental leprosy in three species of monkeys. *Science* 1985;**227**(4686):529–31.

5 Murphey-Corb M, Martin LN, Rangan SR, *et al.* Isolation of an HTLV-III-related retrovirus from macaques with simian AIDS and its possible origin in asymptomatic mangabeys. *Nature* 1986; **321**(6068):435–7.

6 Norton R. In DR Henderson (Ed.) *The Concise Encyclopedia of Economics*, 2nd edn. Liberty Fund, Indianapolis, 2007.

7 Ambrose Z, Palmer S, Boltz VF, *et al.* Suppression of viremia and evolution of human immunodeficiency virus type 1 drug resistance in a macaque model for antiretroviral therapy. *J Virol* 2007;**81**(22):12145–55.

8 Hirsch VM, Olmsted RA, Murphey-Corb M, Purcell RH, Johnson PR. An African primate lentivirus (SIVsm) closely related to HIV-2. *Nature* 1989;**339**(6223):389–92.

9 Marx PA, Li Y, Lerche NW, *et al.* Isolation of a simian immunodeficiency virus related to human immunodeficiency virus Type 2 from a West African pet sooty mangabey. *J Virol* 1991;**65**:4480–85.

10 Peeters M, Fransen K, Delaporte E, *et al.* Isolation and characterization of a new chimpanzee lentivirus (simian immunodeficiency virus isolate cpz-ant) from a wild-captured chimpanzee *AIDS* 1992;**6**(5):447–51.

11 Baskin GB, Martin LN, Rangan SR, *et al.* Transmissible lymphoma and simian acquired immunodeficiency syndrome in rhesus monkeys. *J Natl Cancer Inst* 1986;**77**(1):127–39.

12 Daniel MD, Letvin NL, King NW, *et al.* Isolation of T-cell tropic HTLV-III-like retrovirus from macaques. *Science* 1985;**228**(4704):1201–4.

13 Chalifoux LV, Ringler DJ, King NW, *et al.* Lymphadenopathy in macaques experimentally infected with the simian immunodeficiency virus (SIV). *Am J Pathol* 1987;**128**(1):104–10.

14 Wyand MS, Ringler DJ, Naidu YM, *et al.* Cellular localization of simian immunodeficiency virus in lymphoid tissues. II. In situ hybridization. *Am J Pathol* 1989;**134**(2):385–93.

15 Pantaleo G, Graziosi C, Fauci AS. New concepts in the immunopathogenesis of human immunodeficiency virus infection. *N Engl J Med* 1993;**328**(5):327–35.

16 Veazey RS, DeMaria M, Chalifoux LV, *et al.* Gastrointestinal tract as a major site of CD4$^+$ T cell depletion and viral replication in SIV infection. *Science* 1998;**280**(5362):427–31.

17 Veazey RS, Lackner AA. HIV swiftly guts the immune system. *Nat Med* 2005;**11**(5):469–70.

18 Fauci AS, Johnston MI, Dieffenbach CW, *et al.* HIV vaccine research: the way forward. *Science* 2008;**321**(5888):530–32.

19 Watkins DI, Burton DR, Kallas EG, Moore JP, Koff WC. Nonhuman primate models and the failure of the Merck HIV-1 vaccine in humans. *Nat Med* 2008;**14**(6):617–21.

20 Adachi A, Gendelman HE, Koenig S, *et al.* Production of acquired immunodeficiency syndrome-associated retrovirus in human and non-human cells transfected with an infectious molecular clone, *J Virol* 1986;**59**:284–91.

21 Levy JA, Cheng-Mayer C, Dina D, Luciw PA. AIDS retrovirus (ARV-2) clone replicates in transfected human and animal fibroblasts. *Science* 1986;**232**(4753):998–1001.

22 Morrow WJ, Wharton M, Lau D, Levy JA. Small animals are not susceptible to human immunodeficiency virus infection. *J Gen Virol* 1987;**68**(Pt 8): 2253–7.

23 Fultz PN, McClure HM, Swenson RB, *et al.* Persistent infection of chimpanzees with human T-lymphotropic virus type III/lymphadenopathy-

associated virus: a potential model for acquired immunodeficiency syndrome. *J Virol* 1986;**58**:116–24.

24 Prince AM, Allan J, Andrus L, *et al.* Virulent HIV strains, chimpanzees, and trial vaccines. *Science* 1999;**283**(5405):1117–18.

25 Saksela K, Muchmore E, Girard M, Fultz P, Baltimore D. High viral load in lymph nodes and latent human immunodeficiency virus (HIV) in peripheral blood cells of HIV-1-infected chimpanzees. *J Virol* 1993;**67**(12):7423–7.

26 Kent SJ, Corey L, Agy MB, *et al.* Cytotoxic and proliferative T cell responses in HIV-1-infected *Macaca nemestrina. J Clin Invest* 1995;**95**(1):248–56.

27 Barnett SW, Murthy KK, Herndier BG, Levy JA. An AIDS-like condition induced in baboons by HIV-2. *Science* 1994;**266**(5185):642–6.

28 Looney DJ, McClure J, Kent SJ, *et al.* A minimally replicative HIV-2 live-virus vaccine protects *M. nemestrina* from disease after HIV-2(287) challenge. *Virology* 1998;**242**(1):150–60.

29 Walther-Jallow L, Nilsson C, Söderlund J, *et al.* Cross-protection against mucosal simian immunodeficiency virus (SIVsm) challenge in human immunodeficiency virus type 2-vaccinated cynomolgus monkeys. *J Gen Virol* 2001;**82**, 1601–12.

30 Apetrei C, Kaur A, Lerche NW, *et al.* Molecular epidemiology of simian immunodeficiency virus SIVsm in US primate centers. *J Virol* 2005;**79**(14):8991–9005.

31 Mansfield KG, Lerch NW, Gardner MB, Lackner AA. Origins of simian immunodeficiency virus infection in macaques at the New England Regional Primate Research Center. *J Med Primatol* 1995;**24**(3):116–22.

32 Gibbs CJ, Jr, Gajdusek DC. Transmission of scrapie to the cynomolgus monkey (*Macaca fascicularis*). *Nature* 1972;**236**:73–4.

33 Bonneh-Barkay D, Bissel SJ, Wang G, *et al.* YKL-40, a marker of simian immunodeficiency virus encephalitis, modulates the biological activity of basic fibroblast growth factor. *Am J Pathol* 2008;**173**(1):130–43.

34 Masters CL, Alpers MP, Gajdusek DC, Gibbs CJ, Jr, Kakulas BA. Experimental kuru in the gibbon and sooty mangabey and Creutzefeldt-Jakob disease in the pigtailed macaque. With a summary of the host range of the subacute spongiform virus encephalopathies. *J Med Primatol* 1976;**5**:205–9.

35 Chakrabarti L, Guyader M, Alizon M, *et al.* Sequence of simian immunodeficiency virus from macaque and its relationship to other human and simian retroviruses. *Nature* 1987;**328**(6130):543–7.

36 Hunt RD, Blake BJ, Chalifoux LV, *et al.* Transmission of naturally occurring lymphoma in macaque monkeys. *Proc Natl Acad Sci U S A* 1983;**80**(16):5085–9.

37 Morton WR, Kuller L, Benveniste RE, *et al.* Transmission of the simian immunodeficiency virus SIVmne in macaques and baboons. *J Med Primatol* 1989;**18**(3–4):237–45.

38 Rud EW, Cranage M, Yon J, *et al.* Molecular and biological characterization of simian immunodeficiency virus macaque strain 32H proviral clones containing nef size variants. *J Gen Virol* 1994;**75**(3):529–43.

39 Denesvre C, Le Grand R, Boissin-Cans F, *et al.* Highly attenuated SIVmac142 is immunogenic but does not protect against SIVmac251 challenge. *AIDS Res Hum Retroviruses* 1995;**11**(11):1397–406.

40 Naidu YM, Kestler HW, 3rd, Li Y, *et al.* Characterization of infectious molecular clones of simian immunodeficiency virus (SIVmac) and human immunodeficiency virus type 2: persistent infection of rhesus monkeys with molecularly cloned SIVmac. *J Virol* 1988;**62**(12):4691–6.

41 Fukunishi Y, Meyers WM, Binford CH, *et al.* Electron microscopic study of leprosy in a mangabey monkey (natural infection). *Int J Lepr Other Mycobact Dis* 1984;**52**(2):203–7.

42 Martin LN, Gormus BJ, Wolf RH, *et al.* Depression of lymphocyte responses to mitogens in mangabeys with disseminated experimental leprosy. *Cell Immunol* 1985;**90**(1):115–30.

43 Brown CR, Czapiga M, Kabat J, *et al.* Unique pathology in simian immunodeficiency virus-infected rapid progressor macaques is consistent with a pathogenesis distinct from that of classical AIDS. *J Virol* 2007;**81**(11):5594–606.

44 Hirsch V, Adger-Johnson D, Campbell B, *et al.* A molecularly cloned, pathogenic, neutralization-resistant simian immunodeficiency virus, SIVsmE543-3. *J Virol* 1997;**71**(2):1608–20.

45 Hirsch VM, Fuerst TR, Sutter G, *et al.* Patterns of viral replication correlate with outcome in simian immunodeficiency virus (SIV)-infected macaques: effect of prior immunization with a trivalent SIV vaccine in modified vaccinia virus Ankara. *J Virol* 1996;**70**:3741–52.

46 Hirsch VM, Johnson PR. Pathogenic diversity of simian immunodeficiency viruses. *Virus Res* 1994;**32**:183–203.

47 Fultz PN, McClure HM, Anderson DC, Switzer WM. Identification and biologic characterization of an acutely lethal variant of simian immunodeficiency

virus from sooty mangabeys (SIV/SMM). *AIDS Res Hum Retroviruses* 1989;**5**(4):397–409.

48 Schwiebert R, Fultz PN. Immune activation and viral burden in acute disease induced by simian immunodeficiency virus SIVsmmPBj14: correlation between in vitro and in vivo events. *J Virol* 1994;**68**(9):5538–47.

49 Fultz PN, Zack PM. Unique lentivirus–host interactions: SIVsmmPBj14 infection of macaques. *Virus Res* 1994;**32**(2):205–25.

50 Fultz PN. Isolation of a T-lymphotropic retrovirus from naturally infected sooty mangabey monkeys (*Cercocebus atys*). *Proc Natl Acad Sci U S A* 1986; **83**:5286–90.

51 Ling B, Apetrei C, Pandrea I, *et al*. Classic AIDS in a sooty mangabey after an 18-year natural infection. *J Virol* 2004;**78**(16):8902–8.

52 McClure HM, Anderson DC, Gordon TP, *et al*. Natural simian immunodeficiency virus infections in nonhuman primates. In S Matano, RH Tuttle, H Ishida, M Goodman (Eds) *Topics in Primatology*, vol. **3**: *Evolutionary Biology, Reproductive Endocrinology and Virology*. University of Tokyo Press, Tokyo, 1992, pp. 425–38.

53 Shibata R, Kawamura M, Sakai H, *et al*. Generation of a chimeric human and simian immunodeficiency virus infectious to monkey peripheral blood mononuclear cells. *J Virol* 1991;**65**(7):3514–20.

54 Li J, Lord CI, Haseltine W, Letvin NL, Sodroski J. Infection of cynomolgus monkeys with a chimeric HIV-1/SIVmac virus that expresses the HIV-1 envelope glycoproteins. *J Acquir Immune Defic Syndr* 1992;**5**(7):639–46.

55 Li JT, Halloran M, Lord CI, *et al*. Persistent infection of macaques with simian-human immunodeficiency viruses. *J Virol* 1995;**69**(11):7061–7.

56 Endo Y, Igarashi T, Nishimura Y, *et al*. Short- and long-term clinical outcomes in rhesus monkeys inoculated with a highly pathogenic chimeric simian/human immunodeficiency virus. *J Virol* 2000;**74**(15):6935–45.

57 Harouse JM, Gettie A, Tan RC, Blanchard J, Cheng-Mayer C. Distinct pathogenic sequela in rhesus macaques infected with CCR5 or CXCR4 utilizing SHIVs. *Science* 1999;**284**(5415):816–19.

58 Harouse JM, Tan RC, Gettie A, *et al*. Mucosal transmission of pathogenic CXCR4-utilizing SHIVSF33A variants in rhesus macaques. *Virology* 1998;**248**(1):95–107.

59 Joag SV, Li Z, Foresman L, Stephens EB, *et al*. Chimeric simian/human immunodeficiency virus

that causes progressive loss of CD4$^+$ T cells and AIDS in pig-tailed macaques. *J Virol* 1996;**70**(5): 3189–97.

60 Karlsson GB, Halloran M, Li J, *et al*. Characterization of molecularly cloned simian-human immunodeficiency viruses causing rapid CD4$^+$ lymphocyte depletion in rhesus monkeys. *J Virol* 1997; **71**(6):4218–25.

61 Reimann KA, Li JT, Veazey R, *et al*. A chimeric simian/human immunodeficiency virus expressing a primary patient human immunodeficiency virus type 1 isolate env causes an AIDS-like disease after in vivo passage in rhesus monkeys. *J Virol* 1996; **70**(10):6922–8.

62 Hsu M, Harouse JM, Gettie A, *et al*. Increased mucosal transmission but not enhanced pathogenicity of the CCR5-tropic, simian AIDS-inducing simian/human immunodeficiency virus SHIV$_{SF162P3}$ maps to envelope gp120. *J Virol* 2003; **277**(2):989–98.

63 Tan RC, Harouse JM, Gettie A, Cheng-Mayer C. In vivo adaptation of SHIV(SF162): chimeric virus expressing a NSI, CCR5-specific envelope protein. *J Med Primatol* 1999;**28**(4–5):164–8.

64 Parren PW, Marx PA, Hessell AJ, *et al*. Antibody protects macaques against vaginal challenge with a pathogenic R5 simian/human immunodeficiency virus at serum levels giving complete neutralization in vitro. *J Virol* 2001;**75**(17):8340–47.

65 Wainberg MA. HIV-1 subtype distribution and the problem of drug resistance. *AIDS* 2004;**18**(Suppl 3):S63–8.

66 Ayash-Rashkovsky M, Chenine AL, Steele LN, *et al*. Coinfection with *Schistosoma mansoni* reactivates viremia in rhesus macaques with chronic simian-human immunodeficiency virus clade C infection. *Infect Immun* 2007;**75**(4):1751–6.

67 Chen Z, Huang Y, Zhao X, *et al*. Enhanced infectivity of an R5-tropic simian/human immunodeficiency virus type 1 subtype C envelope after serial passages in pig-tailed macaques (*Macaca nemestrina*). *J Virol* 2000;**74**(14):6501–10.

68 Gruber A, Chalmers AS, Rasmussen RA, *et al*. Dendritic cell-based vaccine strategy against human immunodeficiency virus clade C: skewing the immune response toward a helper T cell type 2 profile. *Viral Immunol* 2007;**20**(1):160–69.

69 Himathongkham S, Halpin NS, Li J, *et al*. Simian-human immunodeficiency virus containing a human immunodeficiency virus type 1 subtype-E

envelope gene: persistent infection, CD4(+) T-cell depletion, and mucosal membrane transmission in macaques. *J Virol* 2000;**74**(17):7851–60.

70 Song RJ, Chenine AL, Rasmussen RA, *et al.* Molecularly cloned SHIV-1157ipd3N4: a highly replication-competent, mucosally transmissible R5 simian-human immunodeficiency virus encoding HIV clade C Env. *J Virol* 2006;**80**(17):8729–38.

71 Ambrose Z, Boltz V, Palmer S, *et al.* In vitro characterization of a simian immunodeficiency virus-human immunodeficiency virus (HIV) chimera expressing HIV type 1 reverse transcriptase to study antiviral resistance in pigtail macaques. *J Virol* 2004;**78**(24):13553–61.

72 Jiang Y, Tian B, Agy MB, Saifuddin M, Tsai C. *Macaca fascicularis* are highly susceptible to an RT-SHIV following intravaginal inoculation: a new model for microbicide evaluation. *J Med Primatol* 2009;**38**(Suppl 1):39–46.

73 Gottlieb MS, Schroff R, Schanker HM, *et al.* Pneumocystis carinii pneumonia and mucosal candidiasis in previously healthy homosexual men: evidence of a new acquired cellular immunodeficiency. *N Engl J Med* 1981;**305**(24):1425–31.

74 Balzarini J, Weeger M, Camarasa MJ, De Clercq E, Uberla K. Sensitivity/resistance profile of a simian immunodeficiency virus containing the reverse transcriptase gene of human immunodeficiency virus type 1 (HIV-1) toward the HIV-1-specific non-nucleoside reverse transcriptase inhibitors. *Biochem Biophys Res Commun* 1995;**211**:850–56.

75 Hofman MJ, Higgins J, Matthews TB, *et al.* Efavirenz therapy in rhesus macaques infected with a chimera of simian immunodeficiency virus containing reverse transcriptase from human immunodeficiency virus type 1. *Antimicrob Agents Chemother* 2004;**48**(9):3483–90.

76 Mori K, Yasutomi Y, Sawada S, *et al.* Suppression of acute viremia by short-term postexposure prophylaxis of simian/human immunodeficiency virus SHIV-RT-infected monkeys with a novel reverse transcriptase inhibitor (GW420867) allows for development of potent antiviral immune responses resulting in efficient containment of infection. *J Virol* 2000;**74**(13):5747–53.

77 North TW, Van Rompay KK, Higgins J, *et al.* Suppression of virus load by highly active antiretroviral therapy in rhesus macaques infected with a recombinant simian immunodeficiency virus containing reverse transcriptase from human immunodeficiency virus type 1. *J Virol* 2005;**79**:7349–54.

78 Soderberg K, Denekamp L, Nikiforow S, *et al.* A nucleotide substitution in the tRNA(Lys) primer binding site dramatically increases replication of recombinant simian immunodeficiency virus containing a human immunodeficiency virus type 1 reverse transcriptase. *J Virol* 2002;**76**(11):5803–6.

79 Van Rompay KK, Johnson JA, Blackwood EJ, *et al.* Sequential emergence and clinical implications of viral mutants with K70E and K65R mutation in reverse transcriptase during prolonged tenofovir monotherapy in rhesus macaques with chronic RT-SHIV infection. *Retrovirology* 2007;**6**(4):25.

80 Akiyama H, Ishimatsu M, Miura T, Hayami M, Ido E. Construction and infection of a new simian/human immunodeficiency chimeric virus (SHIV) containing the integrase gene of the human immunodeficiency virus type 1 genome and analysis of its adaptation to monkey cells. *Microbes Infect* 2008;**10**(5):531–9.

81 Ling, B, Veazey RS, Luckay A, *et al.* SIV(mac) pathogenesis in rhesus macaques of Chinese and Indian origin compared with primary HIV infections in humans. *AIDS* 2002;**16**(11):1489–96.

82 Trichel AM, Rajakumar PA, Murphey-Corb M. Abstract species-specific variation in SIV disease progression between Chinese and Indian subspecies of rhesus macaque. *J Med Primatol* 2002;**31**(4–5):171–8.

83 Alter HJ, Eichberg JW, Masur H, *et al.* Transmission of HTLV-III infection from human plasma to chimpanzees: an animal model for AIDS. *Science* 1984;**226**(4674):549–52.

84 Fultz PN, McClure HM, Daugharty H, *et al.* Vaginal transmission of human immunodeficiency virus (HIV) to a chimpanzee. *J Infect Dis* 1986;**154**(5):896–900.

85 Fultz PN, Wei Q, Yue L. Rectal transmission of human immunodeficiency virus type 1 to chimpanzees. *J Infect Dis* 1999;**179**(Suppl 3):S418–21.

86 Eichberg JW, Zarling JM, Alter HJ, *et al.* T-cell responses to human immunodeficiency virus (HIV) and its recombinant antigens in HIV-infected chimpanzees *J Virol* 1987;**61**; 3804–8.

87 Novembre FJ, Saucier M, Anderson DC, *et al.* Development of AIDS in a chimpanzee infected with human immunodeficiency virus type 1. *J Virol* 1997;**71**(5):4086–91.

88 Girard M, Yue L, Barré-Sinoussi F, *et al.* Failure of a human immunodeficiency virus type 1 (HIV-1) subtype B-derived vaccine to prevent infection of chimpanzees by an HIV-1 subtype E strain. *J Virol* 1996;**70**(11):8229–33.

89 Fultz PN, Yue L, Wei Q, Girard M. Human immunodeficiency virus type 1 intersubtype (B/E) recombination in a superinfected chimpanzee. *J Virol* 1997;**71**(10):7990–95.

90 Agy MB, Frumkin LR, Corey L, *et al.* Infection of *Macaca nemestrina* by human immunodeficiency virus type-1. *Science* 1992;**257**(5066):103–6.

91 Frumkin LR, Agy MB, Coombs RW, *et al.* Acute infection of *Macaca nemestrina* by human immunodeficiency virus type 1. *Virology* 1993;**195**(2):422–31.

92 Miller CJ, Alexander NJ, Sutjipto S, *et al.* Genital mucosal transmission of simian immunodeficiency virus: animal model for heterosexual transmission of human immunodeficiency virus. *J Virol* 1989;**63**(10):1277–84.

93 Marx PA, Spira AI, Gettie A, *et al.* Progesterone implants enhance SIV vaginal transmission and early virus load. *Nat Med* 1996;**2**(10):1084–9.

94 Mascola JR, Stiegler G, VanCott TC, *et al.* Protection of macaques against vaginal transmission of a pathogenic HIV-1/SIV chimeric virus by passive infusion of neutralizing antibodies. *Nat Med* 2000;**6**(2):207–10.

95 Smith SM, Baskin GB, Marx PA. Estrogen protects against vaginal transmission of simian immunodeficiency virus. *J Infect Dis* 2000;**182**(3):708–15.

96 Smith SM, Mefford M, Sodora D, *et al.* Topical estrogen protects against SIV vaginal transmission without evidence of systemic effect. *AIDS* 2004;**18**(12):1637–43.

97 Abel K, Rourke T, Lu D, *et al.* Abrogation of attenuated lentivirus-induced protection in rhesus macaques by administration of Depo-Provera before intravaginal challenge with simian immunodeficiency virus mac239. *J Infect Dis* 2004;**190**(9): 1697–705.

98 Genescà M, Li J, Fritts L, *et al.* Depo-Provera abrogates attenuated lentivirus-induced protection in male rhesus macaques challenged intravenously with pathogenic SIVmac239. *J Med Primatol* 2007; **36**(4-5):266–75.

99 Lu Y, Pauza CD, Lu X, Montefiori DC, Miller CJ. Rhesus macaques that become systemically infected with pathogenic SHIV 89.6-PD after intravenous, rectal, or vaginal inoculation and fail to make an antiviral antibody response rapidly develop AIDS. *J Acquir Immune Defic Syndr Hum Retrovirol* 1998;**19**:6–1.

100 Pauza CD, Emau P, Salvato MS, *et al.* Pathogenesis of SIVmac251 after atraumatic inoculation of the rectal mucosa in rhesus monkeys. *J Med Primatol* 1993;**22**(2–3):154–61.

101 Miller CJ, Vogel P, Alexander NJ, *et al.* Pathology and localization of simian immunodeficiency virus in the reproductive tract of chronically infected male rhesus macaques. *Lab Invest* 1994;**70**(2):255–62.

102 Van de Perre P, Simonon A, Msellati P, *et al.* Postnatal transmission of human immunodeficiency virus type 1 from mother to infant. A prospective cohort study in Kigali, Rwanda. *N Engl J Med* 1991;**325**:593–8.

103 Ziegler JB, Cooper DA, Johnson RO, Gold J. Postnatal transmission of AIDS-associated retrovirus from mother to infant. *Lancet* 1985;**1**(8434):896–8.

104 Amedee AM, Lacour N, Ratterree M. Mother-to-infant transmission of SIV via breast-feeding in rhesus macaques. *J Med Primatol* 2003;**32**(4–5):187–93.

105 Amedee AM, Rychert J, Lacour N, Fresh L, Ratterree M. Viral and immunological factors associated with breast milk transmission of SIV in rhesus macaques. *Retrovirology* 2004;**14**(1):17.

106 Rychert J, Lacour N, Amedee AM. Genetic analysis of simian immunodeficiency virus expressed in milk and selectively transmitted through breastfeeding. *J Virol* 2006;**80**(8):3721–31.

107 Amedee AM, Lacour N, Martin LN, *et al.* Genotypic analysis of infant macaques infected transplacentally and orally. *J Med Primatol* 1996;**25**(3):225–35.

108 Davison-Fairburn B, Blanchard J, Hu FS, *et al.* Experimental infection of timed-pregnant rhesus monkeys with simian immunodeficiency virus (SIV) during early, middle, and late gestation. *J Med Primatol* 1990;**19**(3–4):381–93.

109 Goulder PJ, Watkins DI. HIV and SIV CTL escape: implications for vaccine design. *Nat Rev Immunol* 2004;**4**(8):630–40.

110 Hu SL. Non-human primate models for AIDS vaccine research. *Curr Drug Targets Infect Disord* 2005;**5**(2):193–201.

111 Koff WC, Johnson PR, Watkins DI, *et al.* HIV vaccine design: insights from live attenuated SIV vaccines. *Nat Immunol* 2006;**7**(1):19–23.

112 McMichael AJ. HIV vaccines. *Annu Rev Immunol* 2006;**24**:227–55.

113 Daniel MD, Sehgal PK, Kodama T, *et al.* Use of simian immunodeficiency virus for vaccine research. *J Med Primatol* 1990;**19**(3–4):395–9.

114 Desrosiers RC, Wyand MS, Kodama T, *et al.* Vaccine protection against simian immunodeficiency virus infection. *Proc Natl Acad Sci U S A* 1989;**86**(16):6353–7.

115 Murphey-Corb M, Martin LN, Davison-Fairburn B, *et al.* A formalin-inactivated whole SIV vaccine

confers protection in macaques. *Science* 1989; **246**(4935):1293–7.

116 Sutjipto S, Pedersen NC, Miller CJ, *et al.* Inactivated simian immunodeficiency virus vaccine failed to protect rhesus macaques from intravenous or genital mucosal infection but delayed disease in intravenously exposed animals. *J Virol* 1990;**64**(5):2290–97.

117 Stott EJ. Anti-cell antibody in macaques. *Nature* 1991;**353**(6343):393.

118 Stott EJ, Chan WL, Mills KH, *et al.* Preliminary report: protection of cynomolgus macaques against simian immunodeficiency virus by fixed infected-cell vaccine. *Lancet* 1990;**336**(8730):1538–4.

119 Montefiori DC. Evaluating neutralizing antibodies against HIV, SIV, and SHIV in luciferase reporter gene assays. *Curr Protoc Immunol* 2005;Chapter 12:Unit 12.11.

120 Berman PW, Gregory TJ, Riddle L, *et al.* Protection of chimpanzees from infection by HIV-1 after vaccination with recombinant glycoprotein gp120 but not gp160. *Nature* 1990;**345**(6276):622–5.

121 [No authors listed] VaxGen vaccine trial fails the test but may offer insights. *AIDS Alert* 2003;**18**(4):41, 43–5.

122 Pitisuttithum P, Gilbert P, Gurwith M, *et al.* Randomized, double-blind, placebo-controlled efficacy trial of a bivalent recombinant glycoprotein 120 HIV-1 vaccine among injection drug users in Bangkok, Thailand. *J Infect Dis* 2006;**194**(12):1661–71.

123 Mellman I, Steinman, RM. Dendritic cells: specialized and regulated antigen processing machines. *Cell* 2001;**106**(3):255–8.

124 Kim JJ, Nottingham LK, Tsai A, *et al.* Antigen-specific humoral and cellular immune responses can be modulated in rhesus macaques through the use of IFN-gamma, IL-12, or IL-18 gene adjuvants. *J Med Primatol* 1999;**28**(4–5):214–23.

125 Kim JJ, Yang JS, VanCott TC, *et al.* Modulation of antigen-specific humoral responses in rhesus macaques by using cytokine cDNAs as DNA vaccine adjuvants. *J Virol* 2000;**74**(7):3427–9.

126 Robinson TM, Sidhu MK, Pavlakis GN, *et al.* Macaques co-immunized with SIVgag/pol-HIVenv and IL-12 plasmid have increased cellular responses. *J Med Primatol* 2007;**36**(4–5):276–84.

127 Dubie RA, Maksaereekul S, Shacklett BL, *et al.* Co-immunization with IL-15 enhances cellular immune responses induced by a vif-deleted simian immunodeficiency virus proviral DNA vaccine and confers partial protection against vaginal challenge with SIVmac251. *Virology* 2009;**386**(1):109–21.

128 Muthumani K, Bagarazzi M, Conway D, *et al.* A Gag-Pol/Env-Rev SIV239 DNA vaccine improves CD4 counts, and reduce viral loads after pathogenic intrarectal SIV(mac)251 challenge in rhesus macaques. *Vaccine* 2003;**21**(7–8):629–37.

129 Hu SL, Fultz PN, McClure HM, *et al.* Effect of immunization with a vaccinia-HIV env recombinant on HIV infection of chimpanzees. *Nature* 1987;**328**(6132):721–3.

130 Mackett M, Smith GL, Moss B. Vaccinia virus: a selectable eukaryotic cloning and expression vector. *Proc Natl Acad Sci U S A* 1982;**79**(23):7415–19.

131 Ourmanov I, Bilska M, Hirsch VH, Montefiori DC. Recombinant modified vaccinia virus Ankara expressing the surface gp120 of simian immunodeficiency virus (SIV) primes for a rapid neutralizing antibody response to SIV infection in macaques. *J Virol* 2000;**74**(6):2960–65.

132 Bublot M, Pritchard N, Swayne DE, *et al.* Development and use of fowlpox vectored vaccines for avian influenza. *Ann N Y Acad Sci* 2006;**1081**:193–201.

133 Buge SL, Murty L, Arora K, *et al.* Factors associated with slow disease progression in macaques immunized with an adenovirus-simian immunodeficiency virus (SIV) envelope priming-gp120 boosting regimen and challenged vaginally with SIVmac251. *J Virol* 1999;**73**(9):7430–40.

134 Patterson LJ, Beal J, Demberg T, *et al.* Replicating adenovirus HIV/SIV recombinant priming alone or in combination with a gp140 protein boost results in significant control of viremia following a SHIV89.6P challenge in Mamu-A*01 negative rhesus macaques. *Virology* 2008;**374**(2):322–37.

135 Zhou Q, Hidajat R, Peng B, *et al.* Comparative evaluation of oral and intranasal priming with replication-competent adenovirus 5 host range mutant (Ad5hr)-simian immunodeficiency virus (SIV) recombinant vaccines on immunogenicity and protective efficacy against SIV(mac251). *Vaccine* 2007;**25**(47):8021–35.

136 Ramsburg E, Rose NF, Marx PA, *et al.* Highly effective control of an AIDS virus challenge in macaques by using vesicular stomatitis virus and modified vaccinia virus Ankara vaccine vectors in a single-boost protocol. *J Virol* 2004;**78**(8):3930–40.

137 Rose NF, Marx PA, Luckay A, *et al.* An effective AIDS vaccine based on live attenuated vesicular stomatitis virus recombinants. *Cell* 2001;**106**:539–49.

138 Berglund P, Quesada-Rolander M, Putkonen P, *et al.* Outcome of immunization of cynomolgus monkeys

with recombinant Semliki Forest virus encoding human immunodeficiency virus type 1 envelope protein and challenge with a high dose of SHIV-4 virus. *AIDS Res Hum Retroviruses* 1997;**13**(17):1487–95.

139 Eriksson KK, King NJ, Bublot M, Bukreyev A. Towards a coronavirus-based HIV multigene vaccine. *Clin Dev Immunol.* 2006;**13**(2-4):353–60.

140 King NJ, Getts DR, Getts MT, *et al.* Immunopathology of flavivirus infections. *Immunol Cell Biol* 2007;**85**(1):33–42.

141 Martinon F, Brochard P, Ripaux M, *et al.* Improved protection against simian immunodeficiency virus mucosal challenge in macaques primed with a DNA vaccine and boosted with the recombinant modified vaccinia virus Ankara and recombinant Semliki Forest virus. *Vaccine* 2008;**26**(4):532–45.

142 Demberg T, Boyer JD, Malkevich N, *et al.* Sequential priming with (SIV) DNA vaccines, with or without encoded cytokines, and a replicating Ad-SIV recombinant followed by protein boosting does not control a pathogenic SIVmac251 mucosal challenge. *J Virol* 2008;**82**:10911–21.

143 Gómez-Román VR, Grimes GJ, Jr, Potti GK, *et al.* Oral delivery of replication-competent adenovirus vectors is well tolerated by SIV- and SHIV-infected rhesus macaques. *Vaccine* 2006;**24**(23):5064–72.

144 Gómez-Román VR, Patterson LJ, Venzon D, *et al.* Vaccine-elicited antibodies mediate antibody-dependent cellular cytotoxicity correlated with significantly reduced acute viremia in rhesus macaques challenged with SIVmac251. *J Immunol* 2005;**174**(4):2185–9.

145 Patterson LJ, Malkevitch N, Venzon D, *et al.* Protection against mucosal simian immunodeficiency virus SIV$_{mac251}$ challenge by using replicating adenovirus-SIV multigene vaccine priming and subunit boosting. *J Virol* 2004;**78**(5):2212–21.

146 Peng B, Wang LR, Gómez-Román VR, *et al.* Replicating rather than nonreplicating adenovirus-human immunodeficiency virus recombinant vaccines are better at eliciting potent cellular immunity and priming high-titer antibodies. *J Virol* 2005;**79**(16):10200–209.

147 Hidajat R, Xiao P, Zhou Q, *et al.* Correlation of vaccine-elicited systemic and mucosal nonneutralizing antibody activities with reduced acute viremia following intrarectal simian immunodeficiency virus SIVmac251 challenge of rhesus macaques. *J Virol* 2009;**83**(2):791–801.

148 Evans DT, Bricker JE, Desrosiers RC. A novel approach for producing lentiviruses that are limited to a single cycle of infection. *J Virol* 2004;**78**(21):11715–25.

149 Kuate S, Stahl-Hennig C, ten Haaft P, Heeney J, Uberla K. Single-cycle immunodeficiency viruses provide strategies for uncoupling in vivo expression levels from viral replicative capacity and for mimicking live-attenuated SIV vaccines. *Virology* 2003;**313**(2):653–62.

150 Tang Y, Swanstrom R. Development and characterization of a new single cycle vaccine vector in the simian immunodeficiency virus model system. *Virology* 2008;**372**(1):72–84.

151 Davis NL, West A, Reap E, *et al.* Alphavirus replicon particles as candidate HIV vaccines. *IUBMB Life* 2002;**53**(4–5):209–11.

152 Rose NF, Publicover J, Chattopadhyay A, Rose JK. Hybrid alphavirus-rhabdovirus propagating replicon particles are versatile and potent vaccine vectors. *Proc Natl Acad Sci U S A* 2008;**105**(15):5839–43.

153 Johnston RE, Johnson PR, Connell MJ, *et al.* Vaccination of macaques with SIV immunogens delivered by Venezuelan equine encephalitis virus replicon particle vectors followed by a mucosal challenge with SIVsmE660. *Vaccine* 2005;**23**(42):4969–79.

154 Morrow CD, Porter DC, Ansardi DC, Moldoveanu Z, Fultz PN. New approaches for mucosal vaccines for AIDS: encapsidation and serial passages of poliovirus replicons that express HIV-1 proteins on infection. *AIDS Res Hum Retroviruses* 1994;**10**(2):S61–6.

155 Kent SJ, De Rose R, Mokhonov VV, *et al.* Evaluation of recombinant Kunjin replicon SIV vaccines for protective efficacy in macaques. *Virology* 2008;**374**(2):528–34.

156 Xu R, Srivastava IK, Greer CE, *et al.* Characterization of immune responses elicited in macaques immunized sequentially with chimeric VEE/SIN alphavirus replicon particles expressing SIVGag and/or HIVEnv and with recombinant HIVgp140Env protein. *AIDS Res Hum Retroviruses* 2006;**22**(10):1022–30.

157 Ami Y, Izumi Y, Matsuo K, *et al.* Priming-boosting vaccination with recombinant *Mycobacterium bovis* bacillus Calmette-Guérin and a nonreplicating vaccinia virus recombinant leads to long-lasting and effective immunity. *J Virol* 2005;**79**(20):12871–9.

158 Leung NJ, Aldovini A, Young R, *et al.* The kinetics of specific immune responses in rhesus monkeys inoculated with live recombinant BCG expressing SIV Gag, Pol, Env, and Nef proteins. *Virology* 2000;**268**(1):94–103.

159 Méderlé I, Le Grand R, Vaslin B, *et al.* Mucosal administration of three recombinant *Mycobacterium bovis* BCG-SIVmac251 strains to cynomolgus macaques induces rectal IgAs and boosts systemic cellular immune responses that are primed by intradermal vaccination. *Vaccine* 2003;**21**(27–30):4153–66.

160 Yasutomi Y, Koenig S, Haun SS, *et al.* Immunization with recombinant BCG-SIV elicits SIV-specific cytotoxic T lymphocytes in rhesus monkeys. *J Immunol* 1993;**150**(7):3101–7.

161 Yasutomi Y, Koenig S, Woods RM, *et al.* A vaccine-elicited, single viral epitope-specific cytotoxic T lymphocyte response does not protect against intravenous, cell-free simian immunodeficiency virus challenge. *J Virol* 1995;**69**(4):2279–84.

162 Evans DT, Chen LM, Gillis J, *et al.* Mucosal priming of simian immunodeficiency virus-specific cytotoxic T-lymphocyte responses in rhesus macaques by the Salmonella type III secretion antigen delivery system. *J Virol* 2003;**77**(4):2400–409.

163 Franchini G, Robert-Guroff M, Tartaglia J, *et al.* Highly attenuated HIV type 2 recombinant poxviruses, but not HIV-2 recombinant Salmonella vaccines, induce long-lasting protection in rhesus macaques. *J Virol* 1999;**73**:1853–9.

164 Steger KK, Pauza CD. Immunization of *Macaca mulatta* with aroA attenuated *Salmonella typhimurium* expressing the SIVp27 antigen. *J Med Primatol* 1997;**26**(1–2):44–50.

165 Steger KK, Valentine PJ, Heffron F, So M, Pauza CD. Recombinant, attenuated *Salmonella typhimurium* stimulate lymphoproliferative responses to SIV capsid antigen in rhesus macaques. *Vaccine* 1991;**17**(7–8):923–32.

166 Steger KK, Waterman DPM, Pauza CD. Acute effects of pathogenic simian-human immunodeficiency virus challenge on vaccine-induced cellular and humoral immune responses to Gag in rhesus macaques. *J Virol* 1999;**73**:1853–9.

167 Jiang S, Rasmussen RA, Nolan KM, *et al.* Live attenuated *Listeria monocytogenes* expressing HIV Gag: immunogenicity in rhesus monkeys. *Vaccine* 2007;**25**(42):7470–79.

168 Kestler HW, 3rd, Mori K, Silva DP, *et al.* Nef genes of SIV. *J Med Primatol* 1990;**19**(3–4):421–9.

169 Kestler HW, 3rd,Ringler DJ, Mori K, *et al.* Importance of the *nef* gene for maintenance of high virus loads and for development of AIDS. *Cell* 1991;**65**(4):651–62.

170 Daniel MD, Kirchhoff F, Czajak SC, Sehgal PK, Desrosiers RC. Protective effects of a live attenuated SIV vaccine with a deletion in the *nef* gene. *Science* 1992;**258**(5090):1880–81.

171 Baba TW, Jeong YS, Pennick D, *et al.* Pathogenicity of live, attenuated SIV after mucosal infection of neonatal macaques. *Science* 1995;**267**(5205):1820–25.

172 Baba TW, Liska V, Khimani AH, *et al.* Live attenuated, multiply deleted simian immunodeficiency virus causes AIDS in infant and adult macaques. *Nat Med* 1999;**5**(2):194–20.

173 Hofmann-Lehmann R, Vlasak J, Williams AL, *et al.* Live attenuated, nef-deleted SIV is pathogenic in most adult macaques after prolonged observation. *AIDS* 2003;**17**(2):157–66.

174 Wyand MS, Manson KH, Garcia-Moll M, Montefiori D, Desrosiers RC. Vaccine protection by a triple deletion mutant of simian immunodeficiency virus. *J Virol* 1996;**70**(6):3724–33.

175 Desrosiers RC, Lifson JD, Gibbs JS, *et al.* Identification of highly attenuated mutants of simian immunodeficiency virus. *J Virol* 1998;**72**(2):1431–7.

176 Mansfield K, Lang SM, Gauduin MC, *et al.* Vaccine protection by live, attenuated simian immunodeficiency virus in the absence of high-titer antibody responses and high-frequency cellular immune responses measurable in the periphery. *J Virol* 2008;**82**(8):4135–48.

177 Sharpe SA, Cope A, Dowall S, *et al.* Macaques infected long-term with attenuated simian immunodeficiency virus (SIVmac) remain resistant to wild-type challenge, despite declining cytotoxic T lymphocyte responses to an immunodominant epitope. *J Gen Virol* 2004;**85**(9):2591–602.

178 Stone M, Ma ZM, Genescà M, *et al.* Limited dissemination of pathogenic SIV after vaginal challenge of rhesus monkeys immunized with a live, attenuated lentivirus. *Virology* 2009;**392**(2):260–70.

179 Abel K, Compton L, Rourke T, *et al.* Simian-human immunodeficiency virus SHIV89.6-induced protection against intravaginal challenge with pathogenic SIVmac239 is independent of the route of immunization and is associated with a combination of cytotoxic T-lymphocyte and alpha interferon responses. *J Virol* 2003;**77**(5):3099–118.

180 Genescà M, Rourke T, Li J, *et al.* Live attenuated lentivirus infection elicits polyfunctional simian immunodeficiency virus Gag-specific CD8+ T cells with reduced apoptotic susceptibility in rhesus macaques that control virus replication after

challenge with pathogenic SIVmac239. *J Immunol* 2007;**179**(7):4732–40.

181 LaFranco-Scheuch L, Abel K, Makori N, Rothaeusler K, Miller CJ. High beta-chemokine expression levels in lymphoid tissues of simian/human immunodeficiency virus 89.6-vaccinated rhesus macaques are associated with uncontrolled replication of simian immunodeficiency virus challenge inoculum. *J Virol* 2004;**78**(12):6399–408.

182 Miller CJ, McChesney MB, Lü X, *et al.* Rhesus macaques previously infected with simian/human immunodeficiency virus are protected from vaginal challenge with pathogenic SIVmac239. *J Virol* 1997;**71**(3):1911–21 .

183 Berman NE, Sheffield LG, Purcell J, *et al.* Gradient of microglial activation in the brain of SIV infected macaques. *J NeuroAIDS* 1998;**2**(1):43–54.

184 Fultz PN, Nara P, Barre-Sinoussi F, *et al.* Vaccine protection of chimpanzees against challenge with HIV-1-infected peripheral blood mononuclear cells. *Science* 1992;**256**(5064):1687–90.

185 Putkonen P, Walther L, Zhang YJ, *et al.* Long-term protection against SIV-induced disease in macaques vaccinated with a live attenuated HIV-2 vaccine. *Nat Med* 1995;**1**(9):914–18.

186 O'Neill E, Bostik V, Montefiori DC, Kraiselburd E, Villinger F. IL-12/GM-CSF co-administration in an SIV DNA prime/protein boost protocol enhances Gag-specific T cells but not virus-specific neutralizing antibodies in rhesus macaques. *AIDS Res Hum Retroviruses* 2003;**19**:883–90.

187 Notka F, Stahl-Hennig C, Dittmer U, Wolf H, Wagner R. Accelerated clearance of SHIV in rhesus monkeys by virus-like particle vaccines is dependent on induction of neutralizing antibodies. *Vaccine* 1999;**18**(3–4):291–301.

188 Kent SJ, Dale CJ, Ranasinghe C, *et al.* Mucosally-administered human-simian immunodeficiency virus DNA and fowlpoxvirus-based recombinant vaccines reduce acute phase viral replication in macaques following vaginal challenge with CCR5-tropic SHIVSF162P3. *Vaccine* 2005;**23**(42):5009–21.

189 Amara RR, Villinger F, Altman JD, *et al.* Control of a mucosal challenge and prevention of AIDS by a multiprotein DNA/MVA vaccine. *Science* 2001;**292**(5514):69–74.

190 Girard M, van der Ryst E, Barré-Sinoussi F, *et al.* Challenge of chimpanzees immunized with a recombinant canarypox-HIV-1 virus. *Virology* 1997;**232**(1):98–104.

191 Chen ZP, Zhou P, Ho DD, Landau NR, Marx PA. Genetically divergent strains of simian immunodeficiency virus use CCR5 as a co-receptor for entry. *J Virol* 1997;**71**:2705–14.

192 Kestler H, Kodama T, Ringler D, *et al.* Induction of AIDS in rhesus monkeys by molecularly cloned simian immunodeficiency virus. *Science* 1990;**248**(4959):1109–12.

PART 3
Antigen Discovery

CHAPTER 9

Sequence-Based Computational Approaches to Vaccine Discovery and Design

Darrick Carter

Protein Advances, Inc., Seattle, WA, USA
Infectious Disease Research Institute, Seattle, WA, USA

Introduction

As stated in the 2009 Pacific Symposium on Biocomputing, there is "a clear trend: sequence analysis is back!" [1]. The use of computers in vaccine development and discovery is ubiquitous and
it is difficult to draw the distinction between pure
computational approaches, which use computers
for discovery of new lead vaccine candidates, and
computer-supported approaches, where computers
guide decisions and aid in the development of an
established target. This chapter focuses on a sampling of computer guided methods, some of which –
like the homology and basic local alignment search
tool (BLAST) algorithms – aid in selection of new
targets; some, like the epitope prediction methods, both guide development and aid in new target discovery. The selection of methods is based on
the familiarity of the author with these approaches
and should not diminish the contribution of either
other computational approaches to the subjects discussed in the following sections or other computational vaccine design methods. Each section is
designed to provide the reader the means for performing the type of research themselves. To this extent simple examples are chosen to illustrate how
to approach new designs and write programs to expand on published code. Sections dealing with the

nuts and bolts of implementation use alternate font
function notations as in ``Pseudo_Code().''

Designing vaccines based on alignments

Applications

Homology-based positive and negative antigen selection

There are a few scenarios one can envision in
which the use of homology can be a useful tool
for deciding on the utility of a vaccine candidate
for a disease. The first, a positive selector, is the application of candidates in one disease to a different
disease. An example of this is the utility of Bacille
Calmette-Guérin (BCG) in vaccination against leprosy [2]. BCG is an attenuated strain of *Mycobacterium bovis* and is partially protective against tuberculosis [3]. A homology comparison of *Mycobacterium tuberculosis*, *Mycobacterium bovis* BCG, and
Mycobacterium leprae indicates that there is significant homology on the protein level between these
organisms [4] and one would predict that the partial protection for tuberculosis may be reflected in
protection against leprosy. This is indeed the case: a
study in India found in 2007 that protection against

Vaccinology: Principles and Practice, First Edition. Edited by W. John W. Morrow, Nadeem A. Sheikh, Clint S. Schmidt and D. Huw Davies.
© 2012 Blackwell Publishing Ltd. Published 2012 by Blackwell Publishing Ltd.

tuberculosis was 62% and that similar protection (62%) was found against leprosy [5]. Although this vaccine strategy is far from perfect for numerous reasons beyond the scope of this discussion, it does support the assumption that gross homology between genes in a vaccine target from one organism could translate into useful efficacy against another disease. If one is developing a defined protein vaccine for a disease, a homology alignment with family member proteins from a different pathogen may give a clue to the utility of this protein in a second indication. An example of this was published by researchers at the Infectious Disease Research Institute: the sterol 24-c-methyltranferase protein from *Leishmania infantum*, the causative agent of visceral leishmaniasis, shares 96.6% identity with the same protein from *Leishmania major*, which causes a cutaneous form of the disease. When tested in an animal model, the single protein protects animals from both the cutaneous as well as visceral leishmanisis [6].

An altogether different situation exists when researchers are trying to develop vaccines that have a wide safety margin and are highly immunogenic. Here one would look at homology and identity as a negative selector. In this case, if one is designing a vaccine for human use, one would select the antigen from the pathogen by removing protein candidates with high degrees of homology since they could be construed to cause autoimmunity and, due to tolerance, may not be very immunogenic. It is difficult to understand how a protein would break tolerance and induce an autoimmune disease unless very powerful immune stimulatory molecules are co-administered, but even the idea that the protein could be less of an immune target due to tolerance may guide a researcher away from proteins with high degrees of similarity to a human protein.

For this discussion we will assume the user has a model antigen and its sequence in hand and wants to leverage homology searching to make informed decisions on the development of the vaccine. When performing a homology-based search, the following steps would be recommended for the antigen:

1 Use a BLAST search against all organisms to find out if there are potential matches to the antigen.

2 Perform a pairwise sequence alignment to look at the degree of homology to potential matches.

3 Perform a search for small, identical regions that could be significant epitopes.

Selection of antigens using repeat detection

The use of repeat proteins as molecules that contain epitopes for antibody binding is gaining traction. These proteins appear to have properties that make them good targets for antibodies against a foreign organism and therefore have been used as antigens for the development of serologic diagnostic tests. For example, in one study, tandem repeat (TR) proteins from *L. infantum* or *Trypanosoma cruzi* were identified and evaluated as serological antigens in an ELISA format. It was determined that a number of proteins uncovered by this search could be developed as useful serological targets [7, 8]. For example, bioinformatic studies on *T. cruzi* were performed where the top twenty scoring proteins were studied. Five of these proteins were previously described antigens and were excluded from further analysis. Among the remaining fifteen, two were excluded based on homology to *Leishmania* spp. Eight of nine proteins that were successfully expressed and tested were serological antigens for Chagas disease and the responses were disease-specific. Taken together, at least 13 of 20 TR proteins (including the ones previously published) contained dominant B-cell epitopes. When looking for a vaccine candidate based on this selection mechanism, it is likely that candidates can be identified using computational searching. However, there is some evidence that in the arms race in nature, pathogens have evolved to exploit this and specifically create proteins with multiple repeats as a "smokescreen." Nonetheless, they may make diagnostic targets or in combination with powerful adjuvants may direct an appropriate neutralizing response.

Algorithms

String comparisons

For direct comparison of short sequences it is easy to use simple tools to find identical matches. An example where this may be desirable would be to screen for the presence of an important known CD8 T-cell epitope in variant strains of an organism expressing the target antigen with point mutations. Alternately, one may be looking to exclude the possibility of a human autoantigen epitope arising in a powerful vaccine using a recombinant protein. Here one would chop the antigen sequence into short peptides differing in position by one amino acid and compare them using a matching algorithm to a human protein database. The short epitope in both cases would be unlikely to show up in a BLAST search due to the low score such a short match could generate.

Local and global sequence alignments

These alignments are used to compare sequences directly to each other. Two families of alignment algorithm can be used for both proteins and DNA: the Needleman and Wunsch algorithm [9], which yields optimal global sequence alignments, and the Smith-Waterman algorithm [10], which yields local alignments. Implementation of these dynamic programming algorithms is described in detail below. Direct comparison of two sequences could be used to make decisions on the potential for one antigen to be useful in another disease setting with a known homolog; comparison of a sequence to a database could be used as described in the example to pull up a number of antigen leads.

Basic local alignment search tool

While the search with local alignments using the Smith-Waterman algorithm is sensitive and would have yielded interesting vaccine leads, the algorithm is slow to implement for searching very large datasets. Recently, a number of groups have accelerated the search using a variety of methods [11, 12] – including implementation on a Playstation 3 [13] – but even with an order of magnitude acceleration, the full alignment search may not be capable of keeping up with the quantities of sequence data that are being generated and threaten to become torrents as next-generation sequencing technologies come online. To address these searching requirements, faster implementations of database alignment searches like FASTA have been created

[14], but the most familiar tool is likely to be the basic local alignment search tool (BLAST).

BLAST is a tool for searching large databases for sequences with similar regions. Similarity in BLAST is defined by statistically significant matches of aligned regions of a sequence against another found in the database being searched. The algorithm was originally described in 1990 by Altschul *et al.* [15] and has since undergone a number of revisions and refinements.

Table 9.1 shows the search choices and the variations on the BLAST algorithm provided at the NCBI. BLAST provides for two types of searches – nucleotide and protein based – and each of these implements a slightly different variation to find matches. Both searches follow the basic pattern of chopping the initial sequence into a list of "words" that are n-mers derived from the query sequence; searching the database for matches to these "words," and finally extending the alignment around the matches.

Nucleotide-based searches utilize exact matches between the word and the database test sequence. In this case the default length of a word is 11. In the case of protein searches the default word length is 3 and a point score for matches is calculated using a substitution matrix. If a match is found, it is extended in either direction until the matching score falls below a threshold value. The local alignment, a high-scoring segment pair (HSP), can initiate a gapped extension using dynamic programming described above, if it is above a certain threshold information value. The more recent version of BLAST, gapped BLAST, does not extend all hits; it requires two match hits to be within a certain distance of each other (40 characters by default) before attempting to extend [15–18]. Once the hits have been found, a statistical analysis takes place to try to sort out matches that may have arisen by chance. The principals of this statistical analysis are essentially the ones in the local and global alignments described before. The web-based tool can be found at the National Center for Biotechnology Information (www.ncbi.nlm.nih.gov), where the user can choose to search databases using either a protein sequence or a nucleotide sequence.

Table 9.1 BLAST program variations.

Program name	Query format	Database format	Notes
blastn	Nucleotide sequence	Nucleotide database	Variations include megablast and discontiguous megablast
blastp	Protein sequence	Protein database	Variations include psi-blast and phi-blast
blastx	Nucleotide sequence[a]	Protein database	The nucleotide sequence is translated prior to searching
tblastn	Protein sequence	Nucleotide database[a]	The protein is used to search a translated nucleotide database
tblastx	Nucleotide sequence[a]	Nucleotide database[a]	The nucleotide sequence is translated, then the protein sequence is used to search a translated nucleotide database

[a] A translation is performed prior to searching.

Implementation

In the following example a program is written to align sequences and is used to design a leprosy vaccine based on homology to the tuberculosis ESAT6 vaccine candidate.

Writing the alignment program

Alignments between nucleotide or protein sequences are a useful tool in discovering genetic and structural conservation. Because it is difficult to manually align sequences and since – due to the possibility of insertions – the number of possible alignments quickly grows intractable, algorithms have been developed to reliably generate optimal alignment solutions. Needleman and Wunsch described the use of dynamic programming to align two sequences that gives an optimal global alignment in 1970 [9]. Smith and Waterman later published an algorithm similar to the Needleman and Wunsch approach, which yields the highest scoring local alignments [10].

For the discovery tool we will initialize a scoring matrix and then create alignments using this matrix followed by writing out the score of each alignment.

Substitution Table

For any computed alignment not all changes are equal. While nucleotide alignments often go with

an "all or nothing" scoring system where each change is penalized by the same factor, this approach is not well suited for proteins. The reason for this is that in a nucleotide a change from one base to another often results in the same change in information, while in a protein there may be a reason to preserve functional or structural similarity. Various scoring systems are used for alignments based on a point score for substitution. These systems are usually represented as a 20 by 20 matrix for proteins from which the score for finding two amino acids together can be derived. The most commonly used substitution matrices are the point accepted mutations (PAM) [19] and BLOCKS substitution matrix (BLOSUM) [20] matrices. PAM is based on the rate of mutation of amino acids while BLOSUM is based on frequencies of substitution within the BLOCKS aligned protein data. Table 9.2 shows a section of the BLOSUM62 matrix. Programmatically, initializing the scoring matrix involves reading a matrix from a file [void ReadSubstitution Table (String file)] and exposing a function that, given a pair of amino acids, returns the score given by the matrix [double ValueFromPair(char A, char B)]. Using this table we can now calculate what score to assign a pair in which a proline, P, has changed to a cysteine, C: ValueFromPair (C,P) returns -3 in

Table 9.2 Abbreviated BLOSUM62 scoring matrix.

	C	S	T	P	A	G	W	
C	9							C
S	−1	4						S
T	−1	1	5					T
P	−3	−1	−1	7				P
A	0	1	0	−1	4			A
G	−3	0	−2	−2	0	6		G
W	−2	−3	−2	−4	−3	−2	11	W
	C	S	T	P	A	G	W	

line with the expectation that a change from the helical breaker proline is not a conservative change to the disulfide bond-forming cysteine.

Sequence Alignment

Now that we have a scoring system, we use the dynamic programming algorithm to create the alignment. The alignment accepts two strings that represent the protein sequences to align. In the example we are going to use PPW and PPTW. First, we initialize a score matrix that has dimensions of one greater than each sequence has residues. Sequence one, PPW, forms a column, and sequence two, PPTW, forms a row. In the upper right-hand corner we put a zero as the starting score and we step right (inserting a gap into the top sequence) and score this with a gap penalty (−9); we step right again and add a new gap penalty to the one just scored (−9 +−9 = −18); this continues until the first row is initialized. Similarly, we go down and fill out the first column with gap penalty scores for inserting gaps in the second sequence. While the scoring matrix is initialized, the trace matrix is initialized: we write "Finished" in the upper left-hand corner, "Left" in the rest of the first row, and "Up" in the first column (Figure 9.1, Step 1). After

Step 1: Initializing matrices

		P	P	T	W
	0	−9	−18	−27	−36
P	−9				
P	−18				
W	−27				

		P	P	T	W
	Finished	Left	Left	Left	Left
P	Up				
P	Up				
W	Up				

Step 2: Scoring and tracing the full matrices

		P	P	T	W
	0	−9	−18	−27	−36
P	−9	7	−2	−11	−20
P	−18	−2	14	5	−4
W	−27	−11	5	12	16

		P	P	T	W
	Finished	Left	Left	Left	Left
P	Up	Diag.	Left	Left	Left
P	Up	Up	Diag.	Left	Left
W	Up	Up	Up	Diag.	Diag.

Step 3: Creating the alignment

		P	P	T	W
	Finished	Left	Left	Left	Left
P	Up	Diag.	Left	Left	Left
P	Up	Up	Diag.	Left	Left
W	Up	Up	Up	Diag.	Diag.

Sequence one: PP-W
Sequence two: PPTW

Applying the same algorithm to a larger protein

```
TB ESAT6  :  WLGSAADKYAGQNRKRVDIFQELAELDKELIELIHNQANSVQTTRGILDG
             |  ||    |  |    ||       |    |      |      | ||  |
ML0405    :  WGGSGSEAYQGVQQKWDATATELNNALQNLARTISEAGQAMASTEGNVTG
```

Figure 9.1 Dynamic programming alignment procedure.

initialization, the rest of the cells are filled in using the following algorithm:

1 A score is determined for each move: `score_diagonal` is the score for keeping the sequence pair aligned plus the last score from the diagonal; `score_left` and `score_up` are the scores resulting from inserting a gap in sequence one or sequence two plus their respective last scores for inserting a gap; that is:

```
i.    score_diagonal = ScoreMatrix[y-1][x-1] +
      ValueFromPair(Sequence1[y],
      Sequence2[x]);
ii.   score_up       = ScoreMatrix[y - 1][x] +
      Gap_Penalty;
iii.  score_left     = ScoreMatrix[y][x - 1] +
      Gap_Penalty;
```

2 The maximum score for each move is determined; if two top scores are the same, the move that gave the highest score in the last iteration is chosen.

3 The score is written into the current cell and the move that gave that score written into the corresponding cell of the trace matrix.

The table is shown in Figure 9.1, step 2 after being filled out. For a global alignment, the score is now in the bottom right-hand corner of the table.

In the final step the trace matrix is now used to create the alignment. We start in the lower right-hand corner and read "Diagonal" – this means the last amino acids are left together: "W,W" and we take a diagonal step. Now we are on the field "Left." We insert a gap in sequence one and leave the amino acid in sequence two ("−W, TW"). The next two steps are both diagonal and we have landed on the "Finished" field. The alignment is completed (Figure 9.1, step 3: "PP-W, PPTW").

For implementation of a local alignment, the same pattern is used as described above, but the score is set to 0 if it is negative when the score matrix is filled. Now the highest score within the matrix is used as a starting point and traced back until a "0" is reached. This alignment is reported as the best local alignment.

Using the alignment software to search a database

Now that we have written a tool to perform and score alignments, we use it to search a database for new vaccine targets. The known antigen from *Mycobacterium tuberculosis*, ESAT6, is downloaded from the PubMed database and used as a template to search for a new vaccine candidate in the *Mycobacterium leprae* protein database. Next, the sequence of the ESAT6 protein is shuffled so that the amino acid composition stays the same, but the order is random. The search is then repeated to get a baseline for what may be significant alignments. The result of both searches is shown in Figure 9.2.

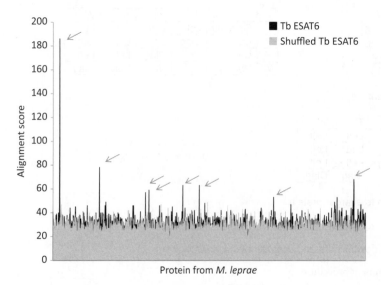

■ Tb ESAT6
■ Shuffled Tb ESAT6

Protein from *M. leprae*

Figure 9.2 Alignment scores for the search of the leprosy proteome using the sequence for TB ESAT6. The protein sequence for ESAT6 was downloaded from PubMed and used to search the leprosy proteome (black). Next, the amino acids of the sequence were placed in random positions and the random protein was used to search the leprosy database (gray).

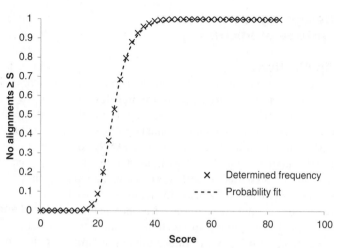

Figure 9.3 The determined frequency of hits and a probability function fit to the determined data. Plotted are the determined frequency (X) and the calculated probability (- - - -) of not having an alignment with score ≥ S using a sequence length of $n = 70$ for the probe and an average length of $m = 317$ for the database. In this case we get $K = 0.016$ and $\lambda = 0.245$.

Visually, the arrows point to possible high scoring matches for this search, but it would be of great utility to be able to objectively determine which hits are highly significant and which ones simply arose by chance.

Determining significance of the output

As mentioned above, an objective measure of significance would be useful for picking out hits that are noteworthy. There have been a lot of treatments of this problem [21–24] and we will focus on the one used for ungapped local alignments, which can also be used in good approximation for gapped local alignments, as we will see using the data generated for this discussion. Because local alignment scores can be modeled as Poisson distributed, one can derive a function for the expectation value E that is dependent on the score S and proportional to the length of the sequences m and n being compared (Equation 9.1). The factors K and λ are scaling and location factors, which depend on the amino acid composition of the database and the scoring matrix being used. The E value can be converted to a p value (Equation 9.2) and is the one reported by alignment programs and the BLAST algorithm. The p value describes the probability that a score S would be found by random chance.

$$E = Kmne^{-\lambda S} \qquad (9.1)$$

$$p = 1 - e^{-E} \qquad (9.2)$$

For our specific application, runs with random sequences were performed to yield scores for searching the database with meaningless sequences. These were grouped into bins and the frequency of sequences in each bin was calculated by dividing the number of sequences scoring below the bin by the total number of sequences (Figure 9.3). In Equation 9.2 we found the probability of at least one score being generated by random chance. Therefore, the probability of no alignment with score ≥ S being generated by chance is:

$$\begin{aligned} y &= 1 - p \\ \Leftrightarrow y &= 1 - (1 - e^{-E}) \\ \Leftrightarrow y &= 1 - \left(1 - e^{-Kmne^{-\lambda S}}\right) \\ \Leftrightarrow y &= e^{-Kmne^{-\lambda S}} \end{aligned} \qquad (9.3)$$

We can fit Equation 9.3 to the data derived from our simulations (Figure 9.3). In this case we get $K = 0.016$ and $\lambda = 0.245$ for our scaling constants. Now we can go back and evaluate the scores in Figure 9.2 and determine the significant hits. With a cutoff of $p < 0.0001$ we collect 11 significant hits from our search, including the known ESAT6 and CFP-10 protein homologs of *M. leprae*. A literature search in PubMed using the protein names and the term "vaccine AND antigen" yields thirteen independent results covering six of the proteins. In comparison, choosing eleven random proteins and performing the same search yields no results.

Designing vaccines using epitope prediction

Applications

Epitope prediction either relies on structural considerations such as surface exposure and flexibility of the backbone residues, used mainly for B-cell epitopes, or is based on machine learning principals such as in artificial neural nets (ANNs) or hidden markov models (HMMs), used primarily for epitopes presented on MHCs. Any combination of these methods can be used to create combined scores, or "voting" mechanisms. The idea behind using predicted epitopes to create a vaccine is to know that the protein can induce the desired immune response in the target population and to be able to trim antigens to the important components involved in immunity to organisms carrying the antigen. Additionally, for some delivery and presentation system, such as virus-like particles, only a certain amount of antigen sequence can be exposed in the context of the delivery framework, and decisions need to be made as to which portions are cloned into the presentation sites.

MHC class I epitopes

Major histocompatibility complex (MHC) class I epitopes arise from a cell processing of antigens made within the cell such as those found in viruses and mutated proteins in cancer. The class I pathway proceeds by cleaving the epitopes into peptides in the proteosome, followed by loading and presentation on the MHC class I. The epitope/MHC-I complexes are presented on the surface of the cell and can be recognized by T cells capable of inducing cytotoxicity. Normal healthy cells present only complexes that should not be recognized by cytotoxic T cells, while abnormal cells, such as infected or cancerous cells, present epitopes derived from viral and mutated proteins, leading to the killing of these cells by cytotoxic T cells and the suppression of further viral replication and avoidance of tumors. Class I epitopes are presented to CD8$^+$ T cells.

MHC class II epitopes

Class II epitopes arise from processing of antigens by professional antigen-presenting cells, which take up the antigens from outside the cell through endocytosis. Once processed, the peptides are loaded into MHC class II molecules and presented on the cell surface to CD4$^+$ T cells. Extracellular antigens such as those arising from bacteria, shed and secreted antigens, and proteins from certain extracellular parasites are processed and presented by MHC II. Class II MHC molecules are more pliable in their binding motifs, making accurate prediction of these epitopes more difficult than prediction of class I epitopes.

B-cell epitopes

There are a number of reasons to attempt to compute and predict epitopes for vaccines that mediate protection via humoral immunity. One may need to string numerous epitopes together to create a polyprotein that elicits responses to variant chains of a single antigen, or one may want to enhance the immune response to a pathogen by having multiple antigens – each of which could be a target for antibody-dependent neutralization. Finally, there is an advantage to designing an immune scaffold that elicits a particular neutralizing antibody response. An example of this is found in HIV, where the CD4 binding protein, gp120, assumes a certain conformation when associated with CD4. Antibodies that recognize this conformation are capable of broad neutralization of HIV [25].

Algorithms

A recent survey of prediction methods for MHC epitopes found that of the thirty approaches surveyed, 43% of the algorithms were based on scoring matrices and 37% used machine learning in the form of ANNs and support vector machines [26,27]. The rest were structure-based calculations, HMMs, or combination methods. Because of the success of machine learning in class I predictions, we will use an ANN method in the programming example. Below is a brief description of each approach.

Position-specific scoring matrices

In the simplest form, the matrix contains a score for each position depending on the prevalence of certain amino acids for each allele at that position.

The score could be a frequency or any other scoring system adopted to optimize epitope recognition. By creating a product of the scores for a test peptide, a total score is calculated that can be compared to a threshold that optimizes the number of correctly classified epitopes. Since using frequencies can lead to the product becoming so small that many computational platforms will underflow, the log of the frequencies is taken and the score calculated using the sum of logs. Much more information can be gleaned by creating a two-dimensional matrix containing information that incorporates relative positions of amino acids to each other and scoring the sequence using the full matrix [17].

Artificial neural nets

An ANN is a system of units that each simulate a neuron by being able to be excited, followed by the ability to decide to "fire," and excite other neurons downstream. In a typical embodiment, there is a "visual" layer of neurons that get presented with data. These neurons are connected to others in a "hidden" layer and, depending on the weights of each connection, can excite all or a subset of the ones they are connected to. The "hidden" layer is then again connected with an "output" layer, which can consist of only a single neuron that integrates the signal of the hidden layer into a final output. The weights between each neuron unit are randomized to small values at the start and the network is trained by presenting the visual layer with data and adjusting the weights until the er-

ror of the output is below a threshold. Machines of this architecture are referred to as multilayered perceptrons. For applications to epitope prediction the visual layer can be the size of the desired input peptide or contain position-specific or mutual position information; the hidden layer is then chosen based on performance of different neuron architectures, and the output layer can be a single neuron with an output of "0" for a nonbinder and "1" for a binder, or an arbitrary score that can be related to binding affinity. The training set is from a known binder/nonbinder database. A step-by-step description is found below in the methodology example.

Support vector machine

Support vector machines (SVMs) attempt to split n-dimensional data into two classes by providing a hyperplane of dimension $n - 1$, which forms a boundary between the two data points. Any point on one side of the plane is of class 1 and data points on the other are of class 2. In the event that the plane cannot linearly separate the classes, one uses a kernel function to map data into a space in which a single hyperplane can distinguish two classes of points. In Figure 9.4, the initial dataset is mapped to a space where the linear hyperplane can easily separate binders from nonbinders. The input vectors used can simply be the presence of an amino acid in binary form (in this case a 20-dimensional vector where all amino acids except the one present are encoded by "0"), the position-specific BLOSUM number for each amino acid, or, in more complex

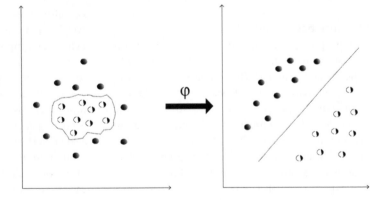

Figure 9.4 Kernel mapping for support vector machine classification. Points in the left graph are mapped using the kernel trick to a space in which a single plane can divide the gray classed points from the open classed points. Although the example shows two-dimensional vectors being split by a one-dimensional hyperplane, the same principals are usually employed in higher dimensional spaces.

cases, a vector indicating both the position as well as the similarity properties extracted from the substitution table, which gives better discrimination for binders and nonbinders [28,29]. When developing an SVM, the choice of a kernel mapping function and the number of vectors to use is important for generalized training. In analogy to an ANN, using too many examples and overmapping the training set can lead to excellent recognition within the training set but poor performance when the SVM encounters new test sets.

Hidden markov model

In an HMM a matrix of transition probabilities is calculated and the probability of a state can be related to the events leading up to that state. In the case of binding to T-cell or B-cell epitopes the HMM states are "epitope" or "non-epitope" and the sequence can be fed to the model in a number of ways to lead up to the state.

HMMs can be powerful in decoding complex information and are commonly used in speech recognition. In the theory behind HMMs there are a few assumptions about the probabilities:

1 Each state has a defined probability with $0 < p_i <= 1$.
2 The sum of all states in the model equals 1.
3 The transition probability between states is dependent on only the previous state.

This last assumption is the most problematic for many applications; in sequence analysis if a sliding window is fed into the model the probabilities of the window as they approach the transition from non-epitope to epitope could give the model information on when the transition is going to happen.

Structure-based methods

Epitope prediction can also rely on comparisons against known three-dimensional structures of antigens and peptide-MHC complexes. In the case of a B-cell antigen, the 3D structure will demonstrate which epitopes lie on the surface of the molecule and allow prediction of epitopes that are discontinuous; that is, where the linear peptide sequence would not be sufficient to predict which regions are adjacent to each other. Predicted surface exposure can also be used on linear sequences

where the hydrophilicity of a stretch and its predicted flexibility may give clues on whether the stretch will be solvent and thus possibly exposed. Since motifs are not easily found for B-cell epitopes, these are most commonly predicted using the structure-based approaches [30,31]. Finally, the computed energies of binding models on an MHC/peptide complex can be used to predict if a peptide will bind with reasonable affinity to a given MHC.

Combinations

Each of the above methods can be combined to either form a joint score on an epitope, or to create a consensus prediction. Since different approaches to prediction leverage different types of data, the combined approach can be more sensitive than using just a single algorithm. An example of this would be the approach used in CTLPred, where voting on the epitope by an ANN and an SVM is used to determine an epitope. If either one or both predict the peptide is an epitope, it is designated an epitope; otherwise, if both vote against, it is designated "non-epitope." This type of combined voting has been shown to improve performance [30].

Implementation

The network

An ANN is created by individual units that are connected to each other by weights. A standard feedforward backpropagation neural net consists of a visual layer, a hidden layer, and an output layer. Figure 9.5 shows a simple neural net. This figure can also be used as a reference for the activation, weight, and output symbols used in the discussion below. The input layer is connected with weights to the hidden layer. This layer is then connected to the output layer. This three-layer arrangement is sufficient to model nonlinear data where a single input vector is connected to a single output vector. Modeling data with higher solution dimensions can also be performed using multiple hidden layers, although there are few problems where this is necessary. The similarity to biological neuron systems is easy to see: the units are the equivalent of neurons

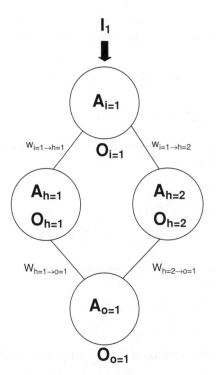

Figure 9.5 A simple neural net architecture. A very simple multilayered ANN is shown above. The input, I_1, is encoded into the activation of the input layer. The output, O_i, is then propagated to the two hidden neurons, where the output O_i is multiplied by the weight to form the activation, A_h. A_h is then transformed with the sigmoid function to form O_h, which is then further propagated forward to activate the output neuron with A_o. The output of the neural net O_o is then again computed by applying the activation function to A_o.

and the weights simulate the strength of connection between neurons at synapses.

In our example below, we will map a nine-dimensional input vector representing the sequence to a one-dimensional output representing a score for "binder" and "nonbinder." Selecting the number of "neurons" in the hidden layer is often achieved by trial and error, but often a good basis is to use about 85% of the number of neurons in the input layer. The danger of adding many neurons to the hidden layer is that the network will be easily overtrained and may not be able to generalize the training to examples it has not yet seen. Having too few neurons in the hidden layer may not allow the net to encode enough information to learn the dataset.

Each "neuron"

Each neuron contains inputs from all its incoming weights, a threshold value, and an activation function to integrate the inputs. A common activation function is the sigmoidal function below:

$$f(x) = \frac{1}{(1 + e^{-x})}$$

Activation Function

Upon firing, a neuron distributes its output to each connected neuron in the next layer.

Feedforward

The input neurons (A_i) are activated by numeric inputs (I) into the input layer:

$$A_i = I$$

Input layer activation

The activation of each neuron in the first hidden layer (A_h) is computed by summing the activation of each input neuron multiplied with the weights connecting the two ($w_{i \to h}$).

$$A_h = \sum_i A_i w_{i \to h}$$

Hidden layer activation

The output of each neuron is calculated by subtracting a threshold t from the activation and applying the activation function to the result:

$$O_h = f(A_h - t)$$

Output function

Finally, the activation of the output layer (A_o) is computed by multiplying the output of the connected hidden neurons O_h by the weight between the connected hidden neuron and output neuron ($w_{h \to o}$). For networks with multiple hidden layers the same processes are performed to pass the results to intervening hidden layers.

$$A_o = \sum_h O_h w_{h \to o}$$

Output layer activation

The output of the neural net is then calculated in the same manner as the output from the hidden layers.

Backpropagation

While in the feedforward mode, the activation propagates through the network from visual to hidden to output in backpropagation learning, and the adjustments are calculated and made from the output to the hidden layer up to the input layer. There are numerous methods to adjust learning. In this example we will use the steepest descent method, which simply adjusts the weights between neurons by multiplying the computed difference by a learning rate.

First, the error of the output layer is calculated simply as the difference between the output layer's output and the desired output:

$$\varepsilon_o = O_o - d$$

Output error

The gradient of error as a function of the weights between the hidden and output layer is given by:

$$\Delta \varepsilon_o (w_{h \to o}) = \frac{\partial \varepsilon_o}{\partial w_{h \to o}} = O_h f'(A_o - t)\varepsilon_o$$

Gradient of output error as a function of weights

The derivative here is one of the reasons the choice of the sigmoidal activation function is practical:

$$f'(x) = f(x)(1 - f(x))$$

Notice that $(A_o - t)$ is equal to the output of the output layer:

$$f'(A_o - t) = O_o(1 - O_o)$$

Finally, combining these equations, the weights can be adjusted by taking a step against the gradient of the error. The size of this step is determined by the learning rate, L_R, which is typically in the range of 0.05 to 0.1:

$$\Delta w_{h \to o} = -L_R \nabla \varepsilon_o (w_{h \to o})$$

$$\Delta w_{h \to o} = -L_R O_h O_o (1 - O_o)\varepsilon_o$$

Weight updates for the hidden to output neurons

In the same manner, the weights between the hidden layer and the input layer can now be updated:

$$\Delta \varepsilon_h (w_{i \to h}) = \frac{\partial \varepsilon_h}{\partial w_{i \to h}} = O_i f'(A_h - t)$$

$$\times \sum_o \varepsilon_o O_o (1 - O_o) w_{h \to o}$$

Gradient of hidden error as a function of weights

Yielding:

$$\Delta w_{i \to h} = -L_R \nabla \varepsilon_h (w_{i \to h})$$

$$\Delta w_{i \to h} = -L_R O_i O_h (1 - O_h) \sum_o \varepsilon_o O_o (1 - O_o) w_{h \to o}$$

Weight updates for the input to hidden neurons

Finally, the thresholds are updated:

$$\Delta t_o = L_R O_o (1 - O_o)\varepsilon_o$$

Threshold updates for the output neurons

$$\Delta t_h = L_R O_h (1 - O_h) \sum_o \varepsilon_o O_o (1 - O_o) w_{h \to o}$$

Threshold updates for the hidden neurons

Notice that the threshold updates are equivalent to the weight updates for a connected neuron with a fixed -1 input. Once the updates have been applied to the neurons in the net, the network activations are cleared and the network is activated with new inputs. These are fed forward, the errors calculated, and the weights adjusted again by backpropagation. The cycle is repeated until the network gives acceptable performance.

Some things to keep in mind

When implementing a network such as the one described above, the number of input neurons depends on the form of the data being fed to the network and the number of output neurons depends on the desired output. However, the number of hidden neurons can be chosen freely. This presents a problem in selecting the network architecture. Having lots of hidden neurons will allow the network to encode a lot of information and likely will give good performance on any given dataset. The drawback to this is that such a network will easily become overtrained and specialized, and will only perform well on the dataset it was trained on. The choice of the number of hidden neurons really depends on what is being learned and is achieved by trial and error. A reasonable starting point is to use about 85% of the number of input neurons and then decrease the number of neurons until the network's performance drops steeply.

Another problem can be if one wants outputs that go beyond classification from zero to one. In the given examples it works quite well to transform the desired outputs using:

$$d_{\text{transformed}} = \frac{d_{\text{original}} - d_{\text{min}}}{d_{\text{max}} - d_{\text{min}}}$$

This normalizes the desired outputs to between zero and one and gives good performance when training the neural net. To read the outputs of the neural net the equation is simply solved for d_{original}.

Finally, due to the way in which the steepest descent algorithm works, it can get "stuck" in local minima. For this reason it is good to train a few versions of the neural net to see if they all converge at the same spot or if by chance one can shake out of a local minimum and try to find a global minimum. Numerous minimization algorithms have been developed to address this problem; when implementing these, the reader should look for algorithms such as momentum, Qprop, RProp, and Delta-bar-delta to more rapidly and robustly converge the network.

Creating the artificial neural net program

In this example we will create a simple ANN, train it on a dataset of known binders using a randomly selected training set, and create predicted output using a model organism. The success of the prediction will be evaluated at the end using known epitopes from this organism.

Dataset

To create a test database, 10000 "HLA-A2* 201" peptides were downloaded from www.immuneepitope.org [32]. For training, 50 strong positive 9-mers were selected at random and 50 negative 9-mers were downloaded. Similarly, 1000 positives and 1000 negatives were selected as 9-mers at random as a test dataset.

Encoding

The data were encoded as comma-separated values (csv) in a text file. Each amino acid is represented as a "1" on a 20-dimensional vector with the other values set to "0"; that is, Alanine (A) is encoded as "1,0,0, ... $n = 14$ ... 0,0,0" and Tyrosine (Y) is encoded as "0,0,0, ... $n = 14$ ... 0,0,1". Since there are 9 amino acids in the epitopes selected in the first step, the inputs are $20 \times 9 = 180$ digits long. The next line in each file is one digit long, encoding if the sequence preceding it is an epitope. The strong binders are given a "1," the negatives from the database a "0." At the end of the encoding process we have two csv files, one with 100 sequences of known binders and nonbinders to be used to train the neural net (Training Set.csv) and one with 2000 sequences of epitopes that the net should then classify (Test Set.csv) [33].

A neuron class

The principals discussed for a feedforward/backpropagation neural net can be used directly to program the net. First, the code for a Neuron class is created that has an Activation, which is simply a number that sums the activations the neuron receives. It has a Threshold, which is a numeric threshold as discussed above. It also has an Activation_Function() (in our case the sigmoid function above) and an Output, which is its Activation if it is an Input_Neuron or is the Activation_Function() applied to the Activation minus the Threshold. For simplicity it is useful to define the Derivative of the Neuron as well, as described above, as being Output * (1 - Output). Finally, the Neuron encodes a set of weights as a numeric array, the size of the array being chosen to be how many neurons in the following layer the individual Neuron is connected to.

A network class

The network can then be designed. It is constructed by defining the amount of Input_Neurons,

`Hidden_Neurons`, and `Output_Neurons`. For our network we will use 180 `Input_Neurons`, one for each digit in the encoded epitope. We can vary the number of `Hidden_Neurons` depending on performance, and we will have one `Output_Neuron`, where an output of "0" indicates the input is not an epitope and an output of "1" indicates the input is predicated to be an epitope.

The layers are initialized using an `Init_Layers()` function, which sets the weights and thresholds of all `Neurons` to small random numbers between −0.05 and 0.05.

The `FeedForward()` function first clears the `Activation` of all `Neurons` and then activates the `Input_Neurons` with the `Inputs`. It then computes the activation of each `Hidden_Neuron` by multiplying the `Output` of the `Input_Neuron` with the weight connecting that `Neuron` to the `Hidden_Neuron` and adding the result to the current `Activation` of the `Hidden_Neuron`; this is repeated for each `Input_Neuron`. Similarly, the `Output` of each `Hidden_Neuron` is then multiplied by the weight connecting that `Neuron` to the `Output_Neuron`. The function finally returns the `Output` of the `Output_Neuron`.

The `Backpropagate()` function starts by calculating the error in the `Output_Neurons Output`, computing the changes in weight for the `Hidden_Neurons`, then computing the changes in weight for the `Input_Neurons`. It then computes and updates the `Thresholds` for each `Neuron`. Finally, it applies the updates to all `Neurons`.

Finally, for ease of use, two functions are made accessible: `Train()` and `Analyze_Input()`. The `Train()` function accepts the `Inputs` and the desired result and goes through one cycle of `FeedForward()` and `Backpropagate()`. It returns the current error in the output. The `Analyze_Input()` function accepts the inputs, applies `FeedForward()`, and returns the `Output_Neuron`'s `Output`.

Using the network

Now that everything is set up, the network is trained with the 100 examples in the training set and quickly learns the dataset as seen in the rapid drop in error (Figure 9.6). We quickly arrive at

a classification rate that correctly identifies 87.7% of the 1000 true epitopes using a cutoff of 0.5. The same network correctly assigns a low value to 72.9% of the negatives.

Evaluating the performance of the network

ANNs and diagnostic determinations are commonly evaluated using receiver operating characteristic (ROC) curves. In this analysis, the true positive proportion (also the sensitivity) of the dataset is computed as the ratio of detected positives that are truly positive to the total number of known positives in the dataset. In the example, 877 of the known positives were assigned to be positive while the test dataset contained 1000 positives. The true positive proportion here is 0.877. Next, the false positive proportion is calculated as 1 − the ratio of the correctly identified negatives divided by the total number of known negatives. In our case this is 1 − 729 negatives identified over 1000 negatives known, or 1 − 0.729 = 0.271. The plot is then constructed by plotting the true positive proportion as a function of the false positive proportion. The individual points are created by shifting the cutoff value. Our neural net gives an `Output_Neuron.Output` value of > 0.99 for epitopes it classifies as such and of < 0.1 for negatives. However, some are in between, with values of 0.4 or 0.12. Sliding the threshold value starts capturing some of these as either epitopes or negatives. For example, if the cutoff is 0 then all outputs are classified as epitopes. This captures all the true positives, and our true positive proportion (TPP) is 1. The drawback of this, of course, is that now all the negatives are classified as epitopes and the false positive proportion (FPP) is also 1. The opposite happens when the cutoff is 1: all epitopes are classified as negatives (TPP and FPP = 0). By sliding the cutoff from 0 to 1 and plotting the resulting values for TPP versus FPP, one can create a ROC curve. If the neural net is guessing values between 0 and 1, the curve will be a 45 degree line through the graph from (0,0) to (1,1). If the neural net is a perfect classifier, all negatives will receive a value of 0 and all positives a value of 1, making the curve a 90 degree wedge – that is, as soon as the threshold exceeds 0 the FPP is 0 and the TPP is 1

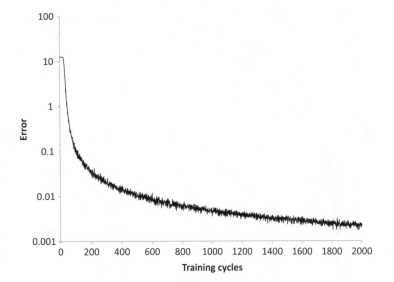

Figure 9.6 The artificial neural net learns the dataset minimizing error in the training set. The error over the training set, calculated as: $\frac{1}{2}\sum_i^n(O_i - d_i)^2$, begins close to the expected 12.5 ($1/2 * 100 * 0.5^2$) And rapidly decreases as the net learns the dataset.

until the threshold is 1, when the FPP is 1 and the TPP is 1.

To quantify the degree of proper classification one can calculate the area under the ROC curve. This A_{ROC} figure is commonly used to compare methods of classification and variables within a method. The perfect scenario is depicted by a curve with a line from (0,0) to (0,1) and from (0,1) to (1,1). The area under this curve is 1. The 45 degree line for random guesses encloses an area of 0.5. This can give boundaries to set for evaluating performance: $A_{ROC} = 1$ is perfect performance. $A_{ROC} = 0.5$ is random performance. Any system with a value above that has learned some information about classifying the dataset. In real systems, $A_{ROC} > 0.7$ is performing satisfactorily and a system with an $A_{ROC} > 0.85$ is performing well. Figure 9.7 shows the results of three training approaches, one with low training cycles, one with few examples, and one with a reasonable number of training cycles and many examples. Too few training cycles did not allow the neural net to learn the data and the $A_{ROC} = 0.5$ for the 20 cycles of training. The neural net with good training conditions performs well, with an $A_{ROC} = 0.895$. The matrix that was only presented 20 examples did a reasonable job of generalizing its training to the 2000 samples in the test set with an A_{ROC} of 0.834 as seen in Figure 9.7 [34].

Designing an epitope-based vaccine using the network

Having completed the validation of the network, we now want to use our simple neural net to create a vaccine. Since CD8[+] T-cells are involved in control of herpes simplex virus (HSV), we will choose a protein from HSV, run the trained neural net on it, and see how it performs against a known epitope group. There are eight reported HLA-A2*201 epitopes from the envelope glycoprotein D of HSV in the immune epitope database. The protein was downloaded from the NCBI (gi|81984907) and split into 386 9-mers each overlapping by 8 amino acids with the previous 9-mer in Excel. The 9-mers were encoded with the sparse matrix encoding described above and tested with the neural net trained for 2000 cycles.

Using the cutoff from above, 0.5, five out of eight (62.5%) of the known epitopes would have been identified. The neural net was able to significantly differentiate epitopes from non-epitopes ($p < 0.001$). This strategy of using the neural net to narrow down peptides would also have had significant cost cutting effects: from the nearly 400 peptides to be synthesized for the whole set, 48 off-target peptides would have been synthesized and the researcher would have captured 62.5% of the on-target epitopes. This was achieved despite

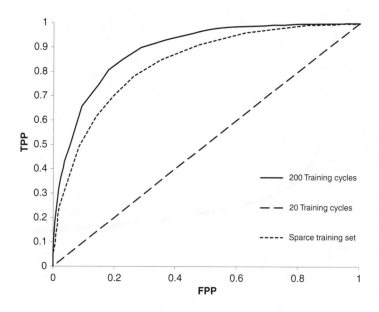

Figure 9.7 ROC curve for the training set and test set described in the text. After 20 training cycles the neural net is still giving random results. After 200 training cycles it has learned the dataset and 2000 or 20 000 cycles do not improve the ROC curve. A sparse training set of 20 examples gives reasonable performance in this setting that is far better than random, but worse than the 200 examples in the training set used.

the fact that we used straightforward encoding and performed little optimization of the neural net.

Conclusions

We have covered the use of sequence analysis as a decision tool using alignments and as a predictor for various types of epitopes. In the examples the reader should have gleaned how to implement sequence alignments and how to write software for both alignments and ANNs. The success of these simple examples in being powerful tools for creating new vaccines using homology in the first segment and in predicting epitopes in the second makes it clear that further development of these methods has the potential to cut laboratory costs and to accelerate scientific vaccine discovery. It is hoped that the predictive power of these applications will be sufficient at one point to make the use of computational approaches the first step in most vaccine discovery efforts.

References

1 Altman RB, Dunker AK, Hunter L, Klein TE. Preface. In RB ALltman, AK Dunker, Hunter L, *et al.* (Eds) *Pa-cific Symposium on Biocomputing 2009*. World Scientific, Hackensack, NJ, 2009.

2 Zodpey SP, Ambadekar NN, Thakur A. Effectiveness of Bacillus Calmette Guerin (BCG) vaccination in the prevention of leprosy: a population-based case-control study in Yavatmal District, India. *Public Health* 2005;**119**(3):209–16.

3 McShane H. Vaccine strategies against tuberculosis. *Swiss Med Wkly* 2009;**139**(11–12):156–60.

4 Smith DR, Richterich P, Rubenfield M, *et al.* Multiplex sequencing of 1.5 Mb of the *Mycobacterium leprae* genome. *Genome Res* 1997;**7**(8):802–19.

5 Zodpey SP, Shrikhande SN, Kulkarni SW, Maldhure BR. Scar size and effectiveness of Bacillus Calmette Guerin (BCG) vaccination in the prevention of tuberculosis and leprosy: a case-control study. *Indian J Public Health* 2007;**51**(3):184–9.

6 Goto Y, Bhatia A, Raman VS, *et al. Leishmania infantum* sterol 24-c-methyltransferase formulated with MPL-SE induces cross-protection against *L. major* infection. *Vaccine* 2009;**27**(21):2884–90.

7 Goto Y, Carter D, Reed SG. Immunological dominance of *Trypanosoma cruzi* tandem repeat proteins. *Infect Immun* 2008;**76**(9):3967–74.

8 Goto Y, Coler RN, Reed SG. Bioinformatic identification of tandem repeat antigens of the *Leishmania donovani* complex. *Infect Immun* 2007;**75**(2):846–51.

9 Needleman SB, Wunsch CD. A general method applicable to the search for similarities in the amino

acid sequence of two proteins. *J Mol Biol* 1970;**48**(3): 443–53.

10 Smith TF, Waterman MS. Identification of common molecular subsequences. *J Mol Biol* 1981;**147**(1): 195–7.

11 Farrar M. Striped Smith-Waterman speeds database searches six times over other SIMD implementations. *Bioinformatics* 2007;**23**(2):156–61.

12 Liu Y, Maskell DL, Schmidt B. CUDASW++: optimizing Smith-Waterman sequence database searches for CUDA-enabled graphics processing units. *BMC Res Notes* 2009;**2**: 73.

13 Wirawan A, Kwoh CK, Hieu NT, Schmidt B. CBESW: sequence alignment on the Playstation 3. *BMC Bioinformatics* 2008;**9**: 377.

14 Lipman DJ, Pearson WR. Rapid and sensitive protein similarity searches. *Science* 1985;**227**(4693):1435–41.

15 Altschul SF, Gish W, Miller W, Myers EW, Lipman DJ. Basic local alignment search tool. *J Mol Biol* 1990; **215**(3):403–10.

16 Altschul SF, Madden TL, Schaffer AA, *et al.* Gapped BLAST and PSI-BLAST: a new generation of protein database search programs. *Nucleic Acids Res* 1997; **25**(17):3389–402.

17 Lund O. Immunological bioinformatics. In *Computational Molecular Biology.* MIT Press, Cambridge, MA, 2005.

18 Vlček Č. Methods in Molecular Biology 395 and 396: Comparative Genomics. *Folia Microbiologica* 2008; **53**(3):271–2.

19 Eck RV, Dayhoff MO. *Atlas of Protein Sequence and Structure.* National Biomedical Research Foundation, 1966.

20 Henikoff S, Henikoff JG. Amino acid substitution matrices from protein blocks. *Proc Natl Acad Sci U S A* 1992;**89**(22):10915–19.

21 Agrawal A, Huang X. Pairwise statistical significance of local sequence alignment using multiple parameter sets and empirical justification of parameter set change penalty. *BMC Bioinformatics* 2009;**10** (Suppl 3):S1.

22 Altschul SF, Gish W. Local alignment statistics. *Methods Enzymol* 1996;**266**:460–80.

23 Mitrophanov AY, Borodovsky M. Statistical significance in biological sequence analysis. *Brief Bioinform* 2006;**7**(1):2–24.

24 Waterman MS, Vingron M. Rapid and accurate estimates of statistical significance for sequence data base searches. *Proc Natl Acad Sci U S A* 1994;**91**(11): 4625–8.

25 Burton DR, Stanfield RL, Wilson IA. Antibody vs. HIV in a clash of evolutionary titans. *Proc Natl Acad Sci U S A* 2005;**102**(42):14943–8.

26 Lin HH, Ray S, Tongchusak S, Reinherz EL, Brusic V. Evaluation of MHC class I peptide binding prediction servers: applications for vaccine research. *BMC Immunol* 2008;**9**: 8.

27 Lin HH, Zhang GL, Tongchusak S, Reinherz EL, Brusic V. Evaluation of MHC-II peptide binding prediction servers: applications for vaccine research. *BMC Bioinformatics* 2008;**9**(Suppl 12):S22.

28 Li S, Yao X, Liu H, Li J, Fan B. Prediction of T-cell epitopes based on least squares support vector machines and amino acid properties. *Anal Chim Acta* 2007;**584**(1):37–42.

29 Yang ZR, Johnson FC. Prediction of T-cell epitopes using biosupport vector machines. *J Chem Inf Model* 2005;**45**(5):1424–8.

30 Ponomarenko J, Bui HH, Li W, *et al.* ElliPro: a new structure-based tool for the prediction of antibody epitopes. *BMC Bioinformatics* 2008;**9**: 514.

31 Rubinstein ND, Mayrose I, Martz E, Pupko T. Epitopia: a web-server for predicting B-cell epitopes. *BMC Bioinformatics* 2009;**10**: 287.

32 Peters B, Sidney J, Bourne P, *et al.* The immune epitope database and analysis resource: from vision to blueprint. *PLoS Biol* 2005;**3**(3):e91.

33 Nielsen M, Lundegaard C, Worning P, *et al.* Reliable prediction of T-cell epitopes using neural networks with novel sequence representations. *Protein Sci* 2003;**12**(5):1007–17.

34 Posavad CM, Koelle D, Corey, L. High frequency of CD8$^+$ cytotoxic T-lymphocyte precursors specific for herpes simplex viruses in persons with genital herpes. *J Virol* 1996;**70**(11):8165–8.

CHAPTER 10

Antigen Discovery for Vaccines Using High-throughput Proteomic Screening Technologies

D. Huw Davies

School of Medicine, University of California at Irvine, Irvine, CA, USA

Introduction

A major aim of systems biology is the development of high-throughput (HT) technologies to determine functions of genome-encoded proteins. Such functions may be mediated through protein-protein, protein-carbohydrate, and protein-nucleic acid interactions. In the context of vaccine design I will focus on HT screening methods for antibody profiling of immune sera and identification of T-cell antigens, with emphasis on synthetic proteomes produced from expression libraries, or "ORFeomes." "High throughput" in this context can refer to any of the different stages in the antigen discovery process, including bioinformatic analysis, library construction, protein expression, antigen screening, patient sample analysis, and testing of vaccine candidates in preclinical studies.

The natural proteome is that obtained from a living cell, and is distinct from synthetic proteomes obtained in the laboratory from combinatorial polypeptide libraries (Figure 10.1). Natural proteomes do not comprise all of the proteins encoded in the genome. Instead only those genes that are expressed *in vivo* are represented. Inactive genes or those expressed at low levels may not be represented. For some applications this may be an advantage, whereas synthetic proteomes may be required where more comprehensive coverage of the proteome is required. The quantities of individual proteins in the natural proteome are also highly variable, and depend on several factors, including mRNA levels, translation efficiency, and protein degradation rate [1,2].

"Synthetic" proteomes

An alternative to the natural proteome is expression of individual genes directly from genomic nucleic acid. There are essentially three approaches to library construction:

1 *Genomic libraries.* In the genomic library approach, a genome is cleaved with restriction enzymes and the fragments cloned into a vector. As a rule the fragments are randomly generated from the genomic DNA. Genome libraries have been used for the direct production of synthetic proteomes (see for example [3]) although they are more widely used as the starting material for other, gene-specific cloning approaches.

2 *cDNA libraries.* Here, mRNA transcripts (the "transcriptome") are reverse transcribed into complementary DNA (cDNA) using a generic primer against the poly-(A) tail. This kind of library represents only the genes that are expressed in the

Vaccinology: Principles and Practice, First Edition. Edited by W. John W. Morrow, Nadeem A. Sheikh, Clint S. Schmidt and D. Huw Davies.
© 2012 Blackwell Publishing Ltd. Published 2012 by Blackwell Publishing Ltd.

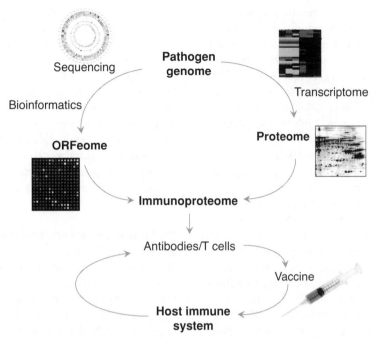

Figure 10.1 Overview of high-throughput (HT) approaches to antigen discovery for vaccines. The pre-genomic era approaches combined traditional biochemical and immunologic techniques that were slow and piecemeal. In the post-genomic era, available genomic sequence information has allowed essentially two complementary paths toward the development of vaccines. In one (right), the naturally expressed genome forms the starting material, which can be probed for gene expression levels (mRNA transcripts), or the proteome itself interrogated with antibodies or T cells from immune humans or animals, followed by mass spectrometry to identify recognized antigens (for example, see [84,115,116]). Sequence data is required to construct DNA arrays and to interpret the results of mass spectrometry. HT alternatives (left) use sequence data as the starting point. Individual open reading frames (ORFs) are cloned and expressed separately as a synthetic proteome. Whole antigens can also be substituted by synthetic peptide libraries for T-cell studies, although currently not suitable for proteome-wide approaches. Bioinformatic filtering to identify proteins with predicted antigenic properties is often used to refine larger libraries. This may include prediction of membrane proteins for antibody recognition or possession of MHC-binding motifs for T-cell recognition. Unlike the natural proteome where only those genes that were expressed are represented, levels of individual proteins in the ORFeome are independent of transcription levels. Synthetic proteomes are also interrogated with antibodies or T cells to identify recognized antigens. Candidate antigens are then tested in animal models for protection against challenge, although this still represents a bottleneck to HT screening for antigen discovery. Images credits as follows: genome sequence map [117]; 2D SDS PAGE [118]; transcriptome heat map [119]; proteome microarray (author].

pathogen, and is particularly suited to eukaryotic organisms as introns are spliced from fully transcribed eukaryotic mRNA. The cDNA library can then be readily expressed in a bacterial expression system.

3 *ORFeome libraries.* The third approach is the so-called "ORFeome" library approach, in which individual open reading frames (ORFs) in the pathogen are amplified from genomic template by PCR (or RT-PCR in the case of RNA viruses). Unlike the two former approaches, the ORFeome approach is unbiased (independent of the transcriptome) but does require knowledge of the genome sequence in order to design gene-specific primers.

The main advantage of cDNA and ORFeome expression libraries over the natural proteome is that the gene products can be resolved at the clonal level (colony picking). Therefore each protein can be analyzed at a level of purity that can rarely be matched by fractionation of the natural proteome on two-dimensional (2D) gels or by other biochemical means. It is conventional to assay synthetic proteomes in indexed matrices – for example, microarrays for antibody screening, and 96-well plates for T cells.

At the heart of any synthetic ORFeome approach is the need to rapidly obtain transcriptionally active ORFs that can be expressed into protein. PCR is the method of choice provided genomic sequence and template for PCR is available. The amplicons are then expressed into protein directly after cloning into a suitable expression vector by an HT ligase-free recombination cloning such as the commercially available systems (e.g., Gateway from Invitrogen) [4], or homologous recombination *in vivo* [5] or *in vitro* [6]. PCR amplicons can also be expressed directly without cloning, so-called "transcriptionally active PCR" (TAP) [5,7]. This increases throughput but in most cases a plasmid library is preferable as this can be replicated.

Both the cDNA and ORFeome approaches have their pros and cons. The cDNA library approach has the advantage that it focuses on expressed genes only, and because it provides a way to express eukaryotic proteomes in prokaryotic cells. The cons are related to the variable representation of different cDNA species according to transcript abundance. High-level mRNA expression does not automatically correlate with protein abundance in the proteome because of post-translational regulatory mechanisms [1]. This variability is overcome by the ORFeome library approach, in which each ORF in the genome is obtained by PCR using gene-specific primers. Because the identity of each gene is known before the library is constructed, the ORFeome can also be refined before construction. For example, it may be desirable to focus only on genes whose products have a predicted surface location in the organism. Limitations of the ORFeome approach include the requirement for genomic sequence for the design of PCR primers and the availability of good quality genomic DNA for the PCR template (or RNA for RT-PCR). These conditions

may be unmet, particularly for new or emerging pathogens. Larger genes (>2–3 kb) are difficult to amplify and usually have to be cloned in fragments. Moreover, DNA with high G+C content has a higher *Tm* and is inherently more difficult to amplify by PCR. Also problematic are eukaryotic pathogens whose coding sequences are interrupted by introns. Here, individual exons can be amplified and cloned, although this considerably increases the number of "ORFs." For example, the apicomplexan parasite *Toxoplasma gondii* has 8155 genes, although this represents >43 000 individual exons [8].

Protein expression: cell-based versus cell-free

Once the expression library is obtained, it is necessary to translate each gene into protein so that they can then be interrogated for recognition by antibodies or T cells. Cell-based expression systems are well established and indeed form the foundation for much of the biotechnology industry. *E. coli* is the cell of choice, although yeast and other eukaryotic cells are available if glycosylation is required. The main advantages of cell-based expression versus cell-free are low cost and high yield. However, not all proteins are "expressible" *in vivo* and the genes may need modifying, such as by codon optimization or removal of hydrophobic transmembrane and signal sequences. Proteins that do express *in vivo* may also be unstable or rapidly degraded, or insoluble and form inclusion bodies, particularly those with hydrophobic features. Inclusion bodies then need to be solubilized in some way (usually in urea, which then needs to be gradually removed by dialysis) before they can be used in functional assays.

Cell-free protein synthesis is an *in vitro* system that rapidly converts template DNA into functional proteins in a few hours. The speed and convenience of cell-free expression provides an attractive alternative to more time consuming cell-based methods. Cell-free synthesis is commonly based on the transcription and translation machinery of *E. coli* and is available in kit form from commercial suppliers (such as Expressway™ by Invitrogen and *E. coli* HY RTS from 5 Prime). For eukaryotic expression, lysates derived from rabbit reticulocytes (TNT® Reticulocyte Lysate from Promega) and wheat germ (RTS Wheat from 5 Prime, TNT® Wheat Germ Extract from Promega) are also available. Most allow the transcription and translation reactions to be conducted in the same reaction tube, so-called "coupled" *in vitro* transcription/translation (IVTT). A major advantage is that the proteins that are expressed in cell-free systems are usually soluble, which is especially important for proteins with hydrophobic signal sequences and transmembrane domains such as membrane proteins. In one laboratory where ORFeomes have been expressed in cell-free *E. coli* lysates for several pathogens, expression rates, determined using monoclonal antibodies to N- and C-terminal epitope tags, are consistently in excess of 95% for bacteria [9–11], although somewhat lower for eukaryotic parasites [8,12–14]. The main disadvantages preventing wider adoption of cell-free expression systems are high cost and low yield, although this is less significant for miniaturized HT platforms such as microarrays where reactions of only a few microliters are required.

Protein purification

Once expressed, recombinant proteins then need to be configured into an immunologic screening assay in an HT fashion. This usually requires some form of purification because contaminants may have nonspecific reactivity that interferes with an immunologic screen. For example, *E. coli* contaminants are readily recognized by human sera, which overwhelm any specific reactivity to the recombinant protein of interest. *E. coli* contaminants are also powerful T-cell mitogens and have an analogous effect on T-cell assays. Protein purification still remains a bottleneck that will hinder most HT immunologic screening [15].

Affinity column chromatography

Proteins expressed from ORFeomes are engineered at the cloning stage to express C- and/or N-terminal tags, such as polyhistidine or fusion partners such as glutathione *S*-transferase (GST), to facilitate purification by traditional nickel-chelate or glutathione affinity chromatography, respectively.

For nickel columns, optimal purity and yield is achieved by using custom-designed protocols for each protein with optimized binding and elution conditions. This approach can be used for virtually any organism with significant investments of time and resources, as has been accomplished for *E. coli* [16], yeast [17], and human [18] proteomes. However, such resources are often beyond the reach of most research laboratories. HT purification on nickel-chelate resins can be achieved in 96-well plates (www.nature.com/protocolexchange/protocols/402), which are also available as kits (such as Ni-NTA Superflow from Qiagen, or His-Pur* Ni-NTA Spin Plates from Thermo). Ultimately, such methods use generic protocols, and purity and yield will inevitably be suboptimal. GST-fusion proteins, which can be purified using a standardized glutathione capture method, is probably preferable for HT purification since the binding requirements are more uniform between different proteins. Glutathione resins are also available in HT format (such as Glutathione Spin Plates from Pierce). Purifying ORFeomes semi-manually can be a *tour de force*, but has been accomplished for a few pathogens, including severe acute respiratory syndrome (SARS) virus [19], and the plague organism *Yersinia pestis* [20]. Automated HT protein purification is under development [21–23] and is likely to have a major impact on this field in the near future.

In situ tag capture

True proteome-wide screening is best achieved by circumventing traditional purification methods altogether. HT expression *in vitro* by IVTT or *in vivo* is often conducted in small volumes [10–100 μL]. These small quantities are sufficient for sensitive antibody and T-cell screens, particularly in miniaturized formats such as microarrays (discussed below). However, these volumes are too small to be purified by conventional column-based purification approaches. Instead, tag capture can be used to purify the antigen *in situ*, within the immunoassay platform itself. For example, nickel-coated substrates, such as ELISA plates or polystyrene beads, can be used to capture recombinant antigens with engineered polyhistidine tags present in IVTT reactions or lysates of cells expressing the protein *in vivo*, and washed free of contaminants. Similarly, GST fusion proteins can be captured with immobilized glutathione. Proteins can also be captured using immobilized antibodies against specific epitope tags or fusion partners translated in-frame with the recombinant antigen. The affinity of the antibody-antigen interaction (10^{-6}–10^{-9} M) is generally higher than the nickel-polyhistidine interaction (10^{-6} M).

Unpurified proteins

Challenges that currently exist to HT protein purification have spawned the development of antigen-screening methods that use the crude protein mixtures (whole IVTT, whole cells), thereby completely obviating the purification bottleneck. This introduces special challenges for antigen discovery, in particular the mitogenic effect of crude bacterial lysates for T cells, and nonspecific antibody reactivity. The solutions to these challenges are discussed in the relevant sections below.

HT antibody screening

Antibodies are exquisitely specific for particular antigens, are rapidly amplified after initial exposure to antigen, and are sustained for long periods. Serum (or plasma) itself can be collected and stored for long periods and shipped with ease. For these reasons antibodies represent versatile biomarkers for diagnosing exposure to infectious agents and for monitoring vaccination. Proteomic approaches enable sera to be probed against hundreds or thousands of proteins simultaneously, and considerably increase the rate of antigen discovery compared to traditional immunologic methods. Below is an overview of proteomic approaches.

2D gel electrophoresis and peptide mass fingerprinting

The ability to resolve protein mixtures according to molecular weight on sodium dodecyl sulfate poly-acrylamide electrophoresis (SDS PAGE) has been available since the 1970s [24]. While adequate for simple mixtures, natural proteomes that may comprise thousands of different proteins need to be resolved on large 2D gels, using isoelectric focusing in the first dimension followed by separation according to molecular weight in the second. Resolved proteins can then be transferred to nitrocellulose membranes and probed with immune sera to identify immunoreactive spots, so-called "western" or immunoblotting [25]. In the early 1990s 2D gel technology, coupled with the technique of peptide mass fingerprinting, forged much of the early progress in proteomics in the post-genomic era. Individual immunoreactive proteins of unknown identity are cut from the 2D blot, trypsinized into peptides, and their masses accurately measured using a matrix-assisted laser desorption ionization – time of flight (MALDI-TOF) mass spectrometer. The masses are then compared to protein databases such as Swiss-Prot and GenBank using software that generates lists of the masses of theoretical fragments and matches the experimental and predicted peptides. This is a mature technique and has been applied to immunoproteome mapping of several pathogens, including *Bordetella pertussis* (whooping cough) [26], *Bacillus anthracis* (anthrax) [27], and *Treponema pallidum* (syphilis) [28].

An advantage of the 2D gel approach is that it can resolve different isoforms of a single protein, such as proteins within cells that have multiple phosphorylation states. The presence of such isoforms cannot be easily determined from the gene sequence alone. Disadvantages include the requirement for proteins to be denatured in the SDS-PAGE dimension, which will alter the native conformation and will influence detection by conformation-dependent antibodies. Fortunately, there seem to be plenty of antibodies that recognize non-native epitopes in a typical antibody response.

Ultimately, 2D PAGE gels coupled to MALDI-TOF microscopy is a technique that is unsuitable for screening large numbers of sera. For this, miniaturization onto microarrays is more appropriate. In lieu of synthetic ORFeome libraries, there have been attempts to fractionate the natural proteome by biochemical methods and print fractions onto arrays. For example, Sartain and colleagues [29] used sequential rounds of ammonium sulfate precipitation and anion exchange chromatography to resolve the native *M. tuberculosis* cytosol and culture filtrate protein mixtures into 960 unique fractions. The fractions, which comprised mostly simple protein mixtures, were then printed onto protein microarrays and probed with several human TB-immune sera. This approach, which revealed several novel antibody targets, increased the throughput of sera that could be screened over conventional 2D gel methods. However, it is not a widely used technique and, like the 2D gels, the proteins displayed on the arrays are reflective of expression levels *in vivo*.

ELISA

The enzyme-linked immunosorbant assay is another mature technology for which the expertise and necessary equipment, such as ELISA plate readers, are present in virtually all diagnostic laboratories. The ELISA is conventionally used for assaying multiple samples against single purified antigens and does not immediately come to mind when discussing HT screening technologies. However, in the post-genomic era the ELISA format can be used as a convenient substrate to immobilize ORFeomes expressed in cell-free or cell-based systems, for example SARS corona virus [19] and *Treponema pallidum* [30].

Bead arrays

Small latex beads can be coated with different antigens, and cocktails of differently coated beads can be incubated in a serum sample. Provided the beads can be distinguished in some way, this approach can be used as a multi-antigen screening system. The Luminex Corp. has a proprietary fluorescent bead system in which beads are labeled with two (or more) different flurophores. When present in different ratios these fluorophores provide many different colors (up to 500 are possible) that can be distinguished using a flow cytometer or a dedicated Luminex® machine. It is a true HT multi-antigen (multiplex) platform, in that multiple antigens can be screened with many samples simultaneously. Luminex is well suited to multiplex diagnostic applications, and defined serodiagnostic antigens from several pathogens, including *Streptococcus pneumoniae* [31–33], *Haemophilus influenzae*

and *Neisseria meningitides* [34], human papilloma viruses (HPV) [35], and *Bordetella pertussis* [36], among others, have been developed into diagnostic tests. In theory, small proteome mining studies (<500 antigens) are also possible using the Luminex platform, although it is less suitable for larger screens.

Protein microarrays

Protein microarrays consist of individual proteins immobilized onto a substrate in an indexed high-density format (generally several thousand per cm^2) using a mechanical printer. In many respects they are like miniature ELISAs. The development of protein microarrays has followed on from the DNA microarrays before them, and in most cases the printers, scanners, and analysis software used are identical to those used for DNA arrays. While different oligonucleotides have uniform stability and binding properties, proteins have widely different biochemical properties according to the primary amino acid sequence. Consequently, different proteins have differing solubility and substrate binding properties, which need to be accommodated in an HT fashion. Ideally this should be achieved without resorting to custom protocols for each protein, which would otherwise impede throughput. The main advantages of the microarray come from miniaturization. Multiple replicate arrays each consisting of several hundred or thousand proteins can be accommodated on a single slide, allowing multiple sera samples to be probed simultaneously. For example, a slide may have 16, 8, 3, or 1 array(s), which can display approximately 256, 1156, 4624, or >13,872 unique spots, respectively. The small size of each array also means only a few microliters of sera are required. For these reasons, the array has found preference over the ELISA for HT antigen discovery.

The original protein microarrays were antibody arrays, such as the anti-cytokine antibody arrays widely used to identify cytokines present in cell culture supernatants or in sera (Figure 10.2). Monoclonal antibodies against cytokines have been available for many years, and although each antibody is technically a different protein, different antibodies have very similar and predictable biochemical

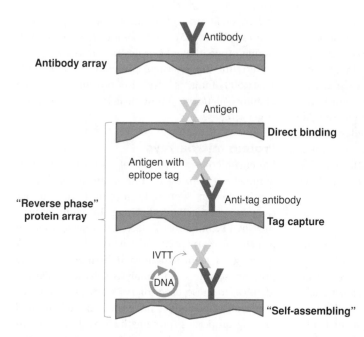

Figure 10.2 Different protein microarray formats. The first protein arrays were antibodies immobilized onto glass or other substrates. Antigen (or "reverse phase") arrays can be produced by direct binding of antigen to the substrate, for example to nitrocellulose, or via tag capture, such as nickel-polyhistidine or antibody-epitope interactions. Arrays can also be assembled *in situ* using immobilized DNA template-directed expression of protein in IVTT and simultaneous tag capture. See text for details.

properties. For this reason, antibody arrays were among the first to be produced. More recently, arrays of divergent proteins have been produced, such as natural proteomes from cell lysates [29], and synthetic proteomes from expression libraries expressed in IVTT [37–39]. Such arrays have many applications but here we focus on the discovery of the antigen targets of antibodies. This kind of array is traditionally termed a "reverse-phase" protein microarray to distinguish it from the original antibody arrays. The specific challenges of producing large numbers of biochemically disparate proteins and immobilizing them on arrays in an efficient HT way has been addressed in different ways.

Tag capture

Proteins expressed in IVTT reactions or cells *in vivo* can be immobilized to a substrate as they are translated via capture of tags in-frame with the antigen polypeptide (e.g., polyhistidine, GST). Sometimes referred to as protein *in situ* arrays (PISA) [40], these have the advantage that the protein is semipurified in the process and provides an HT alternative to traditional purification methods. As discussed above, the efficiency of the capture process is dependent on the affinity of the interaction

and the accessibility of the tag in the synthesized protein.

Self-assembling arrays or nucleic acid programmable protein arrays

Pioneered by J. LaBaer and colleagues, this approach uses a combination of DNA array and *in situ* protein expression and purification by tag capture. Protein-encoding expression plasmids are first printed on microarrays and co-printed with protein-capturing antibody. When required, the arrays are then incubated in IVTT reaction mix and newly synthesized proteins are captured in the vicinity of the arrayed DNA template [41–44]. In addition to the benefit of protein purification *in situ*, other advantages of this approach include the ability to generate the proteins immediately prior to use, and the relatively consistent protein concentrations captured on the array. The nucleic acid programmable protein array (NAPPA) approach has been used to profile the antibody response to pathogens, including varicella zoster virus [45] and *Pseudomonas aeruginosa* [46], as well as the autoimmune antibody profile to discover markers for autoimmune disease [47] and cancer [48]. This self-assembling approach can also be used to prepare antigen-coated Luminex beads [49,50].

Nitrocellulose substrate arrays

Nitrocellulose membrane, which has been in use for decades for immunoblotting applications, is particularly efficient at binding soluble proteins regardless of their size, charge, hydrophobicity, conformation, or presence of signal sequences or transmembrane helices. Because of this universal protein-binding property, no *in situ* purification is afforded by nitrocellulose and any contaminants will also be displayed. This substrate is ideal for antibody arrays where pure monoclonals are available. For ORFeome arrays, however, the bottleneck of protein purification has limited its popularity. Nevertheless, printing of *E. coli*-based IVTT directly onto nitrocellulose without any purification circumvents this, provided steps are taken to remove any antibodies to the IVTT reaction components in the sera tested. In particular, human serum has antibodies to *E. coli*, which will mask specific antibody expressed in *E. coli*-based expression systems. This reactivity can be readily blocked using *E. coli* lysate, thereby revealing the antigen-specific signal. This relatively simple approach has been successfully applied to the discovery of antibody targets in the ORFeomes of several pathogens, including vaccinia virus [51–54], *M. tuberculosis* [11], *Plasmodium falciparum* [13,55,56], *Brucella melitensis* [57], *Chlamydia trachomatis* [58], *Francisella tularensis* [59,60], *Burkholderia pseudomallei* [9], *Coxiella burnetii* [61–63], *Borrelia burgdorferi* [64], *Bartonella henselae* [65], *Toxoplasma gondii* [66], *Candida albicans* [67], *Schistosoma mansoni* [14] *Schistosoma japonicum* [14], and HPV [68].

Conformation issues

Proteins expressed in *E. coli* are often assumed to be non-native and lack conformation-dependent epitopes. However, a protein molecule folds spontaneously during synthesis into a shape that is the most thermodynamically stable. This process is usually driven by forces that maximize exposure of hydrophilic groups and minimize exposure of hydrophobic groups, and no input energy is needed. In contrast, denaturation is not a spontaneous process, and requires input of energy in the form of heat, radiation, shearing, or chemical denaturants. Thus, proteins expressed in *E. coli*-based IVTT reactions or *in vivo* may not automatically become non-native. Regardless, such proteins are very effective for detecting antibodies, despite the lack of any post-translational modification, such as glycosylation, disulfide-bond formation, or assembly into higher-order structures. Production in prokaryotes also facilitates manufacturing. Antigens that are bound directly to solid substrates, such as nitrocellulose, may also adopt non-native configurations. If this is a concern, recombinant proteins can be assayed in solution, such as the liquid phase LIPS microbead assay [38], or captured via a linker or fusion partner such as GST to help preserve the native conformation.

T-cell screening platforms

T-cell assays require both live T cells as responders and antigen-presenting cells (APCs) to present antigenic peptide in the context of surface-expressed major histocompatibility complex (MHC) molecules (see Chapter 3). These requirements considerably increase the complexity of T-cell assay compared to antibody screening. Tissue culture equipment is thus required. A limiting step on the number of antigens that can be screened is the availability of T cells, which may necessitate the expansion of polyclonal T-cell cultures or "lines" *in vitro* to obtain sufficient numbers prior to screening, or miniaturization of the assay. Moreover, certain microbial components such as LPS or prokaryotic DNA may be found contaminating antigens expressed in *E. coli* or in IVTT reactions typically used for HT applications, even in ostensibly highly purified proteins. Such components are powerful mitogens (i.e., cause antigen-independent, polyclonal T-cell activation) and completely overwhelm any antigen-specific responses being measured. Overall, these problems make proteome-wide T-cell antigen discovery challenging. Fortunately, T cells are insensitive to the original conformation of the antigen prior to enzymatic cleavage (or antigen "processing"), thereby obviating many of the conformation issues that face antibody screening.

Different T-cell responses can be measured according to the type of T cell, and include proliferation, cytotoxicity, and release of cytokines such as IFN-γ and IL2 into the culture medium. Some of the older, more cumbersome assays for measuring cytotoxicity (^{51}Cr-release) and proliferation (^{3}H-thymidine uptake) have been replaced with more convenient, nonradioactive methods such as CFSE staining for proliferation [69], and lactate dehydrogenase release from killed cells for cytotoxicity. These in turn are gradually being superseded by cell-surface activation markers that can be quantified by flow cytometry. For example, CD154 [70, 71] and co-expression of CD25 and CD134 are useful markers of CD4 T-cell activation [72,73]. CD137 is proving a useful marker for activated CD8 T cells [74,75].

The measurement of cytokine released into culture medium, previously performed by ELISA or bioassay, is now routinely performed by intracellular cytokine staining (ICS) using flow cytometry. This technique, coupled with surface phenotyping, is simpler, higher throughput, and provides significantly more information than traditional methods. Automated loading of samples from tubes or 96-well plates allows rapid sampling. Most modern flow cytometers can measure many different fluorophores simultaneously. The upper limit to the number of cytokines that can be measured depends on the number of different lasers, although 6, 8, and 10 color flow is common. If the simultaneous measurement of more cytokines is important, the fluorescent Luminex bead approach can accomplish this. Antibodies against individual cytokines attached to beads of a particular color signature are available from vendors, and are used by researchers to assay cytokines from culture supernatants. Panels of beads are available that measure 30 or more different cytokines simultaneously, and can be used to measure panels of proinflammatory cytokines, immunomodulatory cytokines, panels characteristic of different T-cell subsets (e.g., Th1 and Th2 cells), and other applications. All of these developments open up the opportunity for HT T-cell screening that was hitherto impossible.

Peptide libraries and predictive algorithms

The use of synthetic peptides to fine map T-cell epitopes is a technology that has been in existence since the mid-1980s, when it was first recognized that synthetic peptides could substitute for the products of natural antigen processing displayed on the surface of APCs [76]. Conventionally, overlapping synthetic peptides are constructed spanning the antigen(s) of interest, which are then incubated with APCs and used in assays with MHC-matched responder T cells. In addition to the availability of T cells, the main constraint to HT peptide screening is the cost of peptide synthesis. This effectively precludes proteome-wide searches, but can be addressed in two ways. First, computational prediction of epitopes from primary amino acid sequences can be utilized. Algorithms based on a combination of properties (MHC allele-specific binding motifs, TAP transporter binding motifs, and known processing enzyme cleavage sites) are used to identify candidate epitopes, which can then be prioritized for synthesis based on the prediction score [77,78]. Curated databases of experimentally defined epitopes help refine these algorithms [79–81]. The second approach is by miniaturization of existing assays to minimize peptide quantities needed and/or to allow more peptides to be screened with the same number of T cells [82]. Downsizing T-cell cultures will reduce the sensitivity of the assay, since clones with the lowest responder frequencies will approach undetectable numbers or be lost altogether.

MHC-peptide elution

A more direct approach to identifying potential T-cell epitopes is to elute MHC-bound peptides at low pH from infected cells and sequence the eluted peptides using mass spectrometry [83,84]. In the absence of any infectious agent, MHC class I and II molecules present a vast number of different "self" peptides to the outside world. The T-cell receptor repertoire is essentially blind to these peptides owing to the mechanisms of central and peripheral tolerance. During an infection, however, foreign peptides are displayed to which T cells will respond. The analysis of naturally processed peptides has been applied to a number of pathogens, including vaccinia [85] and *Chlamydia* [86].

ORFeome expression libraries

In practice, expression libraries are probably the most suitable approach for HT and comprehensive (proteome-wide) screening of T-cell antigens. For CD4 T cells, antigens are usually delivered exogenously to APCs so that soluble protein is taken in by endocytosis and delivered to the MHC class II export pathway (see Chapter 3). True proteome-wide CD4 T-cell antigen mapping has been accomplished in a few cases using ORFeome expression libraries expressed in IVTT reactions or in *E. coli in vivo*. To circumvent the protein purification bottleneck, whole IVTT or fixed bacteria can be used, but in each case the mitogenicity of the bacterial components present has to be mitigated. Jing and colleagues, using IVTT to identify antigens in OR-Feome libraries of HSV and vaccinia, accomplish this by diluting the IVTT to submitogenic concentrations [87,88]. Co-dilution of the antigen is compensated by the use of enriched T-cell lines to increase the T-cell responder frequency. ORFeomes expressed in bacteria have also been used directly to map antigens recognized by Th17 cells in *Streptococcus pneumoniae* [89]. Here, mitogencity is mitigated by a two-step procedure in which the recombinant bacteria (chemically fixed to sterilize them) are first incubated with APCs separately from the responder T cells. The bacteria, containing the recombinant antigen cargo, are internalized and processed within the APC. After processing (~4 h) the cells are washed, fixed, and presented to the T cells and the cytokine response measured.

Antigens can also be purified *in situ* by tag capture and used to deliver antigen to APC, where it is processed and presented to T cells in a conventional T-cell assay. For example, Turner and colleagues developed a bead capture system using polyhistidine tag [90,91]. This method has recently been demonstrated to have utility for T-cell antigen discovery using a small (45 ORF) *Francisella tularensis* expression library [92,93]. HT T-cell screening of proteomes is a new field, and similar studies are in the pipeline.

For CD8 T cells the antigen needs to be introduced into the cytosol, either as preformed protein using a lipid delivery vehicle, or via an expression plasmid or recombinant virus that instructs the transcription and translation of the antigen within the cytosol. This route ensures the antigen is delivered to the class I MHC processing pathway for presentation to CD8 T cells. Koelle and colleagues have pioneered the use HT transfection of expression vectors in 96-well plates to deliver the HSV ORFeome and map reactive antigens recognized by human cytotoxic T cells [94–96].

Strategies for identification of protective antigens

Once a proteome has been interrogated, one or more of the antigens discovered must be selected for testing in animal models for protection. The number of candidates to test can be large and downselection based on a rational system is needed. For antibody-inducing vaccines, precedence is normally given to candidates that are related to known protective antigens in other pathogens. In bacterial pathogens these might be surface structures such as membrane proteins, flagellins, pili proteins, secretion system components, or heat shock proteins. In viruses, these may be membrane, capsid, or tegument proteins. Any overlap between antibody and T-cell target antigens may also be used to prioritize candidates [92, 97]. In contrast, a T-cell vaccine is required to eliminate intracellular infections or tumor cells. This can be mediated by both CD4 (Th1-mediated respiratory burst) and CD8 (cytotoxic) T cells. There are many more potential epitopes encoded than are actually displayed, and additional methods are needed to determine which of these immunodominant epitopes are protective [98]. Unlike antibodies, which need to access surface structures, protective T-cell epitopes could be expressed anywhere in the proteome of the pathogen. In practice, this is determined by immunizing animals with selected antigens or peptide epitopes and evaluating protection.

DNA vaccination

Another challenge is whether to administer single antigens, or whether multiple antigens are required. Single antigens can confer complete or partial protection against many pathogens, which can be improved by combining into cocktails, for example in vaccinia [99] or meningococcus [100]. For testing very large numbers of experimental vaccines, purification of proteins in *E. coli* or other expression systems presents a bottleneck. For this, DNA vaccination is an expeditious alternative route to primary screening without the need to purify protein and formulate in adjuvant. DNA vaccination is discussed in detail elsewhere in this book (Chapter 18). Most animals (with the notable exception of humans) respond well to naked DNA vaccines. Thus, the testing of candidates discovered from antibody or T-cell screening of expression libraries can be made directly from the DNA.

Discovery of protective antigens

Extracting the best information from a proteomic screening platform requires careful choice of the source of antibodies or T cells that are screened. A simple comparison of disease cases with disease-free controls is likely to reveal both protective antigens and other antigens that play no role in protection. In the context of vaccine design, it is desirable to compare disease cases that are protected or unprotected. For example, probing a *P. falciparum* partial proteome microarray with sera from children in Mali revealed IgG responses to hundreds of different parasite antigens [13]. The magnitude and breadth of the parasite-specific antibody profile increases incrementally with each malaria season, so that after several years of exposure, immunity to malaria is gradually acquired. Interestingly, infected children who were free of malaria had responses to 49 antigens that were significantly higher than in age-matched children who suffered from malaria. These antigens may represent a significant part of the protective response.

Similar protected and unprotected states can also be achieved by successful and unsuccessful vaccination, such as against malaria using the irradiated sporozoite vaccine [12,55]. In *F. tularensis* infection,

some mice strains are protected by the live vaccine stain (LVS) of *F. holarctica* while other strains are not [101]. Probing sera from protected mice on 2D gels revealed antibodies to at least six proteins that were not recognized by sera from unprotected mice. Asymptomatic and symptomatic herpes simplex infections represent another example of naturally occurring protection [102]. Proteomic screening of T- and B-cell responses of these two disease states is yet to be performed, but should reveal interesting insights into acquired immunity that could be emulated by vaccination.

In addition to the discovery of protective vaccine candidates, large-scale protein analyses can also be used to tease out other useful antigens with diagnostic applications. IVTT protein microarrays alone have helped in the discovery of markers that distinguish acute and chronic infection in *Toxoplasmosis* [66], latent and active tuberculosis [11], wild-type and attenuated or killed smallpox and *Chlamydia* vaccines [54,58], and human and animal hosts of *Borrelia burgdorferi* [64], vaccinia [51], and *Brucella melitensis* [57]. Clearly there is much scope for a new generation of diagnostics able to assess disease status and monitor vaccination.

Translation of HT screening into protective vaccines

While reports describing proteome-wide antigen discovery continue to increase, translating these data into successful new vaccines is more challenging. Often multiple antigens may be required, particularly in complex organisms such as bacteria. Particular adjuvants may also be required to elicit the appropriate response. Moreover, as discussed in Chapter 1, the relationship between responses to specific antigens that can be measured, and responses that mediate protection, is not well understood. Many antibody or T-cell targets detected may be misleading. Consequently the list of such examples is relatively small but growing. Below are just a few examples that show that even some basic understanding of the nature of protective immunity should be used to design the most relevant readout for screening.

Neisseria meningitides

This organism was among the first bacterial genomes to be fully sequenced and mined for vaccine candidate antigens *in silico* [103,104]. This landmark study ushered in the post-genomic era of vaccinology, where traditional crude live preparations were to be replaced by genome-based approaches, a process termed "reverse vaccinology" by Rappuoli [105]. *N. meningitidis* causes meningococcal meningitis and bacterial septicemia, and is particularly lethal in children and young adults. One of the main challenges for vaccine development is the antigenic variability of surface proteins. Even while the sequencing of *N. meningitidis* was in progress, the unassembled DNA sequences were being searched for membrane proteins and other surface-exposed structures using predictive algorithms [104]. Antibodies were raised to 350 candidate antigens expressed in *E. coli*, and each screened for binding to *N. meningitidis* bacteria in ELISA or flow cytometry and in complement fixation assays. Genome mining in this way revealed many candidate vaccine antigens, some variable and others conserved. Currently a lead candidate is the variable factor H binding protein (fHBP) [106], whereas a 5-mer cocktail of antigens discovered by reverse vaccinology provides protection against ~90% of 85 different global strains [100]. Progress with developing meningococcal vaccines since this breakthrough study has been reviewed recently [107].

Treponema pallidum

This organism is the causative agent of syphilis. A library of GST fusion proteins representing 85% of the *T. palladium* proteome was purified *in situ* on ELISA plates coated with glutathione and probed with immune rabbit [30] or human sera [108]. Over 140 reactive antigens were discovered; some were previously known but many were novel antigens. A candidate vaccine antigen that reacted well against human and rabbit sera, TP0136, was selected on the basis of predicted type II secretion signal sequence and relative abundance of transcripts in infected cells, and was subsequently found to confer protection in the rabbit model [109].

Streptococcus pneumoniae

S. pneumoniae causes pneumococcal pneumonia, and is a leading cause of mortality in the very young. The elderly or individuals who are immunocompromised are also particularly at risk. IL17-secreting CD4 T cells (Th17 cells) are believed to play a major role in mucosal immunity against several different bacteria, including *S. pneumoniae*. Recombinant-protein vaccines are particularly attractive for cost effective control in resource-poor countries, although the main candidate antigens have been chosen on the basis of surface location on the bacterium and generation of antibody. Protective T-cell antigens, however, are likely to be represented throughout the proteome. Moffitt and colleagues developed an HT CD4 T-cell screening system to identify antigens in *S. pneumoniae* that stimulate Th17 [89]. An expression library representing >96% of the proteome was expressed in *E. coli* BL21 cells and the cells fixed in paraformaldehyde. To assay the library, the fixed *E. coli* were "fed" to APCs for 2 hours prior to fixation and adding to purified CD4 T cells from mice immunized with killed unencapsulated pneumococcal whole-cell antigen vaccine. After 3 days, IL17 was assayed by ELISA. The large number of "hits" was refined to 17 antigens by bioinformatic filtering to eliminate antigens related to other bacteria or human antigens. Five were purified on nickel-chelate columns, of which two showed significant protection in mice against pneumococcal colonization that was CD4- and IL17-dependent. This study nicely demonstrates the power of expression libraries for T-cell screening and may open up opportunities for similar studies in other mucosal bacteria.

Chlamydia trachomatis

Chlamydia is a sexually transmitted bacterial infection and a leading cause of pelvic inflammatory disease and ectopic pregnancy in women, and infertility in both men and women. In developing countries, *C. trachomatis* is also the leading cause of infection-related blindness. Since the bacterium adopts a predominantly intracellular infection, it is likely both antibodies and T cells will be required to mediate protective immunity from vaccines. In one recent study [97], a subset of 120 antigens (representing ~13% of the proteome), which had been prioritized previously by bioinformatic filtering for peripherally located proteins [110], was cloned and expressed in *E. coli*, and recombinant proteins purified on nickel chelate or glutathione columns. These purified proteins were then used to produce protein microarrays to screen sera from *C. trachomatis*-infected patients. In parallel, the same protein library was screened in IFN-γ release assays with spleen cells from infected mice. A total of 42 antigens were recognized by human sera and/or mouse T cells, with 5 of them overlapping. Protection studies were performed in mouse with adjuvanted proteins, which identified several partially protective antigens. More robust protection was achieved by combining antigens, which was shown by antibody ablation experiments to be CD4 T-cell mediated. In other studies, full proteome arrays have been produced by using the HT IVTT approach to obviate protein purification. For example, an array of 921 different gene products (approximately 99% of the ORFs encoded in *C. trachomatis*) were expressed in IVTT and printed, and probed with sera from mice infected with live or UV-irradiated organisms [10]. A total of 185 proteins were reactive in mice. Several of these were familiar from studies from other groups, while many new antigens were also discovered, although the protective efficacy of these needs to be determined.

Bacillus anthracis

Anthrax is lethal in humans, and because of the environmental stability and ease of transmission of spores, *B. anthracis* is considered a biodefense priority organism. Several hundred proteins are secreted by growing bacilli into growth medium, which include toxins, hemolysins, proteases, lecithinases, and other pathogenic proteins. In the wake of sequencing of the *B. anthracis* genome [111] and associated virulence plasmids [112], considerable effort has been invested in developing vaccines and diagnostics, particularly against the secreted components of the proteome (the "secretome") where much of the pathogenicity resides. In one study, culture-conditioned media were resolved on 2D

gels and probed with antisera from *B. anthracis*-infected animals [27]. Tryptic digests of spots were subjected to mass spectrometry to identify the antigens. These were tested in animal (guinea pig) challenge studies using DNA vaccines [113], which circumvented the need to purify each protein for vaccination.

Dengue virus

Dengue is a small virus with a genome that encodes only 10 polypeptides. However, there are four distinct serotypes (DEN1–4), each comprised of multiple individual genetic variants. Infection causes dengue fever, and virus neutralization is engendered by antibodies directed predominantly against the envelope (E) protein. Antibodies to one serotype protect against secondary exposure to the same serotype, whereas secondary exposure to a different serotype may cause more severe dengue hemorrhagic fever or dengue-shock syndrome. How antibody can mediate protection verses more severe infections is not clear but may relate to the avidity of the cross-reactive antibodies for E or its precursor, preM [114]. To this end, proteome microarrays with representatives of all four serotypes were recently used to profile sera from several macaques receiving live attenuated or inactivated vaccines both boosted with live attenuated vaccine, and compared them with profiles from animals infected with wild-type strains [89]. Qualitatively different profiles are seen with the two vaccines although both skewed the response toward structural antigens. In contrast, wild-type infection engenders a more balanced response to both structural and nonstructural proteins. This begins to help understand the complex serology of dengue, although much larger arrays will be needed to help understand the importance of the genetic variation within each serotype in protection verses antibody-dependent enhancement.

Future challenges

We can assume that in the not too distant future, the proteomes of most human pathogens will be fully mapped for reactive antigens using both predictive and experimentally derived approaches. This data set will clearly improve the accuracy of existing predictive approaches, but will also facilitate the development of new predictive algorithms. The Holy Grail is the accurate prediction of protective antigens. The main challenges, as they are today, are (i) translating antigen profiles from HT antigen discovery into effective vaccines, particularly against rapidly evolving pathogens; and (ii) the lengthy process of validating candidates *in vitro* (for neutralization, complement fixation, phagocytosis, and so on in the case of antibody; cytokine production and other cell-mediated responses in the case of T cells), and *in vivo* in preclinical animal toxicity and protection studies. Genome-wide comparisons of different pathogen strains will help reveal conserved antigens or regions within antigens that may enable a vaccine to be designed to target all strains and serotypes. These hurdles will require the development of new HT screens for *in vitro* and *in vivo* antigen validation, and for the computational processing that will be required to mine these databases.

References

1 Tian Q, Stepaniants SB, Mao M, *et al.* Integrated genomic and proteomic analyses of gene expression in mammalian cells. *Mol Cell Proteomics* 2004; **3**(10):960–69.

2 Dressaire C, Gitton C, Loubiere P, *et al.* Transcriptome and proteome exploration to model translation efficiency and protein stability in *Lactococcus lactis*. *PLoS Comput Biol* 2009;**5**(12):e1000606.

3 Etz H, Minh DB, Henics T, *et al.* Identification of in vivo expressed vaccine candidate antigens from *Staphylococcus aureus*. *Proc Natl Acad Sci U S A* 2002; **99**(10):6573–8.

4 Park J, Labaer J. Recombinational cloning. *Curr Protoc Mol Biol* 2006;Chapter **3**:Unit 3.20.

5 Liang X, Teng A, Braun DM, *et al.* Transcriptionally active polymerase chain reaction (TAP): high throughput gene expression using genome sequence data. *J Biol Chem* 2002;**277**(5):3593–8.

6 Li MZ, Elledge SJ. Harnessing homologous recombination in vitro to generate recombinant DNA via SLIC. *Nat Methods* 2007;**4**(3):251–6.

7 Regis DP, Dobano C, Quinones-Olson P, *et al.* Transcriptionally active PCR for antigen identification and vaccine development: in vitro genome-wide screening and in vivo immunogenicity. *Mol Biochem Parasitol* 2008;**158**(1):32–45.

8 Liang L, Doskaya M, Juarez S, *et al.* Identification of potential serodiagnostic and subunit vaccine antigens by antibody profiling of toxoplasmosis cases in Turkey. *Mol Cell Proteomics* 2011;**10**(7): M110.006916.

9 Felgner PL, Kayala MA, Vigil A, *et al.* A *Burkholderia pseudomallei* protein microarray reveals serodiagnostic and cross-reactive antigens. *Proc Natl Acad Sci U S A* 2009;**106**(32):13499–504.

10 Cruz-Fisher MI, Cheng C, Sun G, *et al.* Identification of immunodominant antigens by probing a whole *Chlamydia trachomatis* open reading frame proteome microarray using sera from immunized mice. *Infect Immun* 2011;**79**(1):246–57.

11 Kunnath-Velayudhan S, Salamon H, Wang HY, *et al.* Dynamic antibody responses to the *Mycobacterium tuberculosis* proteome. *Proc Natl Acad Sci U S A* 2010;**107**(33):14703–8.

12 Trieu A, Kayala MA, Burk C, *et al.* Sterile protective immunity to malaria is associated with a panel of novel *P. falciparum* antigens. *Mol Cell Proteomics* 2011;**10**(9):M111.007948.

13 Crompton PD, Kayala MA, Traore B, *et al.* A prospective analysis of the Ab response to *Plasmodium falciparum* before and after a malaria season by protein microarray. *Proc Natl Acad Sci U S A* 2010; **107**(15):6958–63.

14 Driguez P, Doolan DL, Loukas A, Felgner PL, McManus DP. Schistosomiasis vaccine discovery using immunomics. *Parasit Vectors* 2010;**3**:4.

15 Mehlin C, Boni E, Buckner FS, *et al.* Heterologous expression of proteins from *Plasmodium falciparum*: results from 1000 genes. *Mol Biochem Parasitol* 2006;**148**(2):144–60.

16 Chen CS, Korobkova E, Chen H, *et al.* A proteome chip approach reveals new DNA damage recognition activities in *Escherichia coli. Nat Methods* 2008;**5**(1):69–74.

17 Gelperin DM, White MA, Wilkinson ML, *et al.* Biochemical and genetic analysis of the yeast proteome with a movable ORF collection. *Genes Dev* 2005; **19**(23):2816–26.

18 Lueking A, Possling A, Huber O, *et al.* A nonredundant human protein chip for antibody screening and serum profiling. *Mol Cell Proteomics* 2003; **2**(12):1342–9.

19 Zhu H, Hu S, Jona G, *et al.* Severe acute respiratory syndrome diagnostics using a coronavirus protein microarray. *Proc Natl Acad Sci U S A* 2006; **103**(11):4011–16.

20 Keasey SL, Schmid KE, Lee MS, *et al.* Extensive antibody cross-reactivity among infectious gram-negative bacteria revealed by proteome microarray analysis. *Mol Cell Proteomics* 2009;**8**(5):924–35.

21 Steen J, Uhlen M, Hober S, Ottosson J. High-throughput protein purification using an automated set-up for high-yield affinity chromatography. *Protein Expr Purif* 2006;**46**(2):173–8.

22 Tegel H, Steen J, Konrad A, *et al.* High-throughput protein production – lessons from scaling up from 10 to 288 recombinant proteins per week. *Biotechnol J* 2009;**4**(1):51–7.

23 Scheich C, Sievert V, Bussow K. An automated method for high-throughput protein purification applied to a comparison of His-tag and GST-tag affinity chromatography. *BMC Biotechnol* 2003; **3**:12.

24 Laemmli UK. Cleavage of structural proteins during the assembly of the head of bacteriophage T4. *Nature* 1970;**227**(5259):680–85.

25 Towbin H, Staehelin T, Gordon J. Electrophoretic transfer of proteins from polyacrylamide gels to nitrocellulose sheets: procedure and some applications. *Proc Natl Acad Sci U S A* 1979;**76**(9):4350–54.

26 Tefon BE, Maass S, Ozcengiz E, *et al.* A comprehensive analysis of *Bordetella pertussis* surface proteome and identification of new immunogenic proteins. *Vaccine* 2011;**29**(19):3583–95.

27 Chitlaru T, Gat O, Gozlan Y, Ariel N, Shafferman A. Differential proteomic analysis of the *Bacillus anthracis* secretome: distinct plasmid and chromosome CO_2-dependent cross talk mechanisms modulate extracellular proteolytic activities. *J Bacteriol* 2006;**188**(10):3551–71.

28 McGill MA, Edmondson DG, Carroll JA, *et al.* Characterization and serologic analysis of the *Treponema pallidum* proteome. *Infect Immun* 2010; **78**(6):2631–43.

29 Sartain MJ, Slayden RA, Singh KK, Laal S, Belisle JT. Disease state differentiation and identification of tuberculosis biomarkers via native antigen array profiling. *Mol Cell Proteomics* 2006;**5**(11):2102–13.

30 McKevitt M, Brinkman MB, McLoughlin M, *et al.* Genome scale identification of *Treponema pallidum* antigens. *Infect Immun* 2005;**73**(7):4445–50.

31 Pickering JW, Larson MT, Martins TB, Copple SS, Hill HR. Elimination of false-positive results in a Luminex assay for pneumococcal antibodies. *Clin Vaccine Immunol* 2009;**17**(1):185–9.

32 Pickering JW, Martins TB, Greer RW, *et al.* A multiplexed fluorescent microsphere immunoassay for antibodies to pneumococcal capsular polysaccharides. *Am J Clin Pathol* 2002;**117**(4):589–96.

33 Pickering JW, Martins TB, Schroder MC, Hill HR. Comparison of a multiplex flow cytometric assay with enzyme-linked immunosorbent assay for quantitation of antibodies to tetanus, diphtheria, and *Haemophilus influenzae* type b. *Clin Diagn Lab Immunol* 2002;**9**(4):872–6.

34 de Voer RM, Schepp RM, Versteegh FG, van der Klis FR, Berbers GA. Simultaneous detection of *Haemophilus influenzae* type b polysaccharide-specific antibodies and *Neisseria meningitidis* serogroup A, C, Y, and W-135 polysaccharide-specific antibodies in a fluorescent-bead-based multiplex immunoassay. *Clin Vaccine Immunol* 2009;**16**(3):433–6.

35 Dias D, Van Doren J, Schlottmann S, *et al.* Optimization and validation of a multiplexed Luminex assay to quantify antibodies to neutralizing epitopes on human papillomaviruses 6, 11, 16, and 18. *Clin Diagn Lab Immunol* 2005;**12**(8):959–69.

36 Prince HE, Lape-Nixon M, Matud J. Evaluation of a tetraplex microsphere assay for *Bordetella pertussis* antibodies. *Clin Vaccine Immunol* 2006;**13**(2):266–70.

37 He M, Wang MW. Arraying proteins by cell-free synthesis. *Biomol Eng* 2007;**24**(4):375–80.

38 Burbelo PD, Ching KH, Bush ER, Han BL, Iadarola MJ. Antibody-profiling technologies for studying humoral responses to infectious agents. *Expert Rev Vaccines* 2010;**9**(6):567–78.

39 Vigil A, Davies DH, Felgner PL. Defining the humoral immune response to infectious agents using high-density protein microarrays. *Future Microbiol* 2010;**5**(2):241–51.

40 He M, Taussig MJ. Single step generation of protein arrays from DNA by cell-free expression and in situ immobilisation (PISA method). *Nucleic Acids Res* 2001;**29**(15):E73–3.

41 Ramachandran N, Anderson KS, Raphael JV, *et al.* Tracking humoral responses using self assembling protein microarrays. *Proteomics Clin Appl* 2008; **2**(10–11):1518–27.

42 Ramachandran N, Hainsworth E, Bhullar B, *et al.* Self-assembling protein microarrays. *Science* 2004;**305**(5680):86–90.

43 Ramachandran N, Hainsworth E, Demirkan G, LaBaer J. On-chip protein synthesis for making microarrays. *Methods Mol Biol* 2006;**328**: 1–14.

44 Qiu J, LaBaer J. Nucleic acid programmable protein array a just-in-time multiplexed protein expression and purification platform. *Methods Enzymol* 2011;**500**: 151–63.

45 Ceroni A, Sibani S, Baiker A, *et al.* Systematic analysis of the IgG antibody immune response against varicella zoster virus (VZV) using a self-assembled protein microarray. *Mol Biosyst* 2010;**6**(9):1604–10.

46 Montor WR, Huang J, Hu Y, *et al.* Genome-wide study of *Pseudomonas aeruginosa* outer membrane protein immunogenicity using self-assembling protein microarrays. *Infect Immun* 2009;**77**(11): 4877–86.

47 Wright C, Sibani S, Trudgian D, *et al.* Detection of multiple autoantibodies in patients with ankylosing spondylitis using nucleic acid programmable protein arrays. *Mol Cell Proteomics* 2010;Feb 1 (Epub ahead of print).

48 Anderson KS, Sibani S, Wallstrom G, *et al.* Protein microarray signature of autoantibody biomarkers for the early detection of breast cancer. *J Proteome Res* 2010;**10**(1):85–96.

49 Wong J, Sibani S, Lokko NN, LaBaer J, Anderson KS. Rapid detection of antibodies in sera using multiplexed self-assembling bead arrays. *J Immunol Methods* 2009;**350**(1–2):171–82.

50 Wong SJ, Demarest VL, Boyle RH, *et al.* Detection of human anti-flavivirus antibodies with a West Nile virus recombinant antigen microsphere immunoassay. *J Clin Microbiol* 2004;**42**(1):65–72.

51 Davies DH, Liang X, Hernandez JE, *et al.* Profiling the humoral immune response to infection by using proteome microarrays: high-throughput vaccine and diagnostic antigen discovery. *Proc Natl Acad Sci U S A* 2005;**102**(3):547–52.

52 Davies DH, McCausland MM, Valdez C, *et al.* Vaccinia virus H3L envelope protein is a major target of neutralizing antibodies in humans and elicits protection against lethal challenge in mice. *J Virol* 2005;**79**(18):11724–33.

53 Davies DH, Molina DM, Wrammert J, *et al.* Proteome-wide analysis of the serological response to vaccinia and smallpox. *Proteomics* 2007; **7**(10):1678–86.

54 Davies DH, Wyatt LS, Newman FK, *et al.* Antibody profiling by proteome microarray reveals the immunogenicity of the attenuated smallpox vaccine modified vaccinia virus Ankara is comparable to that of Dryvax. *J Virol* 2008;**82**(2):652–63.

55 Doolan DL, Mu Y, Unal B, *et al.* Profiling humoral immune responses to *P. falciparum* infec-tion with protein microarrays. *Proteomics* 2008;**8**(22): 4680–94.

56 Sundaresh S, Doolan DL, Hirst S, *et al.* Identification of humoral immune responses in protein microarrays using DNA microarray data analysis techniques. *Bioinformatics* 2006;**22**(14):1760–66.

57 Liang L, Leng D, Burk C, *et al.* Large scale immune profiling of infected humans and goats reveals differential recognition of *Brucella melitensis* antigens. *PLoS Negl Trop Dis* 2010;**4**(5):e673.

58 Molina DM, Pal S, Kayala MA, *et al.* Identification of immunodominant antigens of *Chlamydia trachomatis* using proteome microarrays. *Vaccine* 2010; **28**(17):3014–24.

59 Eyles JE, Unal B, Hartley MG, *et al.* Immunodominant *Francisella tularensis* antigens identified using proteome microarray. *Proteomics* 2007; **7**(13):2172–83.

60 Sundaresh S, Randall A, Unal B, *et al.* From protein microarrays to diagnostic antigen discovery: a study of the pathogen *Francisella tularensis*. *Bioinformatics* 2007;**23**(13):i508–18.

61 Beare PA, Chen C, Bouman T, *et al.* Candidate antigens for Q fever serodiagnosis revealed by immunoscreening of a *Coxiella burnetii* protein microarray. *Clin Vaccine Immunol* 2008;**15**(12):1771–9.

62 Vigil A, Ortega R, Nakajima-Sasaki R, *et al.* Genome-wide profiling of humoral immune response to *Coxiella burnetii* infection by protein microarray. *Proteomics* 2010;**10**(12):2259–69.

63 Chen C, Bouman TJ, Beare PA, *et al.* A systematic approach to evaluate humoral and cellular immune responses to *Coxiella burnetii* immunoreactive antigens. *Clin Microbiol Infect* 2009;**15**(Suppl 2):156–7.

64 Barbour AG, Jasinskas A, Kayala MA, *et al.* A genome-wide proteome array reveals a limited set of immunogens in natural infections of humans and white-footed mice with *Borrelia burgdorferi*. *Infect Immun* 2008;**76**(8):3374–89.

65 Vigil A, Ortega R, Jain A, *et al.* Identification of the feline humoral immune response to *Bartonella henselae* infection by protein microarray. *PLoS One* 2010;**5**(7):e11447.

66 Liang L, Döşkaya M, Juarez S, *et al.* Identification of potential serodiagnostic and subunit vaccine antigens by antibody profiling of toxoplasmosis cases in Turkey. *Molec Cell Proteomics* 2011; **10**(7):M110.006916.

67 Mochon AB, Jin Y, Kayala MA, *et al.* Serological profiling of a *Candida albicans* protein microarray reveals permanent host-pathogen interplay and

stage-specific responses during candidemia. *PLoS Pathog* 2010;**6**(3):e1000827.

68 Luevano M, Bernard HU, Barrera-Saldana HA, *et al.* High-throughput profiling of the humoral immune responses against thirteen human papillomavirus types by proteome microarrays. *Virology* 2010; **405**(1):31–40.

69 Lyons AB. Analysing cell division in vivo and in vitro using flow cytometric measurement of CFSE dye dilution. *J Immunol Methods* 2000;**243**(1–2): 147–54.

70 Chattopadhyay PK, Yu J, Roederer M. A live-cell assay to detect antigen-specific CD4$^+$ T cells with diverse cytokine profiles. *Nat Med* 2005;**11**(10): 1113–17.

71 Chattopadhyay PK, Yu J, Roederer M. Live-cell assay to detect antigen-specific CD4$^+$ T-cell responses by CD154 expression. *Nat Protoc* 2006;**1**(1):1–6.

72 Zaunders JJ, Munier ML, Seddiki N, *et al.* High levels of human antigen-specific CD4$^+$ T cells in peripheral blood revealed by stimulated coexpression of CD25 and CD134 (OX40). *J Immunol* 2009; **183**(4):2827–36.

73 Keoshkerian E, Helbig K, Beard M, *et al.* A novel assay for detection of hepatitis C virus-specific effector CD4(+) T cells via co-expression of CD25 and CD134. *J Immunol Methods* 2012;**375**(1–2): 148–58.

74 Wehler TC, Karg M, Distler E, *et al.* Rapid identification and sorting of viable virus-reactive CD4(+) and CD8(+) T cells based on antigen-triggered CD137 expression. *J Immunol Methods* 2008;**339**(1):23–37.

75 Wolfl M, Kuball J, Eyrich M, Schlegel PG, Greenberg PD. Use of CD137 to study the full repertoire of CD8$^+$ T cells without the need to know epitope specificities. *Cytometry A* 2008;**73**(11):1043–9.

76 Townsend AR, Rothbard J, Gotch FM, *et al.* The epitopes of influenza nucleoprotein recognized by cytotoxic T lymphocytes can be defined with short synthetic peptides. *Cell* 1986;**44**(6):959–68.

77 Lundegaard C, Lund O, Buus S, Nielsen M. Major histocompatibility complex class I binding predictions as a tool in epitope discovery. *Immunology* 2010;**130**(3):309–18.

78 Stern LJ, Calvo-Calle JM. HLA-DR: molecular insights and vaccine design. *Curr Pharm Des* 2009; **15**(28):3249–61.

79 Kim Y, Sette A, Peters B. Applications for T-cell epitope queries and tools in the Immune Epitope Database and Analysis Resource. *J Immunol Methods* 2011;**374**(1-2):62–9.

80 Vita R, Peters B, Josephs Z, *et al.* A model for collaborative curation, the IEDB and ChEBI Curation of Non-peptidic Epitopes. *Immunome Res* 2011; **7**(1):1–8.

81 Vita R, Zarebski L, Greenbaum JA, *et al.* The immune epitope database 2.0. *Nucleic Acids Res* 2009;**38**: D854–62.

82 Li Pira G, Ivaldi F, Moretti P, Manca F. High throughput T epitope mapping and vaccine development. *J Biomed Biotechnol* 2010;**2010**: 325720.

83 Purcell AW, Gorman JJ. Immunoproteomics: mass spectrometry-based methods to study the targets of the immune response. *Mol Cell Proteomics* 2004; **3**(3):193–208.

84 Hillen N, Stevanovic S. Contribution of mass spectrometry-based proteomics to immunology. *Expert Rev Proteomics* 2006;**3**(6):653–64.

85 Johnson KL, Ovsyannikova IG, Mason CJ, Bergen HR, 3rd, Poland GA. Discovery of naturally processed and HLA-presented class I peptides from vaccinia virus infection using mass spectrometry for vaccine development. *Vaccine* 2009;**28**(1):38–47.

86 Karunakaran KP, Yu H, Foster LJ, Brunham RC. Development of a *Chlamydia trachomatis* T cell vaccine. *Hum Vaccin* 2010;**6**(8):676–80.

87 Jing L, Davies DH, Chong TM, *et al.* An extremely diverse CD4 response to vaccinia virus in humans is revealed by proteome-wide T cell profiling. *J Virol* 2008;**82**(14):7120–34.

88 Jing L, McCaughey SM, Davies DH, *et al.* ORFeome approach to the clonal, HLA allele-specific CD4 T-cell response to a complex pathogen in humans. *J Immunol Methods* 2009;**347**(1–2):36–45.

89 Moffitt KL, Gierahn TM, Lu YJ, *et al.* T(H)17-based vaccine design for prevention of *Streptococcus pneumoniae* colonization. *Cell Host Microbe* 2011;**9**(2):158–65.

90 Turner MJ, Abdul-Alim CS, Willis RA, *et al.* T-cell antigen discovery (T-CAD) assay: a novel technique for identifying T cell epitopes. *J Immunol Methods* 2001;**256**(1–2):107–19.

91 Valentino M, Frelinger J. An approach to the identification of T cell epitopes in the genomic era: application to *Francisella tularensis*. *Immunol Res* 2009;**45**(2–3):218–28.

92 Valentino MD, Maben ZJ, Hensley LL, *et al.* Identification of T-cell epitopes in *Francisella tularensis* using an ordered protein array of serological targets. *Immunology* 2011;**132**(3):348–60.

93 Valentino MD, Abdul-Alim CS, Maben ZJ, *et al.* A broadly applicable approach to T cell epitope identification: application to improving tumor

associated epitopes and identifying epitopes in complex pathogens. *J Immunol Methods* 2011; **373**(1–2):111–26.

94 Koelle DM. Expression cloning for the discovery of viral antigens and epitopes recognized by T cells. *Methods* 2003;**29**(3):213–26.

95 Koelle DM, Chen HB, Gavin MA, *et al*. CD8 CTL from genital herpes simplex lesions: recognition of viral tegument and immediate early proteins and lysis of infected cutaneous cells. *J Immunol* 2001;**166**(6):4049–58.

96 Koelle DM, Corey L. Recent progress in herpes simplex virus immunobiology and vaccine research. *Clin Microbiol Rev* 2003;**16**(1):96–113.

97 Finco O, Frigimelica E, Buricchi F, *et al*. Approach to discover T- and B-cell antigens of intracellular pathogens applied to the design of *Chlamydia trachomatis* vaccines. *Proc Natl Acad Sci U S A* 2011; **108**(24):9969–74.

98 Sette A, Peters B. Immune epitope mapping in the post-genomic era: lessons for vaccine development. *Curr Opin Immunol* 2007;**19**(1):106–10.

99 Hooper JW, Custer DM, Thompson E. Four-gene-combination DNA vaccine protects mice against a lethal vaccinia virus challenge and elicits appropriate antibody responses in nonhuman primates. *Virology* 2003;**306**(1):181–95.

100 Giuliani MM, Adu-Bobie J, Comanducci M, *et al*. A universal vaccine for serogroup B meningococcus. *Proc Natl Acad Sci U S A* 2006;**103**(29):10834–9.

101 Twine SM, Petit MD, Shen H, *et al*. Immunoproteomic analysis of the murine antibody response to successful and failed immunization with live anti-Francisella vaccines. *Biochem Biophys Res Commun* 2006;**346**(3):999–1008.

102 Dasgupta G, Chentoufi AA, Nesburn AB, Wechsler SL, BenMohamed L. New concepts in herpes simplex virus vaccine development: notes from the battlefield. *Expert Rev Vaccines* 2009;**8**(8):1023–35.

103 Tettelin H, Saunders NJ, Heidelberg J, *et al*. Complete genome sequence of *Neisseria meningitidis* serogroup B strain MC58. *Science* 2000; **287**(5459):1809–15.

104 Pizza M, Scarlato V, Masignani V, *et al*. Identification of vaccine candidates against serogroup B meningococcus by whole-genome sequencing. *Science* 2000;**287**(5459):1816–20.

105 Rappuoli R, Covacci A. Reverse vaccinology and genomics. *Science* 2003;**302**(5645):602.

106 Scarselli M, Arico B, Brunelli B, *et al*. Rational design of a meningococcal antigen inducing broad protective immunity. *Sci Transl Med* 2011;**3**(91): 91ra62.

107 Granoff DM. Review of meningococcal group B vaccines. *Clin Infect Dis* 2010;**50**(Suppl 2):S54–65.

108 Brinkman MB, McKevitt M, McLoughlin M, *et al*. Reactivity of antibodies from syphilis patients to a protein array representing the *Treponema pallidum* proteome. *J Clin Microbiol* 2006;**44**(3):888–91.

109 Brinkman MB, McGill MA, Pettersson J, *et al*. A novel *Treponema pallidum* antigen, TP0136, is an outer membrane protein that binds human fibronectin. *Infect Immun* 2008;**76**(5):1848–57.

110 Montigiani S, Falugi F, Scarselli M, *et al*. Genomic approach for analysis of surface proteins in *Chlamydia pneumoniae*. *Infect Immun* 2002;**70**(1):368–79.

111 Read TD, Peterson SN, Tourasse N, *et al*. The genome sequence of *Bacillus anthracis* Ames and comparison to closely related bacteria. *Nature* 2003;**423**(6935):81–6.

112 Okinaka R, Cloud K, Hampton O, *et al*. Sequence, assembly and analysis of pX01 and pX02. *J Appl Microbiol* 1999;**87**(2):261–2.

113 Chitlaru T, Gat O, Grosfeld H, *et al*. Identification of in vivo-expressed immunogenic proteins by serological proteome analysis of the *Bacillus anthracis* secretome. *Infect Immun* 2007;**75**(6):2841–52.

114 Dejnirattisai W, Jumnainsong A, Onsirisakul N, *et al*. Cross-reacting antibodies enhance dengue virus infection in humans. *Science* 2010;**328**(5979):745–8.

115 Gupta MK, Subramanian V, Yadav JS. Immuno-proteomic identification of secretory and subcellular protein antigens and functional evaluation of the secretome fraction of *Mycobacterium immunogenum*, a newly recognized species of the *Mycobacterium chelonae-Mycobacterium abscessus* group. *J Proteome Res* 2009;**8**(5):2319–30.

116 Lock RA, Coombs GW, McWilliams TM, *et al*. Proteome analysis of highly immunoreactive proteins of *Helicobacter pylori*. *Helicobacter* 2002;**7**(3):175–82.

117 Pagani I, Chertkov O, Lapidus A, *et al*. Complete genome sequence of *Marivirga tractuosa* type strain (H-43). *Stand Genomic Sci* 201; **4**(2):154–62.

118 Wu Y, Craig A. Comparative proteomic analysis of metabolically labelled proteins from *Plasmodium falciparum* isolates with different adhesion properties. *Malar J* 2006;**5**:67.

119 Galindo CL, Sha J, Moen ST, *et al*. Comparative global gene expression profiles of wild-type *Yersinia pestis* CO92 and its Braun lipoprotein mutant at flea and human body temperatures. *Comp Funct Genomics* 2010: 342168.

CHAPTER 11
Phage Libraries

Aaron K. Sato
OncoMed Pharmaceuticals, Redwood City, CA, USA

Introduction

In this chapter, the goal is to review the work of those skilled in the art of using phage display for vaccine discovery. The author is not an expert in this area, but rather an avid user of the technology and has applied it to a number of fields (therapeutics [1,2], imaging agents [3,4], and affinity media [5]) and display formats (peptides, small proteins, Fab). With this in mind, the author will provide an objective review and highlight how phage display has empowered the field of vaccinology.

Peptide mimotopes

Using peptide phage display (PPD) technology, peptide mimotopes can be generated that mimic protein, carbohydrates, or lipid antigen epitopes. A monoclonal antibody or polyclonal sera is selected against a highly diverse PPD library and binders to the antibody-antigen interface are discovered (Figure 11.1). In the antibody field, these mimotopes are similar in function to anti-idiotype antibodies. The displayed peptides are either random or derived from a cDNA source, such as fragments of the antibody antigen. For random peptide libraries, many laboratories use either peptide libraries donated from academic laboratories [6] or libraries available from New England Biolabs [7]. They are conformational B-cell epitopes and usually do not participate in T-cell activation, although several groups have shown that mimotopes can partici-

pate in such processes [8]. When coupled to carriers, expressed with a plasmid vector along with a helper T-cell epitope, or displayed on phage, mimotopes can be immunogenic and induce antibody responses to their parental antigen. In such cases, the mimotope mimics the antigen at the antibody interface (antigenicity) as well as immunogenic properties of the parental antigen, which is characterized as being "immunologically fit" by Mathews *et al.* [9]. Although most laboratories use random PPD libraries, Mathews *et al.* showed that natural fragment libraries yield more immunologically fit mimotopes in a comparative study [9]. Besides using peptide libraries to generate mimotopes, antibody libraries have also been used to generate anti-idiotype antibodies that mimic their parental antigen and induce immunogenicity to them [10]. As you will see in the upcoming sections, the process of discovering an immunologically fit mimotope is incredibly difficult. Literature examples from several fields will be reviewed and for each example, the mimotope properties will be scrutinized to determine their level of immunologic fitness.

Infectious disease mimotopes

Infectious diseases are caused by the presence of pathogenic viruses, pathogenic bacteria, fungi, protozoa, multicellular parasites, and aberrant proteins known as prions. Since these organisms are foreign to the human immune system, traditional infectious disease vaccines, such as recombinant

---

Vaccinology: Principles and Practice, First Edition. Edited by W. John W. Morrow, Nadeem A. Sheikh, Clint S. Schmidt and D. Huw Davies.
© 2012 Blackwell Publishing Ltd. Published 2012 by Blackwell Publishing Ltd.

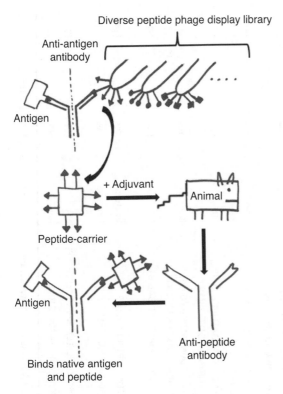

Diverse peptide phage display library

Anti-antigen antibody

Antigen

+ Adjuvant

Animal

Peptide-carrier

Antigen

Anti-peptide antibody

Binds native antigen and peptide

Figure 11.1 Mimetope discovery process. An anti-antigen antibody (monoclonal antibody or polyclonal sera) is selected against a highly diverse PPD library and binders to the antibody-antigen interface are discovered. When coupled to carriers (or in other formats), the peptides can be immunogenic and induce an anti-peptide response in animals. If the peptide mimetope is a good mimic of the original antigen epitope, then the anti-peptide antibody should also cross-react with the parental antigen.

coat proteins, have typically been very successful in protecting individuals from these agents. In some cases, however, these approaches have not yielded a robust, protective immune response against the pathogen. As an alternative approach, peptide mimotopes have been employed to increase the robustness of the immune response.

The mimotope approach has been very successful against infectious diseases, with nearly half of the surveyed mimotope publications focused in this area (see Tables 11.1–11.4). Numerous peptide mimotopes have been discovered for carbohydrate and protein antigens. Since carbohydrates have his-

torically been less immunogenic than their protein counterparts on the same pathogen, peptide-based mimotopes are often discovered in an attempt to boost the immune response against the parental carbohydrate antigen.

Capsular polysaccharide antigen (CPA) is a common target for bacterial vaccines and in the mimotope discovery literature. Pathogenic bacteria commonly coat themselves in a thick layer of polysaccharide (capsule) that hides antigenic proteins from the host immune system. The capsular polysaccharides are water soluble, usually acidic, and have molecular weights between 100 and 1000 kDa. These polysaccharides are highly diverse within the same organism, with *E. coli* having nearly two hundred different ones. Mixtures of capsular polysaccharides are often used for vaccines in either conjugated or native format. Although a large number of publications are focused on this antigen in multiple organisms, six from the literature are reviewed in Table 11.1 [11–16]. Of these publications, four of them discovered an immunologically fit mimotope that elicited a response to the parental CPA [12–15]. In all cases, the mimotopes were conjugated either to a carrier protein (Ova, KLH, BSA, TT, proteosomes) [12,13,15] or expressed with a plasmid vector along with a helper T-cell epitope [14]. Only one immunologically fit mimotope had a possible disulfide constraint [13] and the rest were linear. Since the parental antigen is a carbohydrate, the discovered mimotopes did not bear any resemblance to the CPA.

Lipopolysaccharide (LPS) O-chain is another carbohydrate antigen that has been the focus of mimotope discovery. LPS is a significant component of Gram-negative bacteria and helps maintain the structural integrity of the outer membrane. It is composed of three domains: O-antigen (also known as O-chain or O-polysaccharide), core oligosaccharide, and lipid A. O antigen connects to the core oligosaccharide, and comprises the outermost domain of the LPS molecule. Four O-chain mimotope discovery projects were found in the literature [17–20], as shown in Table 11.1. Of these, three mimotopes were immunologically fit [17–19] and elicited a response to their parental antigen. In all cases, the mimotopes were conjugated to

Table 11.1 Infectious disease mimotopes (bacteria/parasites).

Antigen	Type	Disease	Sequence	Format	Immunologically fit?	Ref.
O-chain Brucella LPS	Carb	Brucellosis	WTEIHDWEAAME (MB1.3)	DNA	Yes	[17]
O-chain Brucella LPS	Carb	Brucellosis	GPGQCNTRNPCPRPM (6B3[6]), CHHSPEEYQPC (2C8[7])	Phage	Yes (weak)	[18]
O-antigen	Carb	Bacillary dysentery	YLQDWIKYNNQK	Phage, BSA	No	[20]
O-antigen	Carb	*Vibrio cholerae*	NHNYPPLSLLTF (4P-8)	KLH	Yes	[19]
CPA	Carb	Group B *Streptococcal type III*	FDTGAFDPDWPAC	Ova, KLH, BSA	Yes	[15]
GXM/CPA	Carb	Meningoencephalitis	FGGETFTPDWMMEVAIDNE (P206.1)	TT, MAP	No	[11]
GXM/CPA	Carb	Meningoencephalitis	GMDGTQLDRW (peptide 13)	NA	NA	[16]
MAPS/CPA	Carb	Meningoencephalitis	GEASGLCCRWSSLKGC	Proteosome	Yes	[13]
CPA	Carb	Meningococcal disease, serotype B	DYAWDQTHQDPAK (9M)	DNA	Yes	[14]
CPA	Carb	*Streptococcus pneumoniae*	FHLPYNHNWFAL (PUB1)	TT	Yes	[12]
ViCPS	Carb	*Salmonella enterica*	TSHHDSHGLHRV (NP4.01), ENHSPVNIAHKL (NP4.16)	NA	NA	[56]
Surface protein 1	Protein	*Plasmodium vivax* malaria	YSPELE (C4), GRVCLR (C15)	Phage	Yes	[22]
Multiple	Protein	*Plasmodium falciparum* malaria	CTGDARHRC (M1)	KLH	Yes	[23]
RESA	Protein	*Plasmodium falciparum* malaria	GLKNCTVQPWDATDVCD (17(3)), CFDYAPYVSAVDDIC(15(1))	NA	NA	[57]
AMA1	Protein	*Plasmodium falciparum* malaria	IPSTAFTDIAWVRLPNHYG (J1), LASLRKAFADTVPVRPPSNYG (J7)	KLH	Yes	[21]
Chlamydophila pneumoniae	Unknown	*Chlamydophila pneumoniae*	PNEPDDLALMRIIRI (CP-8A6-B1)	NA	NA	[58]
TRAP	Protein	*Staphylococcus aureus* infection	SWFDNFLYPTHD (TA21)	Bacteria	Yes	[24]
RAP	Protein	*Streptococcus pneumoniae* pneumonia	GGSGTSRTPILG (13)	Bacteria	Yes	[25]
Colicin A	Protein	*E. coli* infection	LRCPEPGCLL (LL), ERVREYYPEP (EP)	NA	NA	[59]
EG95	Protein	Hydatid disease	HYKWLNDPLAAAW (E100)	NA	NA	[60]

CPA, Capsular polysaccharide antigen; Carb, Carbohydrate; Ova, ovalbumin; KLH, keyhole limpet hemocyanin; TT, tetanus toxin; BSA, bovine serum albumin; MAP, multiple antigen peptide; NA, not applicable.

Table 11.2 Infectious disease mimotopes (viruses).

Antigen	Type	Disease	Sequence	Format	Immunologically fit?	Ref.
LOS	Carb	Nontypeable *Haemophilus influenzae*	NMMNYIMDPRTH (P2)	KLH	Yes	[28]
Hepatitis A virus	Protein	Hepatitis A	SHSVTKSLRVFGGPP (BA1-56)	Phage	Yes	[30]
HBsAg	Protein	Hepatitis B	TSNTHACRTCSNPSR (φD1)	Phage	Yes	[31]
HCV c100 NS4	Protein	Hepatitis C	ANLINEFDDLAS (X43)	NA	NA	[26]
RABVG	Protein	Rabies	CKRDSTWC	Phage	Yes	[29]

KLH, Keyhole limpet hemocyanin; NA, not applicable.

either a carrier protein (keyhole limpet hemocyanin, KLH) [19], expressed with a plasmid vector along with a helper T-cell epitope [17], or used the peptide displayed on phage directly [18]. Only one publication had disulfide-constrained peptides [18] and the others had linear ones. Since the parental antigen is a carbohydrate, the discovered mimotopes did not bear any resemblance to O-chain.

Numerous protein antigen mimotopes were discovered against a variety of bacterial and parasitic disease antigens (Table 11.1), of which five were immunologically fit. Three of them were mimotope discovery projects against malaria antigens (either *Plasmodium falciparum* or *Plasmodium vivax*) [21–23]. In each publication, nearly all of the mimotopes had sequence similarity to the parental antigen or antigens expressed in that organism. Peptides were either displayed on phage [22] or conjugated to tetanus toxin [21,23] to stimulate an immune response to the parental antigen or organism. Only one publication had a disulfide-constrained peptide [23], whereas the others had linear ones.

From Table 11.1, the remaining two immunologically fit protein antigen mimotope projects were against *Staphylococcus aureus* and *Streptococcus pneumoniae* [24,25]. Of the two mimotopes, only the TRAP mimotope displayed sequence similarity to the parental antigen. Both peptide mimotopes were linear peptides and were displayed on the surface of bacteria to elicit an immune response against the parental antigen.

Similar to bacteria and parasite antigens, viruses are recognized as foreign by the immune system. Viruses, however, are dependent on the host system for propagation and survival. Five viral mimotope projects (Table 11.2) were found in the literature [26–31] and four of them yielded immunologically fit mimotopes [27–31]. Of these, all had to be immunized as peptide on phage [29–31] or conjugated to KLH [28] to elicit an immune response. One publication yielded an immunologically fit mimotope to lipo-oligosaccharide (LOS) [28]. All three hepatitis papers [26,30,31] discovered immunologically fit mimotopes with sequence similarity to the parental protein antigen. Two hepatitis mimotopes were linear [26,30] and the other was disulfide constrained [31].

For infectious diseases, many groups successfully generated immunologically fit mimotopes for their parental antigens. In several cases, mimotopes were discovered for carbohydrate antigens, which have traditionally been very difficult to use as vaccines. Those mimotopes mimicking protein antigens often resemble their parental protein counterparts. Linear peptides were as successful as their disulfide-constrained counterparts as mimotopes, suggesting that structural constraint is not an absolute prerequisite for mimotope development. The immunologically fit peptide mimotopes were displayed on phage/bacteria, conjugated to carrier proteins, or expressed from DNA expression vectors. As infectious disease antigens are foreign to the human immune system and do not have to compete with tolerance to self-antigen, these mimotopes potentially hold great promise in serving as a new source of potent vaccines against infectious disease agents.

Cancer mimotopes

Most anti-cancer antibodies can be broken down into two basic classes. Overexpressed cancer antigens can be targeted and killed with antibodies utilizing the host's immune system (ADCC, CDC). Functional antibodies are also generated that block or promote cancer cell functions. For example, some functional antibodies block receptor-ligand interactions critical for cancer cell survival/proliferation, for example, anti-EGFR therapy. Others activate apoptosis pathways and enhance cancer cell death.

GD2 is a disialoganglioside expressed on human neuroblastoma and melanoma tumors and shows highly restricted expression on normal human tissues (cerebellum and peripheral nerves). It is composed of five carbohydrate residues linked to a ceramide chain that anchors the ganglioside in the cell membrane. Since GD2 is highly tumor specific, it has been the target of both active and passive immunotherapy. Three GD2 mimotope discovery projects were found in the literature [27,32–34] and all of them yielded immunologically fit mimotopes (Table 11.3). Both disulfide-constrained [27, 33] and linear peptides [32,34] were discovered. Peptides were conjugated to KLH [27,33,34], synthesized in as a multiple antigenic peptide (MAP) [34], or immunized in a DNA vector [32]. Since the parental antigen is a carbohydrate, the discovered mimotopes bore no resemblance to GD2.

The human high molecular weight melanoma-associated antigen (HMW-MAA) is a membrane-bound protein of 2322 residues that is overexpressed on benign nevi and melanoma lesions. Besides tumors of melanocytic origin, HMW-MAA is also expressed by squamous and basal cell carcinomas. Since the antigen shows little to no expression in normal tissues, HMW-MAA is an attractive target for both active and passive immunotherapy. Two immunologically fit mimotopes were discovered against HMW-MAA in the literature [35,36]. Peptides were conjugated to either TT [35] or ABP [36]. Even though HMW-MAA is a protein antigen, the peptide mimotopes bore no primary sequence similarity to it.

Cetuximab (anti-EGFR/ErbB1) and trastuzumab (anti-Her2/ErbB2) are marketed antibodies against members of the ErbB family. Cetuximab targets EGFR and blocks ligand (EGF, TGF-α) binding to the receptor and is approved for the treatment of metastatic colon cancer. Trastuzumab initiates internalization of the Her2 receptor, which inhibits downstream receptor signaling, and is approved for the treatment of advanced Her2-positive breast cancer. Although passive immunotherapy is successful against both of these targets, an active immunotherapy approach may provide a sustained and ongoing production of antibodies in patients without the need for multiple infusions. Riemer et al. [37,38] generated immunologically fit mimotopes against both approved antibodies, and Jiang et al. [39] discovered an immunologically fit mimotope to trastuzumab alone. In all three publications, the discovered mimotopes elicited an immune response that mimicked the functional activity of the parental antibodies as described. Riemer et al. generated disulfide-constrained mimotopes conjugated to KLH, whereas Jiang et al. discovered linear mimotopes conjugated to GST. The mimotopes also did not have any primary sequence homology to either EGFR or Her2.

Two other publications were found that discovered anti-cancer mimotopes to carbohydrate antigens. Hoess et al. discovered a peptide that mimicked Lewis Y antigen [40]. Heimburg-Molinaro et al. generated an immunologically fit peptide mimotope to Thomsen-Friedenreich (TF) carbohydrate antigen [41]. The peptide was immunized as a MAP and bore no resemblance to TF antigen.

From this overview of cancer mimotopes (Table 11.3), nearly all of them yielded immunologically fit mimotopes in their initial publication. Unlike the infectious disease mimotopes, none of the cancer mimotopes had any sequence similarity to their parental antigen and were either conjugated to carrier proteins or used as a MAP. Some peptides were disulfide constrained, but the majority

Table 11.3 Cancer mimotopes.

Antigen	Type	Disease	Sequence	Format	Immunologically fit?	Ref.
Disialoganglioside GD2	Carb	Cancer	CDGGWLSKGSWC, CGRLKMVPDLEC	KLH	Yes	[27,33]
Disialoganglioside GD2	Carb	Cancer	EDPSHSLGLDAALFM (47-LDA)	DNA	Yes	[32]
Disialoganglioside GD2	Carb	Cancer	LDVVLAWRDGLSGAS (P9), GVVWRYTAPVHLGDG (P10)	KLH, MAP	Yes	[34]
Lewis Y antigen	Carb	Cancer	APWLYGPA	NA	NA	[40]
TF-Ag	Carb	Cancer	HIHGWKSPLSSLGGG (D2)	MAP	Yes	[41]
HMW-MAA	Protein	Cancer	RPSSNFNPL (K11)	ABP	Yes	[35]
HMW-MAA	Protein	Cancer	TRTNPWPAL (225D9.2)	TT	Yes	[36]
HER-2	Protein	Cancer	LLGPYELWELSH (H98)	GST	Yes	[39]
HER-2	Protein	Cancer	CQMWAPQWGPDC	TT	Yes	[37]
EGFR	Protein	Cancer	CQYNLSSRALKC, CVWQRWQKSYVC	KLH	Yes	[38]

Carb, Carbohydrate; KLH, keyhole limpet hemocyanin; MAP, multiple antigen peptide; TF-Ag, Thomsen-Friedenreich antigen; HMW-MAA, high molecular weight melanoma-associated antigen; TT, tetanus toxin; ABP, albumin binding protein; GST, glutathione S-transferase; NA, not applicable.

was linear. As exemplified by these publications, it may be possible to replace many passive immunotherapy approaches with active immunization using either the parental antigen or mimotopes to them.

Other mimotope applications

Besides infectious diseases and cancer, the mimotope approach has been applied to a number of other fields (Table 11.4). In the allergy field, some IgG antibodies block IgE binding to allergens and inhibit the allergic response, while others enhance this and support the anaphylactic reaction. Three mimotopes were discovered that mimicked their parental antigen [42–44], but only one was immunologically fit [43]. Rudolf et al. [43] discovered a mimotope to IgE and showed that immunization with the mimotope in rabbits elicited an anti-IgE response. Unlike allergy immunizations, which promote removal of specific IgE antigen specificities, anti-IgE therapy clears the body of all IgE so

that the overall allergic response is minimized and is used in allergy patients with life-threatening disease.

In another example, Laman et al. discovered peptide mimotopes to N-acetylglucosaminyl-1-4-N-acetylmuramyl-alanyl-d-isoglutamine (GMDP), which is a fragment of bacterial cell wall peptidoglycan murein and can substitute for killed mycobacteria in complete Freund's adjuvant (CFA) [45]. Unlike other projects, where the anti-mimotope response is the primary driver of the vaccine response, these peptides were discovered to augment the immune response to other vaccines and replace GMDP or CFA in adjuvants. The mimotopes augmented the response to Ova, but were nonimmunogenic by themselves.

Two mimotope discovery projects were found in the area of transplantation [46,47]. Of them, Chiang et al. [46] established that their mimotope to histone H1 was immunologically fit with a KLH-peptide conjugate. Primary sequence similarity to the parent antigen was noted for some of the mimotopes.

Table 11.4 Other mimotope applications.

Antigen	Type	Disease	Sequence	Format	Immunologically fit?	Ref.
GMNDP	Carb	Adjuvant	RVPPRYHAKISPMVN (RN-peptide)	Peptide/ Ova	Yes	[45]
α-Gal	Carb	Xenotransplantation	FHENWPS (1), SMLDTPT (16)	NA	NA	[47]
Histone H1	Protein	Organ transplant	SSVLYGGPPSAA (SSV)	KLH	Yes	[46]
Pru p 3	Protein	Peach allergy	PRSTPRPWAXL (OAS-IgE), TSRPALLNDQGH (SYS-IgE)	NA	NA	[42]
Parvalbumin	Protein	Fish allergy	CYRGVTLAGHRC (Clone 1), CAREYGTNRWVC (Clone 4)	NA	NA	[44]
IgE	Protein	Allergy	EFCRRHNYGFWVCGD (PhBSW.6-9), EFCINHRGYWVCGD (PhBSW.29-8)	Phage	Yes	[43]

Carb, Carbohydrate; Ova, ovalbumin; KLH, keyhole limpet hemocyanin; NA, not applicable.

Phage vaccines

As reviewed, peptides displayed on bacteriophage can serve as vehicles for immunizing animals to generate a robust immune response [18,20,22,29–31,43]. This approach is not a new one [48] and has been used for the past several decades to replace traditional protein conjugation approaches, for example KLH, TT, GST, BSA, and ABP. In one of the earliest reports, de la Cruz *et al.* [48] demonstrated that a scarce malaria protein (circumsporozoite protein) could be displayed on the pIII coat protein and immunized in rabbits to generate a specific anti-malaria protein response. Unlike many animal viruses, bacteriophage are well understood on both a genetic and structural level. The viruses are highly immunogenic and contain multiple T-cell epitope peptides within the coat proteins. Since they are produced in bacteria, it is also possible to scale up production of the viruses and make large quantities for less cost than a traditional conjugated peptide.

The displayed peptide can also be displayed on multiple coat proteins to modulate the immune response. Greenwood *et al.* [49], for example, constructed multiple display systems for encoding peptides on the more abundant pVIII coat protein (versus pIII coat protein) in combination with wild-type pVIII. Using circumsporozoite protein peptides [(NANP)$_3$] as a model, the hybrid phage particle elicited a strong immune response in rabbits that cross-reacted with the synthetic peptide. The majority of the response was against the displayed peptide and not to the wild-type phage coat proteins. Greenwood *et al.* determined that pVIII display may be more robust than pIII display (limited to 5 copies) because greater copy numbers are possible (up to 2700) and pVIII displayed peptides may be masked less than their pIII displayed counterparts.

As an extension of this work, the same laboratory used multidimensional solution NMR to determine the structure of the modified pVIII proteins in lipid micelles [50]. In the context of the pVIII coat protein, the 12-residue peptide [(NANP)$_3$] adopts a single, stable conformation. Peptides fused to pVIII (or any other coat protein), therefore, may have a greater propensity to adopt their native structure relative to the free synthetic peptide alone. As a result, the stable, native-like structures are capable of eliciting a pronounced immune response to the displayed peptide and native antigen.

Phage-based vaccines have been used successfully in a multitude of different vaccine approaches.

For the advantages cited here, they hold much promise and should be considered as one strategy for immunizing animals with candidate peptides.

Antigen discovery and epitope mapping

The organisms and diseases described so far often elicit an immune response to multiple targets and epitopes. In cases where they are not known, PPD libraries are often used to discover what antigens are targeted by the immune system and, more specifically, what epitopes dominate the immune response. Like the mimotope approach described previously, monoclonal antibodies or polyclonal sera are selected against either random or cDNA fragment PPD libraries. In the case of random PPD libraries, the resulting sequences are analyzed for homology to known proteins in the organism and then binding is confirmed to the homologous peptide sequence. For cDNA fragment libraries, one only needs to determine which antigen the fragment is derived from to determine the antibody specificity. The antibody epitope is often further refined through additional PPD libraries that mutate residues within the sequence, for example, alanine scanning, or truncate the sequence (N- or C-terminal) to find the epitope boundaries.

Several laboratories have shown that cDNA fragment libraries are often more robust and yield more antibody-binding peptides than their random library counterparts. Already cited previously for mimotope discovery, Mathews et al. compared the performance of a whole genome fragment library (T4 bacteriophage) to a random peptide library for finding peptide mimotopes to several T4 antisera derived from Balb/c mice [9]. The fragment library yielded more robust mimotopes to the target antigens as compared to the random peptide libraries. Even though both libraries had equivalent diversity, the natural peptide libraries presumably contained self-folding domains that more closely resemble the native antigen structure, whereas the random libraries must rely on chance to adopt such structures. From an epitope mapping and antigen discovery perspective, this publication demonstrates that fragment libraries (if available) work well for antigen and epitope ID and are also robust sources of peptide mimotopes.

Fack et al. also compared cDNA fragment versus random PPD libraries for epitope mapping [51]. In their study, four antibodies to different antigens (RNA polymerase II, p53, Hantaan virus glycoprotein G2, and nucleocapsid protein) were selected against both antigen-specific fragment libraries and two random peptide libraries (6-mer and 15-mer). 10-mer synthetic peptide scans were also conducted against each antibody. After a single round of selection, the fragment libraries yield epitope-specific binders to each antibody, whereas only two of the antibodies (anti-p53, anti-G2) proved successful against the random peptide libraries with three to four selection rounds. The peptide scan approach yielded epitope-specific binder to three of the four antibodies and, therefore, also proved more successful than the random peptide libraries.

In a similar approach, Coley et al. employed a combined PPD approach using both fragment and random PPD libraries to epitope map anti-AMA1 antibodies (*Plasmodium falciparum*) [52]. First, anti-AMA1 antibodies were selected against an AMA1 fragment library and the epitopes identified. One antibody (MAb5G8) recognized a short linear epitope (with AYP sequence) with the prodomain and another antibody (MAb1F9) recognized a subdomain (57 amino acids) of domain one. With this information in hand, they followed up each epitope and determined the fine epitope specificity with additional PPD libraries. In a parallel approach, a random PPD library was also selected against MAb5G8 and the same AYP sequence motif was discovered in the mimotopes. This study and the others cited demonstrate that both fragment and random libraries can be used successfully to epitope map candidate antibodies and mimotope discovery.

Conclusion and future direction

Currently, recombinant protein approaches constitute the bulk of vaccine discovery and development in the pharmaceutical industry. Phage display derived mimotope vaccines, however, should be considered as replacements for recombinant vaccines when they do not elicit a pronounced immune response – for example, carbohydrate antigens – or cannot be produced in an economic manner. Mimotope vaccines could be developed in concert with other more validated computational (Chapter 9) and proteomic/microarray approaches (Chapter 10). They should also be considered for follow-on approaches for well-validated, expensive vaccines on the market. Since mimotopes are not restricted to peptides, other small protein/peptide scaffolds that present amino acids in a stable uniform manner should be considered, such as phylomers [53], protein A, lipocalins, fibronectin [54], ankyrins, and thioredoxin [55]. These mutant scaffolds may have increased immunogenicity compared to small peptide mimotopes, which can adopt multiple conformations, and could serve as a rich source of immunologically fit mimotopes. Overall, phage display libraries have the capacity to have a major impact on the field of vaccinology and should be considered as one arm of future vaccine development programs.

References

1 Ladner RC, Sato AK, Gorzelany J, de Souza M. Phage display-derived peptides as therapeutic alternatives to antibodies. *Drug Discov Today* 2004;**9**(12):525–9.

2 Sato AK, Viswanathan M, Kent RB, Wood CR. Therapeutic peptides: technological advances driving peptides into development. *Curr Opin Biotechnol* 2006;**17**(6):638–42.

3 Liu G, Wescott C, Sato A, et al. Nitriles form mixed-coligand complexes with (99m)Tc-HYNIC-peptide. *Nucl Med Biol* 2002;**29**(1):107–13.

4 Shrivastava A, von Wronski MA, Sato AK, et al. A distinct strategy to generate high-affinity peptide binders to receptor tyrosine kinases. *Protein Eng Des Sel* 2005;**18**(9):417–24.

5 Sato AK, Sexton DJ, Morganelli LA, et al. Development of mammalian serum albumin affinity purification media by peptide phage display. *Biotechnol Prog* 2002;**18**(2):182–92.

6 Smith GP, Scott JK. Libraries of peptides and proteins displayed on filamentous phage. *Methods Enzymol* 1993;**217**:228–57.

7 Noren KA, Noren CJ. Construction of high-complexity combinatorial phage display peptide libraries. *Methods* 2001;**23**(2):169–78.

8 Wierzbicki A, Gil M, Ciesielski M, et al. Immunization with a mimotope of GD2 ganglioside induces CD8+ T cells that recognize cell adhesion molecules on tumor cells. *J Immunol* 2008;**181**(9):6644–53.

9 Matthews LJ, Davis R, Smith GP. Immunogenically fit subunit vaccine components via epitope discovery from natural peptide libraries. *J Immunol* 2002;**169**(2):837–46.

10 Uttenreuther-Fischer MM, Kruger JA, Fischer P. Molecular characterization of the anti-idiotypic immune response of a relapse-free neuroblastoma patient following antibody therapy: a possible vaccine against tumors of neuroectodermal origin? *J Immunol* 2006;**176**(12):7775–86.

11 Beenhouwer DO, May RJ, Valadon P, Scharff MD. High affinity mimotope of the polysaccharide capsule of *Cryptococcus neoformans* identified from an evolutionary phage peptide library. *J Immunol* 2002;**169**(12):6992–9.

12 Buchwald UK, Lees A, Steinitz M, Pirofski LA. A peptide mimotope of type 8 pneumococcal capsular polysaccharide induces a protective immune response in mice. *Infect Immun* 2005;**73**(1):325–33.

13 Grothaus MC, Srivastava N, Smithson SL, et al. Selection of an immunogenic peptide mimic of the capsular polysaccharide of *Neisseria meningitidis* serogroup A using a peptide display library. *Vaccine* 2000;**18**(13):1253–63.

14 Lo Passo C, Romeo A, Pernice I, et al. Peptide mimics of the group B meningococcal capsule induce bactericidal and protective antibodies after immunization. *J Immunol* 2007;**178**(7):4417–23.

15 Pincus SH, Smith MJ, Jennings HJ, Burritt JB, Glee PM. Peptides that mimic the group B streptococcal type III capsular polysaccharide antigen. *J Immunol* 1998;**160**(1):293–8.

16 Zhang H, Zhong Z, Pirofski LA. Peptide epitopes recognized by a human anti-cryptococcal glucuronoxylomannan antibody. *Infect Immun* 1997;**65**(4):1158–64.

17 Beninati C, Garibaldi M, Passo CL, et al. Immunogenic mimics of *Brucella* lipopolysaccharide epitopes. *Peptides* 2009;**30**(10):1936–9.

18 De Bolle X, Laurent T, Tibor A, et al. Antigenic properties of peptidic mimics for epitopes of the lipopolysaccharide from Brucella. *J Mol Biol* 1999;**294**(1): 181–91.

19 Dharmasena MN, Jewell DA, Taylor RK. Development of peptide mimics of a protective epitope of

Vibrio cholerae Ogawa O-antigen and investigation of the structural basis of peptide mimicry. *J Biol Chem* 2007;**282**(46):33805–16.

20 Theillet FX, Saul FA, Vulliez-Le Normand B, *et al.* Structural mimicry of O-antigen by a peptide revealed in a complex with an antibody raised against *Shigella flexneri* serotype 2a. *J Mol Biol* 2009;**388**(4):839–50.

21 Casey JL, Coley AM, Anders RF, *et al.* Antibodies to malaria peptide mimics inhibit *Plasmodium falciparum* invasion of erythrocytes. *Infect Immun* 2004;**72**(2):1126–34.

22 Demangel C, Lafaye P, Mazie JC. Reproducing the immune response against the *Plasmodium vivax* merozoite surface protein 1 with mimotopes selected from a phage-displayed peptide library. *Mol Immunol* 1996;**33**(11–12):909–16.

23 Eda S, Sherman IW. Selection of peptides recognized by human antibodies against the surface of *Plasmodium falciparum*-infected erythrocytes. *Parasitology* 2005;**130**(Pt 1):1–11.

24 Yang G, Gao Y, Dong J, *et al.* A novel peptide screened by phage display can mimic TRAP antigen epitope against *Staphylococcus aureus* infections. *J Biol Chem* 2005;**280**(29):27431–5.

25 Yang G, Gao Y, Dong J, *et al.* A novel peptide isolated from phage library to substitute a complex system for a vaccine against staphylococci infection. *Vaccine* 2006;**24**(8):1117–23.

26 Ferrieu-Weisbuch C, Bettsworth F, Becquart L, *et al.* Usefulness of the phage display technology for the identification of a hepatitis C virus NS4A epitope recognized early in the course of the disease. *J Virol Methods* 2006;**131**(2):175–83.

27 Forster-Waldl E, Riemer AB, Dehof AK, *et al.* Isolation and structural analysis of peptide mimotopes for the disialoganglioside GD2, a neuroblastoma tumor antigen. *Mol Immunol* 2005;**42**(3):319–25.

28 Hou Y, Gu XX. Development of peptide mimotopes of lipooligosaccharide from nontypeable *Haemophilus influenzae* as vaccine candidates. *J Immunol* 2003;**170**(8):4373–9.

29 Houimel M, Dellagi K. Peptide mimotopes of rabies virus glycoprotein with immunogenic activity. *Vaccine* 2009;**27**(34):4648–55.

30 Larralde OG, Martinez R, Camacho F, *et al.* Identification of hepatitis A virus mimotopes by phage display, antigenicity and immunogenicity. *J Virol Methods* 2007;**140**(1–2):49–58.

31 Motti C, Nuzzo M, Meola A, *et al.* Recognition by human sera and immunogenicity of HBsAg mimo-

topes selected from an M13 phage display library. *Gene* 1994;**146**(2):191–8.

32 Bolesta E, Kowalczyk A, Wierzbicki A, *et al.* DNA vaccine expressing the mimotope of GD2 ganglioside induces protective GD2 cross-reactive antibody responses. *Cancer Res* 2005;**65**(8):3410–18.

33 Riemer AB, Forster-Waldl E, Bramswig KH, *et al.* Induction of IgG antibodies against the GD2 carbohydrate tumor antigen by vaccination with peptide mimotopes. *Eur J Immunol* 2006;**36**(5):1267–74.

34 Wondimu A, Zhang T, Kieber-Emmons T, *et al.* Peptides mimicking GD2 ganglioside elicit cellular, humoral and tumor-protective immune responses in mice. *Cancer Immunol Immunother* 2008;**57**(7):1079–89.

35 Riemer AB, Hantusch B, Sponer B, *et al.* High-molecular-weight melanoma-associated antigen mimotope immunizations induce antibodies recognizing melanoma cells. *Cancer Immunol Immunother* 2005;**54**(7):677–84.

36 Wagner S, Hafner C, Allwardt D, *et al.* Vaccination with a human high molecular weight melanoma-associated antigen mimotope induces a humoral response inhibiting melanoma cell growth in vitro. *J Immunol* 2005;**174**(2):976–82.

37 Riemer AB, Klinger M, Wagner S, *et al.* Generation of peptide mimics of the epitope recognized by trastuzumab on the oncogenic protein Her-2/neu. *J Immunol* 2004;**173**(1):394–401.

38 Riemer AB, Kurz H, Klinger M, *et al.* Vaccination with cetuximab mimotopes and biological properties of induced anti-epidermal growth factor receptor antibodies. *J Natl Cancer Inst* 2005;**97**(22):1663–70.

39 Jiang B, Liu W, Qu H, *et al.* A novel peptide isolated from a phage display peptide library with trastuzumab can mimic antigen epitope of HER-2. *J Biol Chem* 2005;**280**(6):4656–62.

40 Hoess R, Brinkmann U, Handel T, Pastan I. Identification of a peptide which binds to the carbohydrate-specific monoclonal antibody B3. *Gene* 1993;**128**(1):43–9.

41 Heimburg-Molinaro J, Almogren A, Morey S, *et al.* Development, characterization, and immunotherapeutic use of peptide mimics of the Thomsen-Friedenreich carbohydrate antigen. *Neoplasia* 2009;**11**(8):780–92.

42 Pacios LF, Tordesillas L, Cuesta-Herranz J, *et al.* Mimotope mapping as a complementary strategy to define allergen IgE-epitopes: peach Pru p 3 allergen as a model. *Mol Immunol* 2008;**45**(8):2269–76.

43 Rudolf MP, Vogel M, Kricek F, *et al*. Epitope-specific antibody response to IgE by mimotope immunization. *J Immunol* 1998;**160**(7):3315–21.

44 Untersmayr E, Szalai K, Riemer AB, *et al*. Mimotopes identify conformational epitopes on parvalbumin, the major fish allergen. *Mol Immunol* 2006;**43**(9):1454–61.

45 Laman AG, Shepelyakovskaya AO, Berezin IA, *et al*. Identification of pentadecapeptide mimicking muramyl peptide. *Vaccine* 2007;**25**(15):2900–906.

46 Chiang KC, Shimada Y, Nakano T, *et al*. A novel peptide mimotope identified as a potential immunosuppressive vaccine for organ transplantation. *J Immunol* 2009;**182**(7):4282–8.

47 Lang J, Zhan J, Xu L, Yan Z. Identification of peptide mimetics of xenoreactive alpha-Gal antigenic epitope by phage display. *Biochem Biophys Res Commun* 2006;**344**(1):214–20.

48 de la Cruz VF, Lal AA, McCutchan TF. Immunogenicity and epitope mapping of foreign sequences via genetically engineered filamentous phage. *J Biol Chem* 1988;**263**(9):4318–22.

49 Greenwood J, Willis AE, Perham RN. Multiple display of foreign peptides on a filamentous bacteriophage. Peptides from *Plasmodium falciparum* circumsporozoite protein as antigens. *J Mol Biol* 1991;**220**(4):821–7.

50 Monette M, Opella SJ, Greenwood J, Willis AE, Perham RN. Structure of a malaria parasite antigenic determinant displayed on filamentous bacteriophage determined by NMR spectroscopy: implications for the structure of continuous peptide epitopes of proteins. *Protein Sci* 2001;**10**(6):1150–59.

51 Fack F, Hugle-Dorr B, Song D, *et al*. Epitope mapping by phage display: random versus gene-fragment libraries. *J Immunol Methods* 1997;**206**(1–2):43–52.

52 Coley AM, Campanale NV, Casey JL, *et al*. Rapid and precise epitope mapping of monoclonal antibodies against *Plasmodium falciparum* AMA1 by combined phage display of fragments and random peptides. *Protein Eng* 2001;**14**(9):691–8.

53 Watt PM. Screening for peptide drugs from the natural repertoire of biodiverse protein folds. *Nat Biotechnol* 2006;**24**(2):177–83.

54 Koide A, Bailey CW, Huang X, Koide S. The fibronectin type III domain as a scaffold for novel binding proteins. *J Mol Biol* 1998;**284**(4):1141–51.

55 Skerra A. Alternative non-antibody scaffolds for molecular recognition. *Curr Opin Biotechnol* 2007; **18**(4):295–304.

56 Tang SS, Tan WS, Devi S, *et al*. Mimotopes of the Vi antigen of *Salmonella enterica* serovar *typhi* identified from phage display peptide library. *Clin Diagn Lab Immunol* 2003;**10**(6):1078–84.

57 Adda CG, Tilley L, Anders RF, Foley M. Isolation of peptides that mimic epitopes on a malarial antigen from random peptide libraries displayed on phage. *Infect Immun* 1999;**67**(9):4679–88.

58 Marston EL, James AV, Parker JT, *et al*. Newly characterized species-specific immunogenic *Chlamydophila pneumoniae* peptide reactive with murine monoclonal and human serum antibodies. *Clin Diagn Lab Immunol* 2002;**9**(2):446–52.

59 Coulon S, Metais JY, Chartier M, Briand JP, Baty D. Cyclic peptides selected by phage display mimic the natural epitope recognized by a monoclonal anticolicin A antibody. *J Pept Sci* 2004;**10**(11):648–58.

60 Read AJ, Casey JL, Coley AM, *et al*. Isolation of antibodies specific to a single conformation-dependant antigenic determinant on the EG95 hydatid vaccine. *Vaccine* 2009;**27**(7):1024–31.

PART 4
Antigen Engineering

CHAPTER 12

Attenuated Bacterial Vaccines

Richard W. Titball[1] & Helen S. Atkins[2]
[1] School of Biosciences, University of Exeter, Exeter, UK
[2] Department of Biomedical Sciences, Defence Science and Technology Laboratory, Porton Down, UK

Introduction

Live attenuated vaccines strike a fine balance between being sufficiently disabled to eliminate the potential to cause disease and being able to survive in the host to evoke protective immune responses. If the appropriate balance can be achieved then live attenuated vaccines are often highly effective, inducing long-lasting protective immunity after a single dose of the vaccine. Many of the live attenuated vaccines that are in use today protect against viral infections. These vaccines have been extremely effective in controlling diseases such as smallpox, polio, and yellow fever. In contrast, although there are a number of live attenuated bacterial vaccines that are either in use today or have been widely used in the past (Table 12.1), the performance of these vaccines is generally poor. These vaccines have usually been generated using empirical methods and in general the basis of attenuation is not known.

Over the past two decades new approaches to the generation of live attenuated vaccines have been intensively researched. These vaccines are not generated empirically but rather by interrupting specific biosynthetic or regulatory pathways. These vaccines are often referred to as rationally attenuated live vaccines. These approaches offer the potential to resolve many of the problems and limitations that exist with historical vaccines. In addition, the next generation of live attenuated vaccines offers the potential to be used to deliver heterologous antigens.

Live attenuated, killed, or subunit vaccines?

Killed or subunit vaccines against bacterial diseases are in widespread use and are generally given by parenteral routes, stimulating mainly systemic immune responses. However, many bacteria gain entry to the host via mucosal surfaces. Thus, parenterally administered vaccines, which may be limited in their capacity to induce mucosal immune responses, may not provide optimal protection against many bacterial infections.

In contrast, live attenuated vaccines offer the potential advantage of administration via the natural route of infection to stimulate appropriate immune responses, often mucosal delivery inducing both systemic and mucosal immunity. Unlike killed and subunit vaccines, which are generally poor at inducing cellular immune responses, live attenuated vaccines are able to induce cellular immune responses, which may be important for protection against intracellular bacterial pathogens. Such vaccines may also offer the further advantage of being easier and safer to administer than killed or subunit vaccines, which are given by injection.

However, live attenuated vaccines do have some limitations when compared to killed or sub-unit

Vaccinology: Principles and Practice, First Edition. Edited by W. John W. Morrow, Nadeem A. Sheikh, Clint S. Schmidt and D. Huw Davies.
© The contents include material subject to Crown Copyright 2012/DSTL – published with the permission of the Controller of Her Majesty's Stationery Office. Published 2012 by Blackwell Publishing Ltd.

Table 12.1 Live attenuated bacterial vaccines that have been used or are currently in use.

Pathogen	Vaccine designation	Attenuating lesion	Target population	Ref.
Shigella flexneri	FS	Not known	Humans	[94]
Francisella tularensis	LVS	Not known	Human	[95]
Bacillus anthracis	ST-I	Plasmid pXO2⁻ (capsule negative) mutant	Humans	[96]
Bacillus anthracis	Sterne	Plasmid pXO2⁻ (capsule negative) mutant	Livestock	[96]
Salmonella enterica serovar Typhi	TY21a	Not certain	Humans	[3]
Yersinia pestis	EV76	Pigmentation mutant	Humans	[97]
Brucella abortus	S19	Not known	Livestock	[98]
Mycobacterium tuberculosis	BCG	Not certain	Humans	[99]
Vibrio cholera	CVD103 HgR	Lacks cholera toxin A-subunit	Humans	[100]
Aeromonas salmonicida	644Rb aroA	*aroA* mutant	Farmed fish	[31]

vaccines. Because they are live, they often require storage under carefully controlled conditions, and have limited shelf lives. More importantly, the ability of live attenuated vaccines to induce protective immunity is dependent on a fine balance between ensuring the vaccine strain is able to survive in the host for a sufficient length of time and ensuring that the vaccine is sufficiently disabled that it is not able to cause disease. This latter consideration is especially important when the vaccine might be used in immunocompromised hosts. Newer approaches to the development of live attenuated vaccines can help to minimize this problem, but some of the existing live attenuated bacterial vaccines are not considered to be safe for use in immunocompromised hosts.

Existing live attenuated vaccines

Many of the live attenuated bacterial vaccines in use today have been generated using empirical approaches, and the reasons why these particular approaches were followed to generate the vaccines seems quite obscure. At the time of their discovery the genetic basis of attenuation was not known and for many live bacterial vaccines the molecular basis of attenuation is still not clear.

It might be assumed that the availability of genome sequencing methodologies would now

make the characterization and identification of attenuating mutations possible. In some cases this has proven to be the case, but for others the reasons for attenuation are still only partially understood. For example, although the genome sequence of the Bacille Calmette-Guérin (BCG) strain of *Mycobacterium bovis* has now been determined, and can be compared to the sequences of virulent strains, the exact identity of the mutations introduced during passaging is not known because the original virulent strain is not available [1].

This chapter does not aim to cover all of the existing live attenuated vaccines, but rather, highlights specific vaccines that have been used in humans, describing the performance and limitations of these vaccines. The Ty21a and BCG vaccines against typhoid and tuberculosis, respectively, are examples of vaccines of limited efficacy while the EV76 and S19 vaccines against plague and brucellosis are not considered to be safe for use in humans. Finally, the LVS vaccine is effective in preventing tularemia and is not reactogenic but the lack of data on the reasons for attenuation of the strain contributes to the difficulties of licensing this vaccine for use in humans.

S. *enterica* serovar Typhi

A live attenuated oral typhoid fever vaccine based on the Ty21a strain of *S. enterica* serovar Typhi [2] has been used widely to immunize against typhoid fever. This mutant, derived by ni-trosoguanidine treatment of the TY2 strain [3], is a *galE* (galactose epimerase) mutant [4] deficient in O antigen production and is also unable to synthesize the Vi capsular antigen. Although attenuation was originally thought to be attributable to the *galE* mutation, it has since been shown that a genetically defined *S. enterica* serovar Typhi *galE* and Vi-negative mutant was not as highly attenuated as TY21a when tested in human volunteers [5]. Thus, it seems likely that additional mutations contribute to the attenuation of Ty21a. A theoretical problem associated with Ty21a is reversion to virulence, although no such revertants have been isolated to date [6]. Ty21a has been evaluated as a typhoid vaccine in several efficacy trials and shown to be safe and effective [3]. However, Ty21a is only modestly immunogenic and requires three or four initial doses [3]. Therefore the vaccine is usually administered initially as 3–4 capsules containing bacteria on alternate days, and requires boosters every 5 years [4], although a liquid formulation of Ty21a vaccines has been developed, which has been shown to further improve the protection afforded [7,8].

M. bovis BCG

The BCG strain was generated early in the 20th century by continuous passage of a virulent bovine isolate every 3 weeks for 13 years – a total of 231 cycles [1]. The BCG vaccine is used worldwide as a vaccine against tuberculosis, caused by *M. tuberculosis*. However, its efficacy remains controversial since BCG is effective in protecting infants from tuberculosis but immunity declines with age and fails to protect adults against pulmonary tuberculosis, the primary source of dissemination [9]. Surprisingly, the mechanisms by which BCG generates protective immunity remain largely undefined. There are several variants of BCG available, all of which have undergone two distinct phases of attenuation: the *in vitro* passages conducted by Albert Calmette and Camille Guérin at the Institute Pasteur, France, in 1908–1921, followed by subsequent attenuation during widespread use and worldwide distribution prior to the establishment of frozen seed lots [10]. Comparison of the genomes of BCG strains has uncovered several individual components likely to contribute to the attenuation of BCG, including mutations in the PhoP-PhoR system [11].

Y. pestis EV76

Live attenuated *Y. pestis* vaccines have been used mainly in the former Soviet Union (FSU) and the former French colonies and are still in use in the FSU and in Mongolia. These are based on pigmentation mutants of fully virulent strains [12,13]. The inability of *Y. pestis* to appear pigmented when grown on certain solid media (for example, containing congo red dye) is a consequence of the deletion of a region of the chromosome that includes the hemin storage locus and high pathogenicity island. *Y. pestis* strain EV76 is the most widely used and best characterized pigmentation mutant that has been used as a vaccine. In the murine model, vaccination with EV76 induces protection against subsequent subcutaneous and inhalation challenges with *Y. pestis* [14]. Live *Y. pestis* vaccines are not licensed or commercially available in Europe or in the USA mainly because there are significant concerns over the safety of this vaccine. The vaccination of mice or vervets with this strain can result in fatalities [12,14]. Of greater concern, studies in the FSU have reported that some human vaccinees (1–20% depending on the route of vaccine administration) develop a febrile response, with headache, weakness, and general malaise, and individuals with severe reactions required hospitalization [12].

B. abortus S19

The *B. abortus* S19 live vaccine strain has been used extensively to prevent bovine brucellosis, and efficacy studies have demonstrated that approximately 70% of vaccinated cattle are protected [15]. In this situation, S19 typically shows low virulence, although the vaccine causes abortions when administered to 1–2.5% of pregnant animals [16]. In humans, S19 is not considered a safe vaccine candidate. In the FSU, live S19 was used to immunize over 3 million people [17]. S19 was immunogenic and human vaccination was associated with a reduction in cases of brucellosis. However, S19 caused localized hypersensitivity reactions and, in a controlled experimental trial, the live strain persisted in 2 of 16 vaccinates [18].

F. tularensis LVS

The *F. tularensis* live vaccine strain (LVS) or progenitors of this strain have been used extensively in humans to immunize against tularemia. In spite of this there are few reports of controlled studies to evaluate the efficacy of the LVS vaccine. In one study in the USA, both individuals immunized with a live attenuated vaccine and naïve individuals were exposed to airborne virulent *F. tularensis* [19]. Good protection against a challenge of 10 infectious doses (IDs) was reported but when challenged with 1000 IDs the degree of protection was marginal [19]. In another study, the incidence of laboratory-acquired tularemia at Fort Detrick in Maryland was shown to reduce markedly following the immunization of laboratory workers [20]. Live attenuated tularemia vaccines have generally been given by the intradermal or subcutaneous routes, but there is evidence that oral, aerogenic, and intranasal immunization are also effective [21,22]. Indeed, some studies suggest that the aerogenic rather than intradermal route of immunization provided a higher level of protection against a subsequent respiratory challenge [23]. This finding might be in accordance with more recent studies, which have shown that mice immunized with the LVS strain by the intranasal route are better protected against a subsequent challenge than mice immunized by the intradermal or subcutaneous route [24,25].

While in the past the LVS vaccine has been used in humans as an investigational new drug, currently the vaccine is not available for use in humans. The principal reasons preventing licensing for use in humans include the potential for batch-to-batch variation of vaccine lots and the lack of information on the molecular or biochemical basis of attenuation. It has been suggested [26] that any future work to license this vaccine should especially focus on characterizing the LVS strain and identifying the genetic or biochemical basis of attenuation of the LVS strain.

Rationally attenuated live vaccines

As highlighted above, the genetic basis of attenuation of many live attenuated vaccines is not known – these vaccines have been generated using empirical approaches often involving the selection of spontaneous mutants. Thus, the acceptability of some of these vaccines lies in their history of widespread use. However, the methods used to generate these vaccines are not acceptable nowadays and it is unlikely that vaccines devised in this way would be licensable. In addition, as highlighted above, many of these vaccines are of limited efficacy or are highly reactogenic in humans. Against this background, research over the past two decades has focused on the introduction of defined and attenuating genetic lesions into bacteria. A wide range of genes and pathways have been targeted in these studies and an overview of these is provided in the following sections.

Auxotrophs

Shikimate pathway auxotrophs

The shikimate pathway is the common pathway for the biosynthesis of chorismate in bacteria (Figure 12.1). Chorismate is the precursor for the generation of aromatic amino acids (phenylalanine, tryptophan, and tyrosine), folate, coenzymes, vitamins (such as the benzenoid and naphthenoid coenzymes Q and vitamin K), and aromatic secondary metabolites, including the 2,3-dihydroxybenzoate-containing siderophores required for iron uptake and accumulation [27]. The inactivation of genes in the shikimate pathway has resulted in attenuation of many pathogens, including *S. enterica* serovar Typhimurium [28], *S. enterica* serovar Typhi [29], *Neisseria gonorrhoeae* [30], *A. salmonicida* [31], and *Pasteurella multocida* [32]. However, the mechanism of attenuation has not been fully defined although it seems likely to involve the inability of the bacteria to produce siderophores.

Most of the detailed studies on attenuation consequent to the disruption of the shikimate pathway

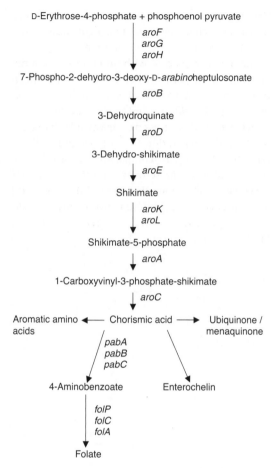

D-Erythrose-4-phosphate + phosphoenol pyruvate

↓ *aroF*
↓ *aroG*
↓ *aroH*

7-Phospho-2-dehydro-3-deoxy-D-*arabino*heptulosonate

↓ *aroB*

3-Dehydroquinate

↓ *aroD*

3-Dehydro-shikimate

↓ *aroE*

Shikimate

↓ *aroK*
↓ *aroL*

Shikimate-5-phosphate

↓ *aroA*

1-Carboxyvinyl-3-phosphate-shikimate

↓ *aroC*

Aromatic amino ← Chorismic acid → Ubiquinone /
acids   menaquinone

pabA
pabB
pabC

4-Aminobenzoate   Enterochelin

folP
folC
folA

Folate

Figure 12.1 The shikimate pathway in bacteria. Chorismic acid is the starting point for the biosynthesis of aromatic amino acids, *p*-aminobenzoic acid and folic acid, enterochelin, and ubiquinone and menaquinone.

have been carried out in *S. enterica*. The first reported study demonstrated attenuation of *S. enterica* serovar Typhimurium following inactivation of the *aroA* gene (encoding 5-*enol*pyruvylshikimate-3-phosphate synthase) [28]. The *aroA* mutant was able to undergo limited replication in mice, but unable to cause disease and was therefore attenuated [33]. The immunization of mice with the *aroA* mutant stimulated protective immunity to a subsequent challenge with wild-type bacteria [28,33]. Additionally, the inactivation of other genes in the shikimate pathway, including *aroB*, *aroC* (encod-

ing chorismate synthase), and *aroD* (encoding 3-dehydroquinase), has been shown to attenuate *S. enterica* [34–36]. For the development of rationally attenuated *S. enterica* serovar Typhi as typhoid fever vaccines, multiple mutations have been introduced into the shikimate pathway. These double mutants have been constructed by combining the *aroA* deletion with deletions in other genes in the shikimate pathway genes such as *aroC* or *aroD* (encoding 3-dehydroquinase) [34,36]. This minimizes the possibility of reversion, and the restoration of wild-type virulence.

Although *aro* mutants of *S. enterica* have been extensively tested in animal models of disease, and shown to be attenuated and to induce protective immunity [37], volunteer studies and clinical trials in humans have revealed that *S. enterica* serovar Typhi *aro* (CVD 908) mutants can cause vaccinemias [37,38]. Two approaches have been proposed to resolve this problem. First, an additional mutation has been introduced into the *htrA* gene [39,40]. In phase I clinical trials, doses of 5×10^7–5×10^9 colony forming units (cfu) of CVD 908-*htrA* have been well tolerated, with only one case of fever and three cases of diarrhea in 36 subjects following high doses of the vaccines [40]. There were no cases of vaccinemia. More recently CVD 908-*htrA* has completed phase II clinical trials [39].

An alternative approach involves the introduction of an additional mutation into the *ssaV* gene of the SPI-2 type III system that is required for *S. enterica* survival and growth within macrophages. The resultant strain (*S. enterica* var. Typhi ZH9 (Ty2 *aroC ssaV*) does not cause vaccinemias at doses of up to 10^9 cfu but retains immunogenicity [41]. These mutants may be alternatives to the *aro htrA* mutants as typhoid fever vaccines, but the results of controlled trials with *S. enterica* var Typhi *aroC ssaV* mutants have yet to be reported.

Purine biosynthetic pathway auxotrophs

Attenuation can also be achieved by blocking the *de novo* synthesis of purines and has been shown to attenuate several pathogens, including *Y. pestis* [42,43], *B. anthracis* [44], *Brucella melitensis* [45], *M. tuberculosis* [46], *F. tularensis* [47,48], *S. enterica* serovar Dublin and serovar Typhimurium [49], and *Shigella flexneri* [50].

In general, the level of attenuation depends on the position at which the pathway is blocked (Figure 12.2). Strains with a mutation in the *purA* gene encoding the enzyme adenylosuccinate synthetase, involved in the first step of the conversion of inosine monophosphate (IMP) to adenosine monophosphate (AMP) in the synthesis of purines, and resulting in a requirement for adenosine, are the most widely studied. Of these, *S. enterica* serovar Typhimurium strains harboring either the *purA* mutation or an *aroA purA* double mutation are poorly immunogenic in mice [51] and humans [52]. Conversely, immunization with an

Edwardsiella ictaluri purA mutant provided protection against challenge with a virulent strain [53].

Differences in the degree of attenuation are also found between species, with mutations in different positions of the pathway being more attenuating in one species than another. For example, mutations in *purE* in *B. melitensis* and *purC* in *M. tuberculosis*, which act earlier in the enzyme cascade than *purA*, blocking the generation of IMP, are markedly attenuating [45,46]. In comparison, *Y. pestis*, *B. anthracis*, and *S. enterica* serovar Typhimurium are less sensitive to mutations that block IMP [33,42,49]. Thus, it is clear that different pathogens have different requirements for purine precursors that can limit their ability to cause disease.

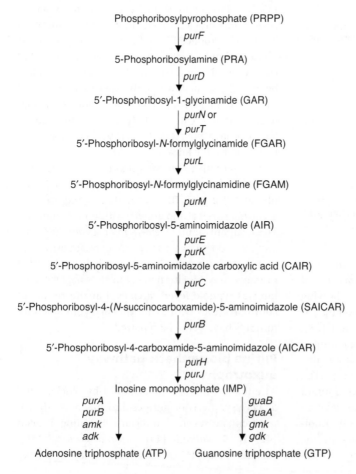

Figure 12.2 The *de novo* pathway of purine biosynthesis in bacteria.

Branched-chain amino acid biosynthesis auxotrophs

The pathway responsible for the synthesis of branched-chain amino acids has rarely been targeted for attenuation. However, several studies have reported the attenuation of *M. bovis* and *M. tuberculosis* branched-chain amino acid biosynthesis mutants [54–56]. The attenuating mutations were in the *leuD* gene, which encodes a protein in the branch of the pathway specific to leucine biosynthesis [54,55]. These mycobacteria are unable to survive and multiply within mononuclear phagocytes. The exact mechanism of stimulation of the specific immune response by the *leuD* mycobacterial mutant, protective against challenge with wild-type mycobacteria, has not been determined.

A branched-chain amino acid biosynthesis mutant of *Burkholderia pseudomallei* has also been reported [57]. In contrast to the mycobacterial mutants, this mutant was defective in the biosynthesis of leucine, isoleucine, and valine, and the attenuating mutation was shown to be in the *ilvB* gene. Immunization with the *ilvB* mutant provided good protection against a subsequent challenge with 6×10^3 median lethal doses of the wild type [57].

In both of these cases it seems unlikely that the inability to synthesize branched-chain amino acids is responsible for attenuation since these amino acids would be freely available in mammals. Like the aromatic amino acid pathway, it is possible that products of this pathway other than the amino acid are necessary for growth *in vivo*, although the identity of these products has yet to be established.

Regulatory mutants

Adenylate cyclase (*cya*) and camp receptor protein (*crp*) mutants

The inactivation of genes that regulate virulence of pathogens is an attractive option for the generation of attenuated mutants as vaccines. If regulatory systems play roles after the initial invasion of the host then the ability of the attenuated mutant to colonize the host is not impaired. However, the ability to become established and to cause disease is severely compromised. *Salmonella* vaccine candidates with deletions in adenylate cyclase (*cya*) and cAMP receptor protein (*crp*) genes have received some attention. These genes play roles in the regulation of *Salmonella* virulence, affecting the expression of genes involved in carbohydrate and amino acid metabolism and in the expression of fimbrae and flagella [58,59]. *S. enterica* serovar Typhimurium single mutants of *cya* or *crp*, or a double mutant of *cya* and *crp*, all show attenuated virulence and can protect mice against oral challenge with the wild-type strain [58]. *S. enterica* serovar Typhi Ty2 ΔcyA Δcrp Δcdt (strain $\chi 4073$) has also yielded promising results [60]. Following inoculation with a single dose of up to 5×10^8 cfu of $\chi 4073$, most healthy adult volunteers tolerated the vaccine well and developed *S. enterica* serovar Typhi-specific serum antibody responses and serovar Typhi-specific antibody secreting cells.

PhoP/Q mutants

The phoP/Q two-component regulatory system has also received attention as a target for rational attenuation. This system is associated with the ability of bacteria to survive within host cells, and in *S. enterica* phoP/Q regulated genes play roles in the invasion of epithelial cells, survival within macrophages, resistance to antimicrobial peptides, and resistance to low pH.

The inactivation of the phoP/Q two-component regulatory system has been shown to attenuate a number of pathogens, including *S. enterica*, *Neisseria meningitidis* [61], *Y. pestis* [62], and *M. tuberculosis* [63,64]. In the case of *Y. pestis* the bacterium was not sufficiently attenuated to warrant further consideration as a vaccine but the *S. enterica* mutants have progressed to human volunteer studies. Strain Ty445, an *aroA phoP phoQ* mutant, was nonreactogenic in human volunteers given a high dose of 5×10^{10} cfu, but was poorly immunogenic [65]. In an attempt to provide a better compromise between attenuation and immunogenicity, strain Ty800, a *phoP/Q* mutant, was produced. In a dose escalation trial, this vaccine was shown to be safe and immunogenic. Only volunteers receiving a dose of 1×10^{10} CFU of Ty800 showed mild adverse effects. Those receiving lower doses were not affected and, importantly, no Ty800 was detected in blood cultures following vaccination [66].

The *M. tuberculosis phoP* mutant is widely considered to be the most promising vaccine candidate of a range of live attenuated mutants that have been constructed and tested as possible replacements for the BCG vaccine [63]. In guinea pig models of disease a *phoP* mutant has proven to be safe (it is more highly attenuated than BCG) and to induce immunity that protects against inhalation challenge [64]. It seems likely that this vaccine will be trialled in humans in the near future.

Immune responses to live attenuated vaccines

The use of live attenuated bacteria as vaccines takes advantage of the natural properties of the organisms, including cell invasion and tissue tropism, natural presentation of immunogens, and the ability to induce appropriate immune responses. For example, attenuated strains of *S. enterica* serovar Typhi may be delivered via the oral route of infection and are capable of eliciting both humoral and cellular immune responses, both systemically and at mucosal surfaces. The attenuated strains may be fine-tuned to enable modulation of the immune responses generated. For example, *S. enterica* serovar Typhimurium strains carrying different mutations but resulting in similar levels of attenuation stimulate distinct immune responses [67]. This ability of live attenuated bacteria to generate the full repertoire of immune responses, which are likely to be required for controlling infection of many pathogens, is a significant advantage to their use as vaccines in comparison to killed or subunit vaccines, which are likely to require the development of delivery platforms in order to stimulate protective immunity to prevent disease.

A number of studies have characterized the diversity of the immune response elicited by live attenuated vaccines. The types of responses that are elicited are best described from studies with rationally attenuated mutants of *S. enterica* serovar Typhimurium. It is likely that other live attenuated vaccines that have life cycles similar to *S. enterica*

would elicit similar immune responses. Oral immunization with *aro* mutants of *S. enterica* serovar Typhimurium is able to elicit serum and mucosal antibody responses to lipopolysaccharide [68]. Serum antibody is characterized by high levels of IgG2a, suggesting a Th1-type response [68]. Both CD4$^+$ and CD8$^+$ T-cell responses are induced after immunization with *aro* mutants of *S. enterica* serovar Typhimurium, and both responses appear to play roles in protection against disease [69,70].

Safety of live attenuated vaccines

The balance between the attenuation and immunogenicity of live attenuated bacteria is critical for the development of safe, efficacious vaccines. In general, the extensive use of the existing live attenuated vaccines in healthy individuals has enabled a high level of confidence in the safety of these vaccines. However, the use of the existing vaccines in those who are immunocompromised may be problematic. Recently, the Global Advisory Committee on Vaccine Safety established by the World Health Organization has recommended that the BCG vaccine should not be administered to children known to be HIV infected [71], highlighting the problem. This may present a significant obstacle to the development of new and effective vaccines since subunit-based vaccines alone are unlikely to be superior to live vaccines for a range of diseases, including those caused by intracellular pathogens.

The development of new live attenuated vaccines is facilitated by the safety data derived from many years of experience with the existing live vaccine strains. However, for a new live attenuated vaccine to be considered safe for use in humans it is generally considered necessary for at least two defined mutations to be introduced to reduce the risk of the bacterium reverting to a virulent form. The strains need to be well-defined strains with characterized mutations and safe and effective for use in all populations, including the immunocompromised. Finding the right balance between attenuation and immunogenicity is a key challenge.

There have been some studies in animals to assess how safe rationally attenuated vaccines are likely to be in humans. Burns-Guydish *et al.* have shown that *aroA* mutants of *S. enterica* var Typhimurium are unable to cause disease in young mice (though *phoP* mutants were not attenuated) [72]. The evidence is that rationally attenuated mutants such as *aro* mutants of *S. enterica* var Typhimurium can be safe in moderately immunosuppressed mice [73] and *htrA* mutants are reportedly unable to cause disease in irradiated mice or mice with B-cell defects [74]. In severely immunocompromised mice (e.g., nude mice) even *aroA* mutants are able to cause slowly progressing lethal infections [75].

Live attenuated vaccines as vaccine carriers

Live attenuated vaccines have attracted considerable attention as delivery systems for heterologous vaccine antigens. In principle, the use of live attenuated vaccines in this way is simple. The gene encoding the heterologous antigen of interest is expressed in a live vaccine, and immunization with the recombinant live vaccine then results in the induction of immunity to both the vaccine carrier and the heterologous antigen. Most work on the delivery of heterologous antigens has been carried out with attenuated *S. enterica* strains that have been developed as candidate typhoid vaccines. In addition to oral administration and the ability to generate a range of immune responses, *Salmonella* are easily genetically manipulated and are able to express heterologous antigens of bacterial, viral, and eukaryotic origin.

The drive to develop new recombinant vector vaccines in *S. enterica* has led to the use of a range of technologies that have provided solutions to some of the problems associated with effective immunization [76].

Stable antigen expression

The expression of heterologous antigens, at sufficient levels to elicit protective immune responses, is a significant challenge for live recombinant vaccine development. Under some circumstances, constitutive high-level expression of a heterologous

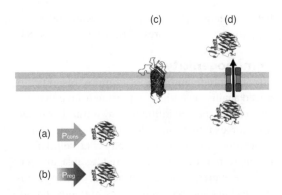

Figure 12.3 Generalized representation of the strategies employed to express heterologous antigens in *S. enterica*. Protein antigens can be expressed from a strong unregulated (a) or a regulated (b) promoter that is active only *in vivo*. Fragments (epitopes) of the heterologous antigen can be inserted into permissive outer membrane proteins such as MalE, OmpA, or LamB, resulting in the display of an epitope from the protein on the bacterial cell surface (c). They may be fused to signals (e.g., HlyA or ClyA) that result in export of the proteins via secretion systems (d).

antigen may be toxic to the live vaccine carrier (Figure 12.3a). One strategy to overcome this problem involves the use of *in vivo*-inducible promoters (Figure 12.3b) that maintain a low level of antigen expression until the vaccine carrier recognizes an appropriate environmental stimulus, which then results in increased antigen expression. Additionally, problems associated with unstable expression of heterologous antigens may be encountered, particularly when the vaccine carriers are used *in vivo*. To address the instability of heterologous antigen-encoding plasmids within the bacterial cells, systems have been developed to allow the heterologous antigen-encoding DNA to be incorporated in the chromosome of the bacterial carrier [77,78]. However, using this approach, antigen will be expressed from only a single copy of the foreign gene, compared to multiple copies of the gene present in vaccine carriers harboring a multicopy expression plasmid. This may result in low expression of the antigen and, as a result, poor immunogenicity. Thus, approaches to solve the instability and segregational loss of the multicopy antigen-encoding plasmids are being sought, including balanced-lethal [79–82], post-segregational killing [83], and operator-repressor titration systems [84].

Immunogenicity

The magnitude and type of immune response induced against an antigen expressed from a live vaccine carrier may be influenced by a number of factors, for example, the cellular location of antigen expression. Since both antibody and cellular immune responses may be elicited against antigens that are expressed on the surfaces of carrier strains, studies have focused on directing antigens that are normally expressed in the cytoplasm onto the cell surface. Typically this is achieved by inserting peptides derived from the protein of interest into permissive sites in the periplasmic binding protein, MalE [85], or outer membrane proteins such as OmpA [86] or LamB [85] (Figure 12.3c). Additionally, the secretion of proteins from *Salmonella* (Figure 12.3d) may improve the protective immunogenicity of antigens, as shown for the Hly and p60 proteins of *Listeria monocytogenes*, which were protective against subsequent *L. monocytogenes* infection when secreted, but were not protective when displayed somatically [87]. The secretion of heterologous antigens from *Salmonella* vaccine strains has been achieved, for example, using the type III secretion system of *Salmonella* [88] or the *E. coli* Hly haemolysin secretion system [89]. Despite these studies, numerous reports have confirmed that induction of a broad spectrum of immune responses could be elicited against heterologous antigens expressed in the *Salmonella* cytoplasm. Thus it appears that cell-surface expression is not a prerequisite for induction of both cellular and humoral immunity against heterologous antigens, although it is possible that some naturally secreted antigens may require cell-surface expression in order to fold correctly and to adopt a conformation that is immunogenic.

The immunogenicity of antigens expressed from vaccine carriers may also be improved by fusion to proven carrier antigens, such as TetC. For example, expression in *Salmonella* of the *Schistosoma mansoni* [90] or *Schistosoma haematobium* [91] 28 kDa glutathione *S*-transferases as fusions to TetC enhanced their immunogenicity. It is thought that TetC pro-

motes the immune response against fused antigens by providing additional T-cell helper epitopes. In other studies, *Streptococcus sobrinus* antigens [92] or the *E. coli* heat-stable enterotoxin [93] were expressed in *Salmonella* as fusions to the *E. coli* heat-labile toxin subunit B (LT-B), which is also known to have immune-enhancing effects. LT-B and CT-B, the cholera toxin B subunit, are well-known nontoxic adjuvants containing structural features that provide adjuvant and immunogenic stimulation in the intestinal mucosa. Similarly, it may also be possible to modulate the immune response generated against heterologous antigens expressed by carriers by the co-expression or fusion to cytokines.

The value of such technical approaches to improve vaccines remains to be proved in clinical trials. To date a limited number of recombinant live vector vaccines have been evaluated in clinical trials. The lack of immunogenicity of recombinant vaccines based on the licensed *Salmonella* vaccine strain Ty21a is likely due to high attenuation by multiple mutations in the strain. Disappointingly, recombinant vaccines based on more immunogenic strains such as CVD908 and CVD908-*htrA* are also relatively ineffective, demonstrating the technical challenge in achieving the correct balance between antigen expression and immunogenicity, in addition to the correct level of attenuation of the carrier strain.

Conclusions

Live attenuated mutants of bacteria continue to be used widely as vaccines against a range of diseases. However, the genetic basis of attenuation of some of these vaccines is not known, and some are not considered to be safe for use in immunocompromised hosts. Rationally attenuated mutants, created by deleting one or more genes required for the growth of bacteria *in vivo*, have been extensively investigated over the past two decades. These mutants fall broadly into two groups: auxotrophs and virulence regulatory mutants. Most of the pioneering work with these mutants has been carried out in *S. enterica*, and information from these studies has informed much of the subsequent work to devise rationally attenuated mutants of other pathogens. It is clear from studies in *S. enterica* that mutations in more than one pathway may be required to ensure safety in human volunteers.

In spite of the intensive research to develop rationally attenuated vaccines, and the large body of information on the testing of these mutants in animal models of disease, none of these rationally attenuated mutants is currently licensed for use in humans. In part this reflects the problems associated with the licensing of any live vaccine and ensuring safety in individuals with differing degrees of immunocompetence.

In spite of these challenges, live attenuated bacterial vaccines offer a number of important advantages over killed or subunit vaccines. They are often single-dose vaccines, and many can be given non-invasively. More importantly, live vaccines have the potential to induce a wide range of immune responses ranging from the induction of mucosal antibody to the stimulation of cytotoxic T-cells. In addition, live vaccines can be used to deliver heterologous antigens, allowing multivalent vaccines to be devised. Collectively, these advantages highlight the reasons for continuing to develop live vaccines against a range of diseases caused by bacterial pathogens.

References

1 Smith KC, Orme IM, Starke JR. Tuberculosis vaccines. In S Plotkin, W Orenstein, P Offit (Eds) *Vaccines*. Elsevier Saunders, Oxford, 2008, pp. 857–86.

2 Germanier R, Fuer E. Isolation and characterization of Gal E mutant Ty 21a of *Salmonella typhi*: a candidate strain for a live, oral typhoid vaccine. *J Infect Dis* 1975;**131**:53–8.

3 Levine MM. Typhoid fever vaccines. In S Plotkin, W Orenstein, P Offit (Eds) *Vaccines*. Elsevier Saunders, Oxford, 2008, pp. 887–914.

4 Merican I. Typhoid fever: present and future. *Med J. Malaysia* 1997;**52**:299–308; quiz 309.

5 Hone DM, Attridge SR, Forrest B, *et al*. A *galE* via (Vi antigen-negative) mutant of *Salmonella typhi* Ty2 retains virulence in humans. *Infect Immun* 1988; **56**:1326–33.

6 McKenna AJ, Bygraves JA, Maiden MC, *et al*. Attenuated typhoid vaccine *Salmonella typhi* Ty21a: fingerprinting and quality control. *Microbiology* 1995; **141**:1993–2002.

7 Levine MM, Ferreccio C, Cryz S, *et al*. Comparison of enteric-coated capsules and liquid formulation of Ty21a typhoid vaccine in randomised controlled field trial. *Lancet* 1990;**336**:891–4.

8 Levine MM, Ferreccio C, Abrego P, *et al*. Duration of efficacy of Ty21a, attenuated *Salmonella typhi* live oral vaccine. *Vaccine* 1999;**17**(Suppl 2):S22–7.

9 Colditz GA, Brewer TF, Berkey CS, *et al*. Efficacy of BCG vaccine in the prevention of tuberculosis. Meta-analysis of the published literature. *JAMA* 1994;**271**: 698–702.

10 Liu J, Tran V, Leung AS, *et al*. BCG vaccines: their mechanisms of attenuation and impact on safety and protective efficacy. *Hum Vaccin* 2009;**5**:70–78.

11 Leung AS, Tran V, Wu Z, *et al*. Novel genome polymorphisms in BCG vaccine strains and impact on efficacy. *BMC Genomics* 2008;**9**:413.

12 Meyer KF, Cavanaugh DC, Bartelloni PJ, *et al*. Plague immunization. I. Past and present trends. *J Infect Dis* 1974;**129**, S13–18.

13 Brubaker RR. Mutation rate to non-pigmentation in *Pasturella pestis*. *J Bacteriol* 1969;**98**:1404–6.

14 Russell P, Eley SM, Hibbs SE, *et al*. A comparison of plague vaccine, USP and EV76 vaccine induced protection against *Yersinia pestis* in a murine model. *Vaccine* 1995;**13**:1551–6.

15 Nicoletti P. Vaccination against *Brucella*. *Adv Biotechnol Processes* 1990;**13**:147–68.

16 Schurig GG, Sriranganathan N, Corbel MJ. Brucellosis vaccines: past, present and future. *Vet Microbiol* 2002;**90**:479–96.

17 Vershilova PA. The use of live vaccination for vaccination of human beings against brucellosis in the USSR. *Bull World Health Organ* 1961;**24**:85–9.

18 Spink WW, Hall JW, 3rd, Finstad J, *et al*. Immunization with viable *Brucella* organisms. Results of a safety test in humans. *Bull World Health Organ* 1962; **26**:409–19.

19 McCrumb FR. Aerosol infection of man with *Pasteurella tularensis*. *Bacteriol Rev* 1961;**25**:262–7.

20 Burke DS. Immunization against tularemia: analysis of the effectiveness of live *Francisella tularensis* vaccine in prevention of laboratory acquired tularemia. *J Infect Dis* 1977;**135**:55–60.

21 Eigelsbach HT, Tulis JJ. Aerogenic immunization of the monkey and the guinea pig with live tularemia vaccine. *Proc Soc Exp Biol Med* 1961;**108**:732–4.

22 Eigelsbach HT, Tulis JJ, McGavran MH, *et al.* Live tularemia vaccine. I. Host-parasite relationship in monkeys vaccinated intracutaneously or aerogenically. *J Bacteriol* 1962;**84**:1020–27.

23 Hornick RB, Eigelsbach HT. Aerogenic immunization of man with live tularemia vaccine. *Bacteriol Rev* 1966;**30**:532–8.

24 Conlan JW, Shen H, Kuolee R, *et al.* Aerosol-, but not intradermal-immunization with the live vaccine strain of *Francisella tularensis* protects mice against subsequent aerosol challenge with a highly virulent type A strain of the pathogen by an alphabeta T cell- and interferon gamma-dependent mechanism. *Vaccine* 2005;**23**:2477–85.

25 Wu TH, Hutt JA, Garrison KA, *et al.* Intranasal vaccination induces protective immunity against intranasal infection with virulent *Francisella tularensis* biovar A. *Infect Immun* 2005;**73**:2644–54.

26 Ellis J, Oyston PCF, Green M, *et al.* Tularemia. *Clin Microbiol Rev* 2002;**15**:631–46.

27 Liu J, Quinn N, Berchtold GA, *et al.* Overexpression, purification, and characterization of isochorismate synthase (EntC), the first enzyme involved in the biosynthesis of enterobactin from chorismate. *Biochemistry* 1990;**29**:1417–25.

28 Hoiseth SK, Stocker BAD. Aromatic-dependent *Salmonella typhimurium* are non-virulent and effective as live vaccines. *Nature* 1981;**291**:238–9.

29 Stocker BA. Auxotrophic *Salmonella typhi* as live vaccine. *Vaccine* 1988;**6**:141–5.

30 Chamberlain LM, Strugnell R, Dougan G, *et al.* *Neisseria gonorrhoeae* strain MS11 harbouring a mutation in gene *aroA* is attenuated and immunogenic. *Microb Pathog* 1993;**15**:51–63.

31 Vaughan LM, Smith PR, Foster TJ. An aromatic-dependent mutant of the fish pathogen *Aeromonas salmonicida* is attenuated in fish and is effective as a live vaccine against the salmonid disease furunculosis. *Infect Immun* 1993;**61**:2172–81.

32 Homchampa P, Strugnell RA, Adler B. Molecular analysis of the *aroA* gene of *Pasteurella multocida* and vaccine potential of a constructed *aroA* mutant. *Mol Microbiol* 1992;**6**:3585–93.

33 O'Callaghan D, Maskell D, Liew FY, *et al.* Characterization of aromatic- and purine-dependent *Salmonella typhimurium*: attention, persistence, and ability to induce protective immunity in BALB/c mice. *Infect Immun* 1988;**56**:419–23.

34 Hone DM, Harris AM, Chatfield S, *et al.* Construction of genetically defined double aro mutants of *Salmonella typhi*. *Vaccine* 1991;**9**:810–16.

35 Gunel-Ozcan A, Brown KA, Allen AG, *et al.* *Salmonella typhimurium aroB* mutants are attentuated in BALB/c mice. *Microb Pathog* 1997;**23**:311–16.

36 Dougan G, Chatfield S, Pickard D, *et al.* Construction and characterization of vaccine strains of *Salmonella* harboring mutations in two different aro genes. *J Infect Dis* 1988;**158**:1329–35.

37 Tacket CO, Hone DM, Losonsky GA, *et al.* Clinical acceptability and immunogenicity of CVD 908 *Salmonella typhi* vaccine strain. *Vaccine* 1992;**10**:443–6.

38 Hone DM, Tackett CO, Harris AM, *et al.* Evaluation in volunteers of a candidate live oral attenuated *Salmonella typhi* vector vaccine. *J Clin Invest* 1992;**90**:412–20.

39 Tacket CO, Sztein MB, Wasserman SS, *et al.* Phase 2 clinical trial of attenuated *Salmonella enterica* serovar *typhi* oral live vector vaccine CVD 908-*htrA* in US volunteers. *Infect Immun* 2000;**68**:1196–201.

40 Tacket CO, Sztein MB, Losonsky GA, *et al.* Safety of live oral *Salmonella typhi* vaccine strains with deletions in *htrA* and *aroC aroD* and immune response in humans. *Infect Immun* 1997;**65**:452–6.

41 Hindle Z, Chatfield SN, Phillimore J, *et al.* Characterization of *Salmonella enterica* derivatives harboring defined *aroC* and Salmonella pathogenicity island 2 type III secretion system (*ssaV*) mutations by immunization of healthy volunteers. *Infect Immun* 2002;**70**:3457–67.

42 Brubaker RR. The genus *Yersinia*: biochemistry and genetics of virulence. *Curr Top Microbiol Immunol* 1972;**57**:111–58.

43 Oyston PCF, Mellado G, Pasetti MF, *et al.* A *Yersinia pestis guaBA* mutant is attenuated in virulence and provides protection against plague in a mouse model of infection. *Microb Pathog* 2010;**48**(5):191–5.

44 Ivanovics G, Marjai E, Dobozy A. The growth of purine mutants of *Bacillus anthracis* in the body of the mouse. *J Gen Microbiol* 1968;**53**:147–62.

45 Crawford RM, Van De Verg L, Yuan L, *et al.* Deletion of *purE* attenuates *Brucella melitensis* infection in mice. *Infect Immun* 1996;**64**:2188–92.

46 Jackson M, Phalen SW, Lagranderie M, *et al.* Persistence and protective efficacy of a *Mycobacterium tuberculosis* auxotroph vaccine. *Infect Immun* 1999;**67**:2867–73.

47 Quarry JE, Isherwood KE, Michell SL, *et al.* A *Francisella tularensis* subspecies *novicida purF* mutant, but not a *purA* mutant, induces protective immunity to tularemia in mice. *Vaccine* 2007;**25**:2011–18.

48 Santiago AE, Cole LE, Franco A, *et al.* Characterization of rationally attenuated *Francisella tularensis* vaccine strains that harbor deletions in the *guaA* and *guaB* genes. *Vaccine* 2009;**27**:2426–36.

49 McFarland WC, Stocker BA. Effect of different purine auxotrophic mutations on mouse-virulence of a Vi-positive strain of *Salmonella dublin* and of two strains of *Salmonella typhimurium. Microb Pathog* 1987;**3**:129–41.

50 Noriega FR, Losonsky G, Lauderbaugh C, *et al.* Engineered delta*guaB-A* delta*virG Shigella flexneri* 2a strain CVD 1205: construction, safety, immunogenicity, and potential efficacy as a mucosal vaccine. *Infect Immun* 1996;**64**:3055–61.

51 O'Callaghan D, Maskell D, Tite J, *et al.* Immune responses in BALB/c mice following immunization with aromatic compound or purine-dependent *Salmonella typhimurium* strains. *Immunology* 1990; **69**:184–9.

52 Levine MM, Herrington D, Murphy JR, *et al.* Safety, infectivity, immunogenicity, and in vivo stability of two attenuated auxotrophic mutant strains of *Salmonella typhi*, 541Ty and 543Ty, as live oral vaccines in humans. *J Clin Invest* 1987;**79**:888–902.

53 Lawrence ML, Cooper RK, Thune RL. Attenuation, persistence, and vaccine potential of an *Edwardsiella ictaluri purA* mutant. *Infect Immun* 1997;**65**:4642–51.

54 Hondalus MK, Bardarov S, Russell R, *et al.* Attenuation of and protection induced by a leucine auxotroph of *Mycobacterium tuberculosis. Infect Immun* 2000;**68**:2888–98.

55 McAdam RA, Weisbrod TR, Martin J, *et al.* In vivo growth characteristics of leucine and methionine auxotrophic mutants of *Mycobacterium bovis* BCG generated by transposon mutagenesis. *Infect Immun* 1995;**63**:1004–12.

56 Bange FC, Brown AM, Jacobs WR, Jr. Leucine auxotrophy restricts growth of *Mycobacterium bovis* BCG in macrophages. *Infect Immun* 1996;**64**:1794–9.

57 Atkins T, Prior RG, Mack K, *et al.* A mutant of *Burkholderia pseudomallei*, auxotrophic in the branched chain amino acid biosynthetic pathway, is attenuated and protective in a murine model of melioidosis. *Infect Immun* 2002;**70**:5290–94.

58 Curtiss R, 3rd, Kelly SM. *Salmonella typhimurium* deletion mutants lacking adenylate cyclase and cyclic AMP receptor protein are avirulent and immunogenic. *Infect Immun* 1987;**55**:3035–43.

59 Curtiss R, 3rd, Goldschmidt RM, Fletchall NB, *et al.* Avirulent *Salmonella typhimurium* delta *cya* delta *crp* oral vaccine strains expressing a strepto-coccal colonization and virulence antigen. *Vaccine* 1988;**6**:155–60.

60 Tacket CO, Kelly SM, Schodel F, *et al.* Safety and immunogenicity in humans of an attenuated *Salmonella typhi* vaccine vector strain expressing plasmid-encoded hepatitis B antigens stabilized by the Asd-balanced lethal vector system. *Infect Immun* 1997;**65**:3381–5.

61 Newcombe J, Eales-Reynolds LJ, Wootton L, *et al.* Infection with an avirulent *phoP* mutant of *Neisseria meningitidis* confers broad cross-reactive immunity. *Infect Immun* 2004;**72**:338–44.

62 Oyston PC, Dorrell N, Williams K, *et al.* The response regulator PhoP is important for survival under conditions of macrophage-induced stress and virulence in *Yersinia pestis. Infect Immun* 2000;**68**:3419–25.

63 Cardona PJ, Asensio JG, Arbues A, *et al.* Extended safety studies of the attenuated live tuberculosis vaccine SO2 based on *phoP* mutant. *Vaccine* 2009;**27**:2499–505.

64 Martin C, Williams A, Hernandez-Pando R, *et al.* The live *Mycobacterium tuberculosis phoP* mutant strain is more attenuated than BCG and confers protective immunity against tuberculosis in mice and guinea pigs. *Vaccine* 2006;**24**:3408–19.

65 Hohmann EL, Oletta CA, Miller SI. Evaluation of a *phoP/phoQ*-deleted, *aroA*-deleted live oral *Salmonella typhi* vaccine strain in human volunteers. *Vaccine* 1996;**14**:19–24.

66 Hohmann EL, Oletta CA, Killeen KP, *et al.* phoP*phoQ*-deleted *Salmonella typhi* (Ty800) is a safe and immunogenic single-dose typhoid fever vaccine in volunteers. *J Infect Dis* 1996;**173**:1408–14.

67 Raupach B, Kurth N, Pfeffer K, *et al. Salmonella typhimurium* strains carrying independent mutations display similar virulence phenotypes yet are controlled by distinct host defense mechanisms. *J Immunol* 2003;**170**:6133–40.

68 Harrison JA, Villarreal-Ramos B, Mastroeni P, *et al.* Correlates of protection induced by live *aro⁻ Salmonella typhimurium* vaccines in the murine typhoid model. *Immunology* 1997;**90**:618–25.

69 Mastroeni P, Villarreal-Ramos B, Hormaeche CE. Role of T cells, TNF alpha and IFN gamma in recall of immunity to oral challenge with virulent salmonellae in mice vaccinated with live attenuated *aro Salmonella* vaccines. *Microb Pathog* 1992;**13**:477–91.

70 Mastroeni P, Villarreal-Ramos B, Hormaeche CE. Adoptive transfer of immunity to oral challenge with virulent salmonellae in innately susceptible BALB/c

mice requires both immune serum and T cells. *Infect Immun* 1993;**61**:3981–4.

71 World Health Organization. Global Advisory Committee on Vaccine Safety, 29–30 November 2006. *Wkly Epidemiol Rec* 2007;**82**:18–24.

72 Burns-Guydish SM, Zhao H, Stevenson DK, *et al.* The potential *Salmonella aroA*⁻ vaccine strain is safe and effective in young BALB/c mice. *Neonatol.* 2007;**91**:114–20.

73 Izhar M, DeSilva L, Joysey HS, *et al.* Moderate immunodeficiency does not increase susceptibility to *Salmonella typhimurium aroA* live vaccines in mice. *Infect Immun* 1990;**58**:2258–61.

74 Strahan K, Chatfield SN, Tite J, *et al.* Impaired resistance to infection does not increase the virulence of Salmonella htrA live vaccines for mice *Microb Pathog* 1992;**12**:311–17.

75 Coynault C, Norel F. Comparison of the abilities of *Salmonella typhimurium rpoS, aroA* and *rpoS aroA* strains to elicit humoral immune responses in BALB/c mice and to cause lethal infection in athymic BALB/c mice. *Microb Pathog* 1999;**26**:299–305.

76 Garmory HS, Brown KA, Titball RW. *Salmonella* vaccines for use in humans: present and future perspectives. *FEMS Microbiol Rev* 2002;**26**:339–53.

77 Lee E, Platt R, Kang S, *et al.* Chromosomal integration and expression of the *Escherichia coli* K88 gene cluster in *Salmonella enterica* ser. Choleraesuis strain 54 (SC54). *Vet Microbiol* 2001;**83**:177–83.

78 Strugnell RA, Maskell D, Fairweather N, *et al.* Stable expression of foreign antigens from the chromosome of *Salmonella typhimurium* vaccine strains. *Gene* 1990;**88**:57–63.

79 Ryan ET, Crean TI, Kochi SK, *et al.* Development of a DeltaglnA balanced lethal plasmid system for expression of heterologous antigens by attenuated vaccine vector strains of *Vibrio cholerae*. *Infect Immun* 2000;**68**:221–6.

80 Galan JE, Nakayama K, Curtiss R, 3rd. Cloning and characterization of the *asd* gene of *Salmonella typhimurium*: use in stable maintenance of recombinant plasmids in *Salmonella* vaccine strains. *Gene* 1990;**94**:29–35.

81 Nakayama K, Kelly SM, Curtiss IR. Construction of an Asd⁺ expression cloning vector: stable maintenance and high level expression of cloned genes in a *Salmonella* vaccine strain. *Biotechnology* 1988; **6**:693–7.

82 McNeill HV, Sinha KA, Hormaeche CE, *et al.* Development of a nonantibiotic dominant marker for positively selecting expression plasmids in multivalent *Salmonella* vaccines. *Appl Environ Microbiol* 2000;**66**:1216–19.

83 Galen JE, Nair J, Wang JY, *et al.* Optimization of plasmid maintenance in the attenuated live vector vaccine strain *Salmonella typhi* CVD 908-*htrA*. *Infect Immun* 1999;**67**:6424–33.

84 Garmory HS, Leckenby MW, Griffin KF, *et al.* Antibiotic-free plasmid stabilization by operator-repressor titration for vaccine delivery by using live *Salmonella enterica* serovar typhimurium. *Infect Immun* 2005;**73**:2005–11.

85 O'Callaghan D, Charbit A, Martineau P, *et al.* Immunogenicity of foreign peptide epitopes expressed in bacterial envelope proteins. *Res Microbiol* 1990;**141**:963–9.

86 Pistor S, Hobom G. OmpA-haemagglutinin fusion proteins for oral immunization with live attenuated *Salmonella*. *Res Microbiol* 1990;**141**:879–81.

87 Hess J, Gentschev I, Miko D, *et al.* Superior efficacy of secreted over somatic antigen display in recombinant *Salmonella* vaccine induced protection against listeriosis. *Proc Natl Acad Sci U S A* 1996;**93**:1458–63.

88 Russmann H, Shams H, Poblete F, *et al.* Delivery of epitopes by the *Salmonella* type III secretion system for vaccine development. *Science* 1998;**281**:565–8.

89 Gentschev I, Sokolovic Z, Kohler S, *et al.* Identification of p60 antibodies in human sera and presentation of this listerial antigen on the surface of attenuated salmonellae by the HlyB-HlyD secretion system *Infect Immun* 1992;**60**:5091–8.

90 Khan CM, Villarreal-Ramos B, Pierce RJ, *et al.* Construction, expression, and immunogenicity of the *Schistosoma mansoni* P28 glutathione *S*-transferase as a genetic fusion to tetanus toxin fragment C in a live Aro attenuated vaccine strain of *Salmonella*. *Proc Natl Acad Sci U S A* 1994;**91**:11261–5.

91 Lee JJ, Sinha KA, Harrison JA, *et al.* Tetanus toxin fragment C expressed in live *Salmonella* vaccines enhances antibody responses to its fusion partner *Schistosoma haematobium* glutathione *S*-transferase. *Infect Immun* 2000;**68**:2503–12.

92 Jagusztyn-Krynicka EK, Clark-Curtiss JE, Curtiss R, 3rd. *Escherichia coli* heat-labile toxin subunit B fusions with *Streptococcus sobrinus* antigens expressed by *Salmonella typhimurium* oral vaccine strains: importance of the linker for antigenicity and biological activities of the hybrid proteins. *Infect Immun* 1993;**61**:1004–15.

93 Cardenas L, Clements JD. Development of mucosal protection against the heat-stable enterotoxin (ST)

of *Escherichia coli* by oral immunization with a genetic fusion delivered by a bacterial vector. *Infect Immun* 1993;**61**:4629–36.

94 Venkatesan M, Kaminski RW, Ranallo RT. Shigellosis. In ADT Barrett, LR Stanberry LR (Eds) *Vaccines for Biodefense and Emerging and Neglected Diseases*. Elsevier/Academic Press, Oxford, 2009, pp. 1163–92.

95 Oyston PCF, Titball RW. *Francisella tularensis*. In ADT Barrett, LR Stanberry LR (Eds) *Vaccines for Biodefense and Emerging and Neglected Diseases*. Elsevier/Academic Press, Oxford, 2009, pp. 1242–57.

96 Comer JE, Peterson JW. Anthrax. In ADT Barrett, LR Stanberry LR (Eds) *Vaccines for Biodefense and Emerging and Neglected Diseases*. Elsevier/Academic Press, Oxford, 2009, pp. 790–807.

97 Williamson ED, Simpson AJ, Titball RW. Plague vaccines. In S Plotkin, W Orenstein, P Offit (Eds) *Vaccines*. Elsevier Saunders, Oxford, 2008, pp. 519–30.

98 Ficht TA, Adams GL. *Brucella*. In ADT Barrett, LR Stanberry LR (Eds) *Vaccines for Biodefense and Emerging and Neglected Diseases*. Elsevier/Academic Press, Oxford, 2009, pp. 808–31.

99 Conelly-Smith K, Orme IM, Starke JR. Tuberculosis vaccines. In S Plotkin, W Orenstein, P Offit (Eds) *Vaccines*. Elsevier Saunders, Oxford, 2008, pp. 857–86.

100 Tacket CO, Sack DA. Cholera vaccines. In S Plotkin, W Orenstein, P Offit (Eds) *Vaccines*. Elsevier Saunders, Oxford, 2008, pp. 127–38.

CHAPTER 13

Virus-like Particles as Antigen Scaffolds

Bryce Chackerian[1] & John T. Schiller[2]

[1]Department of Molecular Genetics and Microbiology, University of New Mexico School of Medicine, Albuquerque, NM, USA
[2]Laboratory of Cellular Oncology, National Cancer Institute, Bethesda, MD, USA

Virus-like particles, a new class of vaccines

Viral vaccines have traditionally been based on attenuated or inactivated virus preparations, and many of the most successful vaccines on the market today are based on these technologies. Attenuated vaccines are typically highly immunogenic and can stimulate broad humoral and cell-mediated responses against multiple viral antigens, usually upon a single dose. However, attenuated viruses can be dangerous in immunodeficient or pregnant individuals. Reversion to a more virulent form of the virus can also occur, leading to the risk of vaccine-related outbreaks (such as a 2007 vaccine-related polio outbreak in Nigeria [1]). In the current regulatory climate, even rare or minimal vaccine-related side effects may be unacceptable (one example is the withdrawal of the Rotashield vaccine due to the rare, but statistically significant, association with intussusception). Inactivated virus can also form the basis for effective vaccines. However, manufacturing of inactivated vaccines requires handling of large volumes of a virulent pathogen, there is a risk of incomplete inactivation, and there is also the risk that inactivation, particularly with chemical agents, may alter the structure of the virus, affecting the quality of the immune response. Moreover, the manufacture of both attenuated and inactivated vaccines relies on an ability to produce large quantities of virus, and, for many viruses, the lack of tissue culture systems that allow for efficient propagation is a substantial barrier to using either of these methods.

The advent of recombinant techniques has allowed the preparation of subunit vaccines that consist of isolated viral antigens. Although these vaccines generally have good safety profiles, subunit vaccines are often poorly immunogenic without the use of large doses of antigen in combination with potent adjuvants. In addition, it can be challenging to generate subunit vaccines that are structurally similar to the native antigen and induce antibody responses against physiologically relevant epitopes.

Virus-like particle (VLP) vaccines combine many of the advantages of subunit and whole-virus vaccines. Like subunit vaccines, VLPs can be produced using recombinant technologies, using expression systems (such as bacteria, yeast, or insect cells) that can generate large amounts of recombinant protein without relying on the ability of the parental virus to replicate. Because VLPs lack viral nucleic acid, they cannot replicate and are therefore intrinsically safer than attenuated virus. Most importantly, VLPs structurally and antigenically resemble infectious virus and their multivalent, particulate structure is highly immunogenic.

Vaccinology: Principles and Practice, First Edition. Edited by W. John W. Morrow, Nadeem A. Sheikh, Clint S. Schmidt and D. Huw Davies.
© 2012 Blackwell Publishing Ltd. Published 2012 by Blackwell Publishing Ltd.

Properties of VLPs that promote immune responses

VLPs have structural properties that enhance interactions with immune cell types such as antigen-presenting cells (APCs) and B cells. These interactions form the basis for the ability of VLPs to elicit strong cellular and humoral immune responses. In this section, we will give an overview of these features.

Interactions with antigen-presenting cells

The uptake of antigens by phagocytic APCs depends on many different characteristics, including the shape, charge, and hydrophobicity of the antigen complex. Antigen size is also a key determinant of uptake. Macrophages, for example, efficiently take up larger antigens, such as bacteria or parasites, whereas dendritic cells (DCs) have been shown to most efficiently take up particles between 20 and 100 nm in diameter (optimally 40 nm), which is the size of most viruses and VLPs [2]. Once taken up by DCs, VLPs, like most exogenous antigens, are processed and presented by major histocompatibility complex (MHC) class II molecules for activation of T helper cells. However, unlike nonparticulate exogenous antigens, VLPs are also trafficked to the cytosol of certain DC lineages and, through cross-presentation or direct endosomal loading, can be processed and presented by MHC class I [3–6]. This enables the priming of CD8$^+$ T cells and induction of cytotoxic T lymphocyte (CTL) responses by DCs in the absence of viral replication. Thus, immunization with VLPs can prime both helper and cytotoxic T cells.

Although this is not a common property of all VLPs, some VLP types can also directly induce the phenotypic and functional maturation of DCs, leading to the upregulation of co-stimulatory molecules and cytokines that enhance activation of CD8$^+$ T cells. VLPs derived from human papillomavirus (HPV), Ebola virus, papaya mosaic virus (PapMV), and HIV gag, for example, can directly stimulate DC maturation [7–11]. For most of these examples the molecular basis of VLP activation of DCs is not well understood. However, the ability of HPV VLPs to stimulate DCs is MyD88-dependent, indicating that Toll-like receptor (TLR) recognition of VLPs is critical for this process [12].

VLPs are often combined with an exogenous adjuvant. However, VLPs can also be directly modified to include adjuvants that promote APC stimulation. This linkage allows adjuvants to be delivered alongside of VLPs to APCs in a more directed manner than simple co-administration. VLPs are essentially empty shells and can be loaded with a variety of substances with immunostimulatory properties. For example, nonmethylated CpG DNA, a TLR9 agonist, can be packaged into different VLPs types, including VLPs derived from the hepatitis B core antigen or the bacteriophage Qβ (shown in Figure 13.1). VLPs loaded with CpG oligonucleotides elicit higher frequencies of antigen-specific CD8$^+$ T cells than empty VLPs [4]. VLPs derived from RNA viruses naturally encapsidate single- or double-stranded RNA, which are recognized

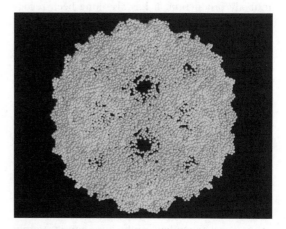

Figure 13.1 The structure of the bacteriophage Qβ capsid. The 24 nm diameter capsid of bacteriophage Qβ consists of a single protein, called coat protein. Coat protein forms a homodimer and 90 dimers form the T = 3 particle. Coat protein exists in three slightly different conformations, here shown using different shades. As described in the text, the immunogenicity of Qβ and other VLPs is conferred by its particulate nature and highly repetitive structure. This structure was generated using Jmol (www.rcsb.org/pdb/explore/jmol. do?structureId=1QBE&bionumber=1) from the X-ray crystal structure data of Golmohammadi *et al.* [81].

by TLR3 and TLR7/8, respectively, on APCs [13]. Molecules with adjuvanting properties can also be linked to the surface of VLPs or incorporated into particles. For example, cholera toxin B can be chemically linked to the surface of SIV VLPs, enhancing mucosal immune responses [14]. VLPs of enveloped viruses can also be modified so that stimulatory molecules are imbedded into the lipid bilayer of the particle. For example, incorporation of CD40L or GPI-anchored GM-CSF into SIV VLPs enhanced maturation and functional activation of DCs and increased CD4+ and CD8+ T-cell responses to SIV Env, compared to standard SIV VLPs [15].

Interactions with B cells

Antibody production is initiated by interactions between antigen and its cognate B-cell receptor (BCR) on the surface of naïve B cells. The magnitude of B-cell response to antigen stimulation can vary dramatically and is influenced by several factors. Co-engagement of the complement receptor CR2 or stimulation of TLRs can enhance antibody production. It has also long been recognized that antigen density influences the magnitude of an antibody response [16]. Antigens that have highly dense, multivalent structures, such as VLPs, can activate B cells at much lower concentrations than monomeric antigens and without the use of exogenous adjuvants [17–20]. These studies have consistently shown that epitopes that have a spacing of 5–10 nm, a spacing that is common to most virus particles, optimally induce B-cell responses [21–23]. Many VLPs are so strongly activating that they can rapidly induce T-cell independent production of IgM antibodies. In addition, VLPs contain T helper epitopes, and can induce strong T-cell dependent antibody responses. Highly multivalent antigens can provoke extensive cross-linking of the BCR, leading to the formation of stable lipid raft microdomains that are associated with enhanced signaling to the B cell [24]. This signaling stimulates B-cell proliferation and migration, and upregulates the expression of molecules (such as MHC class II, CD80, CD86, and CD40L) that permit subsequent interactions with T helper cells [20]. These interactions with T helper cells, in turn, lead to Ig class switching, antibody affinity maturation, and the generation of long-lived memory B cells. Hence, VLPs are innately immunogenic; they induce high-titer and long-lasting antibody responses at low doses, often without requiring adjuvants.

One of the most extraordinary findings underscoring the potent immunogenicity of VLPs was the observation that VLPs can be used as a platform to induce antibody responses against self-proteins [25]. This ability is seemingly limited by the mechanisms of B-cell tolerance, which eliminate, anergize, or change the specificity of potentially self-reactive B cells [26–30]. However, self-antigens displayed in a highly dense, multivalent format on VLPs can induce strong autoantibody responses [31]. Immunization with highly multivalent self-antigens can actually reverse the effects of B-cell anergy [20] and efficiently induce antibodies against self. VLP display makes a self-antigen as immunogenic as a foreign antigen presented in the same context [32] and the magnitude of the anti-self IgG responses is strictly correlated with the density at which the self-antigen is displayed on the VLP surface [21,22], indicating that B-cell recognition of "foreign-like" multivalent structural elements can overwhelm the mechanisms that normally maintain B-cell tolerance. As described below, these observations have made possible the development of an entirely new class of vaccines that target self-molecules involved in chronic diseases.

Commercial VLP-based vaccines

VLP-based vaccines to prevent infection by two viruses, hepatitis B virus (HBV) and human papilloma virus (HPV), have been approved for human use. Both vaccines are thought to prevent infection by the induction of virion neutralizing antibodies. The ultimate goal of these vaccines is to prevent the cancers caused by the two viruses, liver cancer and predominantly cervical cancer, respectively. However, the compositions of the vaccines are quite different. Current HBV vaccines are monovalent and produced in *Saccharomyces cerevisiae* by several manufacturers. The VLPs are composed of yeast lipid membrane particles into which the HBV S envelope protein (HBsAg) has been incorporated [33]. They morphologically resemble the noninfectious 22 nm particles found in the blood of HBV-infected individuals. These vaccines, which became commercially available in 1986, are the first commercial vaccines generated via recombinant DNA technology and so represent a hallmark in the translation of modern molecular biology into public health interventions [34]. A course of three intramuscular injections over six months generates protective antibody responses in more than 95% of healthy infants and adults. HBsAg antibodies remain detectable in the majority of vaccinees even after 20 years and protection is thought to be life long [35]. Rates of acute hepatitis and HBV carrier rates have dramatically decreased in countries with universal vaccination programs [36]. In addition, a recent study in Taiwan has demonstrated a greater than two-thirds reduction in hepatocellular carcinoma in individuals vaccinated at birth [37].

HPV vaccines are composed of naked icosohedral VLPs composed of the L1 major capsid protein [38]. There are two commercial vaccines. Cervarix is a bivalent vaccine that contains the L1 VLPs of types 16 and 18, which are found in about 70% of cancers worldwide. The VLPs are produced in L1 recombinant baculovirus infected insect cells. Gardasil (also marketed as Silgard) is a quadrivalent vaccine that, in addition to HPV16 and HPV18, contains L1 VLPs of types 6 and 11, which cause about 90% of external genital warts. The VLPs for Gardasil are produced in *Saccharomyces cerevisiae*. Both vaccines contain an adjuvant, a simple aluminum salt in the case of Gardasil and an aluminum salt combined with monophosphoryl lipid A, a TLR4 agonist, in the case of Cervarix. Gardasil and Cervarix were first approved for commercial use in young women in 2006 and 2007, respectively, and both are now available in many countries worldwide. Three intramuscular injections over six months induce virtually 100% seroconversion. In women without evidence of previous exposure, both vaccines generated greater than 90% protection against persistent infection and premalignant cervical neoplasia caused by the types targeted by the vaccines [39,40]. Gardasil also induced almost complete protection against genital warts caused by the vaccine-targeted types. There are no indications of waning immunity in the six or more years since the trials began. Thus, there is optimism that the vaccines will induce long-term protection and ultimately be shown to substantially reduce the rates of cervical and other HPV-associated cancers in women. Gardasil has also been approved for vaccination of young men in some countries, including the USA.

The HBV and HPV vaccines clearly demonstrate that VLP-based vaccines can safely and consistently induce high titer and durable antibody responses in humans. Their success encourages the use of similar strategies in the development of other human vaccines. VLP-based vaccines for immunoprophylaxis against a number of other human virus infections are being pursued, but in most cases, efforts remain at the preclinical stage [41]. For example, naked icosohedral VLP vaccine candidates have been generated for rotavirus, Norwalk virus, hepatitis E Virus, and B19 parvovirus. Lipid envelope-containing VLP vaccine candidates have been generated for HIV, hepatitis C Virus, influenza A virus, and SARS coronavirus. In addition, VLP vaccines are under development for a number of important animal pathogens, including bluetongue virus, canine and porcine parvoviruses, Newcastle disease virus, and chicken anemia virus.

Exploiting VLPs as platform for antigenic display of heterologous target molecules

The very features that make VLPs such effective standalone vaccines have been exploited to develop VLP-based platform technologies for targeting heterologous molecules. In the remainder of this chapter we will describe how VLPs can be used as platforms to display practically any antigen in a highly immunogenic, multivalent format. This strategy has been utilized to target diverse molecules, including epitopes derived from pathogens, self-antigens, and chemical agents. VLP display can enhance the immunogenicity of molecules that are poorly immunogenic in their native context. This technique is particularly effective in eliciting

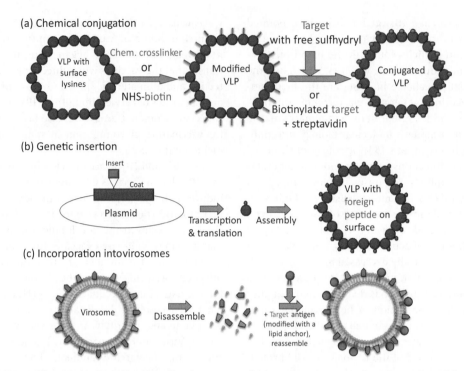

Figure 13.2 Techniques for displaying heterologous antigens on VLPs or virosomes. This figure summarizes the principal techniques for arraying heterologous antigens on the surface of virus structures. In the chemical conjugation approach (a), preformed VLPs are modified with a linking molecule, such as biotin or a chemical cross-linker. These particles are then reacted with target antigen. This technique is highly flexible, allowing for the conjugation of diverse sizes and types of antigen to VLPs. Genetic insertion of peptide epitopes, shown in (b), is dependent on the ability to insert peptide sequences into viral structural proteins such that the insertions are exposed on the surface of the virus particle and do not interfere with the ability of the structural protein to fold correctly and assemble into VLPs. Virosomes, shown in (c), are produced from enveloped viruses through a process that involves detergent solubilization followed by removal of viral internal proteins and nucleic acid. By reconstituting the particles in the presence of target antigens that have been modified to contain a lipid-anchoring domain, target antigens can be incorporated at high density on the surface of the virosome.

antibody responses, but VLP-based vaccines can also be used to induce cell-mediated immune responses.

As described above, the ability of VLPs to elicit strong antibody responses is due to their highly repetitive, multivalent structure. Thus, in order to effectively use VLPs as a display platform, target antigens must also be displayed on the surface of VLPs at high density. The availability of high-resolution viral structural information has facilitated the ability to deliberately modify a diverse collection of VLP types so that they essentially function as molecular scaffolds for antigen presentation.

As shown in Figure 13.2 and as described below, both chemical and genetic approaches have successfully been utilized to array antigens on the surface of VLPs or virosomes.

The use of VLPs as platforms to induce CTL responses against heterologous antigens typically presents less of an engineering challenge. Unlike B-cell epitopes, T-cell epitopes do not need to be exposed on the surface of the particle in their native conformation or presented at high density. Therefore, more flexible approaches can be used to formulate VLPs for this purpose. For example, VLPs can be generated by conjugating or fusing target epitopes to viral major capsid proteins or by making fusions between target antigens and proteins that are minor structural components of VLPs [42].

Recombinant VLPs

Chimeric VLPs can be constructed by genetic insertion of target epitopes into viral structural proteins. Successful incorporation of a target peptide guarantees that the antigen will be displayed in the same conformation and at high density on the VLP surface. In order for a site of insertion to be useful for antibody induction, it must be present on the surface of the VLP and the insertion must not interfere with protein folding and VLP assembly. In many cases, proper folding and presentation can be accomplished by replacing exposed immunodominant viral epitopes (these are predominantly loop structures) with the target epitope (Figure 13.2). Because loop structures are frequently where relevant epitopes are found, this is often a natural location for peptide display. Nevertheless, the generation of chimeric VLPs can be technically challenging. The effects of peptide insertions into viral structural proteins are notoriously difficult to predict, and all too often result in protein folding failures. Peptide length, hydrophobicity, charge, and structure can all influence success rates. As a consequence, the generation of chimeric VLPs in most systems described to date is a largely empirical process of trial and error. However, several VLP display systems have been devised that increase the likelihood of successful peptide insertions.

Numerous VLP platform technologies have been adapted for genetic display of target peptides. These include plant viruses such as tobacco mosaic virus [43], cowpea mosaic virus [44], and papaya mosaic virus [11], insect viruses such as flock house virus [45], bacteriophage [46–48], and animal viruses such as papillomavirus [49], rhinovirus [50], and parvovirus [51]. All of these platforms have their own advantages and limitations that distinguish their individual applicability. These considerations include adaptability to diverse peptide insertions, special immunogenic properties, yield and manufacturing complexity, environmental stabil-

ity, and presence of pre-existing immunity in human populations. To simplify this discussion, we will focus on just two examples of chimeric VLP technologies.

Hepadnavirus core VLPs

VLPs comprised of the HBV core antigen (HBcAg) were among the first particles used for display of a heterologous antigen [52]. The HBcAg particles (and particles from related rodent and duck hepadnaviruses) are well suited for genetic insertion of foreign epitopes into an insertion site in the protein's immunodominant loop or at the N- and C-termini of the protein. Recombinant HBcAg VLPs are highly immunogenic, and can induce strong cellular and humoral immune responses against various targets [53]. Although the peptide insertions in chimeric VLPs are usually limited to 20–30 amino acids or fewer, peptides as large as 55 amino acids have been successfully inserted into HBcAg particles [54]. However, despite this flexibility, anecdotal evidence suggests that more than half of all epitopes inserted into HBcAg prevent the assembly of particles [55]. In some cases, particles can be recovered by flanking the insertions with acidic residues (such as glutamic acid), by altering the specific insertion site, and/or by making additional modifications to the C-terminus of core protein [56].

Notably, two HBcAg VLP-based vaccines have been tested in humans. Malariavax (ICC-1132) consists of a chimeric HBcAg particle that displays the repeat sequences from the circumsporozoite (CS) protein from *Plasmodium falciparum*. Based on promising data in nonhuman primates [57], volunteers were immunized with a single-dose of Malariavax. Although vaccination resulted in moderate levels of anti-CS antibodies, only weak T-cell responses were observed, and the volunteers were not protected from challenge with malarial sporozoites [58]. Since boosting dramatically increased immunity in animal models, it is possible that the study design of this trial may have compromised vaccine efficacy. ACAM-FLU-A is an HBcAg-based vaccine marketed by Acambis (now Sanofi Pasteur) that targets the influenza A M2 protein, which is highly conserved among influenza A strains. Based on favorable animal protection data [59], a human clinical trial was initiated. Although results from the phase I trial have not yet been reported in the literature, Acambis announced that 90% of volunteers had measurable antibodies against M2.

RNA bacteriophage

As described above, the ability to display peptides on VLPs is often limited by structural features of the VLP platform, and the process of designing recombinant VLPs is often an empirical one. However, we have shown that VLPs derived from two related RNA bacteriophage, MS2 and PP7, are widely tolerant of both specific peptide insertions as well as an impressive percentage of random insertions (>95% of random 10 amino acid insertions) [47,60]. In addition, both of these phage VLPs are capable of encapsidating the RNA that encodes their synthesis, raising the possibility that large libraries of VLPs displaying random peptides could be used in affinity selection applications analogous to filamentous phage display (for a thorough discussion of filamentous phage display, see Chapter 11). However, unlike filamentous phage (which do not commonly display heterologous peptides at high density and are poorly immunogenic), selected MS2 or PP7 bacteriophage VLPs could be used directly as immunogens. This coupling of capabilities, affinity selection and epitope presentation, could facilitate epitope discovery and peptide vaccine development, especially for those epitopes where monoclonal antibodies are available but generation or presentation of their epitopes in a useful vaccine format has met with difficulty (summarized in Figure 13.3). Similar random libraries of limited size that are based on live human rhinovirus type 14 [61] and adeno-associated virus [62] have been constructed, but neither of these two systems has been systematically tested for compatibility with diverse peptide insertions.

Display of target antigens by chemical conjugation

Given the difficulties in constructing recombinant VLPs, one alternative has been to chemically link target antigens to preformed VLPs using chemical cross-linkers or bridging molecules. This technique takes advantage of the presence of addressable moieties on the surface of the VLPs and on the target antigens. For example, a bifunctional cross-linker with amine- and sulfhydryl-reactive arms (SMPH) can be used to conjugate cysteine-containing antigens to surface-exposed lysine residues on viral structural proteins (Figure 13.2) [55]. Small peptides and recombinant full-length proteins can be synthesized or engineered to contain terminal cysteine residues and then conjugated to VLPs using SMPH [63]. Conjugation to VLPs using SMPH can result in high-density display of antigens, although the efficiency of conjugation using this method is dependent to a degree on the size of the target antigen. For example, as many as 240 molecules of a 12 amino acid peptide can be linked to bacteriophage Qβ VLPs [55,64], whereas approximately 18 copies of a 34 kDa IL17 homodimer can be linked to Qβ VLPs [63]. Alternatively, bridging molecules can be used to link antigens to VLPs. For example, we have biotinylated papillomavirus VLPs and then conjugated diverse biotinylated antigens to the VLPs through the use of a streptavidin bridging molecule [64]. The ability to target both peptide epitopes and full-length proteins through chemical conjugation allows for a great deal of flexibility in vaccine design. Vaccines that target peptide epitopes allow for precise targeting of critical epitopes involved in target activity. Larger targets increase the likelihood that immunization will induce a broad range of antibodies that recognize both linear and conformational epitopes on the target molecule. Chemical conjugation also allows nonprotein targets, such as glycans or other small haptens, to be attached to VLPs [65].

Although many VLP types can be used as a substrate for chemical conjugation, the RNA bacteriophage Qβ has been used the most extensively. Several Qβ VLP-based vaccines are currently in human clinical trials and many more are in development. We will briefly describe several of these vaccines that are in clinical or preclinical development.

An anti-smoking vaccine

Antibodies against nicotine could potentially help smokers quit by reducing the amount and rate of

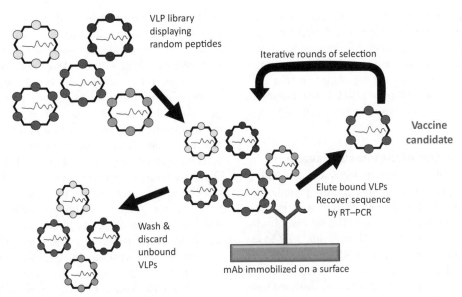

Figure 13.3 Affinity selection using VLPs. The ability to display diverse random sequences on the surface of VLPs or viruses allows these particles to be used in affinity selection schemes that are similar to those employed using filamentous phage display. For example, using the RNA bacteriophage MS2, large libraries of VLPs that display random peptides can be generated. VLPs displaying specific epitopes can be recovered by affinity selection using monoclonal antibodies. Because MS2 VLPs encapsidate the RNA that encodes their expression, selected sequences can be recovered by reverse transcription followed by PCR (RT-PCR) and then be used to regenerate the population of selected VLPs. Through iterative rounds of selection at increasing stringency, followed by amplification, VLPs displaying high-affinity epitopes may be selected. Because VLPs display these selected peptides at high density they can be directly used as immunogens.

nicotine entering the brain. Cytos Biotechnology, a Swiss company, initiated clinical trials of a Qβ VLP-based vaccine targeting nicotine. In a phase I clinical study, the nicotine-conjugated VLPs were well-tolerated and induced nicotine-specific IgG responses in immunized subjects at levels that were expected to be in the range for effective therapeutic use [66]. The vaccine was then tested for efficacy in a double-blind phase II trial in 227 smokers [67]. Subjects were given five injections of 100 μg vaccine formulated with alum at monthly intervals. All of the vaccinated subjects produced antibodies against nicotine, with peak titers approximately one month after the final vaccination. Although vaccination was not associated with a significant increase in smoking abstinence relative to placebo controls, subgroup analysis showed that the third of the vaccinated population with the highest antibody titers showed significantly higher continuous abstinence (about twice that of the placebo group).

These results suggest that a reformulated vaccine (given at a higher dose or with a different adjuvant) may be more effective.

A vaccine for hypertension

Angiotensin II is a key mediator of vasoconstriction of arterioles. Consequently, high angiotensin II levels can lead to hypertension. Based on favorable animal studies [68], Cytos Biotechnology initiated human trials of a vaccine consisting of an 8 amino acid peptide derived from angiotensin II conjugated to Qβ VLPs. A double-blind placebo controlled phase IIa study of 72 patients with mild to moderate hypertension showed that vaccination induced high-affinity antibodies against angiotensin. Statistically significant reductions in blood pressure were observed in the group given the highest dose (300 μg) of vaccine [69]. A subsequent phase II study using an accelerated vaccination schedule failed to show significant reductions in blood pressure [70]. Although the reasons for this failure are not entirely clear, it is thought that the altered regimen resulted in the production of lower affinity antibodies. Despite these mixed results, the angiotensin trials are significant in that they demonstrate the ability of a VLP-based vaccine to induce antibody responses against a self-antigen in humans.

A vaccine for Alzheimer's disease

Antibodies that prevent or decrease the accumulation of aggregated amyloid-β (Aβ) peptide into plaques in the brain are viewed as a potential therapy for Alzheimer's disease (AD). Several groups, including our own, have shown that VLP-based immunogens displaying short Aβ peptides prevent disease in mouse models of AD without inducing T-cell responses against Aβ that are associated with immune pathology [64,71–73]. Novartis has initiated clinical trials of CAD106 in mild to moderate AD patients. CAD106 consists of the N-terminal 6 amino acids of Aβ conjugated to Qβ VLPs. Three doses of 50 μg of the vaccine resulted in a generally favorable safety profile and anti-Aβ antibody responses in 16 of 24 patients [74]. Efficacy trials of this vaccine are ongoing.

Recombinant virosomes

As described previously, virosomes are preformed virus-like liposome-based complexes that display viral surface glycoproteins. Like VLPs, virosomes are highly immunogenic and can be used as a platform to display heterologous antigens. However, in contrast to most other VLPs, virosomes are formed by *in vitro* reconstitution of lipids and virus-derived proteins. Influenza virus virosomes, for example, are produced from influenza virus through a process that involves detergent solubilization, removal of viral internal proteins and nucleic acid, and then reconstitution in the presence of added lipid [75]. Reconstituted virosomes retain the cell binding and membrane fusion properties of the native virus. Virosomes can be engineered to display heterologous antigens. Peptides, whole proteins, or sugar molecules can be incor-porated into virosomes by conjugation to a phosphatidylethanolamine lipid anchor, which is then added to the preparation during the reconstitution step (Figure 12.2). PEV3A, developed by Pevion Biotech, an influenza virosome-based vaccine that combines virosomes that display two peptide antigens from the *Plasmodium falciparum* antigens circumsporozoite (CS) protein and apical membrane antigen 1 (AMA-1). In a phase I/IIa trial, 12 volunteers were given three doses of PEV3A followed by challenge with malaria sporozoites [76]. All 12 vaccinees had high titer and avidity antibodies against both malarial antigens. Although vaccination did not result in sterilizing immunity, vaccinees had significantly lower rates of parasite growth (about twofold lower than controls), suggesting that vaccination provided some protection at the blood stage. The encouraging results of a phase I trial of a virosome-based vaccine targeting Her-2/neu has also been reported [77].

Synthetic multivalent platforms

Virus particles provide a natural platform for antigenic display. However, it is also possible to engineer systems for multivalent display of antigens. Raman *et al.* designed a synthetic polypeptide that contains both a pentameric and a trimeric coiled-coil oligomerization domain [78]. Upon denaturation and refolding, these peptides co-assemble into self-assembling polypeptide nanoparticles (SAPNs), with T = 1 or approximately T = 3 icosahedral symmetry. Because the N- and C-termini are displayed on the surface of the particles, heterologous peptides can be easily displayed in a repetitive fashion on the surface of SAPNs. SAPNs displaying peptides derived from the *Plasmodium berghei* CS protein [79] and the SARS coronavirus spike protein [80] induce high-titer and long-lasting antibody responses without use of adjuvants.

Conclusions

The size, particulate nature, and dense, repetitive structure of VLPs are the basis for their innate immunogenicity. Clinical approval of VLP-based vaccines for HBV and HPV have demonstrated the effectiveness of VLP-based vaccines. Moreover, VLPs can be used as modular display systems to induce potent and broad immune responses against diverse target antigens, including antigens that previously were refractory to vaccine-based approaches, such as self-antigens. Target epitopes can be plugged into a vaccine formats that can be easy to manufacture, safe, well tolerated, and highly immunogenic. Many VLP types have been exploited as vaccine platforms; however, there are technical and practical considerations that distinguish the applicability of different VLP types, including adaptability to display a wide range of targets, special immunogenic properties, yield and manufacturing complexity, and the existence of pre-existing immunity. The continued development of VLP-based immunogens has the potential to rapidly accelerate the development of new vaccines against diverse targets.

Features of VLP-based vaccines

• Highly immunogenic, often without requiring adjuvants.
• The basis of highly effective vaccines for HPV and HBV.
• Can be derived from enveloped and non-enveloped viruses (and even artificial nanoparticles).
• Compatible with a diverse arsenal of display techniques.
• Can be used to deliver internalized TLR ligands.
• Can be used to develop and identify vaccines against pathogens and self-antigens involved in disease.
• A growing number of VLP-based immunogens are currently being evaluated in human clinical trials.

Acknowledgments

The authors would like to thank Dave Peabody for helpful discussions. B.C. is supported by grants from the National Cancer Institute, the National Institute of Allergy and Infectious Diseases, and the Bill and Melinda Gates Foundation. J.T.S. is funded by the intramural program at the National Cancer Institute.

References

1 Roberts L. Infectious disease. Vaccine-related polio outbreak in Nigeria raises concerns. *Science* 2007; **317**(5846):1842.

2 Fifis T, Gamvrellis A, Crimeen-Irwin B, *et al.* Size-dependent immunogenicity: therapeutic and protective properties of nano-vaccines against tumors. *J Immunol* 2004;**173**(5):3148–54.

3 Bachmann MF, Lutz MB, Layton GT, *et al.* Dendritic cells process exogenous viral proteins and virus-like particles for class I presentation to CD8[+] cytotoxic T lymphocytes. *Eur J Immunol* 1996;**26**(11):2595–600.

4 Storni T, Ruedl C, Schwarz K, *et al.* Nonmethylated CG motifs packaged into virus-like particles induce protective cytotoxic T cell responses in the absence of systemic side effects. *J Immunol* 2004; **172**(3):1777–85.

5 Fausch SC, Da Silva DM, Eiben GL, Le Poole IC, Kast WM. HPV protein/peptide vaccines: from animal models to clinical trials. *Front Biosci* 2003;**8**:s81–91.

6 Keller SA, Bauer M, Manolova V, *et al.* Limited specialization of dendritic cell subsets for MHC class II-associated presentation of viral particles. *J Immunol* 2010;**184**(1):26–9.

7 Lenz P, Day PM, Pang YY, *et al.* Papillomavirus-like particles induce acute activation of dendritic cells. *J Immunol* 2001;**166**(9):5346–5.

8 Rudolf MP, Fausch SC, Da Silva DM, Kast WM. Human dendritic cells are activated by chimeric human papillomavirus type-16 virus-like particles and induce epitope-specific human T cell responses in vitro. *J Immunol* 2001;**166**(10):5917–24.

9 Tsunetsugu-Yokota Y, Morikawa Y, Isogai M, *et al.* Yeast-derived human immunodeficiency virus type 1 p55(gag) virus-like particles activate dendritic cells (DCs) and induce perforin expression in Gag-specific CD8(+) T cells by cross-presentation of DCs. *J Virol* 2003;**77**(19):10250–59.

10 Bosio CM, Moore BD, Warfield KL, *et al.* Ebola and Marburg virus-like particles activate human myeloid dendritic cells. *Virology* 2004;**326**(2):280–87.

11 Lacasse P, Denis J, Lapointe R, Leclerc D, Lamarre A. Novel plant virus-based vaccine induces protective cytotoxic T-lymphocyte-mediated antiviral immunity

through dendritic cell maturation. *J Virol* 2008; **82**(2):785–94.

12 Yang R, Murillo FM, Cui H, *et al.* Papillomavirus-like particles stimulate murine bone marrow-derived dendritic cells to produce alpha interferon and Th1 immune responses via MyD88. *J Virol* 2004; **78**(20):11152–60.

13 Lee BO, Tucker A, Frelin L, *et al.* Interaction of the hepatitis B core antigen and the innate immune system. *J Immunol* 2009;**182**(11):6670–81.

14 Kang SM, Yao Q, Guo L, Compans RW. Mucosal immunization with virus-like particles of simian immunodeficiency virus conjugated with cholera toxin subunit B. *J Virol* 2003;**77**(18):9823–30.

15 Skountzou I, Quan FS, Gangadhara S, *et al.* Incorporation of glycosylphosphatidylinositol-anchored granulocyte-macrophage colony-stimulating factor or CD40 ligand enhances immunogenicity of chimeric simian immunodeficiency virus-like particles. *J Virol* 2007;**81**(3):1083–94.

16 Dintzis HM, Dintzis RZ, Vogelstein B. Molecular determinants of immunogenicity: the immunon model of immune response. *Proc Natl Acad Sci U S A* 1976; **73**(10):3671–5.

17 Brunswick M, Finkelman FD, Highet PF, *et al.* Picogram quantities of anti-Ig antibodies coupled to dextran induce B cell proliferation. *J Immunol* 1988; **140**(10):3364–72.

18 Dintzis RZ, Middleton MH, Dintzis HM. Inhibition of anti-DNP antibody formation by high doses of DNP-polyacrylamide molecules; effects of hapten density and hapten valence. *J Immunol* 1985;**135**(1):423–7.

19 Milich DR, Chen M, Schodel F, *et al.* Role of B cells in antigen presentation of the hepatitis B core. *Proc Natl Acad Sci U S A* 1997;**94**(26):14648–53.

20 Chackerian B, Durfee MR, Schiller JT. Virus-like display of a neo-self antigen reverses B cell anergy in a B cell receptor transgenic mouse model. *J Immunol* 2008;**180**(9):5816–25.

21 Jegerlehner A, Storni T, Lipowsky G, *et al.* Regulation of IgG antibody responses by epitope density and CD21-mediated costimulation. *Eur J Immunol* 2002;**32**(11):3305–14.

22 Chackerian B, Lenz P, Lowy DR, Schiller JT. Determinants of autoantibody induction by conjugated papillomavirus virus-like particles. *J Immunol* 2002;**169**(11):6120–26.

23 Dintzis RZ, Vogelstein B, Dintzis HM. Specific cellular stimulation in the primary immune response: experimental test of a quantized model. *Proc Natl Acad Sci U S A* 1982;**79**(3):884–8.

24 Thyagarajan R, Arunkumar N, Song W. Polyvalent antigens stabilize B cell antigen receptor surface signaling microdomains. *J Immunol* 2003;**170**(12): 6099–106.

25 Bachmann MF, Rohrer UH, Kundig TM, *et al.* The influence of antigen organization on B cell responsiveness. *Science* 1993;**262**(5138):1448–51.

26 Hartley SB, Crosbie J, Brink R, *et al.* Elimination from peripheral lymphoid tissues of self-reactive B lymphocytes recognizing membrane-bound antigens. *Nature* 1991;**353**(6346):765–9.

27 Nemazee DA, Burki K. Clonal deletion of B lymphocytes in a transgenic mouse bearing anti-MHC class I antibody genes. *Nature* 1989;**337**(6207): 562–6.

28 Tiegs SL, Russell DM, Nemazee D. Receptor editing in self-reactive bone marrow B cells. *J Exp Med* 1993;**177**(4):1009–20.

29 Gay D, Saunders T, Camper S, Weigert M. Receptor editing: an approach by autoreactive B cells to escape tolerance. *J Exp Med* 1993;**177**(4):999–1008.

30 Goodnow CC, Crosbie J, Adelstein S, *et al.* Altered immunoglobulin expression and functional silencing of self-reactive B lymphocytes in transgenic mice. *Nature* 1988;**334**(6184):676–82.

31 Chackerian B. Virus-like particles: flexible platforms for vaccine development. *Expert Rev Vaccines* 2007;**6**(3):381–90.

32 Chackerian B, Lowy DR, Schiller JT. Conjugation of a self-antigen to papillomavirus-like particles allows for efficient induction of protective autoantibodies. *J Clin Invest* 2001;**108**(3):415–23.

33 Mast EE, Ward JW. Hepatitis B vaccines. In SA Plotkin, WA Orenstei, PA Offit (Eds) *Vaccines*, 5th edn. Saunders, Philadelphia, PA, 2004, pp. 205–42.

34 McAleer WJ, Buynak EB, Maigetter RZ, *et al.* Human hepatitis B vaccine from recombinant yeast. *Nature* 1984;**307**(5947):178–80.

35 Poovorawan Y, Chongsrisawat V, Theamboonlers A, *et al.* Persistence of antibodies and immune memory to hepatitis B vaccine 20 years after infant vaccination in Thailand. *Vaccine* 2010;**28**(3):730–36.

36 Zanetti AR, Van Damme P, Shouval D. The global impact of vaccination against hepatitis B: a historical overview. *Vaccine* 2008;**26**(49):6266–73.

37 Chang MH, You SL, Chen CJ, *et al.* Decreased incidence of hepatocellular carcinoma in hepatitis B vaccinees: a 20-year follow-up study. *J Natl Cancer Inst* 2009;**101**(19):1348–55.

38 Lowy DR, Schiller JT. Prophylactic human papillomavirus vaccines. *J Clin Invest* 2006;**116**(5):1167–73.

39 Munoz N, Kjaer SK, Sigurdsson K, *et al.* Impact of human papillomavirus (HPV)-6/11/16/18 vaccine on all HPV-associated genital diseases in young women. *J Natl Cancer Inst* 2010;**102**(5):325–39.

40 Paavonen J, Naud P, Salmeron J, *et al.* Efficacy of human papillomavirus (HPV)-16/18 AS04-adjuvanted vaccine against cervical infection and precancer caused by oncogenic HPV types (PATRICIA): final analysis of a double-blind, randomised study in young women. *Lancet* 2009;**374**(9686):301–14.

41 Roy P, Noad R. Virus-like particles as a vaccine delivery system: myths and facts. *Hum Vaccin* 2008; **4**(1):5–12.

42 Greenstone HL, Nieland JD, de Visser KE, *et al.* Chimeric papillomavirus virus-like particles elicit antitumor immunity against the E7 oncoprotein in an HPV16 tumor model. *Proc Natl Acad Sci U S A* 1998; **95**(4):1800–805.

43 McCormick AA, Palmer KE. Genetically engineered tobacco mosaic virus as nanoparticle vaccines. *Expert Rev Vaccines* 2008;**7**(1):33–41.

44 Dalsgaard K, Uttenthal A, Jones TD, *et al.* Plant-derived vaccine protects target animals against a viral disease. *Nat Biotechnol* 1997;**15**(3):248–52.

45 Manayani DJ, Thomas D, Dryden KA, *et al.* A viral nanoparticle with dual function as an anthrax antitoxin and vaccine. *PLoS Pathog* 2007;**3**(10): 1422–31.

46 Gupta A, Onda M, Pastan I, Adhya S, Chaudhary VK. High-density functional display of proteins on bacteriophage lambda. *J Mol Biol* 2003;**334**(2):241–54.

47 Peabody DS, Manifold-Wheeler B, Medford A, *et al.* Immunogenic display of diverse peptides on virus-like particles of RNA phage MS2. *J Mol Biol* 2008; **380**(1):252–63.

48 Tissot AC, Renhofa R, Schmitz N, *et al.* Versatile virus-like particle carrier for epitope based vaccines. *PLoS One* 2010;**5**(3):e9809.

49 Chackerian B, Lowy DR, Schiller JT. Induction of autoantibodies to mouse CCR5 with recombinant papillomavirus particles. *Proc Natl Acad Sci U S A* 1999;**96**: 2373–8.

50 Resnick DA, Smith AD, Zhang A, *et al.* Libraries of human rhinovirus-based HIV vaccines generated using random systematic mutagenesis. *AIDS Res Hum Retroviruses* 1994;**10**(Suppl 2):S47–52.

51 Sedlik C, Saron M, Sarraseca J, Casal I, Leclerc C. Recombinant parvovirus-like particles as an antigen carrier: a novel nonreplicative exogenous antigen to elicit protective antiviral cytotoxic T cells. *Proc Natl Acad Sci U S A* 1997;**94**(14):7503–8.

52 Clarke BE, Newton SE, Carroll AR, *et al.* Improved immunogenicity of a peptide epitope after fusion to hepatitis B core protein. *Nature* 1987;**330**(6146):381–4.

53 Whitacre DC, Lee BO, Milich DR. Use of hepadnavirus core proteins as vaccine platforms. *Expert Rev Vaccines* 2009;**8**(11):1565–73.

54 Pumpens P, Grens E. HBV core particles as a carrier for B cell/T cell epitopes. *Intervirology* 2001;**44**(2-3):98–114.

55 Jegerlehner A, Tissot A, Lechner F, *et al.* A molecular assembly system that renders antigens of choice highly repetitive for induction of protective B cell responses. *Vaccine* 2002;**20**(25–26):3104–12.

56 Billaud JN, Peterson D, Barr M, *et al.* Combinatorial approach to hepadnavirus-like particle vaccine design. *J Virol* 2005;**79**(21):13656–66.

57 Birkett A, Lyons K, Schmidt A, *et al.* A modified hepatitis B virus core particle containing multiple epitopes of the *Plasmodium falciparum* circumsporozoite protein provides a highly immunogenic malaria vaccine in preclinical analyses in rodent and primate hosts. *Infect Immun* 2002;**70**(12):6860–70.

58 Walther M, Dunachie S, Keating S, *et al.* Safety, immunogenicity and efficacy of a pre-erythrocytic malaria candidate vaccine, ICC-1132 formulated in Seppic ISA 720. *Vaccine* 2005;**23**(7):857–64.

59 Neirynck S, Deroo T, Saelens X, *et al.* A universal influenza A vaccine based on the extracellular domain of the M2 protein. *Nat Med* 1999;**5**(10): 1157–63.

60 Caldeira Jdo C, Medford A, Kines RC, *et al.* Immunogenic display of diverse peptides, including a broadly cross-type neutralizing human papillomavirus L2 epitope, on virus-like particles of the RNA bacteriophage PP7. *Vaccine* 2010;**28**(27):4384–93.

61 Arnold GF, Velasco PK, Holmes AK, *et al.* Broad neutralization of human immunodeficiency virus type 1 (HIV-1) elicited from human rhinoviruses that display the HIV-1 gp41 ELDKWA epitope. *J Virol* 2009;**83**(10):5087–100.

62 Muller OJ, Kaul F, Weitzman MD, *et al.* Random peptide libraries displayed on adeno-associated virus to select for targeted gene therapy vectors. *Nat Biotechnol* 2003;**21**(9):1040–46.

63 Rohn TA, Jennings GT, Hernandez M, *et al.* Vaccination against IL-17 suppresses autoimmune arthritis and encephalomyelitis. *Eur J Immunol* 2006; **36**(11):2857–67.

64 Chackerian B, Rangel M, Hunter Z, Peabody DS. Virus and virus-like particle-based immunogens for Alzheimer's disease induce antibody responses against

amyloid-beta without concomitant T cell responses. *Vaccine* 2006;**24**(37–39):6321–31.

65 Raja KS, Wang Q, Gonzalez MJ, *et al.* Hybrid virus-polymer materials. 1. Synthesis and properties of PEG-decorated cowpea mosaic virus. *Biomacromolecules* 2003;**4**(3):472–6.

66 Maurer P, Jennings GT, Willers J, *et al.* A therapeutic vaccine for nicotine dependence: preclinical efficacy, and phase I safety and immunogenicity. *Eur J Immunol* 2005;**35**(7):2031–40.

67 Cornuz J, Zwahlen S, Jungi WF, *et al.* A vaccine against nicotine for smoking cessation: a randomized controlled trial. *PLoS One* 2008;**3**(6):e2547.

68 Ambuhl PM, Tissot AC, Fulurija A, *et al.* A vaccine for hypertension based on virus-like particles: preclinical efficacy and phase I safety and immunogenicity. *J Hypertens* 2007;**25**(1):63–72.

69 Tissot AC, Maurer P, Nussberger J, *et al.* Effect of immunisation against angiotensin II with CYT006-AngQb on ambulatory blood pressure: a double-blind, randomised, placebo-controlled phase IIa study. *Lancet* 2008;**371**(9615):821–7.

70 Maurer P, Bachmann MF. Immunization against angiotensins for the treatment of hypertension. *Clin Immunol* 2010;**134**(1):89–95.

71 Li QY, Gordon MN, Chackerian B, *et al.* Virus-like peptide vaccines against Abeta N-terminal or C-terminal domains reduce amyloid deposition in APP transgenic mice without addition of adjuvant. *J Neuroimmune Pharmacol* 2010;**177**(4):2662–70.

72 Zamora E, Handisurya A, Shafti-Keramat S, *et al.* Papillomavirus-like particles are an effective platform for amyloid-beta immunization in rabbits and transgenic mice. *J Immunol* 2006;**177**(4):2662–70.

73 Bach P, Tschape JA, Kopietz F, *et al.* Vaccination with Abeta-displaying virus-like particles reduces soluble and insoluble cerebral Abeta and lowers plaque burden in APP transgenic mice. *J Immunol* 2009;**182**(12):7613–24.

74 Winblad B. Safety, tolerability and immunogenicity of the Aβ immunotherapeutic vaccine CAD106 in a first-in-man study in Alzheimer patients. *Alzheimers Dement* 2008;**4**(4):T128.

75 Moser C, Amacker M, Kammer AR, *et al.* Influenza virosomes as a combined vaccine carrier and adjuvant system for prophylactic and therapeutic immunizations. *Expert Rev Vaccines* 2007;**6**(5):711–21.

76 Thompson FM, Porter DW, Okitsu SL, *et al.* Evidence of blood stage efficacy with a virosomal malaria vaccine in a phase IIa clinical trial. *PLoS One* 2008;**3**(1):e1493.

77 Wiedermann U, Wiltschke C, Jasinska J, *et al.* A virosomal formulated Her-2/neu multi-peptide vaccine induces Her-2/neu-specific immune responses in patients with metastatic breast cancer: a phase I study. *Breast Cancer Res Treat* 2010;**119**(3):673–83.

78 Raman S, Machaidze G, Lustig A, Aebi U, Burkhard P. Structure-based design of peptides that self-assemble into regular polyhedral nanoparticles. *Nanomedicine* 2006;**2**(2):95–102.

79 Kaba SA, Brando C, Guo Q, *et al.* A nonadjuvanted polypeptide nanoparticle vaccine confers long-lasting protection against rodent malaria. *J Immunol* 2009;**183**(11):7268–77.

80 Pimentel TA, Yan Z, Jeffers SA, *et al.* Peptide nanoparticles as novel immunogens: design and analysis of a prototypic severe acute respiratory syndrome vaccine. *Chem Biol Drug Des* 2009;**73**(1):53–61.

81 Golmohammadi R, Fridborg K, Bundule M, Valegard K, Liljas L. The crystal structure of bacteriophage Q beta at 3.5 A resolution. *Structure* 1996;**4**(5):543–54.

CHAPTER 14

Recombinant MVA vaccines: Optimization, Preclinical, and Product Development

Yper Hall & Miles W. Carroll
Microbiology Division, Health Protection Agency, Porton Down, UK

Aims of the chapter

Drawing on over 20 years of experience of developing recombinant vaccinia virus (rVACV) based vaccines in both academia and industry, this chapter aims to review the use of recombinant modified vaccinia Ankara (rMVA) virus as a viral vector for vaccine antigen delivery. Much of the chapter draws on experience devising and then leading preclinical, clinical, and product development of a recombinant MVA expressing tumor-associated antigen 5T4 (TroVax), which was later progressed to phase III in a metastatic renal cancer indication and out-licensed to the pharmaceutical sector. Development of this product confirmed that it is essential for a recombinant to be optimized at the preclinical stage to ensure efficacy, a smooth regulatory path, and an effective intellectual property strategy. Fortuitously, these aspects were sufficiently addressed for TroVax during early preclinical research so that in addition to inducing significant and relevant immunologic responses, the construct was also able to withstand the scrutiny of regulatory authorities and due diligence of pharmaceutical industry technical experts and legal teams. This chapter reviews characteristics of MVA relevant to its use as a recombinant viral vaccine and discusses aspects of recombinant

MVA research that are pertinent to the development of rMVA-based products.

Introduction to MVA

Viral vectors are an efficient and reliable technology with which to deliver and induce effective immune responses to vaccine antigens. MVA exhibits many of the properties required of an optimal viral delivery system, from induction of long-lasting antigen-specific humoral and cell-mediated immune responses, through to ease of construction and manufacture, stability, regulatory acceptance, and relative low cost of goods.

MVA is a highly attenuated, replication-defective derivative of vaccinia virus (VACV) Ankara developed as an alternative for safer vaccination against smallpox. Although effective during the campaign to eradicate smallpox, replication-competent VACV was observed to cause a high rate of complications in specific groups of recipients, such as infants and individuals with immunologic disorders [1]. The attenuated growth characteristics of MVA were achieved through serial passage in primary chick embryo fibroblast (CEF) cells. After more than 500 passages, the starting strain Ankara was found to be replication-defective in human cells and most

Vaccinology: Principles and Practice, First Edition. Edited by W. John W. Morrow, Nadeem A. Sheikh, Clint S. Schmidt and D. Huw Davies.
© 2012 Blackwell Publishing Ltd. Published 2012 by Blackwell Publishing Ltd.

other mammalian cell types, and nonpathogenic in various animal models [2,3]. From 1968 onwards, German authorities safely administered MVA to over 120 000 individuals without the complications associated with VACV. VACV is still in use for smallpox vaccination in select, at-risk populations, such as military and laboratory personnel, using the current vaccine strain, ACAM2000, approved by the FDA in 2007. The protective efficacy of MVA has yet to be accepted by regulatory authorities.

In 1980, at the end of the smallpox vaccination campaign, general use of MVA ceased. Approximately 10 years later, following advances in genetic engineering of recombinant vaccinia virus, MVA was revisited as a potential viral vector with a favorable safety profile for vaccine antigen delivery [4]. This nonreplicating poxvirus vector also possesses the positive attributes of replicating VACV, including high-level transgene expression, theoretical capacity to accommodate >25 kb exogenous DNA [5], and the ability to potentiate both humoral and cell-mediated antigen-specific responses [6]. By the mid-1990s, the properties of rMVA as an optimized viral delivery system were being described [7,8]. In the proceeding 18 years, a multitude of rMVA-based vaccines have since been evaluated for preclinical efficacy against viral, bacterial, parasitic, and cancer-related diseases [9] and there have been in excess of 100 clinical-based studies, some examples of which are shown in Table 14.1.

In addition to its proven clinical safety and ability to elicit protective immunologic responses, the advantages of rMVA as a viral vaccine vector now extend to include established manufacturing processes (compliant with Good Manufacturing Practice; GMP), low costs of goods, ease of storage, and clear requirements for regulatory submission.

As outlined in this chapter, the techniques required to generate rMVA are easy to implement so that novel rMVA can be readily constructed and researched. Numerous publications describe MVA generation; however, we advise the reader to consult a key set of methods developed by Bernie Moss's laboratory at the National Institutes of Health [10–12]. Those requiring expedient progression to the clinic can be made to GMP with relative ease, with a number of contract manufacturing organizations (CMO) available. Recombinant MVA is, therefore, an attractive platform for development of recombinant vaccine-based interventions.

MVA is a member of the *Orthopoxvirus* genus within the *Poxviridae* family. Other poxviruses in use as viral vaccines include fowlpox and canarypox virus, and are discussed in Chapter 16.

MVA molecular biology and replication

Life cycle and gene expression

MVA contains a single copy of double-stranded DNA genome, approximately 178 kb in length [13]. Unlike other DNA viruses, vaccinia replication occurs exclusively in the host cell cytoplasm, operating with relative autonomy from the host-cell nucleus. In common with most other viruses, replication is controlled via tight temporal regulation of gene expression falling into specific categories – early, intermediate, and late [14] – with an additional, intermediate-early class of genes more recently described [15]. The infectious virion has packaged within it enzymes and transcription factors required for early gene expression so that viral mRNA transcripts are detectable within 20 minutes post-infection [16]. Under the tight regulation of vaccinia transcriptional promoters, the first genes to be expressed code for immune modulators and for enzymes and transcriptional factors required for intermediate expression. After viral DNA replication, intermediate gene transcription is activated and viral late gene transcription factors are expressed to enable subsequent late gene expression to occur. The proteins and enzymes required for early transcription are expressed at late times so that they are encapsulated into progeny virus ready for the next round of replication. The majority of virus particles are then released during cell lysis. The tightly regulated cascade of viral early, intermediate, and late transcription is shown in Figure 14.1. Also shown is the point at which replication is defective for MVA infecting nonpermissive cell types. As MVA replication is blocked in the final step of virus particle maturation, authentic gene expression is still able to occur at all stages, a feature

Table 14.1 Examples of recombinant MVA in clinical development.

Target	Vaccine	Antigen	Developer	Clinical phase	Ref.
Cancer: breast	MVA-BN® HER2	HER2	Bavarian Nordic	I/II	[84]
Cancer: colorectal, renal, and prostate	TroVax	5T4	Oxford Biomedica	II/III	[85]
Cancer: lung	TG4010	MUC1 and IL2	Transgene	IIb	[71]
Cancer: prostate	MVA-BN® PRO	PSA and PAP	Bavarian Nordic	I/II	[86]
Hepatitis C	TG4040	NS3, NS4, NS5B	Transgene	II	[87]
HIV	MVA-CMDR	CRF01_AE gag, env, pol	MHRP	I	[88]
HIV	MVA-BN® HIV multiantigen	gag, pol, nef, tat, vpr, vpu, vif, rev	Bavarian Nordic	I/II	[89]
HIV	MVA/HIV62	gag, pol, env	GeoVax	II	[75]
HPV-induced disease	TG4001/RG3484	HPV16 E6, E7, IL2	Transgene/Roche	IIb	[70]
Influenza	MVA-NP+M1	NP+M1	University of Oxford	IIa	[81]
Malaria	MVA ME-TRAP (FP prime)	ME-TRAP	University of Oxford	IIb	[90]
Malaria	MVA ME-TRAP MVA MSP1 MVA AMA1 (Ad prime)	ME-TRAP MSP1 AMA1	University of Oxford	I/IIa	[76]
Tuberculosis	MVA85A	Ag85A	Oxford Emergent Tuberculosis Consortium	IIb	[91]

Abbreviations: Ag85A, mycobacterial mycolyl transferase 85A; AMA1, apical membrane antigen 1; CMDR, Chiang Mai Double Recombinant; HER2, human epidermal growth factor receptor 2; HPV, human papilloma virus; IL2, interleukin 2; M1, matrix 1 protein; ME-TRAP, multiple epitope string fused to thrombospondin-related adhesion protein; MSP1, merozoite surface protein 1; MUC1, mucin 1; NP, nucleoprotein; NS3/NS4/NS5B, HCV nonstructural antigens; PAP, prostate acid phosphatase proteins; PSA, prostate-specific antigen.

confirmed for high-level expression of recombinant genes [4] capable of evoking an effective immune response [6]. That MVA replicates in the host-cell cytoplasm with relative autonomy from the host-cell nucleus represents another favorable characteristic of rMVA-based vaccines from the perspective of GM safety – that is, the lack of opportunity for insertion of viral DNA into the host genome.

Host range restriction

During the course of its attenuation in primary CEF, approximately 30 kb of the parent vaccinia genome was deleted, rendering MVA replication defective in human and most other mammalian cells. While the genetic basis for host range restriction has not been fully elucidated, it is known to involve multiple gene defects [17,18] and those regulatory proteins still present and enabling late transcription continue to be described in the literature [19–22]. Initially, propagation of MVA was thought to require culture in CEF, but later other nonhuman cell lines permissive to MVA growth were identified, and one in particular, baby hamster kidney cells (BHK-21), was found to support efficient replication [23–25] and production of rMVA [23]. The most common cell cultures now in use for *in vitro* manipulation of MVA are primary CEF and BHK-21, although for GMP production of

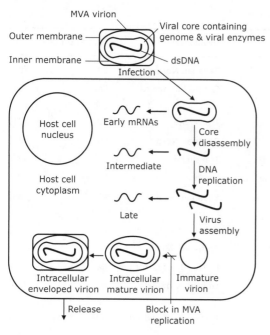

Figure 14.1 MVA life cycle.

MVA, additional designer avian cell lines have been developed for optimized scalability and robustness (discussed below).

Construction and use of recombinant MVA

Background

The first examples of recombinant vaccinia virus used homologous recombination as the mechanism for gene transfer [26,27], and this is still the most widely used technique for generation of rMVA. Other methods, such as bacterial artificial chromosome (BAC) technology, have been described [28, 29], but will not be discussed in detail here. Detailed protocols describing generation of rMVA are available [10–12,30]. Briefly, MVA permissive cells are infected with wild-type virus and then transfected with a transfer plasmid vectoring exogenous DNA. Homologous recombination into a specific site of the MVA genome is mediated by homologous sequences flanking the transgene [12]. In addition to the gene of interest, the transfer plasmid contains a vaccinia promoter for control of its ex-

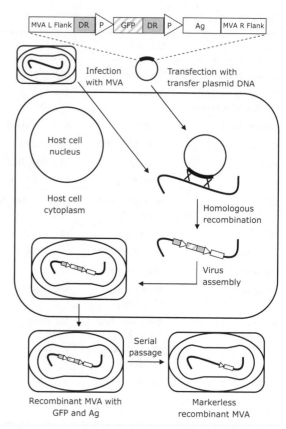

Figure 14.2 Generation of rMVA. L, left; DR, direct repeat; P, vaccinia promoter; GFP, green fluorescent protein; Ag, antigen of interest; R, right.

pression and, dependent upon the precise nature of the protocol, a selection marker to aid isolation of recombinant virus. An example based on transient expression of GFP [31] is shown in Figure 14.2. During MVA replication, homologous recombination between genomic and transfer plasmid DNA occurs at a frequency of approximately 1:1000. Thus, when genomic DNA is repackaged to yield MVA progeny, a proportion of the population, reflective of this frequency, is recombinant. Purified recombinant virus must subsequently be prepared through a process enabling selective enrichment.

Selection markers

Since the first rVACV were generated in the early 1980s, there have been many technical advances relating to construction and isolation of recombinants. Early methodology relied on insertion of the foreign gene into the thymidine kinase (TK) coding sequence via homologous recombination and enrichment on the basis of a TK⁻ phenotype selected by using bromodeoxyuridine (BrdU) [26,27,32]. Later this method was combined with simultaneous insertion of the *E.coli* lac Z gene, coding for β-galactosidase, so that recombinants could be further distinguished from TK⁻ mutants arising under the cytotoxic influence of BrdU; lac Z recombinant plaques turn blue when grown in the presence of X-gal [33]. Other genes added to transfer vectors to improve versatility in recombinant isolation include antibiotic resistance markers such as the *E.coli* neomycin gene [34] and xanthine-guanine phosphoribosyl transferase (*gpt*) gene [35], and additional color markers, green fluorescent protein (GFP) [36] and *E.coli* β-glucuronidase A gene (*gus*) [37].

Where markers are not cross-reactive, it is possible to combine them for improved selection, as in the case of a *gpt-gus* fusion expressed under a single vaccinia promoter [38]. Or they can be used simultaneously in the construction of recombinants containing multiple inserts. Another strategy for the isolation of recombinant vaccinia, developed using VACV, involves use of a modified parent strain with a deficiency restored by a gene included in the transfer vector [39,40].

When making rMVA products destined for clinical use, inclusion of a selection marker is not desirable. Several systems have been designed to allow for transient expression of marker genes, many employing a second recombination event for their removal [31,41,42]. Where recombinant protein is expressed on the surface of infected cells, selection markers may not be required at all if recombinant plaques can be immunostained and plaque purified [12]. A popular approach in the development of rMVA-based vaccines today is the use of transiently expressed fluorescent markers. A transfer plasmid vectoring transient GFP has been described [31] in which recombinant virus is plaque purified and then subjected to serial passage so that the GFP marker, located in between two direct repeat sequences is eventually lost through a second recombination event (Figure 14.2). A system for en-

gineering rMVA using a self-excising BAC has also been developed [43].

Vaccinia promoter selection for optimal expression

The first vaccinia virus promoter inserted upstream of a recombinant gene was the 7.5 kb early/late promoter [26]. In the subsequent 30 years, significant improvements in protein expression resulting in enhanced immune response have been observed using rationally optimized promoters. The significance of an optimized promoter in rMVA vaccine development lies not only in its influence over enhancing the immune response, but also in its potential to lower the dose required for vaccination.

As outlined above, vaccinia promoters are active at one of the three transcriptional stages, early, intermediate, or late, and some, such as the 7.5 kb and H5 promoters, contain both early and late elements in tandem. In-depth mutagenesis studies have identified the promoter elements critical to expression activity and have enabled development of synthetic promoters capable of driving even higher levels of expression [44–46]. In the rational design of rMVA-based vaccines, several factors affect the kinetics desirable for recombinant antigen expression. Intermediate and late promoters can give rise to higher protein levels because they are active at a time when DNA template and transcription factors are relatively abundant. However, early promoters may be preferential when cell types, such as dendritic cells and macrophages, prevent late expression [47–49]. Powerful promoters can also result in cytotoxic effects where, dependent upon the gene being expressed, the recombinant may be unstable and/or a higher incidence of gene truncation is observed. For these reasons, combined early/late promoters are the most commonly used. Intuitively, MVA-based vaccines will strive to achieve high levels of antigen expression while avoiding adverse effects and so an assessment of optimal promoter activity can be undertaken *in vitro*. In one such study, as an alternative to PsynE/L and the weaker 7.5 kb promoter, a novel promoter of intermediate strength, modified H5 (mH5), was generated and proven to provide optimal expression and immunogenicity of the transgene [50]. In the development of TroVax the mH5 promoter was found to give optimal immune response to the transgene 5T4 [51]. Additionally, it is important to ensure the transgene is void of vaccinia virus early transcription termination sites TTTTTNT [52,53]. Furthermore, the use of an optimized Kozak sequence and excision of non-essential DNA between the promoter and transcription start site should further enhance gene expression.

Insertion site

In addition to the TK region described above, other sites within the MVA genome that have been targeted for exogenous DNA insertion are the hemagglutinin (HA) gene [54], the more commonly used deletion (Del) sites formed during the course of MVA's attenuation [3], and, most recently, intergenic regions (IGR) [55]. Insertion into IGRs adjacent to essential MVA genes has been used as a strategy for generating stable rMVA where exogenous DNA has otherwise been observed to promote instability. In the event of a deletion or truncation, the essential genes are affected and the strain rendered unable to replicate, thus only full-length recombinants are propagated [56,57].

Effects of pre-existing immunity

Pre-existing immunity has the potential to limit the efficacy of a viral vector, and following the eradication of smallpox, there was a widespread population with humoral immunity to vaccinia virus. With the cessation of global vaccination, this population has halved [58] and is decreasing, but the effects of pre-existing vector immunity still require consideration in the context of multiple-immunization regimes and in light of the number of rMVA vaccines under clinical study.

Preclinically, MVA has been shown to evoke less potent vector-specific immune responses than replication-competent vaccinia, without compromising the strength of immune response elicited against a foreign antigen [59]. Recombinant MVA has also been shown to be effective under conditions of pre-existing immunity to the vector [60, 61]. There are now clinical examples for immunogenic vaccine antigen delivery by rMVA against a

background of MVA-specific antibody, pre-existing, or induced through repeated rMVA immunization [62]. rMVA's ability to induce transgene responses in the presence of pre-existing MVA immunity in homologous prime-boost regimens may be due in part to the rapid expression kinetics of VACV promoters and a lack of requirement for cell-to-cell spread of the vector. For each novel rMVA product, however, the impact of pre-existing immunity on rMVA efficacy should be evaluated [63].

rMVA development

Basic research

As a measure of their suitability for further research, novel rMVA are required to undergo *in vitro* characterization to confirm identity, purity, stability, and expression [30] (see Table 14.2). Amplification of the insertion site via PCR is commonly used to check for recombinants of the expected size and the absence of parent virus [30]. Western blotting of infected cell lysate enables analysis of the expressed product via immunodetection and a related methodology, or radio-immunoprecipitation can be used for quantification of expressed antigen. Serial passage of purified rMVA followed by retesting for existence of nonrecombinant populations provides a measure of recombinant genetic stability. Sequencing of the recombinant region is required for absolute confirmation of insert fidelity. If an rMVA is difficult to purify, or if testing reveals the insert to be truncated, further optimization of the promoter and/or insertion site may be required (as discussed above). Once confirmation of recombinant purity and expression of authentic gene product has been confirmed, the rMVA can be progressed to *in vivo* evaluation of immunogenicity and efficacy, the specifics of which will be dependent upon the target disease, but will include detection of antigen-specific immunologic responses.

Optimizing the efficacy of rMVA vaccines

Recombinant MVA evoke potent antigen-specific humoral and cell-mediated immune responses to expressed antigens, the strength and bias of which

Table 14.2 Key assays for rMVA identity, characterization, and batch release.

Assay description	Comments	Utility
Titration by TCID50 or PFU	TCID50 is standard titration method accepted by regulatory authorities	Used for setting batch release criteria, virus stability and determining dose for clinical use
Titration/potency: plaque immunostain directed to recombinant gene product	Using a monoclonal antibody (Mab) specific to authentically expressed gene product, this assay identifies all plaques that express the full-length vaccine antigen	Assay can be used as potency read-out if specific titer of rMVA has previously been shown to induce protective efficacy in *in vivo* model
Double immunostain: staining with Mab to transgene followed by immunostain with Mab to MVA protein		The assay demonstrates genetic stability of rMVA by identifying those rMVA plaques that do not express authentic protein product
PCR of inserted gene	Primers designed to bind to MVA sequences directly flanking the inserted full-length gene product	Demonstrates genetic stability of insert; used for product characterization and genetic stability
PCR for wild-type virus	Primers designed to bind to MVA flanking regions	Demonstrates absence of wild-type virus
Western blotting using Mabs to recombinant protein	Using a conformational specific Mab. Also used techniques to quantify intensity of signal	Demonstrates rMVA is expressing authentic gene product. Can also demonstrate quantity of expressed product. Used for virus characterization and identity
Sequencing of inserted genes	Primers designed to bind approximately 1 Kb outside each of the MVA flanking regions	Demonstrates genetic stability of entire region of recombination and that no mutations have occurred. Used for characterization. Note for phase III FDA will expect entire genome to be sequenced

can be influenced through a number of approaches, including promoter kinetics, co-expression of immune co-factors, and inoculation regimen.

As discussed above, vaccinia promoters influence antigen expression levels according to their strength and temporal regulation. In addition, promoter kinetics may also influence the bias of antigen-specific immune responses evoked; early promoters driving expression of the recombinant protein are beneficial for the induction of cytotoxic T lymphocyte responses [48,64,65]. In most instances, a promoter with combined early and late elements, optimized for increased expression, is sufficient for rMVA efficacy, such as the modified H5 promoter (mH5).

The effectiveness of MVA-based vaccines may also be improved through insertion of immune co-factors (ICF), especially where it is important to steer the immune system toward a particular type of T-helper response. A key advantage of MVA as a viral vector for vaccine antigen delivery is its capacity for recombinant DNA; theoretically 30 kb. The first ICF to be co-expressed in rVACV was IL2, which was shown to have an attenuating effect in nude mice [66,67]. Subsequently, rVACV co-expressing a range of immune enhancers have been constructed with a view to creating cytokine microenvironments in which favorable antigen-specific responses are activated. Many cytokines, for example IL2 and IL12, have antiviral and antitumor activity; however, their toxic side effects can be severe when delivered systemically. Reports show that co-expression of a model tumor-associated antigen (TAA) and IL12 by an rVACV can obviate the requirement for systemic delivery of toxic levels of IL12 [68]. That co-expression of immune co-factors offers a further dimension to safe and effective enhancement of rMVA-based vaccines has now been demonstrated in clinical-based studies [69–71].

The potential for heterolgous prime-boosting to enhance rMVA efficacy, particularly for the improvement of immunization strategies pursuing cell-mediated immunity, is now well established. Recombinant MVA administered in prime-boost regimens involving plasmid DNA or alternative viral vectors has been demonstrated to drive strong T-cell responses [72] and appears particularly effective when rMVA boosts non-MVA prime [73]. There is also evidence for enhanced cellular and humoral immunity in response to co-administration of viral vectors and recombinant protein in adjuvant [74]. Heterolgous prime-boost regimens are being pursued in a clinical setting for vaccines targeted against HIV [75], malaria [76], and tuberculosis [77].

Route of administration is sometimes thought to be another feature of the immunization protocol that can influence rMVA efficacy. Intramuscular (i.m.) and intradermal (i.d.) delivery are commonly used for rMVA delivery, with the latter leading to higher immune responses in some preclinical studies, evidently a result of the increased number of professional antigen-presenting cell encountered at this site [78]. However, any benefit conferred by i.d. immunization is outweighed by its reduced practicality in the clinic and tendency for localized reaction. In any event, clinical comparison of rMVA i.d. and i.m. administration demonstrates no significant difference in immunogenicity [79–81].

Developing rMVA for clinical use: GMP manufacture

To date, we have concentrated on "research grade" rMVA that enables the researcher to demonstrate that the rMVA has potential clinical utility by showing *in vivo* efficacy in an established authentic disease model. Furthermore, the researcher has investigated a number of avenues to further enhance the ability of the rMVA to induce an effective immune response relevant for disease protection. A decision now has to be taken, if the data generated to date warrants progression to clinical evaluation. Figure 14.3 summarizes stages involved in the transition from research to preclinical development of rMVA.

Recombinant MVA candidates for clinical study must withstand regulatory scrutiny and so are required to be generated, purified, and amplified under conditions conducive to current Good Manufacturing Practice (cGMP). While the following is not an exhaustive description of MVA development to cGMP manufacture, some key aspects of rMVA methodology and their relevance to clinical grade status are discussed. The regulatory process that the investigator will need to adhere to is dependent on the territory where they anticipate performing the clinical study. EU member states are regulated by the European Medicines Agency (www.ema.europa.eu/ema) and the United States by the Food and Drug Administration (www.fda.gov). Though guidelines are available from the respective agency websites, it may be advisable to recruit the services of an experienced regulatory consultant before embarking on rMVA development at this stage.

When constructing an rMVA for clinical development the virus will need to be reconstructed under appropriate "controlled conditions." This means that the investigator needs to ensure the provenance of all materials used to construct the recombinant and the process is performed in a laboratory environment that is free from other infectious agents; that is, the hood is fumigated, HEPA filters changed, and no other infectious agent is used in the designated laboratory. Animal-derived products must be accompanied with manufacturer's documentation to ensure that materials are derived from a prion-free source, also free of other adventitious agents. Even when non-animal derived materials are used, statements from suppliers to confirm that such materials are of appropriate quality and free from animal products are

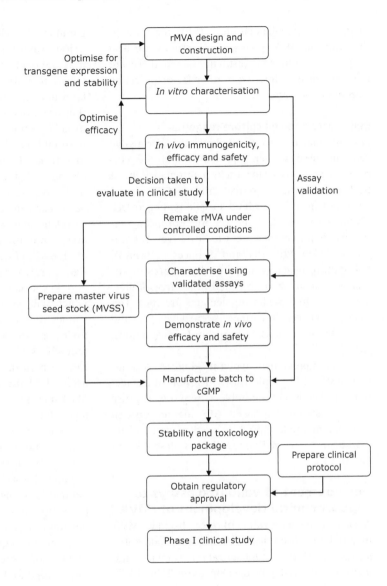

Figure 14.3 Flow chart of rMVA product development.

still required. Batch records of all materials used in the construction and expansion of the rMVA will need to be kept to support regulatory approval. Additionally, activities will need to be performed under a quality management system that controls access to the laboratory area, and ensures laboratory equipment is maintained to the appropriate standards and that effective record keeping is adhered to. Below are a set of key factors to be considered.

MVA provenance

A sample of native MVA can be obtained under Material Transfer Agreement (MTA) from a variety of sources (e.g., ATCC, USA) or collaborating institute. For preclinical research, MVA must be free of contaminants; for use in GMP manufacture and clinical studies, the provenance of the parent strain must enable assurance of prion-free status. Broadly speaking, the FDA accepts samples from 1984 and earlier to be free of transmissible spongiform encephalopathies (TSE). Separate to the issue of MVA quality, MVA strains are also subject to commercial restrictions, and these are discussed below along with other factors affecting freedom to operate.

Cell source and cell culture reagents

For manufacture to GMP, both the permissive cell line used to generate rMVA and the culture reagents used for their maintenance must be from an assured source. Primary CEF can be used, but must be certified specific pathogen free (SPF). A source satisfying US and European regulatory requirements are Charles River Laboratories, Avian Products and Services (SPAFAS). Cell culture reagents, in particular sources of animal serum, must be certified prion free. Preferably serum-free media supplements are used. Designer avian cell lines have been developed and are grown in suspension in serum-free conditions. [82,83].

As stated previously, when making rMVA products destined for clinical use, inclusion of a selection marker is not desirable. Therefore, the use of a transiently expressed GFP marker system, or other method, should be used to prepare the marker-free recombinant MVA, as described in Figure 14.2.

Development of validated assays to support clinical development of rMVA

Assays for characterization of research-grade rMVA material have been discussed. However, additional assays for rMVA characterization, stability, and identity, will need to be developed (see Table 14.2). Additionally, assays will need to undergo a level of "validation" to ensure they are reproducible, sensitive, and fit for purpose. Guidelines on assay validation can be found at the respective European and US regulatory websites (*ICH Topic Q2 (R1): Validation of Analytical Procedures*, www.ema.europa.eu/docs/en_GB/document_library/Scientific_guideline/2009/09/WC500002662.pdf; *Guidance for Industry: Bioanalytical Method Validation* www.fda.gov/downloads/Drugs/GuidanceComplianceRegulatory Information/Guidances/UCM070107.pdf). Assay validation normally involves evaluating assay parameters such as precision, intermediate precision, robustness, linearity, and accuracy, and it is advisable to take advice from a regulatory expert to fully understand which assays need to be validated and to what extent. Those assays that are essential for "release" of cGMP material usually require the highest level of validation. It should also be remembered that the assay the investigator intends to use to evaluate the immune response to the rMVA may also be required to undergo a validation process. Validation of assays is particularly important when attempting to identify correlates of protection or therapy. If the regulators accept immune correlates of efficacy the timelines of phase III efficacy studies and licensure, could be significantly reduced.

A key assay to be validated is virus titration, which will be used to support biological stability studies, define dosing in preclinical efficacy and toxicology studies, define genetic stability, and potentially as a read-out of vaccine potency. Titration can be performed via standard $TCID_{50}$ or plaque assay, the latter requiring an immunostain step as MVA does not form discrete plaques on cell monolayers [10]. If an antibody recognizing the authentic gene product is used then the immunostain plaque titration assay could potentially be used as a potency release assay for the cGMP manufactured product. A specific titer of rMVA may have to be defined previously that has been shown to induce protection in an appropriate *in vivo* model. A double immunostain technique has been developed that can distinguish between rMVA populations that do not express full-length gene product, which can be used to demonstrate a homogeneous rMVA population.

Several assays based on PCR are utilized to sensitively detect the presence of wild-type MVA or rMVA containing truncated transgenes. Sequencing, starting 1 kb outside of the flanking regions used in the homologous recombination event, is used to demonstrate that no individual base mutation has occurred. However, though adequate to support applications to phase II, the FDA will require full genome sequencing for phase III application. Fortuitously, studies show that the MVA genome is extremely stable, thus this level of sequence analysis should not lead to additional regulatory questions.

Manufacture of MVA-based vaccines

Several companies utilize MVA as a recombinant vaccine delivery platform and MVA has also been manufactured to product scale to support the US requirement for their national strategic stockpile of smallpox vaccine. To date, all clinical studies have used material produced in primary CEFs supplied from specific pathogen-free flocks. However, to obviate the requirement of egg supplies and to reduce costs, two companies have derived avian cell lines that should be suitable for the production of clinical-grade MVA material. There are a number of contract manufacturing organizations that can produce rMVA for clinical use. However, IDT (www.idt-biologika.com) have produced rMVA GMP material for numerous clinical studies and have a proven track record for producing material used in both Europe and the USA.

Freedom to operate and intellectual property considerations

It is worth remembering that to develop and license an rMVA-based product will take a significant investment amounting to tens of millions of dollars. A vaccine company will only invest in such an rMVA if it can assure protection of this investment through intellectual property (IP) filings and it has freedom to operate – that is, the use of rMVA does not infringe the IP of others. It is essential, therefore, that before publication of early research stage data that consideration is given to potential patent filings. Additionally, consideration should be given to each component and method used in the construction of the preclinical rMVA. The early patents on recombinant vaccinia virus construction are still valid and are held by the NIH and others; however, non-exclusive access to this IP has been licensed to several organizations.

Though the inventor of MVA, Anton Mayr, issued samples to various laboratories throughout the world over the past 20 years, there are still claims that recently filed patents could dictate its commercial use. Issued and filed patents also exist that cover the use of specific MVA insertion sites, utility of heterologous prime-boost regimens, and immune co-factor genes. A view from a patent expert is always advisable before significant investment is made into a preclinical rMVA programme.

Summary

MVA is immunopotentiating, has a relatively large capacity for foreign DNA, and offers safe clinical use, making it a prime candidate for utility as a recombinant viral vaccine vector.

In less than 20 years, hundreds of rMVA-based products have been generated and evaluated *in vivo*, demonstrating protective efficacy and immunotherapeutic potential against a range of infectious diseases and cancer targets. Those rMVA warranting clinical evaluation have progressed to preclinical and clinical development so that processes for GMP manufacture and regulatory approval are now well established. What is more, rMVA methodology has advanced to enable rapid construction of rationally designed recombinants capable of evoking enhanced protection. Over the past 10 years, optimized rMVA based vaccines co-expressing immunomodulators have been added to the list of rMVA already in clinical studies. As discussed in this chapter, there are intellectual property issues particular to MVA to be considered, but this should not prevent rapid development of rMVA-based products.

Recombinant rMVA technology is now a key product development platform with which to progress novel health-care interventions.

Acknowledgments

The authors are grateful to Sue Marlow of Marlow Associates Ltd for regulatory input.

References

1 Lane JM, Ruben FL, Neff JM, *et al.* Complications of smallpox vaccination, 1968. *N Engl J Med* 1969;**281**:1201–8.

2 Mayr A, Stickl H, Muller HK, *et al.* [The smallpox vaccination strain MVA: marker, genetic structure, experience gained with the parenteral vaccination and behavior in organisms with a debilitated defence mechanism.] *Zentralbl Bakteriol B* 1978;**167**:375–90 (author's transl).

3 Sutter G, Staib C. Vaccinia vectors as candidate vaccines: the development of modified vaccinia virus Ankara for antigen delivery. *Curr Drug Targets Infect Disord* 2003;**3**:263–71.

4 Sutter G, Moss B. Nonreplicating vaccinia vector efficiently expresses recombinant genes. *Proc Natl Acad Sci U S A* 1992;**89**:10847–51.

5 Merchlinsky M, Moss B. Introduction of foreign DNA into the vaccinia virus genome by in vitro ligation: recombination-independent selectable cloning vectors. *Virology* 1992;**190**:522–26.

6 Sutter G, Wyatt LS, Foley PL, *et al.* A recombinant vector derived from the host range-restricted and highly attenuated MVA strain of vaccinia virus stimulates protective immunity in mice to influenza virus. *Vaccine* 1994;**12**:1032–40.

7 Moss B, Carroll MW, Wyatt LS, *et al.* Host range restricted, non-replicating vaccinia virus vectors as vaccine candidates. *Adv Exp Med Biol* 1996;**397**:7–13.

8 Sutter G, Moss B. Novel vaccinia vector derived from the host range restricted and highly attenuated MVA strain of vaccinia virus. *Dev Biol Stand* 1995;**84**:195–200.

9 Gomez CE, Najera JL, Krupa M, *et al.* The poxvirus vectors MVA and NYVAC as gene delivery systems for vaccination against infectious diseases and cancer. *Curr Gene Ther* 2008;**8**:97–120.

10 Earl PL, Cooper N, Wyatt LS, *et al.* Preparation of cell cultures and vaccinia virus stocks. *Curr Protoc Protein Sci* 2001;Chapter 5, Unit 5.12.

11 Earl PL, Moss B. Characterization of recombinant vaccinia viruses and their products. *Curr Protoc Protein Sci* 2001;Chapter 5, Unit 5.14.

12 Earl PL, Moss B, Wyatt LS, *et al.* Generation of recombinant vaccinia viruses. *Curr Protoc Protein Sci* 2001;Chapter 5, Unit 5.13.

13 Antoine G, Scheiflinger F, Dorner F, *et al.* The complete genomic sequence of the modified vaccinia Ankara strain: comparison with other orthopoxviruses. *Virology* 1998;**244**:365–96.

14 Broyles SS. Vaccinia virus transcription. *J Gen Virol* 2003;**84**:2293–303.

15 Assarsson E, Greenbaum JA, Sundstrom M, *et al.* Kinetic analysis of a complete poxvirus transcriptome reveals an immediate-early class of genes. *Proc Natl Acad Sci U S A* 2008;**105**:2140–45.

16 Baldick CJ, Jr, Moss B. Characterization and temporal regulation of mRNAs encoded by vaccinia virus intermediate-stage genes. *J Virol* 1993;**67**:3515–27.

17 Wyatt LS, Carroll MW, Czerny CP, *et al.* Marker rescue of the host range restriction defects of modified vaccinia virus Ankara. *Virology* 1998;**251**: 334–42.

18 Meyer H, Sutter G, Mayr A. Mapping of deletions in the genome of the highly attenuated vaccinia virus MVA and their influence on virulence. *J Gen Virol* 1991;**72**(Pt 5):1031–8.

19 Backes S, Sperling KM, Zwilling J, *et al.* Viral host-range factor C7 or K1 is essential for modified vaccinia virus Ankara late gene expression in human and murine cells, irrespective of their capacity to inhibit protein kinase R-mediated phosphorylation of eukaryotic translation initiation factor 2alpha. *J Gen Virol* 2010;**91**:470–82.

20 Hornemann S, Harlin O, Staib C, *et al.* Replication of modified vaccinia virus Ankara in primary chicken embryo fibroblasts requires expression of the interferon resistance gene E3L. *J Virol* 2003;**77**: 8394–407.

21 Ludwig H, Mages J, Staib C, *et al.* Role of viral factor E3L in modified vaccinia virus Ankara infection of human HeLa cells: regulation of the virus life cycle and identification of differentially expressed host genes. *J Virol* 2005;**79**:2584–96.

22 Sperling KM, Schwantes A, Staib C, *et al.* The orthopoxvirus 68-kilodalton ankyrin-like protein is essential for DNA replication and complete gene expression of modified vaccinia virus Ankara in nonpermissive human and murine cells. *J Virol* 2009;**83**:6029–38.

23 Carroll MW, Moss B. Host range and cytopathogenicity of the highly attenuated MVA strain of vaccinia virus: propagation and generation of recombinant viruses in a nonhuman mammalian cell line. *Virology* 1997;**238**:198–211.

24 Okeke MI, Nilssen O, Traavik T. Modified vaccinia virus Ankara multiplies in rat IEC-6 cells and limited production of mature virions occurs in other mammalian cell lines. *J Gen Virol* 2006;**87**:21–7.

25 Drexler I, Heller K, Wahren B, *et al.* Highly attenuated modified vaccinia virus Ankara replicates in baby hamster kidney cells, a potential host for virus propagation, but not in various human transformed and primary cells. *J Gen Virol* 1998;**79**(Pt 2):347–52.

26 Mackett M, Smith GL, Moss B. Vaccinia virus: a selectable eukaryotic cloning and expression vector. *Proc Natl Acad Sci U S A* 1982;**79**:7415–19.

27 Panicali D, Paoletti E. Construction of poxviruses as cloning vectors: insertion of the thymidine kinase gene from herpes simplex virus into the DNA of infectious vaccinia virus. *Proc Natl Acad Sci U S A* 1982;**79**:4927–31.

28 Cottingham MG, Andersen RF, Spencer AJ, *et al.* Recombination-mediated genetic engineering of a bacterial artificial chromosome clone of modified vaccinia virus Ankara (MVA). *PLoS One* 2008;**3**:e1638.

29 Domi A, Moss B. Cloning the vaccinia virus genome as a bacterial artificial chromosome in *Escherichia coli* and recovery of infectious virus in mammalian cells. *Proc Natl Acad Sci U S A* 2002;**99**:12415–20.

30 Staib C, Drexler I, Sutter G. Construction and isolation of recombinant MVA. *Methods Mol Biol* 2004;**269**: 77–100.

31 Wyatt LS, Earl PL, Vogt J, *et al.* Correlation of immunogenicities and in vitro expression levels of recombinant modified vaccinia virus Ankara HIV vaccines. *Vaccine* 2008;**26**:486–93.

32 Mackett M, Smith GL, Moss B. General method for production and selection of infectious vaccinia virus recombinants expressing foreign genes. *J Virol* 1984;**49**:857–64.

33 Chakrabarti S, Brechling K, Moss B. Vaccinia virus expression vector: coexpression of beta-galactosidase provides visual screening of recombinant virus plaques. *Mol Cell Biol* 1985;**5**:3403–9.

34 Franke CA, Rice CM, Strauss JH, *et al.* Neomycin resistance as a dominant selectable marker for selection and isolation of vaccinia virus recombinants. *Mol Cell Biol* 1985;**5**:1918–24.

35 Falkner FG, Moss B. *Escherichia coli* gpt gene provides dominant selection for vaccinia virus open reading frame expression vectors. *J Virol* 1988;**62**:1849–54.

36 Wu GY, Zou DJ, Koothan T, *et al.* Infection of frog neurons with vaccinia virus permits in vivo expression of foreign proteins. *Neuron* 1995;**14**:681–4.

37 Carroll MW, Moss B. *E. coli* beta-glucuronidase (GUS) as a marker for recombinant vaccinia viruses. *Biotechniques* 1995;**19**:352–4, 356.

38 Cao JX, Upton C. gpt-gus fusion gene for selection and marker in recombinant poxviruses. *Biotechniques* 1997;**22**:276–8.

39 Blasco R, Moss B. Selection of recombinant vaccinia viruses on the basis of plaque formation. *Gene* 1995;**158**:157–62.

40 Perkus ME, Limbach K, Paoletti E. Cloning and expression of foreign genes in vaccinia virus, using a host range selection system. *J Virol* 1989;**63**:3829–36.

41 Falkner FG, Moss B. Transient dominant selection of recombinant vaccinia viruses. *J Virol* 1990;**64**: 3108–11.

42 Scheiflinger F, Dorner F, Falkner FG. Transient marker stabilisation: a general procedure to construct marker-free recombinant vaccinia virus. *Arch Virol* 1998;**143**:467–74.

43 Cottingham MG, Gilbert SC. Rapid generation of markerless recombinant MVA vaccines by en passant recombineering of a self-excising bacterial artificial chromosome. *J Virol Methods* 2010;**168**:233–6.

44 Davison AJ, Moss B. Structure of vaccinia virus late promoters. *J Mol Biol* 1989;**210**:771–84.

45 Davison AJ, Moss B. Structure of vaccinia virus early promoters. *J Mol Biol* 1989;**210**:749–69.

46 Chakrabarti S, Sisler JR, Moss B. Compact, synthetic, vaccinia virus early/late promoter for protein expression. *Biotechniques* 1997;**23**:1094–7.

47 Broder CC, Kennedy PE, Michaels F, *et al.* Expression of foreign genes in cultured human primary macrophages using recombinant vaccinia virus vectors. *Gene* 1994;**142**:167–74.

48 Bronte V, Carroll MW, Goletz TJ, *et al.* Antigen expression by dendritic cells correlates with the therapeutic effectiveness of a model recombinant poxvirus tumor vaccine. *Proc Natl Acad Sci U S A* 1997; **94**:3183–8.

49 Drillien R, Spehner D, Bohbot A, *et al.* Vaccinia virus-related events and phenotypic changes after infection of dendritic cells derived from human monocytes. *Virology* 2000;**268**:471–81.

50 Wyatt LS, Shors ST, Murphy BR, *et al.* Development of a replication-deficient recombinant vaccinia virus vaccine effective against parainfluenza virus 3 infection in an animal model. *Vaccine* 1996;**14**:1451–8.

51 Harrop R, Ryan MG, Myers KA, *et al.* Active treatment of murine tumors with a highly attenuated vaccinia virus expressing the tumor associated antigen 5T4 (TroVax) is CD4$^+$ T cell dependent and antibody mediated. *Cancer Immunol Immunother* 2006;**55**: 1081–90.

52 Earl PL, Hugin AW, Moss B. Removal of cryptic poxvirus transcription termination signals from the human immunodeficiency virus type 1 envelope gene enhances expression and immunogenicity of a recombinant vaccinia virus. *J Virol* 1990;**64**:2448–51.

53 Moss B. Poxviridae: the viruses and their replication. In BN Fields, DM Knipe, PM Howley (Eds) *Fields*

Virology, 5th edn. Lippincott-Raven, Philadelphia, PA, 2007, pp 2905–46.

54 Antoine G, Scheiflinger F, Holzer G, *et al.* Characterization of the vaccinia MVA hemagglutinin gene locus and its evaluation as an insertion site for foreign genes. *Gene* 1996;**177**:43–6.

55 Timm A, Enzinger C, Felder E, *et al.* Genetic stability of recombinant MVA-BN. *Vaccine* 2006;**24**:4618–21.

56 Manuel ER, Wang Z, Li Z, *et al.* Intergenic region 3 of modified vaccinia ankara is a functional site for insert gene expression and allows for potent antigen-specific immune responses. *Virology* 2010;**403**:155–62.

57 Wyatt LS, Earl PL, Xiao W, *et al.* Elucidating and minimizing the loss by recombinant vaccinia virus of human immunodeficiency virus gene expression resulting from spontaneous mutations and positive selection. *J Virol* 2009;**83**:7176–84.

58 Bray M. Pathogenesis and potential antiviral therapy of complications of smallpox vaccination. *Antiviral Res* 2003;**58**:101–14.

59 Ramirez JC, Gherardi MM, Esteban M. Biology of attenuated modified vaccinia virus Ankara recombinant vector in mice: virus fate and activation of B- and T-cell immune responses in comparison with the Western Reserve strain and advantages as a vaccine. *J Virol* 2000;**74**:923–33.

60 Redchenko I, Ryan MG, Carroll MW. Pre-existing immunity to vaccinia virus does not affect efficacy of a recombinant MVA vaccine: poxvirus cross-reactivity. *12th International Congress of Immunology and 4th Annual Conference of FOCIS*, 2004, pp 459–64.

61 Ramirez JC, Gherardi MM, Rodriguez D, *et al.* Attenuated modified vaccinia virus Ankara can be used as an immunizing agent under conditions of preexisting immunity to the vector. *J Virol* 2000;**74**:7651–5.

62 Harrop R, Drury N, Shingler W, *et al.* Vaccination of colorectal cancer patients with modified vaccinia Ankara encoding the tumor antigen 5T4 (TroVax) given alongside chemotherapy induces potent immune responses. *Clin Cancer Res* 2007;**13**:4487–94.

63 Kannanganat S, Nigam P, Velu V, *et al.* Preexisting vaccinia virus immunity decreases SIV-specific cellular immunity but does not diminish humoral immunity and efficacy of a DNA/MVA vaccine. *J Immunol* 2010;**185**:7262–73.

64 Coupar BE, Andrew ME, Both GW, *et al.* Temporal regulation of influenza hemagglutinin expression in vaccinia virus recombinants and effects on the immune response. *Eur J Immunol* 1986;**16**:1479–87.

65 Zhou JA, McIndoe A, Davies H, *et al.* The induction of cytotoxic T-lymphocyte precursor cells by recombi-

nant vaccinia virus expressing human papillomavirus type 16 L1. *Virology* 1991;**181**:203–10.

66 Ramshaw IA, Andrew ME, Phillips SM, *et al.* Recovery of immunodeficient mice from a vaccinia virus/IL-2 recombinant infection. *Nature* 1987;**329**:545–6.

67 Flexner C, Hugin A, Moss B. Prevention of vaccinia virus infection in immunodeficient mice by vector-directed IL-2 expression. *Nature* 1987;**330**:259–62.

68 Carroll MW, Overwijk WW, Surman DR, *et al.* Construction and characterization of a triple-recombinant vaccinia virus encoding B7-1, interleukin 12, and a model tumor antigen. *J Natl Cancer Inst* 1998;**90**:1881–7.

69 Dreicer R, Stadler WM, Ahmann FR, *et al.* MVA-MUC1-IL2 vaccine immunotherapy (TG4010) improves PSA doubling time in patients with prostate cancer with biochemical failure. *Invest New Drugs* 2009;**27**:379–86.

70 Liu M, Acres B, Balloul JM, *et al.* Gene-based vaccines and immunotherapeutics. *Proc Natl Acad Sci U S A* 2004;**101**(Suppl 2):14567–71.

71 Ramlau R, Quoix E, Rolski J, *et al.* A phase II study of Tg4010 (Mva-Muc1-Il2) in association with chemotherapy in patients with stage III/IV non-small cell lung cancer. *J Thorac Oncol* 2008;**3**:735–44.

72 McConkey SJ, Reece WH, Moorthy VS, *et al.* Enhanced T-cell immunogenicity of plasmid DNA vaccines boosted by recombinant modified vaccinia virus Ankara in humans. *Nat Med* 2003;**9**:729–35.

73 Vuola JM, Keating S, Webster DP, *et al.* Differential immunogenicity of various heterologous prime-boost vaccine regimens using DNA and viral vectors in healthy volunteers. *J Immunol* 2005;**174**:449–55.

74 Douglas AD, de Cassan SC, Dicks MD, *et al.* Tailoring subunit vaccine immunogenicity: maximizing antibody and T cell responses by using combinations of adenovirus, poxvirus and protein-adjuvant vaccines against *Plasmodium falciparum* MSP1. *Vaccine* **28**, 7167–78.

75 Robinson HL. Working towards an HIV/AIDS vaccine. *Hum Vaccin* 2009;**5**:436–8.

76 Hill AV, Reyes-Sandoval A, O'Hara G, *et al.* Prime-boost vectored malaria vaccines: progress and prospects. *Hum Vaccin* 2010;**6**:78–83.

77 Beveridge NE, Price DA, Casazza JP, *et al.* Immunisation with BCG and recombinant MVA85A induces long-lasting, polyfunctional *Mycobacterium tuberculosis*-specific CD4[+] memory T lymphocyte populations. *Eur J Immunol* 2007;**37**:3089–100.

78 Abadie V, Bonduelle O, Duffy D, *et al.* Original encounter with antigen determines antigen-presenting cell imprinting of the quality of the immune response in mice. *PLoS One* 2009;**4**:e8159.

79 Harris S, Meyer J, Satti I, et al. A Phase I clinical trial to compare the safety and immunogenicity of candidate TB vaccine MVA85A administered by the intramuscular route and the intradermal route in healthy adult individuals who have been previously vaccinated with BCG. In *TB Vaccines: A Second Global Forum*, Abstracts, 2010, p. 59.

80 Harrop R, Connolly N, Redchenko I, *et al.* Vaccination of colorectal cancer patients with modified vaccinia Ankara delivering the tumor antigen 5T4 (TroVax) induces immune responses which correlate with disease control: a phase I/II trial. *Clin Cancer Res* 2006;**12**:3416–24.

81 Berthoud TK, Hamill M, Lillie PJ, *et al.* Potent CD8$^+$ T-cell immunogenicity in humans of a novel heterosubtypic influenza A vaccine, MVA$^-$NP$^+$M1. *Clin Infect Dis* 2011;**52**:1–7.

82 Guehenneux F, Pain B. Production of poxviruses with adherent or non adherent avian cell lines VIVALIS (Roussay, FR). US patent application 20090239286, 2009.

83 Lohr V, Rath A, Genzel Y, *et al.* New avian suspension cell lines provide production of influenza virus and MVA in serum-free media: studies on growth, metabolism and virus propagation. *Vaccine* 2009;**27**: 4975–82.

84 Mandl SJ, Delcayre A, Curry D, *et al.* MVA-BN-HER2: a novel vaccine for the treatment of breast cancers which overexpress HER-2. *J Immunother* 2006;**29**: 652.

85 Harrop R, Shingler W, Kelleher M, *et al.* Cross-trial analysis of immunologic and clinical data resulting from phase I and II trials of MVA-5T4 (TroVax) in colorectal, renal, and prostate cancer patients. *J Immunother* 2010;**33**:999–1005.

86 Delcayre A, Laus R, Mandl S, et al. Use of MVA to treat prostate cancer. BN Immunotherapeutics, Inc. (Mountain View, CA). US patent application 20090104225, 2009.

87 Fournillier A, Gerossier E, Evlashev A, *et al.* An accelerated vaccine schedule with a poly-antigenic hepatitis C virus MVA-based candidate vaccine induces potent, long lasting and in vivo cross-reactive T cell responses. *Vaccine* 2007;**25**:7339–53.

88 Earl PL, Cotter C, Moss B, *et al.* Design and evaluation of multi-gene, multi-clade HIV-1 MVA vaccines. *Vaccine* 2009;**27**:5885–95.

89 Overton T, Schmidt D, Hain J, *et al.* P18–12 LB. Phase I clinical trial with a new recombinant MVA-BN®-multiantigen vaccine: high responder rate and considerable breadth of immunological response. *Retrovirology* 2009;**6**:P411.

90 Bejon P, Ogada E, Mwangi T, *et al.* Extended follow-up following a phase 2b randomized trial of the candidate malaria vaccines FP9 ME-TRAP and MVA ME-TRAP among children in Kenya. *PLoS One* 2007;**2**:e707.

91 McShane H. Vaccine strategies against tuberculosis. *Swiss Med Wkly* 2009;**139**:156–60.

CHAPTER 15

Recombinant Adenoviruses for Vaccination

Nelson Cesar Di Paolo[1], Dmitry Shayakhmetov[1], & André Lieber[1,2]
[1]Department of Medicine, Division of Medical Genetics
[2]Department of Pathology, University of Washington, Seattle, WA, USA

Adenovirus vectors for vaccination: advantages and problems

In recent years substantial progress has been made with recombinant viral vaccine technologies (for a review, see [1]). Viruses that have been modified for vaccination purposes and tested clinically include human and chimpanzee adenoviruses, vaccinia virus, fowlpox virus, and canarypox virus. The majority of successful clinical trials involved adenovirus (Ad) -based vaccines, usually in a prime-boost regime.

Adenoviruses are non-enveloped viruses possessing a double-stranded DNA genome (Figure 15.1a). To date, 51 different serotypes of human Ad have been identified and they are classified into 6 species (A to F). In general, Ad tropism for different organs and clinical symptoms varies among serotypes. Ad serotypes from all species, except those belonging to species B and some from species D, are able to use the coxsackievirus-Ad receptor (CAR) on the cell surface for primary Ad attachment [2,3]. Species B (serotypes 3, 7, 11, 14, 16, 21, 34, 35, 50) and some species D (serotype 37) use CD46 as a cellular receptor [4–7]. The current two-step paradigm for Ad infection is based on *in vitro* studies with serotypes Ad2 and Ad5 [8]. An initial high-affinity attachment step between the Ad fiber knob domain and its cellular receptor is followed by internalization that requires interaction between RGD motifs within the Ad penton base and cellular integrins [9]. After Ad internalization, endosome acidification induces Ad particle escape from endosomes to the cytosol, where particles use microtubule transport to translocate to the nucleus. Once at the nucleus, partially disassembled Ad capsids dock with nuclear pore complexes and the viral genome translocates into the nucleus. *In vivo*, the two-step model of Ad infection does not always apply. Upon intravenous delivery the majority of virus transduces the liver, and several studies have demonstrated that mutations which abolish CAR and integrin interactions are not sufficient to eliminate liver transduction [10–13]. Recent studies suggest that Ad infection of the liver is mediated, at least in part, by heparin sulfate proteoglycans, which interact with blood coagulation factors that bind to viral hexon and promote Ad uptake [14,15].

Overall, Ads are used as vaccine vectors (i) to express an antigen-encoding gene in antigen-presenting cells (APCs), (ii) to transfer an antigen protein in the context of the Ad capsid into APCs, or (iii) to enhance the effect of another vaccine [16–19].

Most vectors used for vaccination in preclinical studies and all vectors used so far in humans were based on human serotype 5 (Ad5). Recombinant Ad5 vectors for gene transfer were first

Vaccinology: Principles and Practice, First Edition. Edited by W. John W. Morrow, Nadeem A. Sheikh, Clint S. Schmidt and D. Huw Davies.
© 2012 Blackwell Publishing Ltd. Published 2012 by Blackwell Publishing Ltd.

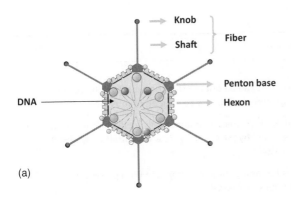

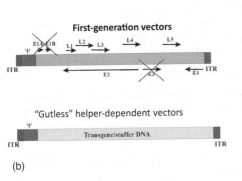

(b)

Figure 15.1 Adenovirus vectors. (a) Scheme of adenovirus particles. The main components of the protein capsid are fiber, penton base, and hexon. The C-terminal fiber domain forms a knob-like structure and mediates high-affinity binding to cellular receptors. A second interaction between penton base and cellular integrins triggers virus internalization. The double-stranded DNA genome is them transported to the nucleus. (b) Genomic structure of Ad vectors. First-generation Ad vectors have the E1A and E1B genes and often the E3 genes deleted. The transgene expression cassette is inserted into the E1 or E3 region. Helper-dependent vectors lack all viral genes. ITR, inverted terminal repeat; ψ, packaging signal; L1–L5, late (structural) viral genes; E1–E4, early (nonstructural) viral genes.

developed in the mid-1980s [20–22]. Advantages of Ad5 vectors include the ease of large-scale production, efficiency of gene transfer, widespread cell tropism, and high transgene DNA insert capacity. For vaccination the vast majority of Ad5 vectors were first-generation vectors – for example, deleted for the viral E1 genes – which renders them replication-deficient (Figure 15.1b). Because

after cell transduction, first-generation vectors still express a number of viral genes, which interfere with cell viability, newer vectors, deleted for all viral genes, have been developed [23]. These vectors require a helper virus for amplification and are therefore called helper-dependent (HD) Ad vectors. While Ad5 vectors are very efficient in conferring high-level, transient transgene expression, several specific features of Ad5 vectors have to be considered for their use in vaccination. See Table 15.1 for a summary of the pros and cons of adenovirus vector vaccines.

Neutralizing anti-Ad5 antibodies

Ad5 is a ubiquitous pathogen and neutralizing antibodies, found in up to 50% of adults in the US, interfere with the efficacy of systemically delivered Ad5 vectors [24]. Notably, most of the neutralizing antibodies are directed against epitopes within the viral hexon. To circumvent this problem associated with Ad5, a more recent approach has been to develop Ad vectors that incorporate fiber, hexon, or penton proteins of alternative Ad serotype, or are based entirely on other, rare Ad serotypes of human or nonhuman origin (for a review, see [18]). For example, Roberts *et al.* [25] mutated the Ad5 hexon capsid proteins in order to evade host neutralizing antibodies. They constructed chimeric Ad5 vectors in which the seven short hypervariable regions (HVRs) within the Ad5 hexon protein were replaced with the corresponding HVRs from the rare Ad serotype Ad48. In the presence of high levels of pre-existing anti-Ad5 immunity, the immunogenicity of HVR-chimeric Ad5/Ad48 vectors was not detectably suppressed, whereas the immunogenicity of parental rAd5 vectors was abrogated. In another study, McCoy *et al.* [26] compared a prime-boost regimen for an HIV vaccine with two serologically distinct Ad vectors derived from chimpanzee serotypes C68 and C1 with a regimen in which human Ad5 vectors were given twice in rhesus macaques that had or had not been pre-exposed to human Ad5 antigens. While pre-existing immunity to human Ad5 completely inhibited induction of transgene product-specific antibodies by the human Ad5 vectors, humoral vaccine responses were not affected when

Table 15.1 Summary of the pros and cons of Ad vectors.

Ads pros and cons	Rationale
Pros	
The vector can be easily modified, both chemically and genetically	Antigens can be displayed in the capsid, or the vector engineered to express an antigen of interest
Ads can enter the cytosol of most cell types	Antigens chemically or genetically loaded in the capsid will be presented by MHC-II or by cross-presentation by MHC-I molecules
Ads can express antigens in almost any cell type	It is the best potential vector for MHC-I presentation of antigens of interest
Several different serotypes exist	It is expected that different serotypes will provide availability of a panel of different vectors with benefits in each particular application needed. A panel of different vectors might also enable serial booster vaccination
Ads do not integrate into the host genome	Reduced risk of insertional mutagenesis
Ads induce a strong local inflammation	Some researchers suggest that this unspecific inflammation will be beneficial for the immune response against the desired antigen
Cons	
Adaptive immunity induced by the vector	Transduced cells are eliminated. Problem partially solved by helper-dependent vectors
Innate acute immune response induced by the vector	Risk of acute toxicity at the doses needed for a therapeutic benefit. This is the major problem that the field has yet to solve
Ads do not integrate into the host genome	The vector is diluted if the target cell divides

chimpanzee Ad vectors were employed. Studies that used alternative Ads focused on serotypes with relatively low serum prevalance of neutralizing antibodies. Magalhaes *et al.* [27] used a human Ad serotype 35 (Ad35) vector for *Mycobacterium tuberculosis* (Mtb) vaccination; Ko *et al.* [28] employed an Ad41 vector for oral T-cell priming against HIV; and Zhang *et al.* [29] developed a new Ad3-based vector. Regarding alternative human or nonhuman Ad serotypes, it has to be noted that the biology of these serotypes is largely unknown, implying that more basic virology work has to be done before these vaccines can be considered for clinical use.

Acute toxicity

Ad5 vector application induces acute vector-mediated toxicity after intravascular delivery,

which is associated with complement activation and the production/release of cytokines (including IL1, IL6, IL10, IL8, TNF-α, and IFN-γ) and chemokines (including MIP-1 and MIP-2) [30–33]. While this is a safety concern if Ad5 is injected intravenously or leaks into the blood circulation after intramuscular injection, the production of proinflammatory cytokines and chemokines can also have a stimulatory effect on vaccination. Several Ad-induced cytokines and chemokines trigger the recruitment of effector cells of the adaptive immune system to the site of Ad injection or activate the functions of immune cells. Recently, several laboratories have provided important insights into the mechanisms of innate immune recognition of Ads. Most of the data on the innate immune recognition of Ad5 has been obtained from *in vitro* systems, and has been recently reviewed [34–36]. The published results allow the conclusion that incoming Ad5 particles are detected by Toll-like receptor (TLR) -dependent [37] and TLR-independent mechanisms, and that type I interferons are key cytokines produced in response to Ad5 vector infections. MyD88, a key molecular adaptor for several receptors involved in pathogen recognition and induction of the innate immune response, has also been implicated in the overall modification of the transcriptome induced by Ad5, both *in vitro* and *in vivo* [38,39]. Our *in vivo* data [40] demonstrated that the very early response to Ad5 vectors is mediated by macrophage recognition of virus through β3 integrin, which mediates induction and maturation of IL1α. In our *in vivo* system, Ad5 recognition is independent of TLRs or the inflammasome. Instead, we found that IL1α signals through the IL1 receptor to induce the amplification of the expression of other important cytokines and chemokines (e.g., MIP-2, KC, MCP-1, IL6). How these findings can be used to modify the outcome of Ad vaccination strategies remains to be studied. In this context, we are currently investigating the interplay of integrin and IL1α-signaling and the induction of cellular and humoral immunity to a transgene.

Transduction of dendritic cells by Ad5 vectors

A critical factor in each vaccination strategy is the efficient uptake of vaccination vectors and antigen expression in professional APCs, such as dendritic cells (DCs). Ad5 vectors are inefficient in transduction of human DCs *in vitro*. The poor transduction of human DCs with Ad5-based vectors is due to low-level expression of CAR. In contrast, a number of studies have shown that Ad vectors containing species B Ad serotype 35 fibers (Ad35 vectors or fiber chimeric Ad5/35) efficiently transduce human DCs *ex vivo* and appear to target APC after intravenous injection into CD46 transgenic mice and baboons [41,42]. Recently, we showed that an Ad5/35 vector expressing a model antigen was able to trigger a stronger T-cell response against the antigen after intramuscular injection than conventional Ad5 vectors [42]. Furthermore, a number of

studies demonstrated the superiority of Ad35 vectors over Ad5 vectors in vaccination against infectious agents [43–46].

Anti-Ad5 T-cell responses

Recent studies have demonstrated that conserved regions within Ad structural proteins can act as specific epitopes for serotype cross-reactive human cytotoxic T lymphocytes (CTLs) [47] and that serotype cross-reactive CD4 and CD8 T-cell responses can be activated in mice and humans [44, 48]. Furthermore, the recent demonstration that anti-Ad memory T cells can be activated at low levels from human peripheral blood mononuclear cells (PBMCs) by canine Ad vectors [49] suggests that conserved antigenic epitopes may stimulate cross-reactive epitopes irrespective of the vector serotype used. Further studies are needed to systematically investigate cross-reactivity of memory T cells between different serotypes of Ad vector. While the impact of this on gene transfer efficiency has been well documented, the effect this might have on Ad-based vaccination therapies has not been properly addressed. Recently Schirmbeck *et al.* [50] investigated whether the immunogenicity of antigens delivered by Ad5 vectors is impaired by the concomitant priming of specific immunity to protein antigens of the vector. They showed that the induced T-cell immunity specific for Ad proteins (either delivered with the Ad capsid or expressed from the Ad genome) is efficiently primed by vaccination with Ad vectors, and can limit the immunogenicity (particularly of subdominant epitopes) of Ad vector-encoded transgenes. It was suggested that the problem of competition between antivirus and vaccination antigen-specific responses could be solved by the use of HD-Ads [51]. More detailed recent studies, however, found that although HD-Ads do indeed show reduced chronic inflammation, Ad-specific cytotoxic T lymphocytes were generated in mice receiving HD Ad5 vectors [52]. We compared first-generation and HD vectors in mice and on human PBMCs *in vitro* and found that there are no differences in the induction of IFN-γ secreting T cells between the two vector platforms (N.C.D.P., A.L., unpublished observations).

Basic concepts of Ad vaccination

Route of administration of Ad-based vaccines

Generally, the route of administration of a vaccine affects its efficacy, and this is also true for Ad-based vaccines. The development of mucosal vaccines is imperative because most infectious agents enter the body at mucosal surfaces. It is therefore thought that vaccination is most effectively induced at the mucosa by immunization through oral, nasal, rectal, or vaginal routes [53]. It is thought that these routes of application circumvent the effect of pre-existing neutralizing antibodies. This concept, however, has recently been challenged by Kaufman et al. [54] for Ad-based vaccines. They showed that intramuscular immunization with recombinant Ad5 vectors expressing SIV Gag resulted in potent, durable, and functional CD8+ T lymphocyte responses at multiple mucosal effectors sites in both mice and rhesus monkeys, demonstrating that the systemic and mucosal immune systems are highly coordinated following vaccination. Li et al. [55], on the other hand, explored a novel prime-boost protocol using attenuated, recombinant L. monocytogenes-gag (rLm-gag) to prime mice followed by a boost with Ad5-gag in different tissues, and found the strongest CD8 T-cell responses in the mucosal vagina after immunization with both vectors through the mucosal vagina. As discussed below, particularly in HIV vaccination, the oral application of Ad vaccines poses risks because it can induce CD4+ T cells within the intestinal mucosa, the preferred targets of early HIV-1 replication. Overall, there is a need for more systematic studies to assess the effect of the route of Ad vaccination for each particular disease.

Heterologous vaccines involving Ads: prime-boost regimens

Clearly, one of the major emerging strategies in Ad-based vaccines in recent years has been their use in heterologous prime-boost regimens. Several groups have demonstrated that Ad-vectors can be used in a vast array of combinations with other peptides, proteins, DNA, and bacterial or viral vaccines, and in most of the cases the results have been encouraging. In all cases, the combination was more immunogenic than the Ad-based vaccine alone. For example, Tatsis et al. [56] demonstrated that heterologous booster immunizations after human Ad5 priming with chimpanzee-derived Ad vectors induced higher T- and B-cell responses than repeated immunizations with the Ad5 vector. McConnell et al. [57] showed that mice primed with plasmid DNA and boosted with an Ad5 vector expressing an anthrax antigen had higher antibody and toxin-neutralizing titers than mice immunized with either single modality alone or with the commercial anthrax vaccine (Anthrax Vaccine Adsorbed).

Ad vaccines in combination with adjuvants

The majority of vaccine antigens are recombinant molecules or subunits of pathogens with little or no inherent immunostimulatory property. Therefore, vaccines often are administered in combination with adjuvants that can boost and direct the vaccine-specific immunity. In the case of Ad-based vaccines, there has been very little effort to use adjuvants because it was thought that the acute innate immune response locally generated by the vector itself would be sufficient to support the priming of adaptive immune responses. However, recent studies indicate that Ad-based vaccination can be enhanced by the use of adjuvants. Wille-Reece et al. [58], for example, assessed the capacity of different TLR-binding compounds to influence the outcome of a recombinant HIV Gag protein/Ad5-Gag vector boost vaccination strategy in nonhuman primates. They found an increase in HIV Gag-specific CD8+ T-cell responses after the boost in all animals that had received a primary immunization with TLR adjuvants. The TLR adjuvants used during primary immunization influenced the magnitude and quality of the Th1 and CD8+ T cell responses after the Ad5-Gag boost. In line with these data, Ophorst et al. [59] increased the immunogenicity of an Ad35-based malaria vaccine by using aluminum phosphate as an adjuvant.

Another adjuvant approach is to express immunostimulatory cytokines or chemokines from Ad vectors together with the vaccination antigen.

A number of cytokines and chemokines that enhance traffic and activity of tumor-specific T cells have been successfully tested in this context, including IL1, IL12, IL18, IL21 [60,61], GM-CSF [62], and Flt3 ligand [63].

Clearly, further studies are required for each particular diseases and antigen to find an optimal adjuvant for each given Ad vaccine.

Depletion of regulatory T cells (Tregs)

Tumor-infiltrating Tregs are present in many human tumors, including ovarian cancer, lung cancer, malignant melanomas, Hodgkin's lymphoma, breast cancer, and cervical cancer. Tregs also represent an important immune escape mechanism for a number of parasites. For example, Tregs are elevated in infected lung areas, draining lymph nodes, and peripheral blood during active Mtb infection in humans [64]. The efficacy of vaccines, including Ad-based vaccines, can therefore be increased by approaches that inactivate or deplete Tregs using antibodies against Treg surface proteins (CD25, GITR, CTLA4) or low-dose cyclophosphamide [65–67].

Peptide incorporation into the Ad capsid

Krause *et al.* [68] compared the anti-antigen immunogenicity of Ad5 vectors with a common epitope of the hemagglutinin (HA) protein of the influenza A virus incorporated into the Ad5 capsid proteins hexon, penton base, fiber knob domain, or protein IX. They showed that the highest primary (immunoglobulin M [IgM]) and secondary (IgG) anti-HA humoral and cellular CD4-γ-interferon and CD4-IL4 response against HA was achieved with the Ad vector carrying the HA epitope in fiber knob domain. The same group [69] went on to develop a new clinical vaccine candidate (AdOprF.RGD.Epi8) against *Pseudomonas aeruginosa* using an Ad5 vector, expressing OprF and incorporating an immune-dominant OprF epitope (Epi8) into loop 1 of the hexon. Intramuscular immunization of C57BL/6 mice with AdOprF.RGD.Epi8 resulted in the generation of anti-OprF antibodies, CD4 and CD8 γ-interferon T-cell responses against OprF, as well as increased survival against

lethal pulmonary challenge with agar-encapsulated *P. aeruginosa*. More recently, Matthews *et al.* [70] were able to produce Ad vectors containing a range of antigenic epitopes within Ad5 hexon hypervariable regions (HVRs) 2 or 5. They defined the maximum peptide size that can be incorporated into HVR2 or HVR5 and suggested that HVR5 is more permissive to a range of insertions. Importantly, in all of these studies, the repeated administration of hexon-modified viruses resulted in a secondary anti-antigen response, whereas minimal secondary effect was present after administration of an Ad5 control vector. Overall, these studies indicate that antigen placement into the Ad capsid is a new approach for vaccination, broadening the possibilities of the Ad-based vaccine platforms.

Ad vaccines against multiple antigens

Many parasites, for example HIV, HCV, and XDR-MTb, replicate through error-prone RNA polymerases and are therefore highly mutagenic, which results in rapid generation of escape mutants to vaccination. Furthermore, a hallmark of tumor cells is their genetic and epigenetic instability, which has the potential to create tumor cell subsets that have lost a particular vaccination epitope. Ad-based vaccines should therefore express and simultaneously display (in the Ad capsid) multiple antigens.

Specific examples for Ad-based vaccination

Ad vaccines for viral pathogens

Ad vaccines are being tested for an array of acute and chronic viral infections. Most of the effort in the field of Ad-based vaccines has been devoted to develop an HIV vaccine. Several years of preclinical studies (reviewed in [71]) with Ad vaccines for HIV in mice and monkeys culminated in the STEP clinical trial sponsored by Merck, a multicenter, randomized, double-blind, placebo-controlled trial in which 3000 participants in North America, South America, the Caribbean, and Australia received three doses of the vaccine (a mixture of three components, each consisting of a first-generation Ad5 vector carrying a synthetic form of either *gag, pol,* or *nef*) or a placebo. The STEP clinical trial was halted, however, in September 2007 after interim analysis indicated that the vaccine failed to reduce both acquisition of HIV infection and viral load in those patients who became infected [72]. Subsequent analyses indicated that the vaccine made some individuals more susceptible to infection with HIV, and more individuals who received the vaccine became infected with HIV than did recipients of the placebo. Although the vaccine itself was not responsible for the increased acquisition of HIV infection, it particularly increased the risk of infection in males who had pre-existing antibodies specific for Ad5 [73]. The National Institute of Allergy and Infectious Diseases (NIAID) decided recently to cancel plans for another large clinical trial of a candidate vaccine against HIV. The canceled clinical trial, known as PAVE 100, was originally proposed in January 2007 and designed to test whether the vaccine, which was developed by the NIAID's Vaccine Research Center (VRC), could reduce acquisition of HIV infection and reduce viral load in those who became infected. However, PAVE 100 was put on hold even before it began enrolling volunteers and was then redesigned in May 2008 to reduce its scope after the failure of a similar vaccine in the STEP trial. The NIAID will consider a much smaller and more focused trial designed to test whether the vaccine can markedly decrease the viral load in individuals who become infected [73]. Mechanistic insight into why in the Merck trial there was a two-fold increase in the incidence of HIV acquisition among vaccinated recipients with increased Ad5-neutralizing antibody titers compared with placebo recipients was published by Perreau and colleagues [74]. Their results indicated that Ad5, in complex with anti-Ad antibodies – that is, Ad5 immunocomplexes (Ad5 IC) – induced significantly higher stimulation of Ad5-specific cytolytic CD8$^+$ T cells, and that Ad5 IC caused significantly enhanced HIV infection in DC/T-cell co-cultures when compared to Ad5 vectors alone. They concluded that Ad5 IC activates a DC/T-cell axis that may set up a permissive environment for HIV-1 infection. But even in the face of this drawback, the field keeps advancing, and new strategies are being applied to overcome the difficulties. Liu *et al.* [75], for example, recently published an improved T-cell-based vaccine prime-boost regimen using two serologically distinct Ad vectors, Ad26 and Ad5 expressing SIV Gag. They found stronger cellular immune responses with augmented magnitude, breadth, and polyfunctionality, compared to the homologous Ad5 regimen, and demonstrated that a durable partial immune control of a pathogenic SIV challenge can be achieved in rhesus monkeys.

Cytomegalovirus (CMV) infections contribute to morbidity and mortality in patients who have received hematopoietic stem cell transplantation. For CMV vaccination, Micklethwaite *et al.* generated CMV-specific T cells *in vitro* by stimulation with dendritic cells transduced with a chimeric Ad5/35 adenoviral vector encoding the CMV-pp65 protein. Patients received a prophylactic infusion of T cells at day 28 after hematopoietic stem cell transplantation, and immune reconstitution to CMV was demonstrated [76]. Ad5-based vaccines have also been developed for rabies [71], encephalitis virus [77,78], and hepatitis C virus [79]. Furthermore, Ad5-based Ebola virus vaccines are being developed and successfully tested in mice [80] and non-human primates [81]. Dengue virus (DENV) infection is a global threat to public health, there is no effective vaccine, and conventional treatment approaches are not optimal. A CD8$^+$ T cell-directed genetic vaccine that could generate cross-serotype protection would be desirable. Promising preclinical results with an Ad5-based Dengue virus vaccine in mice suggested potential cross-serotype protection [82].

Of particular interest is the development of vaccine against influenza. The increasing number and density of the human population, the emergence of lethal influenza strains (avian, swine), the possibility of vaccine shortages, and the potential use of designer influenza virus as a bioweapon collectively highlight a critical need for more rapid production of influenza vaccines and noninvasive methods for vaccine delivery. Because current vaccines require annual updating to protect against the rapidly arising antigenic variations due to antigenic shift and drift, researchers are trying to develop Ad-based influenza vaccines that can be produced without the prerequisite of growing influenza virus. For example, Holman et al. [83] incorporated multiple antigens from influenza viruses into Ad vectors and demonstrated the induction of strong humoral and cellular immune responses against the influenza virus antigens in vaccinated mice. Importantly, vaccinated mice were protected against a lethal H5N1 virus challenge.

Adenovirus serotypes, especially 2, 3, 4, 7, and 21, have been associated with serious chronic sequelae after acute respiratory tract infection, including irreversible atelectasis, bronchiectasis, bronchiolitis obliterans, and unilateral hyperlucent lung, with an estimated 14–60% of children experiencing some degree of permanent lung damage. Live oral Ad4 and Ad7 vaccines have been used for 25 years in military training centers and proven to be highly effective against homologous viruses and Ad3 [84]. Production of these vaccines ceased in 1990. Considering the recent emergence of new pathogenic Ad strains, such as Ad14a [85], the reinstallation of an Ad vaccination program for selected population groups should be considered.

Ad vaccines for bacterial infections

Vaccines against bacterial pathogens are being developed both for the treatment of diseases as well as for defense against bioterrorism.

There is clearly a need for a tuberculosis vaccine that is more potent than the current Bacille Calmette-Guérin (BCG) vaccine. Genetic vaccines, particularly recombinant viral vaccines, are effective in boosting immune activation and protection by BCG vaccination [86]. More recently, improved vectored vaccines using prime-boost regimens combining a recombinant BCG (rBCG) and Ad35 vector showed increased IFN-γ responses and antigen-specific T-cell proliferation in the CD8 T-cell subsets [27]. This and other strategies are paving the way for therapeutic Tb vaccines that would be effective in treating the chronic phase of the disease.

Streptococcus pneumoniae is a major bacterial respiratory pathogen. Current *S. pneumoniae* licensed vaccines are administered by an intramuscular injection. In the search for a new-generation vaccine that can be administered in a needle-free mucosal manner, Arevalo et al. [87] constructed Ad5 vectors expressing antigens from *S. pneumoniae* strain D39. Intranasal vaccination with the Ad vectors in mice resulted in robust antigen-specific serum immunoglobulin G responses, conferring protection against *S. pneumoniae* strain D39 colonization in mouse lungs.

A number of vaccination strategies and monoclonal antibodies have been developed for active and passive vaccination against *Pseudomonas aeruginosa*. Many of these have been tested in preclinical trials and only a few have reached clinical phases, but none of these vaccines has obtained market authorization. Because of this, the field is open to new developments, and Ad-based approaches could be a potential option. In this context, Worgall et al. [69] developed a modified Ad vector expressing the OprF antigen, and detected γ interferon CD4 and CD8 T-cell responses against OprF that protected mice against a lethal pulmonary challenge with agar-encapsulated *P. aeruginosa*.

Ad vaccines for parasitic infections

Without doubt the major focus on vaccines for parasitic infections is on developing a vaccine for malaria. Efforts in this field have been summarized by Li et al. [88]. Reyes-Sandoval et al. [89] recently demonstrated the ability of chimpanzee Ad vectors to generate CD8+ T-cell responses with an effector memory T-cell phenotype, multifunctional CD8+ T-cell responses (co-expressing IFN-γ, TNF-α, and IL2), and induction of sterile protection to *Plasmodium berghei* in a high percentage of treated mice. Furthermore, it was reported that a prime-boost vaccination with an Ad/poxvirus vaccine that expressed the blood-stage malaria antigen merozoite surface protein-1 can induce not only a cellular response to the antigen but also a very high titer of antibodies, which could be enhanced with a simple complement-based adjuvant [90]. The authors also showed that this approach provided protection against *P. yoelii* in mice and strong antibody-mediated growth inhibitory activity in a standardized *in vitro* assay against blood-stage *P. falciparum*.

In addition, Ad-based vaccines have been developed for leishmania [91].

Ad vaccines for cancer

This topic has been extensively reviewed [92,93]. Ad5 has been the platform of choice for several preclinical approaches for both preventive and therapeutic cancer vaccines. Routinely, an Ad-mediated cancer vaccine consists of an Ad vector overexpressing a tumor-associated antigen (TAA) gene(s), which is delivered directly to the host [94,95]. Ad5-based vector vaccines have been tested in preclinical models against a number of TAAs, including MART-1 [96] and carcinoembryonic antigen [97], as well as against tumor virus antigens [42]. A major problem in the development of a successful cancer vaccine is posed by the biology of the tumor itself. With the exception of virus-caused cancers, tumor-associated antigens are often weak "self"-antigens, and malignant cells often escape and survive the surveillance of the immune system by several mechanisms. Significant improvements were achieved by the addition of immunostimulatory genes to the Ad vectors (such as IL2, IL12, TNF-α, and CD40 ligand) or adjuvants [95]. A potent alternative to *in vivo* application of Ad vectors is the *ex vivo* transduction of autologous dendritic cells to express TAA or immune-stimulatory molecules and subsequent transplantation into the cancer patient [98]. A recent study also showed that Ad immunogenicity can be utilized as a means to increase anti-tumor efficacy in *in vivo* settings, where Ad-specific T cells were anti-tumor-reactive even in the presence of regulatory T cells [99]. As has been discussed for other applications, a combination of Ad-based anti-cancer vaccination with other vaccination strategies will probably be the optimal way to induce therapeutic immune response. In this context, Durantez *et al.* [100] showed that heterologous immunization strategies combining peptides, DNA, and Ad vectors was beneficial not only to avoid inducing just a monospecific immune response, but also to broaden the specificity to several epitopes, thus enhancing the efficacy of subunit cancer vaccines. Furthermore, in order to increase the efficacy of anti-TAA immune responses, Ad-based vaccination approaches should be combined with approaches to inhibit immunosuppressive pathways or to express immunostimulatory cytokines and chemokines.

Conclusions and future directions

Ads have emerged as an important player in the arsenal of vaccine delivery systems. Clearly, solving the immunogenicity of the vector is a major concern. Recent efforts in understanding Ad interaction with the host and the development of new Ad vectors can potentially address this problem. Furthermore, recent preclinical studies indicate that the combination of Ad with other vaccine platforms in heterologous prime-boost regimens has the potential to induce protective immunity to infectious agents.

References

1 Draper SJ, Heeney JL. Viruses as vaccine vectors for infectious diseases and cancer. *Nat Rev Microbiol* 2010;**8**:62–73.

2 Bergelson JM, Cunningham JA, Droguett G, *et al.* Isolation of a common receptor for Coxsackie B viruses and adenoviruses 2 and 5. *Science* 1997;**275**: 1320–23.

3 Roelvink PW, Lizonova A, Lee JG, *et al.* The coxsackievirus-adenovirus receptor protein can function as a cellular attachment protein for adenovirus serotypes from subgroups A, C, D, E, and F. *J Virol* 1998;**72**:7909–15.

4 Gaggar A, Shayakhmetov DM, Lieber A. CD46 is a cellular receptor for group B adenoviruses. *Nat Med* 2003;**9**:1408–12.

5 Segerman A, Atkinson JP, Marttila M, *et al.* Adenovirus type 11 uses CD46 as a cellular receptor. *J Virol* 2003;**77**:9183–91.

6 Sirena D, Lilienfeld B, Eisenhut M, *et al.* The human membrane cofactor CD46 is a receptor for species B adenovirus serotype 3. *J Virol* 2004;**78**:4454–62.

7 Wu E, Trauger SA, Pache L, *et al.* Membrane cofactor protein is a receptor for adenoviruses associated with epidemic keratoconjunctivitis. *J Virol* 2004;**78**: 3897–905.

8 Shenk T. Adenoviridae: the viruses and their replication. In BN Fields, DM Knipe, PM Howley (Eds)

Fields Virology, 4th edn. Lippincott-Raven, Philadelphia, PA, 2001, pp. 2265–300.

9 Wickham TJ, Mathias P, Cheresh DA, Nemerow GR. Integrins alpha v beta 3 and alpha v beta 5 promote adenovirus internalization but not virus attachment. *Cell* 1993;**73**:309–19.

10 Smith T, Idamakanti N, Kylefjord H, *et al.* In vivo hepatic adenoviral gene delivery occurs independently of the coxsackievirus-adenovirus receptor. *Mol Ther* 2002;**5**:770–79.

11 Leissner P, Legrand V, Schlesinger Y, *et al.* Influence of adenoviral fiber mutations on viral encapsidation, infectivity and in vivo tropism. *Gene Ther* 2001;**8**:49–57.

12 Alemany R, Curiel DT. CAR-binding ablation does not change biodistribution and toxicity of adenoviral vectors. *Gene Ther* 2001;**8**:1347–53.

13 Martin K, Brie A, Saulnier P, *et al.* Simultaneous CAR- and alpha V integrin-binding ablation fails to reduce Ad5 liver tropism. *Mol Ther* 2003;**8**:485–94.

14 Kalyuzhniy O, Di Paolo NC, Silvestry M, *et al.* Adenovirus serotype 5 hexon is critical for virus infection of hepatocytes in vivo. *Proc Natl Acad Sci U S A* 2008;**105**:5483–8.

15 Waddington SN, McVey JH, Bhella D, *et al.* Adenovirus serotype 5 hexon mediates liver gene transfer. *Cell* 2008;**132**:397–409.

16 Liniger M, Zuniga A, Naim HY. Use of viral vectors for the development of vaccines. *Expert Rev Vaccines* 2007;**6**:255–66.

17 Zhou D, Ertl HC. Therapeutic potential of adenovirus as a vaccine vector for chronic virus infections. *Expert Opin Biol Ther* 2006;**6**:63–72.

18 Stone D, Lieber A. New serotypes of adenoviral vectors. *Curr Opin Mol Ther* 2006;**8**:423–31.

19 Bangari DS, Mittal SK. Development of nonhuman adenoviruses as vaccine vectors. *Vaccine* 2006;**24**:849–62.

20 Berkner KL, Sharp PA. Expression of dihydrofolate reductase, and of the adjacent EIb region, in an Ad5-dihydrofolate reductase recombinant virus. *Nucleic Acids Res* 1984;**12**:1925–41.

21 Van Doren K, Hanahan D, Gluzman Y. Infection of eucaryotic cells by helper-independent recombinant adenoviruses: early region 1 is not obligatory for integration of viral DNA. *J Virol* 1984;**50**:606–14.

22 Ballay A, Levrero M, Buendia MA, Tiollais P, Perricaudet M. In vitro and in vivo synthesis of the hepatitis B virus surface antigen and of the receptor for polymerized human serum albumin from re-

combinant human adenoviruses. *EMBO J* 1985;**4**:3861–5.

23 Kochanek S, Schiedner G, Volpers C. High-capacity "gutless" adenoviral vectors. *Curr Opin Mol Ther* 2001;**3**:454–63.

24 Xiang Z, Li Y, Cun A, *et al.* Chimpanzee adenovirus antibodies in humans, sub-Saharan Africa. *Emerg Infect Dis* 2006;**12**:1596–9.

25 Roberts DM, Nanda A, Havenga MJ, *et al.* Hexon-chimaeric adenovirus serotype 5 vectors circumvent pre-existing anti-vector immunity. *Nature* 2006;**441**:239–43.

26 McCoy K, Tatsis N, Korioth-Schmitz B, *et al.* Effect of preexisting immunity to adenovirus human serotype 5 antigens on the immune responses of nonhuman primates to vaccine regimens based on human- or chimpanzee-derived adenovirus vectors. *J Virol* 2007;**81**(12):6594–604.

27 Magalhaes I, Sizemore DR, Ahmed RK, *et al.* rBCG induces strong antigen-specific T cell responses in rhesus macaques in a prime-boost setting with an adenovirus 35 tuberculosis vaccine vector. *PLoS One* 2008;**3**:e3790.

28 Ko SY, Cheng C, Kong WP, *et al.* Enhanced induction of intestinal cellular immunity by oral priming with enteric adenovirus 41 vectors. *J Virol* 2009;**83**:748–56.

29 Zhang Q, Su X, Seto D, *et al.* Construction and characterization of a replication-competent human adenovirus type 3-based vector as a live-vaccine candidate and a viral delivery vector. *Vaccine* 2009;**27**:1145–53.

30 Lieber A, He CY, Meuse L, *et al.* The role of Kupffer cell activation and viral gene expression in early liver toxicity after infusion of recombinant adenovirus vectors. *J Virol* 1997;**71**:8798–807.

31 Muruve DA. The innate immune response to adenovirus vectors. *Hum Gene Ther* 2004;**15**:1157–66.

32 Muruve DA, Barnes MJ, Stillman IE, Libermann TA. Adenoviral gene therapy leads to rapid induction of multiple chemokines and acute neutrophil-dependent hepatic injury in vivo. *Hum Gene Ther* 1999;**10**:965–76.

33 Shayakhmetov DM, Li ZY, Ni S, Lieber A. Interference with the IL-1-signaling pathway improves the toxicity profile of systemically applied adenovirus vectors. *J Immunol* 2005;**174**:7310–19.

34 Di Paolo N, Shayakhmetov D. Immune responses to adenoviral vectors. In RW Herzog (Ed.) *Gene Therapy Immunology*. John Wiley & Sons, Hoboken, NJ, 2008, pp. 57–84.

35 Huang X, Yang Y. Innate immune recognition of viruses and viral vectors. *Hum Gene Ther* 2009;**20**: 293–301.

36 Hartman ZC, Appledorn DM, Amalfitano A. Adenovirus vector induced innate immune responses: impact upon efficacy and toxicity in gene therapy and vaccine applications. *Virus Res* 2008;**132**:1–14.

37 Muruve DA, Petrilli V, Zaiss AK, *et al.* The inflammasome recognizes cytosolic microbial and host DNA and triggers an innate immune response. *Nature* 2008;**452**:103–7.

38 Appledorn DM, Patial S, McBride A, *et al.* Adenovirus vector-induced innate inflammatory mediators, MAPK signaling, as well as adaptive immune responses are dependent upon both TLR2 and TLR9 in vivo. *J Immunol* 2008;**181**:2134–44.

39 Zhu J, Huang X, Yang Y. Innate immune response to adenoviral vectors is mediated by both Toll-like receptor-dependent and -independent pathways. *J Virol* 2007;**81**:3170–80.

40 Di Paolo NC, Miao EA, Iwakura Y, *et al.* Virus binding to a plasma membrane receptor triggers interleukin-1alpha-mediated proinflammatory macrophage response in vivo. *Immunity* 2009;**31**:1–17.

41 Rea D, Havenga MJ, van Den Assem M, *et al.* Highly efficient transduction of human monocyte-derived dendritic cells with subgroup B fiber-modified adenovirus vectors enhances transgene-encoded antigen presentation to cytotoxic T cells. *J Immunol* 2001;**166**:5236–44.

42 DiPaolo N, Ni S, Gaggar A, *et al.* Evaluation of adenovirus vectors containing serotype 35 fibers for vaccination. *Mol Ther* 2006;**13**:756–65.

43 Barouch DH, Pau MG, Custers JH, *et al.* Immunogenicity of recombinant adenovirus serotype 35 vaccine in the presence of pre-existing anti-Ad5 immunity. *J Immunol* 2004;**172**:6290–97.

44 Lemckert AA, Sumida SM, Holterman L, *et al.* Immunogenicity of heterologous prime-boost regimens involving recombinant adenovirus serotype 11 (Ad11) and Ad35 vaccine vectors in the presence of anti-ad5 immunity. *J Virol* 2005;**79**:9694–701.

45 Ophorst OJ, Radosevic K, Havenga MJ, *et al.* Immunogenicity and protection of a recombinant human adenovirus serotype 35-based malaria vaccine against *Plasmodium yoelii* in mice. *Infect Immun* 2006;**74**:313–20.

46 Nanda A, Lynch DM, Goudsmit J, *et al.* Immunogenicity of recombinant fiber-chimeric adenovirus serotype 35 vector-based vaccines in mice and rhesus monkeys. *J Virol* 2005;**79**:14161–8.

47 Leen AM, Sili U, Vanin EF, *et al.* Conserved CTL epitopes on the adenovirus hexon protein expand subgroup cross-reactive and subgroup-specific CD8+ T cells. *Blood* 2004;**104**:2432–40.

48 Leen AM, Sili U, Savoldo B, *et al.* Fiber-modified adenoviruses generate subgroup cross-reactive, adenovirus-specific cytotoxic T lymphocytes for therapeutic applications. *Blood* 2004;**103**:1011–19.

49 Perreau M, Kremer EJ. Frequency, proliferation, and activation of human memory T cells induced by a nonhuman adenovirus. *J Virol* 2005;**79**: 14595–605.

50 Schirmbeck R, Reimann J, Kochanek S, Kreppel F. The immunogenicity of adenovirus vectors limits the multispecificity of CD8 T-cell responses to vector-encoded transgenic antigens. *Mol Ther* 2008;**16**: 1609–16.

51 Schiedner G, Morral N, Parks RJ, *et al.* Genomic DNA transfer with a high-capacity adenovirus vector results in improved in vivo gene expression and decreased toxicity. *Nat Genet* 1998;**18**:180–83.

52 Muruve DA, Cotter MJ, Zaiss AK, *et al.* Helper-dependent adenovirus vectors elicit intact innate but attenuated adaptive host immune responses in vivo. *J Virol* 2004;**78**:5966–72.

53 Neutra MR, Kozlowski PA. Mucosal vaccines: the promise and the challenge. *Nat Genet* 2006; **6**:148–58.

54 Kaufman DR, Liu J, Carville A, *et al.* Trafficking of antigen-specific CD8+ T lymphocytes to mucosal surfaces following intramuscular vaccination. *J Immunol* 2008;**181**:4188–98.

55 Li Z, Zhang M, Zhou C, *et al.* Novel vaccination protocol with two live mucosal vectors elicits strong cell-mediated immunity in the vagina and protects against vaginal virus challenge. *J Immunol* 2008;**180**:2504–13.

56 Tatsis N, Lasaro MO, Lin SW, *et al.* Adenovirus vector-induced immune responses in nonhuman primates: responses to prime boost regimens. *J Immunol* 2009;**182**:6587–99.

57 McConnell MJ, Hanna PC, Imperiale MJ. Adenovirus-based prime-boost immunization for rapid vaccination against anthrax. *Mol Ther* 2007;**15**: 203–10.

58 Wille-Reece U, Flynn BJ, Lore K, *et al.* Toll-like receptor agonists influence the magnitude and quality of memory T cell responses after prime-boost immunization in nonhuman primates. *J Exp Med* 2006;**203**:1249–58.

59 Ophorst OJ, Radosevic K, Klap JM, *et al.* Increased immunogenicity of recombinant Ad35-based malaria vaccine through formulation with aluminium phosphate adjuvant. *Vaccine* 2007;**25**:6501–10.

60 Chen Y, Emtage P, Zhu Q, *et al.* Induction of ErbB-2/neu-specific protective and therapeutic antitumor immunity using genetically modified dendritic cells: enhanced efficacy by cotransduction of gene encoding IL-12. *Gene Ther* 2001;**8**:316–23.

61 Hoffmann D, Bayer W, Wildner O. Therapeutic immune response induced by intratumoral expression of the fusogenic membrane protein of vesicular stomatitis virus and cytokines encoded by adenoviral vectors. *Int J Mol Med* 2007;**20**:673–81.

62 Tenbusch M, Kuate S, Tippler B, *et al.* Coexpression of GM-CSF and antigen in DNA prime-adenoviral vector boost immunization enhances polyfunctional CD8+ T cell responses, whereas expression of GM-CSF antigen fusion protein induces autoimmunity. *BMC Immunol* 2008;**9**:13.

63 Bernt KM, Ni S, Tieu AT, Lieber A. Assessment of a combined, adenovirus-mediated oncolytic and immunostimulatory tumor therapy. *Cancer Res* 2005;**65**:4343–52.

64 Chen X, Zhou B, Li M, *et al.* CD4(+)CD25(+) FoxP3(+) regulatory T cells suppress *Mycobacterium tuberculosis* immunity in patients with active disease. *Clin Immunol* 2007;**123**:50–59.

65 Tuve S, Chen BM, Liu Y, *et al.* Combination of tumor site-located CTL-associated antigen-4 blockade and systemic regulatory T-cell depletion induces tumor-destructive immune responses. *Cancer Res* 2007;**67**:5929–39.

66 Di Paolo NC, Tuve S, Ni S, *et al.* Effect of adenovirus-mediated heat shock protein expression and oncolysis in combination with low-dose cyclophosphamide treatment on antitumor immune responses. *Cancer Res* 2006;**66**:960–69.

67 Prell RA, Gearin L, Simmons A, Vanroey M, Jooss K. The anti-tumor efficacy of a GM-CSF-secreting tumor cell vaccine is not inhibited by docetaxel administration. *Cancer Immunol Immunother* 2006;**55**:1285–93.

68 Krause A, Joh JH, Hackett NR, *et al.* Epitopes expressed in different adenovirus capsid proteins induce different levels of epitope-specific immunity. *J Virol* 2006;**80**:5523–30.

69 Worgall S, Krause A, Qiu J, *et al.* Protective immunity to *Pseudomonas aeruginosa* induced with a capsid-modified adenovirus expressing *P. aeruginosa* OprF. *J Virol* 2007;**81**:13801–8.

70 Matthews QL, Yang P, Wu Q, *et al.* Optimization of capsid-incorporated antigens for a novel adenovirus vaccine approach. *Virol J* 2008;**5**:98.

71 Tatsis N, Ertl HC. Adenoviruses as vaccine vectors. *Mol Ther* 2004;**10**:616–29.

72 Priddy FH, Brown D, Kublin J, *et al.* Safety and immunogenicity of a replication-incompetent adenovirus type 5 HIV-1 clade B gag/pol/nef vaccine in healthy adults. *Clin Infect Dis* 2008;**46**:1769–81.

73 Honey K. HIV vaccine trial no longer PAVEs the way. *J Clin Invest* 2008;**118**:2989.

74 Perreau M, Pantaleo G, Kremer EJ. Activation of a dendritic cell-T cell axis by Ad5 immune complexes creates an improved environment for replication of HIV in T cells. *J Exp Med* 2008;**205**:2717–25.

75 Liu J, O'Brien KL, Lynch DM, *et al.* Immune control of an SIV challenge by a T-cell-based vaccine in rhesus monkeys. *Nature* 2009;**457**:87–91.

76 Micklethwaite KP, Clancy L, Sandher U, *et al.* Prophylactic infusion of cytomegalovirus-specific cytotoxic T lymphocytes stimulated with Ad5f35pp65 gene-modified dendritic cells after allogeneic hemopoietic stem cell transplantation. *Blood* 2008;**112**:3974–81.

77 Appaiahgari MB, Saini M, Rauthan M, Jyoti, Vrati S. Immunization with recombinant adenovirus synthesizing the secretory form of Japanese encephalitis virus envelope protein protects adenovirus-exposed mice against lethal encephalitis. *Microbes Infect* 2006;**8**:92–104.

78 Phillpotts RJ, O'Brien L, Appleton RE, Carr S, Bennett A. Intranasal immunisation with defective adenovirus serotype 5 expressing the Venezuelan equine encephalitis virus E2 glycoprotein protects against airborne challenge with virulent virus. *Vaccine* 2005;**23**:1615–23.

79 Thammanichanond D, Moneer S, Yotnda P, *et al.* Fiber-modified recombinant adenoviral constructs encoding hepatitis C virus proteins induce potent HCV-specific T cell response. *Clin Immunol* 2008;**128**:329–39.

80 Richardson JS, Yao MK, Tran KN, *et al.* Enhanced protection against Ebola virus mediated by an improved adenovirus-based vaccine. *PLoS One* 2009;**4**:e5308.

81 Sullivan NJ, Geisbert TW, Geisbert JB, *et al.* Immune protection of nonhuman primates against Ebola virus with single low-dose adenovirus vectors encoding modified GPs. *PLoS Med* 2006;**3**:e177.

82 Gao G, Wang Q, Dai Z, *et al.* Adenovirus-based vaccines generate cytotoxic T lymphocytes to epitopes of

NS1 from dengue virus that are present in all major serotypes. *Hum Gene Ther* 2008;**19**:927–36.

83 Holman DH, Wang D, Raviprakash K, *et al.* Two complex, adenovirus-based vaccines that together induce immune responses to all four dengue virus serotypes. *Clin Vaccine Immunol* 2007;**14**:182–9.

84 Sivan AV, Lee T, Binn LN, Gaydos JC. Adenovirus-associated acute respiratory disease in healthy adolescents and adults: a literature review. *Mil Med* 2007;**172**:1198–1203.

85 Wang H, Tuve S, Erdman DD, Lieber A. Receptor usage of a newly emergent adenovirus type 14. *Virology* 2009;**387**:436–41.

86 Xing Z, Santosuosso M, McCormick S, *et al.* Recent advances in the development of adenovirus- and poxvirus-vectored tuberculosis vaccines. *Curr Gene Ther* 2005;**5**:485–92.

87 Arevalo MT, Xu Q, Paton JC, *et al.* Mucosal vaccination with a multicomponent adenovirus-vectored vaccine protects against *Streptococcus pneumoniae* infection in the lung. *FEMS Immunol Med Microbiol* 2009;**55**:346–51.

88 Li S, Locke E, Bruder J, *et al.* Viral vectors for malaria vaccine development. *Vaccine* 2007;**25**:2567–74.

89 Reyes-Sandoval A, Sridhar S, Berthoud T, *et al.* Single-dose immunogenicity and protective efficacy of simian adenoviral vectors against *Plasmodium berghei. Eur J Immunol* 2008;**38**:732–41.

90 Draper SJ, Moore AC, Goodman AL, *et al.* Effective induction of high-titer antibodies by viral vector vaccines. *Nat Med* 2008;**14**:819–21.

91 Resende DM, Caetano BC, Dutra MS, *et al.* Epitope mapping and protective immunity elicited by adenovirus expressing the *Leishmania* amastigote specific A2 antigen: correlation with IFN-gamma and cytolytic activity by CD8+ T cells. *Vaccine* 2008;**26**:4585–93.

92 Yang ZR, Wang HF, Zhao J, *et al.* Recent developments in the use of adenoviruses and immunotoxins in cancer gene therapy. *Cancer Gene Ther* 2007;**14**:599–615.

93 Parato KA, Senger D, Forsyth PA, Bell JC. Recent progress in the battle between oncolytic viruses and tumours. *Nat Rev Cancer* 2005;**5**:965–76.

94 Park JM, Terabe M, Steel JC, *et al.* Therapy of advanced established murine breast cancer with a recombinant adenoviral ErbB-2/neu vaccine. *Cancer Res* 2008;**68**:1979–87.

95 Aurisicchio L, Peruzzi D, Conforti A, *et al.* Treatment of mammary carcinomas in HER-2 transgenic mice through combination of genetic vaccine and an agonist of Toll-like receptor 9. *Clin Cancer Res* 2009;**15**:1575–84.

96 Butterfield LH, Comin-Anduix B, Vujanovic L, *et al.* Adenovirus MART-1-engineered autologous dendritic cell vaccine for metastatic melanoma. *J Immunother* 2008;**31**:294–309.

97 Peruzzi D, Dharmapuri S, Cirillo A, *et al.* A novel chimpanzee serotype-based adenoviral vector as delivery tool for cancer vaccines. *Vaccine* 2009;**27**:1293–1300.

98 Mossoba ME, Medin JA. Cancer immunotherapy using virally transduced dendritic cells: animal studies and human clinical trials. *Expert Rev Vaccines* 2006;**5**:717–32.

99 Tuve S, Liu Y, Tragoolpua K, *et al.* In situ adenovirus vaccination engages T effector cells against cancer. *Vaccine* 2009;**27**:4225–39.

100 Durantez M, Lopez-Vazquez AB, de Cerio AL, *et al.* Induction of multiepitopic and long-lasting immune responses against tumour antigens by immunization with peptides, DNA and recombinant adenoviruses expressing minigenes. *Scand J Immunol* 2009;**69**:80–89.

CHAPTER 16

Recombinant Avipoxviruses

Michael A. Skinner & Stephen M. Laidlaw

Department of Virology, Imperial College London Faculty of Medicine, London, UK

Introduction

The distinctive, common skin lesions found on mature domesticated poultry drew veterinary pathologists to study fowlpox in the early 20th century. Microscopy revealed the characteristic nature of the lesions and the large virion of the causative agent, making fowlpox virus one of the earliest recognized viruses. It therefore played important roles in the development of modern virologic culture techniques during subsequent decades. The same characteristics meant that fowlpox vaccines were some of the earliest veterinary vaccines introduced (in the 1920s). Since then, fowlpox vaccination has become commonplace and extensive, effectively eradicating the disease from developed countries, at least in temperate climates. In most tropical and subtropical regions where poultry are produced, fowlpox remains enzootic, probably because it is spread mechanically by biting insects. Consequently, vaccination is practiced widely among commercial poultry producers. After Newcastle disease, fowlpox is the second largest virus infection of village or backyard poultry in Africa, with considerable socioeconomic impact.

Avipoxvirus phylogeny

Avian poxviruses (or avipoxviruses) are classified in one genus, the *Avipoxviridae*, of the eight genera that comprise the *Chordopoxvirinae* subfamily,

representing poxviruses of vertebrates. Members of all the other seven genera infect only mammals (poxviruses of reptiles, such as crocodilepox virus, have not yet been assigned to a genus). The only other subfamily of the family *Poxviridae* is the *Entomopoxvirinae*, members of which infect insects.

Avipoxvirus infections have been described in more than 230 species of birds [1] but it is as yet unknown how many different species of virus this represents. The single avipoxvirus genus clearly represents a wide range of genome sequence divergence. An early indicator for this was the difficulty of finding *pan*-genus-specific PCR primers that could be used to investigate the molecular phylogeny of viruses isolated from even a relatively small proportion of those 230 species of birds (Jarmin and Skinner, unpublished). Comparison of sequences from fowlpox and canarypox viruses revealed that they were highly diverged [2], comparable to the divergence between some genera of mammalian poxviruses. The data available, from the handful of loci that have yielded sequence across the genus, indicates [3,4] that the genus consists of three deep branches, or clades (themselves equivalent almost to distinct genera), representing fowlpox-like viruses, canarypox-like viruses (infecting mainly passerines), and psittacinepox viruses (infecting parrots, macaws, and lovebirds) (see Figure 16.1).

The epidemiology, host range, and pathogenesis of avipoxviruses are likely to prove complex;

Vaccinology: Principles and Practice, First Edition. Edited by W. John W. Morrow, Nadeem A. Sheikh, Clint S. Schmidt and D. Huw Davies.
© 2012 Blackwell Publishing Ltd. Published 2012 by Blackwell Publishing Ltd.

(a)   Protein: NJ + Bootstrap (1000)

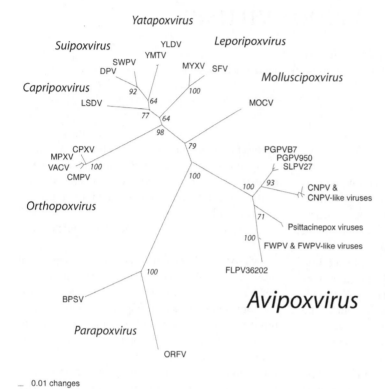

Figure 16.1 Phylogenetic analysis of avipoxvirus P4b orthologs. (a) Unrooted, neighbor-joining phylogram of partial protein sequences for all genera in the subfamily *Chordopoxvirinae*. Bootstrap values (1000 replicates) of >60% are indicated. (b) Neighbor-joining phylogram of DNA sequences from genes encoding avipoxvirus and molluscum contagiosum (MOCV) P4b orthologs, rooted on MOCV. Bootstrap values (1000 replicates) of >80% are shown. Sequences derived as part of this study are indicated by a dot. Avipoxvirus clades A–C and subclades are labeled. Isolates from the same genus of host located in different clades or subclades are as indicated: *, pigeons; +, falcons. SRPVDD1258 and TKPV13401 are not thus marked as it could not be excluded that they were really fowlpox virus (FWPV) [3]. Reproduced from Jarmin *et al.* [4] with permission from Society for General Microbiology.

some types of birds are clearly infected by viruses from the different clades. The picture will only become clearer with more full genome sequences, more species-specific markers, more sampling, and more epidemiologic information to accompany isolates.

Disease control: vaccination and transmission control

Vaccines to control fowlpox infection in poultry were introduced as early as the late 1920s. The derivation and use of these, as well as of vaccines against poxvirus infections of other avian species, was comprehensively described by Beaudette [5] but was reviewed more succinctly,

more recently, and somewhat more accessibly by Hitchner [6].

Commercially available vaccines were often derived from these early vaccines, though some were obtained in the mid-1960s. Unfortunately, commercial confidentiality, coupled with the long history of the vaccines, means that little information on their nature is publicly available. Some were no doubt natural isolates of mild pathogenicity. For instance, pigeonpox virus could be used to vaccinate chickens against fowlpox (in the same way that vaccinia virus could be used to vaccinate humans against the variola virus that causes smallpox). Others were attenuated by passage of field isolates, initially in embryonated eggs, later (as the technology developed) in chicken embryo cell cultures (fibroblast or epithelial, whole embryo, skin, or kidney cells).

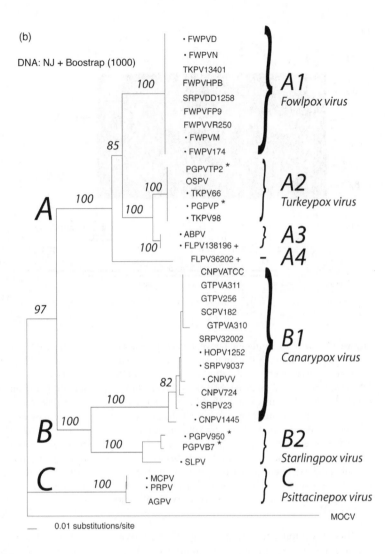

(b)

DNA: NJ + Boostrap (1000)

- FWPVD
- FWPVN
TKPV13401
FWPVHPB   100
SRPVDD1258
FWPVFP9
FWPVVR250
- FWPVM
- FWPV174

A1
Fowlpox virus

PGPVTP2 *
OSPV
- TKPV66   100
- PGPVP *
- TKPV98

A2
Turkeypox virus

- ABPV
- FLPV138196 +   100
FLPV36202 +

A3
A4

CNPVATCC
GTPVA311
GTPV256
SCPV182
GTPVA310
SRPV32002
- HOPV1252
- SRPV9037
- CNPVV   82
CNPV724
- SRPV23
- CNPV1445

B1
Canarypox virus

- PGPV950 *
PGPVB7 *
- SLPV

B2
Starlingpox virus

- MCPV
- PRPV
AGPV

C
Psittacinepox virus

MOCV

A   100   85   100

B   97   100   100   100

C   100

0.01 substitutions/site

Figure 16.1 (*Continued*)

Although some vaccines were labeled as embryo-derived and others as cell-culture-derived, we have little knowledge of the extent of passage of individual vaccines. Generally though, culture-derived vaccines were marketed as milder than embryo-derived. It is clear that some vaccines were capable of inducing considerable residual pathogenicity. For instance, the USDA standard challenge strain of fowlpox virus was "derived from a fowl pox vaccine manufactured by a commercial firm in the early 1960's" [sic]. An ongoing development is the reduction in the range of available commercial vaccines, brought about by the seemingly incessant process of mergers and acquisitions in the veterinary vaccine sector.

Molecular technologies have thus far been able to offer little insight into the origins and nature of the various vaccines. This is because the avipoxvirus genome, though large, is relatively stable so that short-range PCR-based sequencing is generally insufficiently sensitive to discriminate between strains. One study identified an unstable locus that could be used to infer a linked origin for some of the vaccines [7] (Figure 16.2).

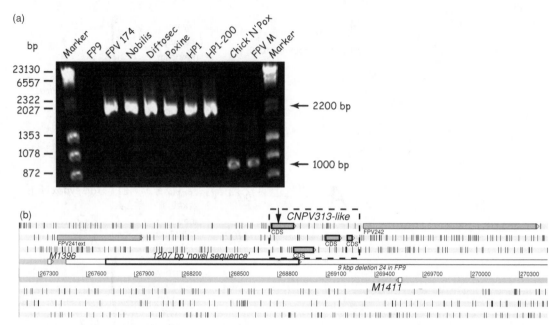

Figure 16.2 (a) Discrimination between vaccine strains of fowlpox virus using PCR at an unstable genomic locus. Products observed were 2.2 kbp (for fowlpox viruses FP9, FPV 174, Nobilis, Diftosec, Poxine, HP1, and HP1-200) and 1 kbp (for Chick'n'Pox and FPV M). No product was seen for FP9. (b) Organization of the H9 locus including 1.2 kbp "novel sequence," shown for HP1 (to scale). Vertical bars represent stop codons in each reading frame (forward above the sequence line; reverse below). ORFs encoding the extended Fpv241 (Fpv241ext) and the N terminus of Fpv242 are shown as shaded boxes, as are four fragments of a canarypox virus (CNPV)313-like ORF (CDS). The binding sites of primers M1396 and M1411 are shown. The bold white box represents the 1207 bp deleted from FPV USDA, FPV M, and Chick'n'Pox, superimposed on a longer white box representing the 9 kbp deletion from FP9. The arrow represents the site of a single-base deletion in Nobilis that would disrupt the upstream CNPV313-like fragment. Sequence coordinates are as for FPV USDA [32], but are adjusted to include the 1207 bp insert. Adapted from a display generated by Artemis [118]. Reproduced from Jarmin *et al.* [7], with permission from Society for General Microbiology.

Further developments will probably have to await the more widespread use of next-generation, high-throughput genome sequencing in the sector, as costs of the technology continue to fall.

Of most relevance to this review is the nature of avipoxviruses used as recombinant vaccine vectors, in particular those used in human clinical trials (as well as those used commercially in other mammals). These will be described in the following section.

Recombinant vector strains

The origins and nature of avipoxvirus strains used as recombinant vaccine vectors are not always thoroughly reported in the literature. The full genome sequence of only one such vector (FP9; see below) is available in the public domain. Some of the strains more extensively used as vectors are described below.

Fowlpox virus vectors

A commercial fowlpox virus vaccine strain called POXVAC-TC (Schering Corporation) was the basis for fowlpox virus recombinants derived by Therion Biologics Corp. [8], including the TRICOM range [9]. Another commercial vaccine strain of fowlpox virus from Ceva (TCP-Blen, Ceva Laboratory, Overland Park, KS) was used as a vector by Tripathy and Schnitzlein [10]. A fowlpox virus strain [11–13] originally obtained from Dr Roland Winterfield (Purdue University, West Lafayette, IN, USA) appears to have been used as a vector by the Nippon Zeon Co.

Fowlpox virus strain FPV-M3, derived from the Australian commercial vaccine FPV-M (Websters), with a detailed restriction enzyme map characterized by Coupar and Boyle [14], has been used as the basis of recombinants for use in poultry and humans (HIV) [15].

The fowlpox virus strain used by the Virogenetics group [16] is a plaque-purified derivative of the "attenuated FPV (FP-1) strain," the origins of which are not further elaborated. This strain formed the basis of the TROVAC range of recombinants marketed by Merial. Fowlpox virus obtained from the Institut Merieux (Lyon, France) was used for making recombinants vFP62 and vFP63 expressing HIV *Env* sequences by Radaelli and De Giuli Morghen [17].

The highly attenuated European fowlpox virus HP1-438 was derived from the pathogenic HP1 strain through 438 passages in chick embryo fibroblasts (CEFs) by Mayr and Malicki [18]. By this stage of passage the virus had lost all residual virulence, even in day-old chicks. It was plaque-purified after two further low-multiplicity passages in CEFs to create strain FP9 [19,20], which has been used extensively to develop recombinants to target diseases of poultry and mammals, including humans. The complete genome sequence of FP9 has been published [21].

In recent years, there has been considerable activity in China in the production of fowlpox virus recombinants for use in the veterinary sector. Two different vector strains are reported. The Harbin group has used a strain called S-FPV-017, described as a less attenuated fowlpox virus strain recommended for use in birds eight weeks of age or older and apparently supplied by T. Yilma (University of California Davis, Davis, CA, USA). This vector has been used to generate recombinant vaccines against avian pathogens such as infectious laryngotracheitis virus [22] and avian influenza virus H5N1 [23]. Groups in Shanghai and Changchun have used strain FPV282E4, an attenuated vaccine produced by the Animal Pharmaceutical Factory

(Nanjing, China). This vector has been used to express HIV gp120 with IL2 [24], chicken anemia VP3 apoptin (as a cancer therapeutic) [25], avian influenza H5 with IL18 [26], FMDV P1/3C (for vaccination of swine) [27,28], porcine reproductive and respiratory syndrome virus GP5/3 with IL18 [29], and the Eimeria chicken parasite rhomboid protein [30].

Canarypox virus vectors

The canarypox virus recombinant vector strain ALVAC, marketed by Merial, was plaque-purified from the live attenuated vaccine strain Kanapox (Rhône-Merieux, Lyon, France) [31]. Canarypox virus obtained from the Institut Merieux (Lyon, France) was used for making recombinants vCP60 and vCP61 expressing HIV *Env* sequences by Radaelli and De Giuli Morghen [17].

Biosafety and environmental safety

Although fowlpox virus causes significant disease in susceptible poultry, it is normally endemic or controlled by vaccination. The disease is not listed as notifiable by the World Organisation for Animal Health (OIE). Because it is unable to cause disease in humans (or other mammals), work on parental virus is generally compatible with the equivalent of biosafety level 1 for human health. Risk assessments based on possible exposure of susceptible poultry should be at a similar level, especially if attenuated strains are used (note that import controls are likely to be in place). Genetically modified viruses will probably require assessment on a case-by-case basis, in line with national guidance, depending on the nature of both the fowlpox virus strain and the genetic insert.

Genome sequences

Complete genome sequences are publicly available for only three avipoxviruses, two fowlpox viruses, and one canarypox virus. The first avipoxvirus genome sequence published [32] was the 288 kbp sequence of a pathogenic fowlpox virus, the standard challenge strain of the US Department of Agriculture (Fowl Pox Challenge Virus; US Department of Agriculture's Animal and Plant Health Inspection Service (APHIS) Veterinary Services Center for Veterinary Biologics, Ames, IA). This is the same strain, developed from a commercial vaccine in the 1960s, as described above. Subsequently we derived the 266 kbp sequence of the highly attenuated, chicken cell culture-adapted, plaque-purified strain FP9 [21].

The 365 kbp sequence of a 1948 pathogenic strain of canarypox virus from New Jersey (Wheatley C93, American Type Culture Collection VR-111, deposited by S. B. Hitchner) has been published [33] but to date there is no publicly available sequence of an attenuated strain, such as ALVAC, for comparative purposes.

Seeing 118 changes (comprising substitutions, deletions, and insertions) between the pathogenic USDA fowlpox challenge strain and attenuated FP9, we therefore partially sequenced the pathogenic European precursor of FP9, HP1, to determine the parental sequence at each of those loci [21]. Analysis showed that 68 of those changes were also present in HP1 and thus represented differences between the geographic lineages. The remaining 50 changes were unique to FP9 and thus represented mutations that occurred during the extensive egg and tissue culture passage history of FP9 and its precursors. These changes, which must together account for the observed attenuation, tended to be more severe (including deletions, insertions, frame-shifts, and nonsense mutations). The specific mechanism(s) of attenuation is (are) not understood though it is interesting that more than a quarter of the genes targeted by these mutations (12 out of 46) represent members of the ankyrin repeat protein family, members of which have been associated with host range restriction in some mammalian poxviruses.

Promoters

Vaccinia virus promoters, whether natural or synthetic and optimized, are functional in the avipox virus-infected cell. It is possible that some avipoxvirus promoters will offer higher levels of expression, particularly in avian cells, but the limited extent of research on avipoxviruses means that there have been no extensive comparative studies of the efficacy of avipoxvirus promoters. As a consequence, most recombinant avipoxviruses carry foreign genes expressed from native (e.g., p7.5, H6) or synthetic vaccinia virus promoters. Some avipoxvirus promoters have been used out of convenience, for instance where they lie upstream of nonessential genes that can serve as useful insertion sites (e.g., FPV030; Laidlaw and Skinner, unpublished).

A particularly useful, compact, bidirectional promoter cassette from fowlpox virus was identified by Kumar and Boyle [34], lying between FPV168 (ortholog of vaccinia virus A4L) and FPV169 (ortholog of vaccina virus A5R). The early/late and late promoters are encompassed within just 42 bp of DNA.

The Therion group has used the (Therion) "C1 promoter" [8], which corresponds to the promoter for the gene FPV090, an ortholog of the vaccinia virus I1L gene (shown to be expressed at intermediate and late times) [35].

Insertion sites

A popular insertion site in vaccinia virus is the thymidine kinase (TK) gene, offering valuable features such as selection for TK$^-$ recombinants carrying inserted gene cassettes and reduced virulence of those recombinants. Although some groups have successfully used the equivalent locus (FPV086, which is relocalized in the avipoxvirus genome compared to the orthopoxvirus genome) in fowlpox virus [10,36,37], others have found that recombinants in fowlpox or pigeonpox viruses with disruptive insertions in this locus are either difficult to isolate or are unstable on passage [38,39]. The different experiences may be due to strain or cell-type differences (some groups use total chick embryo fibroblasts; others use chick embryo skin cells). It is possible that the vectors more adapted to cell culture are more dependent on TK function [40]. Those groups using the FPV282E4 strain commonly use a recombination vector called pUTA2, which also inserts at the TK locus [24,26].

For the FP9 virus, insertions are frequently made in the terminal *Bam*HI fragment of the genome [41], located within the inverted terminal repeat (ITR) region, at unique restriction enzyme sites: *Spe*I (FPV004 and 005), *Nco*I (FPV003), or, most commonly, *Bgl*II (FPV002), in the pEF series of vectors [19,42]. This locus is diploid within the poxvirus genome, offering the benefit of increased expression due to a copy number effect. Although instability of ITRs is a common feature of poxviruses, insertions in this locus in FP9 appear generally stable. This may be due to the extensive passage history of the progenitor of FP9 in tissue culture, leading to a stable vector.

Therion uses an insertion site described as a unique *Bgl*II site in the 7 kbp *Bam*HI-J restriction enzyme fragment [8]. The identity of this site has not yet been documented.

The large gene complement of avipoxviruses means that there are likely to be many nonessential genes that could potentially serve as insertion sites. Indeed, we have isolated fowlpox virus mutants with insertions in about 65 genes, which must therefore be nonessential in culture (Laidlaw and Skinner, unpublished). That is not to say that all would be appropriate as insertion sites. Apart from the issue of insert stability, it is possible that some of the disrupted gene products would, in their native form, have a beneficial effect on induction of immunity to a foreign antigen; these would not be preferred insertion sites. However, others might have a detrimental effect on the induction of immunity; these would therefore represent preferred insertion loci.

It is clear that there is the potential to insert many different antigen expression cassettes in the avipoxvirus genome, offering the ability to generate multivalent expression recombinants, limited only by the availability of promoter sequences, antigen competition, and selection strategies.

Recombination strategies

Recombination is normally allowed to occur between target viral vectors and plasmids, which carry segments of homologous poxviral genomic DNA. The plasmids are transfected into CEFs infected with the vector. The efficiency of transfection of CEFs is relatively low, possibly explaining why strategies that rely on the generation of double crossover events are so inefficient [37]. We now make considerable use of linear DNA recombination substrates, particularly PCR amplicons, for broad-scale strategies. For that reason, we allow recombination to occur in the permanent chicken fibroblast cell line, DF-1 [43], which can be transfected at higher efficiency (but which does not sustain fowlpox virus plaque formation), before applying the recombination products to CEFs for selection, or plaque-screening, and further passage (Laidlaw and Skinner, unpublished).

Boulanger *et al.* [44] inserted into FPV110 (the ortholog of vaccinia virus F11L), and were one of the first groups to use linearized plasmids as recombination substrates for generation of fowlpox virus recombinants. In this case, subsequent removal of the selectable marker by recombination was facilitated by incorporation of direct repeats into the recombination construct.

Bacterial artificial chromosome (BAC) clones of vaccinia virus (including MVA) have been produced, manipulated, and used for recovery of infectious vaccinia virus [45,46]. No such clones have yet been produced for fowlpox virus. They would probably improve the capacity to generate fowlpox virus mutants and recombinants, with a probable increase in speed. Recombination would still be used to generate recombinants but recombination would take place in bacteria, with increased speed and access to novel selection systems. One drawback of using this approach for fowlpox virus in contrast to vaccinia virus is the lack of availability of a suitable rescue virus. Poxvirus genomic DNA is noninfectious. The vaccinia virus BAC clones are rescued by infection of BAC-transfected cells with fowlpox virus. The fowlpox virus can then be eliminated by passage of the rescued virus through mammalian cells, which are nonpermissive for fowlpox virus (BHK-21 cells can even be after the rescue of host-restricted MVA). A fowlpox BAC-clone could be rescued by another fowlpox virus, another avipoxvirus, or a different poxvirus, but a system would need to be developed that would allow elimination of the rescuing virus from the rescued virus.

Recombinant selection and screening

Early recombinants were sometimes selected by plaque hybridization for the presence of the foreign gene or by immunostaining for expression of the foreign protein. These approaches still offer single-step isolation of recombinants and are particularly useful as they do not require the presence of additional selectable markers. However, the low frequency of recombinant generation, coupled with the fact that plaques are not viewed *in situ* in the agarose monolayer, means that these approaches have been superseded by the use of markers for screening or selection, with more complicated procedures for subsequent elimination of marker sequences.

Markers used for screening have included beta-galactosidase (LacZ) [19] and beta-glucuronidase (GUS), though fluorescent markers (such as GFP) now offer attractive options as they allow identification of plaques at an earlier stage. The selection method of choice appears to be use of the *Escherichia coli* xanthine guanine phosphoribosyl transferase (GPT) gene [36], which confers resistance to mycophenolic acid. The use of GPT selection is particularly useful as part of the "transient dominant selection" method [47,48].

Groups using the FPV282E4 strain use a recombination vector called pUTA2 to insert at the TK locus, selecting TK⁻ recombinant viruses using BUdR in chick embryo fibroblasts [24,26]. Isolation of TK⁻ recombinants may be easier with the use of a chicken TK⁻ cell line [49]. No details are given for the cell line (except its source) but it is likely that the line was derived from DU24 cells, which were transformed by retrovirus (MC29 avian leukosis virus; see [50]), making them unsuitable as a vaccine substrate. A TK⁻ quail cell line, QTTK⁻, was derived from QT-35 cells [51], which means that it inherits the same undesirable characteristic, as described below.

Unlike in vaccinia virus, no host range selection methods have yet been devised for avipoxviruses, simply because their host range is restricted to avian cells, and only a few such substrates are readily available. There is potential for development of a plaque size marker following studies on knockout of FPV109, the ortholog of vaccinia virus F12L [11,13].

Propagation of rFWPV

Avipoxviruses are restricted to avian cells for productive replication. They are usually propagated in primary chicken embryo fibroblasts or chicken embryo skin cells. Any strain preference for these substrates is probably attributable to passage history and adaptation. When derived from specific pathogen-free sources, such substrates are suitable for the generation of viruses for clinical trials. There are, however, no finite or permanent cell lines suitable and generally available for such purposes. Fowlpox and canarypox viruses replicate poorly (and do not plaque) in the spontaneously generated chicken fibroblast cell line DF-1. Fowlpox virus can be propagated in transformed quail cell lines such as QT-35 [52], but the presence in these cells of viable endogenous Marek's disease virus (an oncogenic avian herpesvirus) renders them unsuitable for vaccine production [53,54].

The use of avian embryonic stem cell lines (termed EBx cells) for propagation of avipoxviruses was the subject of a 2004 US patent application [55] by a commercial vaccine producer.

Poultry vaccines

Fowlpox virus first came to attention as the obvious candidate recombinant vaccine vector for use in poultry after the development of recombinant technology for vaccinia virus [56]. The genomes of many avian pathogens had been, or were being, sequenced and there was a strong push to exploit the knowledge in practical ways. Early targets were avian influenza virus, Newcastle disease virus, infectious bronchitis virus, Marek's disease virus, and infectious bursal disease virus. In general, more success was obtained with the enveloped viruses, probably because their surface glycoproteins were more readily identified as antigens and more easily expressed in appropriate conformations.

Recombinant fowlpox virus vaccines against Newcastle disease virus (VECTORMUNE FP-ND, Biomune – now Ceva, and TROVAC-NDV, Merial) and avian influenza (TROVAC AI H5, Merial) have been licensed for commercial use. The most successful, indeed the most successful live recombinant vector vaccine in any sector, has been the avian influenza H5 recombinant, with more than 2 billion doses used in Central America against an H5N2 epizootic [57,58]. This same vaccine is part of the APHIS National Veterinary Stockpile, established by Homeland Security Presidential Directive 9 in response to the 9/11 terrorist attack, able to deploy a minimum of 1 million doses anywhere in the continental USA within 24 hours. More recently, recombinants to combat avian influenza H5N1 in poultry have been produced in China, expressing H5 alone or in combination with N1 [23,59,60].

Fowlpox virus vaccine is most effectively and readily applied by wing-web inoculation of young chicks using bifurcated needle inoculators. This is often held as a major disadvantage of recombinant fowlpox virus vaccines. While it is true that distribution would be easier via drinking water or aerosol spray, it is already established practice to vaccinate flocks where endemic fowlpox virus poses a risk, and the use of commercially available, semiautomated inoculators allows higher throughput. The route and throughput of vaccine application becomes a greater disadvantage where fowlpox is not endemic and vaccination is not routine, though application of conventional influenza virus vaccine, for instance, is no less problematic. The routine use of recombinant fowlpox virus vaccines by poultry farmers will always be more cost effective in fowlpox endemic areas, due not only to the cost of application but due to the dual benefit of vaccinating against fowlpox and the "foreign" pathogen.

Mammalian vaccines: background and introduction

It was established in the field that, although fowlpox virus could clearly infect mammalian cells

(causing cytopathic effects at sufficiently high multiplicity of infection), productive infection did not ensue. This no doubt explained, at least in part, why human disease has never been associated with fowlpox infections of poultry, even though there have undoubtedly been countless opportunities for transmission.

It was, nevertheless, seminal work to demonstrate that recombinant fowlpox viruses could not only express foreign antigens in mammalian cells but that they could induce an immune response against the antigen in immunized mammals, a response that could be protective against challenge infection in the case of the rabies [61,62] and measles [63] glycoproteins. At the time, doubts were expressed that the amounts of foreign antigen produced during the abortive poxvirus infection were sufficient to induce a protective response. Instead it was suggested that immunization might be attributed to carry-over of foreign antigen from the permissive avian cells used to propagate the recombinant. We now recognize that even an abortive infection can induce powerful co-stimulatory responses that can induce a relatively strong response despite the low levels of antigen expression within the primarily-infected cells. Indeed, we might even suppose it is just because the infection is abortive that it induces responses out of proportion to the number of cells actually infected. Mismatch between virus immunomodulators and the immune effectors of the nonhomologous host might also contribute to this effect.

The initial observations with fowlpox virus were subsequently reinforced with another avipoxvirus, canarypox virus [64,65], indicating that the phenomenon was a general feature of avipoxviruses and giving rise to the concept of "nonreplicating poxvirus vector vaccines" [66]. The scope of such vaccines was also subsequently extended to include the host-range-restricted and avian cell-adapted vaccinia virus, MVA, which was developed as a vaccine vector following on from the avipoxvirus developments [67,68]. Though MVA shares some features with the avipoxviruses, it lies outside the scope of this chapter and is considered in more detail elsewhere (see Chapter 14).

Little is known specifically of the viral and host factors that limit avipoxvirus replication in mammalian cells, though it is probable that there are multiple hurdles, not all of which may be involved in all cell types and all species [64,69]. Even in Vero cells, which are defective in interferon production, replication is abortive, indicating that tropism is restricted by more than species-specific interferon responses. In interferon-competent cells, however, interferon may play a role; certainly only early fowlpox virus gene expression was observed in HeLa cells [69].

Intriguingly, Vero cells demonstrated fowlpox virus early gene expression, DNA replication, and late gene expression, with the crucial block apparently manifest during early virion morphogenesis [69]. This indicates the involvement of host-specific factors in virion morphogenesis. Similar defects in morphogenesis have been observed for MVA in nonpermissive cells [67,70], which could prove a more tractable model for identifying the responsible virus and host factors.

Patents were filed on the use of avipoxvirus vectors for use as live recombinant vector vaccines in mammals by a commercial company, Virogenetics. Initial reports suggested that canarypox virus vectors induced better humoral responses to the rabies glycoprotein in mammals, so Virogenetics concentrated on the use of its canarypox virus vector (ALVAC™) for the mammalian sectors, leaving its fowlpox virus vector (TROVAC™) for the poultry sector. It has never been demonstrated that this observation applies generally to all antigens nor has it ever been shown to apply to cellular immune responses. Nevertheless, it is generally recognized that, in concentrating on canarypox virus for use in mammals, the company experienced a beneficial intellectual property environment. The boundary may be breaking down, however, as a fowlpox virus H5 recombinant has been trialled in cats by Merial (which licensed the Virogenetics technology and intellectual property) [71] and in pigs [72]. The latter study reported a stronger humoral response in pigs against H5 expressed from NYVAC (an attenuated derivative of vaccinia virus strain Copenhagen made by deliberate deletion of 18 selected genes) [73] or ALVAC than from TROVAC, though curiously these vaccines were adjuvanted (which is not usual practice for the live,

nonreplicating poxvirus vectors). Although data for non-adjuvanted NYVAC and ALVAC are presented, there are none for non-adjuvanted TROVAC.

Especially in the human clinical sector, attempts have often been made to boost the relatively low-level responses to foreign antigens expressed from the live, nonreplicating vector, using prime-boost approaches. Rather than use multiple application of the same poxvirus recombinant, these normally involve application of a second system to deliver the same antigen, focusing the host response on the target antigen. Plasmid DNA vaccines received early attention [74], as did recombinant proteins [75,76], followed by heterologous live, nonreplicating virus vectors [77,78].

Mammalian vaccines: veterinary

As indicated above, licensed, commercial, live, nonreplicating recombinant poxvirus vaccines for the mammalian veterinary sector are dominated by recombinant canarypox viruses, specifically ALVAC recombinants. These include vaccines against equine influenza, equine West Nile virus, rabies, feline leukemia virus, and canine/ferret distemper virus (all marketed by Merial, mainly under the trade names PROTEQ or RECOMBITEK; for review see [79]). More recent developments represent responses to emerging infections of pigs: porcine reproductive and respiratory syndrome virus (PRRSV, an arterivirus), targeted by a recombinant fowlpox virus vaccine [29], and Nipah paramyxovirus (which also represents a zoonotic threat), targeted by an ALVAC recombinant [80]. Foot-and-mouth disease virus (FMDV) recombinant fowlpox viruses have also undergone challenge studies in a guinea pig model and in pigs [27,28].

Preclinical and clinical human vaccine trials

Early targets for human applications of recombinant avipoxviruses were, not surprisingly, HIV-AIDS and cancer. Indeed, a canarypox virus recombinant expressing HIV *Env* sequences is one of the few remaining ongoing HIV vaccine trials (in Thailand), having recently passed a "futility" test [81]. Unfortunately, the lack of immune correlates of protection for HIV-AIDS means that extensive, long-term, clinical trials have to be conducted in "at-risk" populations to demonstrate efficacy. Work on recombinant avipoxvirus vaccines against malaria started somewhat later but progressed much faster, simply because small-scale clinical trials could be conducted to determine efficacy using the chloroquine-sensitive malaria challenge protocol. Early results in small-scale trials in the UK, involving expression of antigens designed to stimulate cellular immunity against liver-stage antigens, were promising [82]. The most successful strategy involved priming with a fowlpox virus recombinant, followed by boosting with an MVA recombinant. Unfortunately, the early promise was not upheld in larger clinical studies in malaria endemic areas, where it became apparent that strong humoral responses were also required to achieve protection [83–89]. However, lessons learnt in the faster progressing field of malaria vaccination may prove useful to the more challenging field of HIV-AIDS vaccination.

A variety of cancers have been targeted using live, nonreplicating recombinant avipoxviruses as candidate therapeutic vaccines, alone or in conjunction with other therapies, especially prostate cancer [90–95], pancreatic cancer [96–98], melanoma [99–101], and colorectal carcinoma [102,103]. Some have been targeted via specific antigens (using, for example, MART-1 or tyrosinase for melanoma), others via common tumor antigens such as carcinoembryonic antigen (CEA) or *Muc*-1.

In general, the approach has not been successful at breaking tolerance and inducing therapeutic immunity against the late-stage cancers targeted in such trials. Approaches to boost such immunity have, however, been trialled, approaches that may have broader utility in vaccination. A fowlpox virus vector called TRICOM [9], expressing a triad of host co-stimulatory molecules (B7.1, ICAM-1, and LFA-3) has been developed and tested in a number of models [93,96,104].

Immune responses induced by avipoxvirus vectors

Many of the agents targeted by recombinant avipoxvirus vaccines have involved the choice of antigens that are known to elicit or require particular types of immune responses. In general, the expected responses have been elicited, though they have often been enhanced by boosting, or by co-expression of cytokines or co-stimulators. There have been relatively few studies to compare the strengths of the different responses to an antigen (or antigens) capable of inducing a full range of responses (this is especially so in birds, with more limited reagents and techniques). Bos *et al.* [105] showed that, in mice, ALVAC induces a mixed Th1/Th2 response against the vector that seems to prevent induction of a CTL response against weak CTL epitopes in CEA but not against the stronger CTL epitope in OVA. The response induced by ALVAC-CEA therefore involved antibody and CD4+ T cells. In clinical trials, ALVAC-CEA expressing B7.1 was shown to induce CEA-specific antibody and T-cells [102] and fowlpox TRICOM virus expressing CEA induced CD8-mediated T-cell responses [104]. Using OVA as a model antigen, Diener *et al.* [106] showed that fowlpox induced low, transient plasmacytoid dendritic cell-mediated type I interferon responses in mice, leading transient CD8 T-cell responses. They suggested these observations might indicate ways that rational modifications could be made to recombinant fowlpox viruses to improve vaccine efficacy.

Enhanced avipoxvirus vectors

Early attempts at improving the efficacy of recombinant avipoxvirus vaccines involved the co-expression of host cytokines. For instance, co-expression of IL6 from a recombinant fowlpox virus enhanced the humoral response to influenza virus HA in a mouse model, while co-expression of IFN-γ suppressed the humoral but not the cellular response in the same model [107]. Although recombinants co-expressing host cytokines have been developed for HIV vaccination, such co-expression has more lately tended to be restricted to cancer immunotherapy. However, porcine IL18 has been co-expressed in fowlpox virus recombinants against PRRSV [29] and FMDV [27], and chicken IL18 has been co-expressed in an avian influenza H5 recombinant fowlpox virus [26].

Kovarik *et al.* found that IL12 could enhance Th1 responses to measles hemagglutinin DNA vaccine but not to ALVAC vaccine expressing the same antigen [108].

The use of recombinants co-expressing host cytokines may be appropriate for use in cancer immunotherapy, where there is strong inherent biological containment of these live, nonreplicating vectors. By that we mean that the nonreplicating virus is unlikely to be shed to a susceptible avian host in which it could replicate. Moreover, even if it did, the therapeutic cytokine (which will be of human origin) is unlikely to have activity in the avian host.

It is, however, more difficult to demonstrate that live recombinant viruses co-expressing homologous host cytokines are appropriate for use in a replication permissive environment, particularly where they will readily come in contact with wild-type field isolates to which the cytokine genes might be transferred by recombination. Under such circumstances, it would be prudent at least to incorporate the cytokine genes into the avipoxvirus genome by inserting into genes where the disruption leads to attenuation. In this way, it is highly improbable that the cytokine gene could be transferred to a wild-type field strain without concomitantly attenuating it. Currently, however, we probably know insufficient about which genes would make appropriate candidates for this to be a viable approach.

Intriguing results have shown that the attenuated strain FP9 is more immunogenic as a recombinant vector background than is a particular commercial vaccine strain (Websters FPV-M). As FP9 is known to have numerous genes deleted or disrupted, this raises the probability that removal of individual genes may induce measurable improvements in the immunogenicity of fowlpox virus. The initial observation was made by Anderson *et al.* [77], using an identical murine malaria anti-

gen expression cassette in single recombinants of FP9 and FPV-M. It was corroborated for multiple recombinants by Cottingham *et al.* [109], who also demonstrated that the observation held for a different (HIV) antigen cassette. The responsible locus(i) has not yet been identified, nor is there currently a publicly available genome sequence for FPV-M to facilitate the comparison.

It is likely that even FP9 retains genes that could be deleted to improve its immunogenicity. In a proof of principle experiment, Eldaghayes [110] showed that deletion from FP9 of a gene encoding a putative IL18 binding protein significantly enhanced cell-mediated protection in chickens against an avian pathogen, infectious bursal disease virus. The enhanced protection, measured by viral load in the bursa, was about half that observed by co-expression of chicken IL18 from the vector. This result is important as it demonstrates an alternative to co-expression of host cytokines – where the virus expresses a binding protein for the cytokine, its deletion is likely to achieve a similar outcome, without the inherent environmental issues.

Clearly, for deletion of virus immunomodulators to enhance immunogenicity of avipoxviruses in a mammalian context, it is a prerequisite that the immunomodulator should be capable of interacting with the mammalian innate immune system, whether by binding a cytokine or by modulating intracellular signaling pathways. Long since diverged from mammalian poxviruses (or rather from the last common ancestral host of avian and mammalian poxviruses), any remaining interactions between avipoxvirus immunomodulators and the mammalian innate immune system must be serendipitous. Discovery of immunomodulators to delete will therefore be somewhat hit-and-miss, unless a more systematic approach is taken. We have established a library of 65 knockout mutants of FP9, each with a lesion in a nonessential gene, which could prove useful in defining immunomodulators with activity in mammalian cells (Laidlaw and Skinner, unpublished). The library could be screened broadscale, using technologies such as expression microarrays, to look for altered host responses. We have already successfully used the library as an approach to identifying genes involved in modulating the avian type I interferon response (Laidlaw and Skinner, unpublished).

Cytokines are not the only host molecules to have been co-expressed from recombinant avipoxviruses in order to enhance their immunogenicity. As described above, the host co-stimulatory molecules B7.1, ICAM-1, and LFA-3 have been expressed together from a fowlpox vector known as TRICOM [9], particularly with the aim of developing therapeutic vaccines against various cancers. The co-stimulatory molecule CD40L has also been co-expressed from recombinant ALVAC in order to stimulate stronger responses to HIV from a *Gag-Pol-Env* construct [111].

A more systematic understanding of the mammalian cellular responses induced by nonreplicating poxviruses should help in design of modifications that will enhance immunogenicity. Early studies demonstrated that FP9 and ALVAC could infect mammalian dendritic cells, inducing their maturation, and that the infected DCs could stimulate an MHC class I restricted response to a foreign antigen [112–115]. For some time afterwards, studies focused on practical attempts at vaccination, measuring outputs of cellular or humoral immunity. Recently, though, attention has returned to changes in host gene expression in potential antigen-presenting cells induced by parental avipoxviruses [106,116,117]. Such studies provide an essential baseline for follow-up with candidates for enhanced vectors. These are likely to be developed following identification and more detailed study of potential avipoxvirus immunomodulators of the innate immune system, particularly of those that modulate the various arms of the type I interferon system.

Acknowledgments

We wish to acknowledge the support of the BBSRC via grants BBS/B/00115/2 and BB/E009956/1.

References

1 Bolte AL, Meurer J, Kaleta EF. Avian host spectrum of avipoxviruses. *Av Path* 1999;**28**:415–32.

2 Amano H, Morikawa S, Shimizu H, *et al*. Identification of the canarypox virus thymidine kinase gene and insertion of foreign genes. *Virology* 1999;**256**:280–90.

3 Luschow D, Hoffmann T, Hafez HM. Differentiation of avian poxvirus strains on the basis of nucleotide sequences of 4b gene fragment. *Avian Dis* 2004;**48**:453–62.

4 Jarmin S, Manvell R, Gough RE, Laidlaw SM, Skinner MA. Avipoxvirus phylogenetics: identification of a PCR length polymorphism that discriminates between the two major clades. *J Gen Virol* 2006;**87**:2191–201.

5 Beaudette FR. Twenty years of progress in immunization against virus diseases of birds. *J Am Vet Med Assoc* 1949;**115**:234–44.

6 Hitchner SB. History of biological control of poultry diseases in the USA. *Avian Dis* 2004;**48**:1–8.

7 Jarmin SA, Manvell R, Gough RE, Laidlaw SM, Skinner MA. Retention of 1.2 kbp of "novel" genomic sequence in two European field isolates and some vaccine strains of fowlpox virus extends open reading frame fpv241. *J Gen Virol* 2006;**87**: 3545–9.

8 Jenkins S, Gritz L, Fedor CH, *et al*. Formation of lentivirus particles by mammalian cells infected with recombinant fowlpox virus. *AIDS Res Hum Retroviruses* 1991;**7**:991–8.

9 Hodge JW, Sabzevari H, Yafal AG, *et al*. A triad of costimulatory molecules synergize to amplify T-cell activation. *Cancer Res* 1999;**59**:5800–807.

10 Tripathy DN, Schnitzlein WM. Expression of avian influenza virus hemagglutinin by recombinant fowlpox virus. *Avian Dis* 1991;**35**:186–91.

11 Calvert JG, Ogawa R, Yanagida N, Nazerian K. Identification and functional analysis of the fowlpox virus homolog of the vaccinia virus p37K major envelope antigen gene. *Virology* 1992;**191**:783–92.

12 Nazerian K, Dhawale S, Payne WS. Structural proteins of two different plaque-size phenotypes of fowlpox virus. *Avian Dis* 1989;**33**:458–65.

13 Ogawa R, Calvert JG, Yanagida N, Nazerian K. Insertional inactivation of a fowlpox virus homologue of the vaccinia virus F12L gene inhibits the release of enveloped virions. *J Gen Virology* 1993;**74**:55–64.

14 Coupar BE, Teo T, Boyle DB. Restriction endonuclease mapping of the fowlpox virus genome. *Virology* 1990;**179**:159–67.

15 Ranasinghe C, Medveczky JC, Woltring D, *et al*. Evaluation of fowlpox-vaccinia virus prime-boost vaccine strategies for high-level mucosal and

systemic immunity against HIV-1. *Vaccine* 2006;**24** (31–2): 5881–95.

16 Taylor J, Weinberg R, Kawaoka Y, Webster RG, Paoletti E. Protective immunity against avian influenza induced by a fowlpox virus recombinant. *Vaccine* 1988;**6**:504–8.

17 Radaelli A, De Giuli Morghen C. Expression of HIV-1 envelope gene by recombinant avipox viruses. *Vaccine* 1994;**12**:1101–9.

18 Mayr A, Malicki K. Attenuierung von virulentem Hühnerpockenvirus in Zellkulturen und Eigenschaften des attenuierten Virus. *Zentralbl Veterinarmed B* 1966;**13**(1):1–13.

19 Boursnell ME, Green PF, Campbell JI, *et al.* Insertion of the fusion gene from Newcastle disease virus into a non-essential region in the terminal repeats of fowlpox virus and demonstration of protective immunity induced by the recombinant. *J Gen Virol* 1990;**71**:621–8.

20 Mockett B, Binns MM, Boursnell MEG, Skinner MA. Comparison of the locations of homologous fowlpox and vaccinia virus genes reveals major genome reorganization. *J Gen Virology* 1992; **73**:2661–8.

21 Laidlaw SM, Skinner MA. Comparison of the genome sequence of FP9, an attenuated, tissue culture-adapted European strain of Fowlpox virus, with those of virulent American and European viruses. *J Gen Virol* 2004;**85**:305–22.

22 Tong GZ, Zhang SJ, Wang L, *et al.* Protection of chickens from infectious laryngotracheitis with a recombinant fowlpox virus expressing glycoprotein B of infectious laryngotracheitis virus. *Avian Pathol* 2001;**30**:143–8.

23 Qiao CL, Yu KZ, Jiang YP, *et al.* Protection of chickens against highly lethal H5N1 and H7N1 avian influenza viruses with a recombinant fowlpox virus co-expressing H5 haemagglutinin and N1 neuraminidase genes. *Avian Pathol* 2003;**32**: 25–32.

24 Jiang W, Jin N, Cui S, *et al.* Construction and characterization of recombinant fowlpox virus coexpressing HIV-1(CN) gp120 and IL-2. *J Virol Methods* 2005;**130**:95–101.

25 Li X, Jin N, Mi Z, *et al.* Antitumor effects of a recombinant fowlpox virus expressing Apoptin in vivo and in vitro. *Int J Cancer* 2006;**119**:2948–57.

26 Mingxiao M, Ningyi J, Zhenguo W, *et al.* Construction and immunogenicity of recombinant fowlpox vaccines coexpressing HA of AIV H5N1 and chicken IL18. *Vaccine* 2006;**24**:4304–11.

27 Ma M, Jin N, Shen G, *et al.* Immune responses of swine inoculated with a recombinant fowlpox virus co-expressing P12A and 3C of FMDV and swine IL-18. *Vet Immunol Immunopathol* 2008;**121**:1–7.

28 Zheng M, Jin N, Zhang H, *et al.* Construction and immunogenicity of a recombinant fowlpox virus containing the capsid and 3C protease coding regions of foot-and-mouth disease virus. *J Virol Methods* 2006;**136**:230–37.

29 Shen G, Jin N, Ma M, *et al.* Immune responses of pigs inoculated with a recombinant fowlpox virus coexpressing GP5/GP3 of porcine reproductive and respiratory syndrome virus and swine IL-18. *Vaccine* 2007;**25**:4193–202.

30 Yang G, Li J, Zhang X, Zhao Q, Liu Q, Gong P. *Eimeria tenella*: construction of a recombinant fowlpox virus expressing rhomboid gene and its protective efficacy against homologous infection. *Exp Parasitol* 2008;**119**:30–36.

31 Cadoz M, Strady A, Meignier B, *et al.* Immunisation with canarypox virus expressing rabies glycoprotein. *Lancet* 1992;**339**:1429–32.

32 Afonso CL, Tulman ER, Lu Z, *et al.* The genome of fowlpox virus. *J Virol* 2000;**74**:3815–31.

33 Tulman ER, Afonso CL, Lu Z, *et al.* The genome of canarypox virus. *J Virol* 2004;**78**:353–66.

34 Kumar S, Boyle DB. A poxvirus bidirectional promoter element with early/late and late functions. *Virology* 1990;**179**:151–8.

35 Assarsson E, Greenbaum JA, Sundstrom M, *et al.* Kinetic analysis of a complete poxvirus transcriptome reveals an immediate-early class of genes. *Proc Natl Acad Sci U S A* 2008;**105**:2140–45.

36 Boyle DB, Coupar BE. Construction of recombinant fowlpox viruses as vectors for poultry vaccines. *Virus Res* 1988;**10**:343–56.

37 Nazerian K, Dhawale S. Structural analysis of unstable intermediate and stable forms of recombinant fowlpox virus. *J Gen Virol* 1991;**72**(Pt 11):2791–5.

38 Letellier C. Role of the TK$^+$ phenotype in the stability of pigeonpox virus recombinant. *Arch Virol* 1993;**131**:431–9.

39 Letellier C, Burny A, Meulemans G. Construction of a pigeonpox virus recombinant: expression of the Newcastle disease virus (NDV) fusion glycoprotein and protection of chickens against NDV challenge. *Arch Virol* 1991;**118**:43–56.

40 Scheiflinger F, Falkner FG, Dorner F. Role of the fowlpox virus thymidine kinase gene for the growth of FPV recombinants in cell culture. *Arch Virol* 1997;**142**:2421–31.

41 Campbell JIA, Binns MM, Tomley FM, Boursnell MEG. Tandem repeated sequences within the terminal region of the fowlpox virus genome. *J Gen Virol* 1989;**70**:145–54.

42 Qingzhong Y, Barrett T, Brown TD, *et al.* Protection against turkey rhinotracheitis pneumovirus (TRTV) induced by a fowlpox virus recombinant expressing the TRTV fusion glycoprotein (F). *Vaccine* 1994;**12**:569–73.

43 Foster DN, Foster LK, inventors; University of Minnesota, assignee. Immortalized cell lines for virus growth. US patent US5672485, 1997.

44 Boulanger D, Baier R, Erfle V, Sutter G. Generation of recombinant fowlpox virus using the non-essential F11L orthologue as insertion site and a rapid transient selection strategy. *J Virol Methods* 2002;**106**:141–51.

45 Domi A, Moss B. Cloning the vaccinia virus genome as a bacterial artificial chromosome in *Escherichia coli* and recovery of infectious virus in mammalian cells. *Proc Natl Acad Sci U S A* 2002;**99**:12415–20.

46 Cottingham MG, Andersen RF, Spencer AJ, *et al.* Recombination-mediated genetic engineering of a bacterial artificial chromosome clone of modified vaccinia virus Ankara (MVA). *PLoS One* 2008; **3**:e1638.

47 Boulanger D, Green P, Smith T, Czerny CP, Skinner MA. The 131-amino-acid repeat region of the essential 39-kilodalton core protein of fowlpox virus FP9, equivalent to vaccinia virus A4L protein, is nonessential and highly immunogenic. *J Virol* 1998;**72**:170–79.

48 Laidlaw SM, Anwar MA, Thomas W, *et al.* Fowlpox virus encodes nonessential homologs of cellular alpha-SNAP, PC-1, and an orphan human homolog of a secreted nematode protein. *J Virol* 1998; **72**:6742–51.

49 Schnitzlein WM, Tripathy DN. Utilization of vaccinia virus promoters by fowlpox virus recombinants. *Anim Biotechnol* 1990;**1**:161–74.

50 Wang H, Morais R. Up-regulation of nuclear genes in response to inhibition of mitochondrial DNA expression in chicken cells. *Biochim Biophys Acta* 1997;**1352**:325–34.

51 Niikura M, Narita T, Mikami T. Establishment and characterization of a thymidine kinase deficient avian fibroblast cell line derived from a Japanese quail cell line, QT35. *J Vet Med Sci* 1991;**53**:439–46.

52 Schnitzlein WM, Ghildyal N, Tripathy DN. Genomic and antigenic characterization of avipoxviruses. *Virus Res* 1988;**10**:65–75.

53 Majerciak V, Valkova A, Szabova D, Geerligs H, Zelnik V. Increased virulence of Marek's disease virus type 1 vaccine strain CV1988 after adaptation to qt35 cells. *Acta Virol* 2001;**45**:101–8.

54 Yamaguchi T, Kaplan SL, Wakenell P, Schat KA. Transactivation of latent Marek's disease herpesvirus genes in QT35, a quail fibroblast cell line, by herpesvirus of turkeys. *J Virol* 2000;**74**:10176–86.

55 Barban V, Aujame L, inventors; Aventis Pasteur, Inc., Swiftwater PA, assignee. Production of ALVAC on avian embryonic stem cells. US patent 2004/0170646A1, 2004.

56 Mackett M, Smith GL, Moss B. General method for production and selection of infectious vaccinia virus recombinants expressing foreign genes. *J Virol* 1984;**49**:857–64.

57 Bublot M, Pritchard N, Cruz JS, *et al.* Efficacy of a fowlpox-vectored avian influenza H5 vaccine against Asian H5N1 highly pathogenic avian influenza virus challenge. *Avian Dis* 2007;**51**:498–500.

58 Bublot M, Pritchard N, Swayne DE, *et al.* Development and use of fowlpox vectored vaccines for avian influenza. *Ann N Y Acad Sci* 2006;**1081**:193–201.

59 Qiao C, Jiang Y, Tian G, *et al.* Recombinant fowlpox virus vector-based vaccine completely protects chickens from H5N1 avian influenza virus. *Antiviral Res* 2009;**81**:234–8.

60 Qiao C, Tian G, Jiang Y, *et al.* Vaccines developed for H5 highly pathogenic avian influenza in China. *Ann N Y Acad Sci* 2006;**1081**:182–92.

61 Taylor J, Paoletti E. Fowlpox virus as a vector in non-avian species. *Vaccine* 1988;**6**:466–8.

62 Taylor J, Weinberg R, Languet B, Desmettre P, Paoletti E. Recombinant fowlpox virus inducing protective immunity in non-avian species. *Vaccine* 1988;**6**:497–503.

63 Wild F, Giraudon P, Spehner D, Drillien R, Lecocq JP. Fowlpox virus recombinant encoding the measles virus fusion protein: protection of mice against fatal measles encephalitis. *Vaccine* 1990; **8**:441–2.

64 Taylor J, Meignier B, Tartaglia J, *et al.* Biological and immunogenic properties of a canarypox-rabies recombinant, ALVAC-RG (vCP65) in non-avian species. *Vaccine* 1995;**13**:539–49.

65 Taylor J, Weinberg R, Tartaglia J, *et al.* Nonreplicating viral vectors as potential vaccines: recombinant canarypox virus expressing measles virus fusion (F) and hemagglutinin (HA) glycoproteins. *Virology* 1992;**187**:321–8.

66 Baxby D, Paoletti E. Potential use of non-replicating vectors as recombinant vaccines. *Vaccine* 1992;**10**:8–9.

67 Sutter G, Moss B. Nonreplicating vaccinia vector efficiently expresses recombinant genes. *Proc Natl Acad Sci U S A* 1992;**89**:10847–51.

68 Moss B, Carroll MW, Wyatt LS, *et al.* Host range restricted, non-replicating vaccinia virus vectors as vaccine candidates. *Adv Exp Med Biol* 1996;**397**:7–13.

69 Somogyi P, Frazier J, Skinner MA. Fowlpox virus host range restriction: gene expression, DNA replication, and morphogenesis in nonpermissive mammalian cells. *Virology* 1993;**197**:439–44.

70 Sancho MC, Schleich S, Griffiths G, Krijnse-Locker J. The block in assembly of modified vaccinia virus Ankara in HeLa cells reveals new insights into vaccinia virus morphogenesis. *J Virol* 2002;**76**:8318–34.

71 Karaca K, Swayne DE, Grosenbaugh D, *et al.* Immunogenicity of fowlpox virus expressing the avian influenza virus H5 gene (TROVAC AIV-H5) in cats. *Clin Diagn Lab Immunol* 2005;**12**:1340–42.

72 Kyriakis CS, De Vleeschauwer A, Barbe F, Bublot M, Van Reeth K. Safety, immunogenicity and efficacy of poxvirus-based vector vaccines expressing the haemagglutinin gene of a highly pathogenic H5N1 avian influenza virus in pigs. *Vaccine* 2009;**27**:2258–64.

73 Tartaglia J, Perkus ME, Taylor J, *et al.* NYVAC: a highly attenuated strain of vaccinia virus. *Virology* 1992;**188**:217–32.

74 Rogers WO, Baird JK, Kumar A, *et al.* Multistage multiantigen heterologous prime boost vaccine for *Plasmodium knowlesi* malaria provides partial protection in rhesus macaques. *Infect Immun* 2001; **69**:5565–72.

75 Kantakamalakul W, Cox J, Kositanont U, *et al.* Cytotoxic T lymphocyte responses to vaccinia virus antigens but not HIV-1 subtype E envelope protein seen in HIV-1 seronegative Thais. *Asian Pac J Allergy Immunol* 2001;**19**:17–22.

76 Kantakamalakul W, De Souza M, Karnasuta C, *et al.* Enhanced sensitivity of detection of cytotoxic T lymphocyte responses to HIV type 1 proteins using an extended in vitro stimulation period for measuring effector function in volunteers enrolled in an ALVAC-HIV phase I/II prime boost vaccine trial in Thailand. *AIDS Res Hum Retroviruses* 2004;**20**:642–4.

77 Anderson RJ, Hannan CM, Gilbert SC, *et al.* Enhanced CD8$^+$ T cell immune responses and protection elicited against *Plasmodium berghei* malaria by prime boost immunization regimens using a novel attenuated fowlpox virus. *J Immunol* 2004; **172**:3094–100.

78 Odin L, Favrot M, Poujol D, *et al.* Canarypox virus expressing wild type p53 for gene therapy in murine tumors mutated in p53. *Cancer Gene Ther* 2001;**8**:87–98.

79 Meeusen EN, Walker J, Peters A, Pastoret PP, Jungersen G. Current status of veterinary vaccines. *Clin Microbiol Rev* 2007;**20**:489–510.

80 Weingartl HM, Berhane Y, Caswell JL, *et al.* Recombinant Nipah virus vaccines protect pigs against challenge. *J Virol* 2006;**80**:7929–38.

81 Plotkin SA. Sang froid in a time of trouble: is a vaccine against HIV possible? *J Int AIDS Soc* 2009;**12**:2.

82 Webster DP, Dunachie S, Vuola JM, *et al.* Enhanced T cell-mediated protection against malaria in human challenges by using the recombinant poxviruses FP9 and modified vaccinia virus Ankara. *Proc Natl Acad Sci U S A* 2005;**102**:4836–41.

83 Bejon P, Kai OK, Mwacharo J, *et al.* Alternating vector immunizations encoding pre-erythrocytic malaria antigens enhance memory responses in a malaria endemic area. *Eur J Immunol* 2006; **36**:2264–72.

84 Bejon P, Mwacharo J, Kai OK, *et al.* Immunogenicity of the candidate malaria vaccines FP9 and modified vaccinia virus Ankara encoding the pre-erythrocytic antigen ME-TRAP in 1–6 year old children in a malaria endemic area. *Vaccine* 2006;**24**:4709–15.

85 Bejon P, Peshu N, Gilbert SC, *et al.* Safety profile of the viral vectors of attenuated fowlpox strain FP9 and modified vaccinia virus Ankara recombinant for either of 2 preerythrocytic malaria antigens, ME-TRAP or the circumsporozoite protein, in children and adults in Kenya. *Clin Infect Dis* 2006;**42**:1102–10.

86 Moore AC, Hill AV. Progress in DNA-based heterologous prime-boost immunization strategies for malaria. *Immunol Rev* 2004;**199**:126–43.

87 Moorthy VS, Imoukhuede EB, Keating S, *et al.* Phase 1 evaluation of 3 highly immunogenic prime-boost regimens, including a 12-month reboosting vaccination, for malaria vaccination in Gambian men. *J Infect Dis* 2004;**189**:2213–19.

88 Vuola JM, Keating S, Webster DP, *et al.* Differential immunogenicity of various heterologous prime-boost vaccine regimens using DNA and viral vectors in healthy volunteers. *J Immunol* 2005;**174**:449–55.

89 Walther M, Thompson FM, Dunachie S, *et al.* Safety, immunogenicity, and efficacy of prime-boost immunization with recombinant poxvirus FP9 and modified vaccinia virus Ankara encoding the full-length

Plasmodium falciparum circumsporozoite protein. *Infect Immun* 2006;**74**:2706–16.

90 Lechleider RJ, Arlen PM, Tsang KY, *et al.* Safety and immunologic response of a viral vaccine to prostate-specific antigen in combination with radiation therapy when metronomic-dose interleukin 2 is used as an adjuvant. *Clin Cancer Res* 2008;**14**:5284–91.

91 Arlen PM, Skarupa L, Pazdur M, *et al.* Clinical safety of a viral vector based prostate cancer vaccine strategy. *J Urol* 2007;**178**:1515–20.

92 Lattouf JB, Arlen PM, Pinto PA, Gulley JL. A phase I feasibility study of an intraprostatic prostate-specific antigen-based vaccine in patients with prostate cancer with local failure after radiation therapy or clinical progression on androgen-deprivation therapy in the absence of local definitive therapy. *Clin Genitourin Cancer* 2006;**5**:89–92.

93 DiPaola RS, Plante M, Kaufman H, *et al.* A phase I trial of pox PSA vaccines (PROSTVAC-VF) with B7-1, ICAM-1, and LFA-3 co-stimulatory molecules (TRICOM) in patients with prostate cancer. *J Transl Med* 2006;**4**:1.

94 Arlen PM, Gulley JL, Parker C, *et al.* A randomized phase II study of concurrent docetaxel plus vaccine versus vaccine alone in metastatic androgen-independent prostate cancer. *Clin Cancer Res* 2006;**12**:1260–69.

95 Kaufman HL, Wang W, Manola J, *et al.* Phase II randomized study of vaccine treatment of advanced prostate cancer (E7897): a trial of the Eastern Cooperative Oncology Group. *J Clin Oncol* 2004; **22**:2122–32.

96 Kaufman HL, Kim-Schulze S, Manson K, *et al.* Poxvirus-based vaccine therapy for patients with advanced pancreatic cancer. *J Transl Med* 2007;**5**:60.

97 Petrulio CA, Kaufman HL. Development of the PANVAC-VF vaccine for pancreatic cancer. *Expert Rev Vaccines* 2006;**5**:9–19.

98 Horig H, Lee DS, Conkright W, *et al.* Phase I clinical trial of a recombinant canarypoxvirus (ALVAC) vaccine expressing human carcinoembryonic antigen and the B7.1 co-stimulatory molecule. *Cancer Immunol Immunother* 2000;**49**:504–14.

99 Lindsey KR, Gritz L, Sherry R, *et al.* Evaluation of prime/boost regimens using recombinant poxvirus/tyrosinase vaccines for the treatment of patients with metastatic melanoma. *Clin Cancer Res* 2006;**12**:2526–37.

100 van Baren N, Bonnet MC, Dreno B, *et al.* Tumoral and immunologic response after vaccination of melanoma patients with an ALVAC virus encoding MAGE antigens recognized by T cells. *J Clin Oncol* 2005;**23**:9008–21.

101 Rosenberg SA, Yang JC, Schwartzentruber DJ, *et al.* Recombinant fowlpox viruses encoding the anchor-modified gp100 melanoma antigen can generate antitumor immune responses in patients with metastatic melanoma. *Clin Cancer Res* 2003; **9**:2973–80.

102 Kaufman HL, Lenz HJ, Marshall J, *et al.* Combination chemotherapy and ALVAC-CEA/B7.1 vaccine in patients with metastatic colorectal cancer. *Clin Cancer Res* 2008;**14**:4843–9.

103 Ullenhag GJ, Frodin JE, Mosolits S, *et al.* Immunization of colorectal carcinoma patients with a recombinant canarypox virus expressing the tumor antigen Ep-CAM/KSA (ALVAC-KSA) and granulocyte macrophage colony-stimulating factor induced a tumor-specific cellular immune response. *Clin Cancer Res* 2003;**9**:2447–56.

104 Gulley JL, Arlen PM, Tsang KY, *et al.* Pilot study of vaccination with recombinant CEA-MUC-1-TRICOM poxviral-based vaccines in patients with metastatic carcinoma. *Clin Cancer Res* 2008; **14**:3060–69.

105 Bos R, van Duikeren S, van Hall T, *et al.* Characterization of antigen-specific immune responses induced by canarypox virus vaccines. *J Immunol* 2007;**179**:6115–22.

106 Diener KR, Lousberg EL, Beukema EL, *et al.* Recombinant fowlpox virus elicits transient cytotoxic T cell responses due to suboptimal innate recognition and recruitment of T cell help. *Vaccine* 2008;**26**:3566–73.

107 Leong KH, Ramsay AJ, Boyle DB, Ramshaw IA. Selective induction of immune responses by cytokines coexpressed in recombinant fowlpox virus. *J Virology* 1994;**68**:8125–30.

108 Kovarik J, Martinez X, Pihlgren M, *et al.* Limitations of in vivo IL-12 supplementation strategies to induce Th1 early life responses to model viral and bacterial vaccine antigens. *Virology* 2000;**268**:122–31.

109 Cottingham MG, van Maurik A, Zago M, *et al.* Different levels of immunogenicity of two strains of fowlpox virus as recombinant vaccine vectors eliciting T-cell responses in heterologous prime-boost vaccination strategies. *Clin Vaccine Immunol* 2006;**13**: 747–57.

110 Eldaghayes I. Use of chicken interleukin-18 as a vaccine adjuvant with a recombinant fowlpox virus fpIBD1, a subunit vaccine giving partial protection against IBDV. PhD thesis, University of Bristol, 2005.

111 Liu J, Yu Q, Stone GW, *et al*. CD40L expressed from the canarypox vector, ALVAC, can boost immunogenicity of HIV-1 canarypox vaccine in mice and enhance the in vitro expansion of viral specific CD8$^+$ T cell memory responses from HIV-1-infected and HIV-1-uninfected individuals. *Vaccine* 2008;**26**:4062–72.

112 Brown M, Davies DH, Skinner MA, *et al*. Antigen gene transfer to cultured human dendritic cells using recombinant avipoxvirus vectors. *Cancer Gene Ther* 1999;**6**:238–45.

113 Brown M, Zhang Y, Dermine S, *et al*. Dendritic cells infected with recombinant fowlpox virus vectors are potent and long-acting stimulators of transgene-specific class I restricted T lymphocyte activity. *Gene Ther* 2000;**7**:1680–89.

114 Ignatius R, Marovich M, Mehlhop E, *et al*. Canarypox virus-induced maturation of dendritic cells is medi-ated by apoptotic cell death and tumor necrosis factor alpha secretion. *J Virol* 2000;**74**:11329–38.

115 Engelmayer J, Larsson M, Lee A, *et al*. Mature dendritic cells infected with canarypox virus elicit strong anti-human immunodeficiency virus CD8$^+$ and CD4$^+$ T-cell responses from chronically infected individuals. *J Virol* 2001;**75**:2142–53.

116 Ryan EJ, Harenberg A, Burdin N. The canarypox-virus vaccine vector ALVAC triggers the release of IFN-gamma by natural killer (NK) cells enhancing Th1 polarization. *Vaccine* 2007;**25**:3380–90.

117 Harenberg A, Guillaume F, Ryan EJ, Burdin N, Spada F. Gene profiling analysis of ALVAC infected human monocyte derived dendritic cells. *Vaccine* 2008;**26**:5004–13.

118 Rutherford K, Parkhill J, Crook J, *et al*. Artemis: sequence visualization and annotation. *Bioinformatics* 2000;**16**:944–5.

CHAPTER 17

Intracellular Facultative Bacterial Vectors for Cancer Immunotherapy

Patrick Guirnalda*, Laurence Wood*, Matthew Seavey, & Yvonne Paterson
Department of Microbiology, University of Pennsylvania, Philadelphia, PA, USA

Patho-biotechnology and the challenge of tumor immunotherapy

The discovery of tumor-associated antigens (TAAs) about three decades ago promoted the development of cancer immunotherapy directed toward them that stimulates the immune system to attack cancer cells. These TAAs are often endogenous antigens, which are either overexpressed or have unregulated expression. As most of these are intracellularly located, it is now believed that tumor regression is highly dependent upon the activities of activated effector cytotoxic T lymphocytes (CTL) directed against TAAs. Thus the latest cancer vaccination strategies are primarily directed toward orchestrating strong anti-tumor-specific T-cell responses and introducing these identified T-cell antigens to the immune system in order to induce immune responses capable of eliminating primary and metastatic cancer. The majority of tumor antigens bear strong homology to self-proteins [1]. In addition, they will have been initially presented to the immune system in the context of tumor cells that are, for the most part, poor antigen-presenting cells (APCs). Such circumstances are likely to induce tolerance to tumor antigens rather than active T-cell responses [1]. The challenge of tumor immunotherapy is to overcome these obstacles; in this chapter we will highlight some advantages that bacterial-based immunotherapeutics may have in "jump-starting" the immune response to poor and/or tolerogenic tumor antigens.

Reliance upon the proinflammatory properties of pathogens in order to overcome tolerance and enhance tumor antigenicity has risen to the forefront of cancer immunotherapy. Pathogen-based immunotherapy for the treatment of cancer finds itself included within the growing field of "patho-biotechnology" [2], which describes the exploitation of the pathogenic characteristics of pathogens for beneficial applications. Of course, the useful application of pathogens for human benefit necessitates their attenuation, mainly through deletion or alteration of their virulence factors.

William Coley was the first investigator to harness bacteria for cancer immunotherapy. A New York City surgeon in the 1880s, he noted tumor regression in cancer patients after they contracted acute bacterial infections [3]. Later, he deliberately injected live bacteria (streptococcus) into a patient with inoperable malignant cancer and ultimately developed a mix of bacterial toxins for use in the early treatment of cancer [3]. Controversies regarding efficacy coupled with support for alternative cancer therapies led to a decline in the use of

*These authors contributed equally to this work.

Vaccinology: Principles and Practice, First Edition. Edited by W. John W. Morrow, Nadeem A. Sheikh, Clint S. Schmidt and D. Huw Davies.
© 2012 Blackwell Publishing Ltd. Published 2012 by Blackwell Publishing Ltd.

Coley's toxins for cancer treatment. The potential use of bacterial products for the treatment of cancer was later resurrected by links to anti-tumor effector immune responses [3].

Attempts to overcome poor antigenicity often associated with tumors have led to the development of a variety of pathogen-based immunotherapies, including viral vectors, such as adenovirus, adeno-associated virus (AAV), vaccinia (see Chapter 14 for a discussion of the development and use of recombinant modified vaccinia virus), avipox, polio, Venezuelan equine encephalitis virus (VEEV), retrovirus, and the bacterial vectors Bacille Calmette-Guérin (BCG), *E. coli*, *Chlamydia*, *Shigella*, *Salmonella*, *L. monocytogenes*, and *Streptococcus*. Microbial strains used for therapy are empirically or rationally attenuated (see Chapter 12 for a discussion of the current state of microbial vaccine attenuation) while retaining their potential adjuvant properties (see Chapter 23 for a review of the history and current use of first- and second-generation adjuvants in immune activation). Moreover, bacterial vaccine strains have the advantage that their infection can be easily treated with antibiotics. Most are also easily and cheaply produced in simple media free from animal products and cells. A select group of bacteria have been developed based on properties inherent in each species. In this chapter we will focus only on the facultative intracellular pathogens, *Listeria*, *Salmonella*, *Shigella*, and BCG.

The biology of intracellular bacterial vectors

Facultative intracellular bacteria are organisms that are free-living but have evolved virulence factors that allow them to infect host animal cells and enable them to survive the microbicidal environment of phagocytic cells. Key to understanding the potential of intracellular bacteria as carriers of passenger antigens to the immune system is knowledge of their cellular localization and mechanisms for inducing immunity. All of the bacteria we will discuss naturally invade the host at mucosal surfaces, usually the gut mucosa in the case of *Listeria*, *Salmonella*, and *Shigella* and the lung mucosa in the case of *Mycobacteria*. Thus, their first encounter with the immune system is most likely to be with phagocytic cells in the Peyer's patches or draining lymph nodes or alveolar macrophages in the case of infection at bronchial surfaces. Bacterial products can signal through Toll-like receptors and induce inflammatory cytokine cascades that drive potent cellular immune responses against pathogens as well as tumors. The burst of innate immunity that precedes the adaptive mucosal immune response must be overcome for a successful infection to take place. In order to survive the microbicidal environment of the phagosome, intracellular bacteria secrete a variety of virulence factors that modify phagolysosomal microbicides such as defensins, reactive oxygen and nitrogen intermediates, and lysosomal enzymes that are active at acid pH. Some mechanisms are common to many intracellular bacteria. Bacterial super-oxide dismutase and catalase, for example, are common virulence factors, which act to neutralize the bactericidal activity of reactive oxygen intermediates. The *Salmonella enterica* serovar Typhimurium *phoP* locus is believed to control the expression of a virulence factor that acts against defensins [4]. The exact mechanisms of many virulence genes are unknown, but there are indeed a large number that testify to the ingenuity of these bacteria in adapting to life inside the cell.

There are other methods that enable intracellular bacteria to survive inside the host cell. Both *M. tuberculosis* [5] and *S. enterica* var. Typhimurium [6] can prevent acidification of the phagosome by inhibition of phagosome-lysosome fusion, thus constructing an innocuous vacuole within which the bacteria can live and replicate. *Mycobacteria* that live and replicate in phagosomes have developed a waxy cell wall that is resistant to lysosomal enzymes and inhibits macrophage activation [7]. *Salmonella* virulence factors encoded in the *phoP* locus induce the formation of spacious vacuoles from phagosomes that allow bacterial persistence and growth in these organelles [8]. Perhaps the most unusual strategy for avoiding destruction in the phagolysosome is that displayed by a small group of intracellular bacteria, including *Listeria* and *Shigella*, which have evolved virulence factors that allow them to escape from this vacuole and live in the less hostile environment of the cell cytoplasm [9,10]. Indeed, the lifestyles of the intracellular bacteria that are currently under investigation as vaccine vectors largely differ by this feature and may be divided into those that persist in a phagosomal compartment and adapt the phagosome for this purpose (*Salmonella* and *Mycobacteria*) and those that escape from this compartment to live in the cytoplasm of the cell, in which they harness the host cell actin to further their passage into neighboring cells (*Listeria* and *Shigella*) (see Figure 17.1).

The uptake of bacteria by macrophages promotes not only changes in the microbicidal properties of the phagolysosomal compartment but also in the antigen-presenting function of these cells to the adaptive arm of the immune system. Bacterial phagocytosis, usually mediated by binding to complement or mannose-binding receptors, stimulates macrophages to secrete a variety of humoral factors. These include chemokines that recruit new cells to the site of infection, inflammatory cytokines that increase vascular permeability, autocrines that

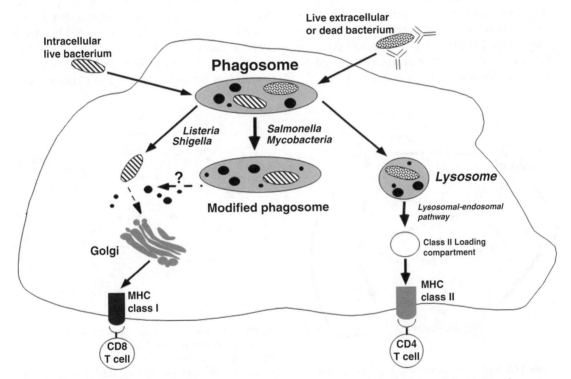

Figure 17.1 Bacterial vector-mediated delivery of recombinant antigens for recognition by T cells. Live and dead bacteria can be phagocytosed by antigen-presenting cells. Dead bacteria remain exclusively in the phagolysosomal vacuole and are targeted to the MHC class II pathway for antigen presentation. Live bacteria are either destroyed within the phagosome or, in the case of *Listeria* and *Shigella*, some may escape into the cytoplasm of the cell. *Salmonella* and *Mycobacteria* can modify this compartment so that they can continue to grow and persist within the vacuole. Fusion of the phagosome with lysosomes directs antigen released by dying bacteria into the endosomal pathway where peptides may be loaded onto MHC class II molecules. In the cytosolic compartment *Listeria* and *Shigella* replicate and any protein they secrete can be processed by proteosomes into peptides, which will be transported to the endoplasmic reticulum (ER) for loading onto MHC class I molecules in the Golgi. *Salmonella* and *Mycobacterial* antigens are also capable of accessing this pathway of antigen presentation but the exact mechanism is still unclear. Modified from Paterson [106] with permission from Wiley-Blackwell.

promote the expression of major histocompatibility complex (MHC) molecules and molecules associated with antigen processing, and lymphokines that act to promote cell-mediated immunity. A key lymphokine in this process is IL12. Macrophages are stimulated by intracellular bacteria to release IL12. This in turn acts on natural killer (NK) cells to release IFN-γ, which further activates macrophages and promotes the destruction of the intracellular bacterium. Indeed, the production of IFN-γ by NK cells, promoted by IL12, has been shown to be a key factor in early host defense mechanisms against *Salmonella, Mycobacteria*, and *Listeria* [11]. In addition to its potent effects on innate immunity, IFN-γ acts to direct the antigen-specific CD4+ T-cell response to the Th1 phenotype required to generate CD8+ T cells and clear bacterial infection via adaptive cell-mediated immunity (see Figure 17.2).

The cytokine-driven activation of macrophages that occurs early in infection will fail to kill those intracellular bacteria such as *L. monocytogenes* and *Shigella* that have retreated into the cytoplasm of the cell. However, the presence of live bacteria in the cytosol facilitates the generation of CD8+ CTL T cells that detect and lyse infected cells displaying antigenic peptides bound to MHC class I molecules. The generation of these peptides takes place in the cytosol of the cell and they are loaded onto MHC class I after transport to the endoplasmic reticulum by specialized chaperone molecules (see Chapter 3 for a review of antigen processing and presentation). Thus bacterial virulence factors that are secreted by these bacteria into the cytosol become a potent source of peptides for the generation of CTL (see Figure 17.3). CD8+ cells are essential for the clearance of listerial infections and CTL have been

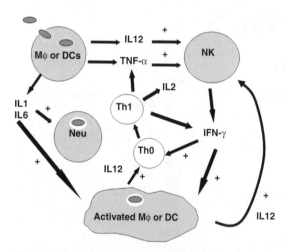

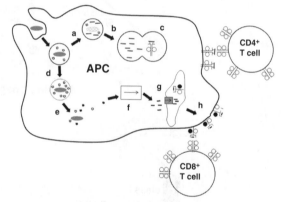

Figure 17.2 Bacterial infection results in strong innate immunity. Bacteria are taken up by phagocytic cells including macrophages (Mφ), dendritic cells (DCs), and neutrophils (Neu). Cell wall and other components activate macrophages to produce IL12 and TNF-α, which activate NK cells, and IL1 and IL6, which activate neutrophils. Activated NK cells produce IFN-γ, which acts on macrophages to upregulate antigen-processing machinery and increase the further production of IL12. This burst of inflammatory innate immunity drives the maturation of Th0 cells to Th1 cells. Adapted from Souders *et al.* [107] with permission from Wiley-Blackwell.

Figure 17.3 Infection with *Listeria monocytogenes* results in cell-mediated immunity. Phagocytosed *L. monocytogenes* that are unable to lyse the phagosomal-lysosomal membrane are degraded (a) and their proteins are broken down into peptides (b) that can be loaded onto MHC class II molecules (c) and presented to CD4+ T cells. Alternatively, if the bacteria succeed in lysing the phagosomal membrane (d), they and their secreted virulence factors are released into the cytoplasm (e). These secreted proteins are cleaved by the proteosome (f) and the resulting peptides are transported into the ER, where they are loaded onto MHC class I molecules (g). The class I MHC molecules are sent to the cell membrane (h), where they present the peptides to CD8+ T cells. Adapted from Souders *et al.* [107] with permission from Wiley-Blackwell.

found that are specific for many of the secreted listerial virulence factors that are required for phagosomal lysis and cell-to-cell spread [12]. The ability of *Listeria* and *Shigella* to target the MHC class I pathway of antigen processing has been a driving force in the exploitation of these bacteria as vaccine vectors [13,14]. Recombinant BCG strains have been constructed that secrete a hemolytic fusion protein containing listeriolysin O (LLO) [15] in an effort to obtain better access to the class I pathway of antigen processing. However, the secretion of LLO did not allow the bacteria to escape from the phagosomal compartment although it did enhance the presentation of co-phagocytosed soluble protein to CD8[+] T cells [15]. To improve the performance of the LLO secreted by BCG, within the context of the acid-modified environment in which it lives, a BCG strain was constructed that could not neutralize the pH in the phagosome. Since LLO is active at acid pH, this superior strain can escape the phagosome and is a more effective immunogen [16].

Bacille Calmette-Guérin

Mycobacteria are usually transmitted through aerosolized droplets via the respiratory tract and typically form granulomas upon lung tissue colonization. The critical resistance to mycobacterial infection is dependent on powerful Th1 cells but there is evidence that CD8[+] T cells may also play a role [17].

BCG is an attenuated mycobacterium of bovine origin that was first developed as a vaccine against *Mycobacterium tuberculosis* by Albert Calmette and Camille Guérin. BCG was found to be an effective vaccine in the prevention of tubercular meningitis in children [18] and is now administered worldwide [19]. However, it is relatively ineffective in preventing pulmonary tuberculosis in adults.

BCG entered the cancer clinic as an unmodified bacterium for the treatment of bladder cancer. After patients have undergone resection of primary bladder surface tumors, targeted administration of BCG to the bladder on a weekly basis can prevent tumor recurrence in almost 60% of patients [20].

The mechanism for this therapeutic effect is believed to be due to the strong immune response triggered by the body's detection of BCG [21]. The proinflammatory cytokines produced during such a response can inhibit tumor growth and new tumor formation. Interestingly, some groups have taken this approach a step further by constructing recombinant BCG (rBCG) vaccines that overexpress proinflammatory cytokines such as IL12, IFN-α-2a, and IFN-α-2b to further increase efficacy [22–24]

More recently, BCG has been used in a more sophisticated fashion to facilitate a specific adaptive immune response against infectious disease. As a vaccine vector, BCG has been engineered to express a wide array of disease-specific genes. Most frequently these strains are utilized as vaccines against other infectious agents such as HIV and hepatitis C virus (HCV) [25–27]. In terms of vaccination against HIV, rBCG vaccines have proven to induce strong adaptive immune responses against HIV-specific antigens that persist over three years post-vaccination [28]. The positive preclinical results for rBCG vaccines against infectious disease paved the way for its application in other diseases such as cancer.

Initial development of rBCG as a cancer vaccine utilized a particular strain that already expressed functional IL2, an important proinflammatory cytokine in the development of effective adaptive immune responses [29]. In addition, the rBCG was engineered to express a tumor-specific antigen known as mucin (MUC1). MUC1 is a heavily glycosylated protein that is aberrantly expressed in a variety of malignancies, including breast cancer [30]. This vaccine, BCG-MUC1-IL2, induced a MUC1-specific adaptive immune response and was capable of providing protection against challenge in a xenografted breast tumor model [29]. In addition, vaccination with BCG-MUC1-IL2 resulted in elevated levels of CD8[+] T cells within the tumor as compared to control vaccine [29]. A recent study has also confirmed the effectiveness of rBCG as a vaccine vector in tumor immunotherapy. In this study, MUC1 was still the target antigen but an rBCG was utilized that secreted GM-CSF instead of IL2 [31]. Similar effectiveness in terms of controlling tumor growth and enhancing CD8 T-cell infiltration into the tumor was again reported after vaccination with this rBCG vaccine [31]. These recent studies along with its current application in the clinic solidify the importance and utility of BCG in tumor immunotherapy.

Shigella flexneri

The intracellular Gram-negative bacterium *Shigella flexneri* is contracted by consumption of contaminated food or contact with infected individuals. *S. flexneri* invades and colonizes the lower intestine. The normal pathology of the infection involves severe gastrointestinal symptoms that frequently lead to death in the developing countries in which it is most commonly found. Due to the urgent need for an *S. flexneri* vaccine, a great deal of effort has been expended in the development of attenuated vaccine strains. While development has been somewhat hampered due to lack of proper experimental models of shigellosis, several promising candidate vaccines are in clinical trials at the moment [32].

As of yet, *S. flexneri* has not been applied as a vector for tumor immunotherapy but numerous studies suggest that it could be effective in this setting. Engineered attenuated vaccine strains have been utilized with success as prophylactic and therapeutic vaccines against numerous other infectious agents, such as HIV and the measles virus [33,34]. Attenuated *S. flexneri* is commonly used in a vaccine setting as a vector for DNA delivery [14,35]. In this context, *S. flexneri* is engineered to deliver plasmid DNA encoding for an antigen to an infected cell. Upon lysis of the bacterium, the plasmid DNA is released into the cytosol and transported to the nucleus, where it is transcribed. Overexpression of the antigen by the host cell along with the inflammatory response to the bacterium then leads to a specific immune response against the antigen. Another avenue of research suggests that *S. flexneri* may be a good vector for delivery of bioactive cytokines [36]. By commandeering the type III secretion system of *S flexneri*, functional IL10 and interleukin-1 receptor antagonist (IL1ra) were efficiently secreted by a recombinant *S. flexneri*. This work opens the door for *S. flexneri* to be utilized as a vaccine vector much like rBCG that can deliver bioactive cytokines along with a tumor antigen to facilitate an anti-tumor response. Collectively, current evidence suggests that while under-studied, *S. flexneri* is a viable vaccine vector for tumor immunotherapy.

Salmonella enterica

Salmonella enterica var. Typhimurium is a facultative anaerobic Gram-negative bacterium that is typically ingested by a human or animal host. Once inside the host *Salmonella* invades the intestinal mucosa and is ultimately captured by phagocytes.

Since the 1970s, the ability of *Salmonella* to elicit strong mucosal immunity has led to extensive research with regard to the development and use of live attenuated strains as vaccine platforms against infectious disease, particularly enteric diseases, for use in a variety of species. In addition to its use as an enteral targeting vehicle for pathogen-derived antigen delivery, *Salmonella* has also shown a propensity for replication within tumors and continues to be investigated for its potential to deliver tumor antigens and induce immune-mediated tumor regression. Subsequently, *Salmonella* has been employed (i) as a tumor-homing bacterium [37–39], (ii) to deliver immune response modulating anti-tumor agents, [40,41], (iii) to deliver DNA vaccines [42–44], and (iv) to deliver protein tumor antigens [45].

The facultative nature of *Salmonella* enables them to colonize small tumors as well as the hypoxic and necrotic portions of large tumors [37]. The earliest bioengineering efforts in developing *Salmonella* as a potential anti-cancer therapeutic focused on attenuating undesirable proinflammatory responses to the wild-type pathogen vector [46,47]. The *msbB⁻* mutant strains of *Salmonella*, in which lipid A biosynthesis was attenuated, still retained the ability to grow *in vivo* [46]. However, a clinical trial using a *purl⁻*, *msbB⁻* strain of *Salmonella* to treat metastatic melanoma showed no clinical responses [39]. Nevertheless, the successful attenuation of *Salmonella* allowed for the development of the bacterium to deliver DNA as well as useful proteins

Table 17.1 *Salmonella*-based anti-tumor vaccine efficacy in *in vivo* animal models of cancer.

Payload	Model/effect	Vaccine type	Vaccine name	Ref.
mAFP	Hepatocellular and colon/prevention	DNA	*S. typhimurium*-mAFP	[48]
HPV-16 L1	C3 cervical tumor/reduction	Protein	GL01/HPV16L1	[49]
gP100	B16 melanoma/reduction	DNA	SL-gp100/li	[50]
gp100/TRP-2	B16 melanoma/growth suppression	DNA	*S. typhimurium*-pUb-M	[41]
CEA	MC38 colon carcinoma/suppression and rejection	DNA	SL7202-CEA	[42]
CD40L/CEA	MC38-CEA-KSA colon adenocarcinoma/growth prevention	DNA	pCD40LT-CEA	[51]
MDR-1	CT-26-MDR-1 colon carcinoma/growth reduction	DNA	mMDR-1	[52]
CCL21	D121 lung carcinoma/protection against growth and metastasis	DNA	RE88-pBud-survivin/CCL21	[43]
CCL21	CT-26 colon and D2F2 breast carcinoma/growth suppression	Protein	*S. typhimurium*-CCL21	[53]
CD105	D2F2 breast/metastatic suppression	DNA	mEndoglin	[54]
FLK-1	B16G3.26 melanoma, D121 lung carcinoma and colon carcinoma/protection and reduced growth of metastases	DNA	pcDNA3.1-Flk-1	[55]
NY-ESO-1	CMS5a/regression	Protein	*S. typhimurium*-NY-ESO-1	[44]
PSA	P815 PSA clone 18/protection	Protein	*SL7207/pMKhly*-CtxB-PSA	[56]

directly to the tumor with reduced deleterious side effects to the patient.

Attenuated *Salmonella*-based vaccines that can be administered orally have received a considerable amount of attention during the past 10 years as DNA vaccines (see Table 17.1). *Salmonella* has also been used to express proteins designed to stimulate anti-tumor immune responses via bacterial processing and presentation to the immune system (Table 17.1). *Salmonella*-based vaccine efficacy has been shown in a variety of cancer models, including melanoma [57], prostate cancer [56,58], renal carcinoma [59], and breast cancer [60]. Efforts continue to refine *Salmonella* colonization of

tumors [57] and are focused on enhancing the ability of *Salmonella* to selectively colonize viable areas of tumors. One current strategy involves optimizing *Salmonella* targeting to live tumor cells rather than necrotic areas of tumors [38]. *Salmonella* has been shown to infiltrate and colonize the tumor microenvironment in response to chemical stimuli and nutrient release from dying tumor cells [38]. Tumor infiltration and accumulation of *Salmonella* depend upon both chemotaxis and preferential proliferation mechanisms [38]. Tumor-infiltrating, nonpathogenic *S. Enterica* var. Typhimurium have also been shown to inhibit tumor growth and increase survival time in mice [37,47]. *In vitro* tumor model systems show that *Salmonella* movement and redistribution to necrotic areas of tumors are based on the activities of a number of chemoreceptors [38]. This same study used *Salmonella* that lacked the ribose/galactose receptor and observed bacterial accumulation in areas of quiescence rather than necrosis with greater apoptotic induction. The natural propensity of the bacterium to home to and infiltrate otherwise inaccessible areas of tumors has led researchers to adapt *Salmonella* for possible drug delivery.

Research continues to hone the targeting capability of *Salmonella*, while other groups are focused on equipping invasive, attenuated *Salmonella* for tumor killing. Recent examples of the use of tumor-targeting bacteria include the development and use of bioengineered recombinant strains of *Salmonella* that produce human cytokines capable of inhibiting tumor growth by facilitating tumor-infiltrating lymphocyte (TIL) entry [39,40].

Salmonella have also been used extensively to deliver a variety of DNA vaccines encoding tumor antigens as well as the proteins themselves (Table 17.1). Indeed, *Salmonella*-based vaccine strategies, like other bacterial-based vaccines, are heavily reliant upon the elevated expression of certain tumor-associated antigens (Table 17.1).

Similar results in alternative bacterial adjuvant-antigen fusion constructs have been observed in other bacterial vector strategies, notably *Listeria monocytogenes*. A major advantage in using *Salmonella* is its ability to deliver genes and protein antigens orally [61]. As efforts continue to refine current vaccines and develop new targets, *Salmonella* vaccines that deliver protein antigens using their type III secretion system are about to enter clinical trials [62].

Listeria monocytogenes

Listeria monocytogenes is a facultative, intracellular, food-borne, Gram-positive rod that is resistant to adverse environmental conditions and capable of avoiding innate and humoral immune responses during the intracellular stages of its infectious cycle. *Listeria* initially bind to host cells via proteins, including internalins, and are phagocytosed. Once inside the phagosome, *Listeria* releases LLO and phospholipase C (PLC), degrading the phagolysosome. *Listeria* are then released into the cytoplasm, where they multiply and become motile via the expression of ActA, a bacterial protein that enables actin mobilization. Motile bacteria then protrude out of the host cell and are subsequently phagocytosed by additional phagocytes, after which they repeat the process (see Figure 17.4 for details). The intracellular localization of the bacterium necessitates cellular immune responses with a vital role for cytotoxic T cells for clearance of infection. *Listeria* can cause serious disease (listeriosis) in immune-compromised people. The bacterium is a well-studied model organism within the context of CD8+ T cell responses. *Listeria* has also received a great deal of attention as a potential anti-cancer vaccine therapeutic.

For nearly two decades, *Listeria* has been viewed as an otherwise pathogenic organism that possesses potential therapeutic value as a vaccine vector. The intracellular lifestyle of *Listeria* ultimately leads to the activation of both CD4+ and CD8+ T-cell mediated adaptive immune responses as well as innate, proinflammatory cytokine responses (see Figures 17.1–17.3). The first attempt to use *Listeria* as a vector to target antigens to the immune system was published by our laboratory in 1992 [63]. Although this paper demonstrated that a CD8+ T-cell response to a passenger antigen could be induced by *Listeria*, its utility in cancer was not established until 1995, when the first demonstration occurred that *Listeria* expressing and secreting a tumor-specific antigen could control tumor growth through a CD8+ T cell mechanism [64]. Importantly, this was the first paper to show that an induced immune response against a tumor-associated antigen could eliminate established tumors without other adjunctive therapy. This groundbreaking experiment is shown in Figure 17.5. Since then, a number of investigators have used *Listeria* to target several different cancers [65,66]. Here we will describe more recent studies focused on overcoming a variety of physiological barriers against efficacious immunotherapeutic treatments of cancer. Specifically, protein products produced and secreted by

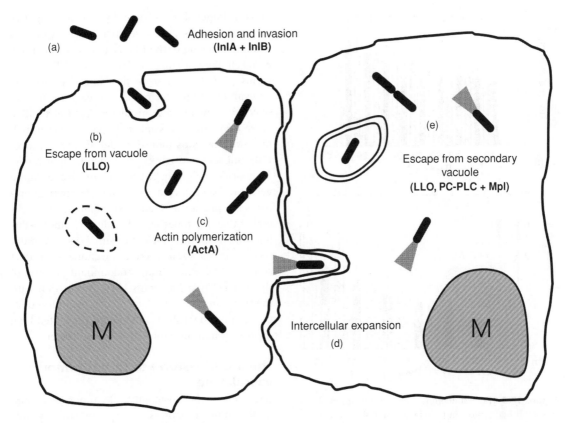

Figure 17.4 How *Listeria monocytogenes* invades host cells. The major steps in cellular infection by *L. monocytogenes* are: (a) adhesion and invasion, mediated by phagocytosis by phagocytic cells or through interaction of InlA or InlB; with cadherins on epithelial cells or hepatocytes; (b) escape from the phagosomal vacuole, mediated by LLO; (c) motility within the host cell cytosol, mediated by ActA, which nucleates actin at one pole of the bacterium; (d) cell-to-cell spread; and (e) escape from the secondary vacuole, which requires LLO, PC-PLC, and metalloprotease. Reproduced from Seavey *et al.* [65] with permission from CRC Press.

the bacterium, such as LLO and ActA, have been fused to tumor antigens in order to increase the antigenicity of otherwise poorly immunogenic tumor antigens [67] in animal models of cervical and thyroid cancer.

The primary cellular targets for *Listeria* are phagocytic cells; however, *Listeria* can also infect epithelial cells and some reports suggest that *Listeria* can also infect tumor cells directly [68,69]. The ability of *Listeria* to infect phagocytic cells, including APCs such as macrophages and dendritic cells (DCs), is of particular interest since *Listeria* engineered to express TAAs could prime or re-activate tumor-specific T cells that are capable of killing tumors. After phagocytosis by an APC, *Listeria* escapes the phagosome via the hemolytic virulence factor LLO and enters the cytoplasm. In our laboratory, we engineered *Listeria* to express our genes of interest under the LLO (*hly*) promoter. In addition to delivering our antigen in a bacterial vector that will drive strong inflammatory responses, we fuse our gene of interest to LLO. In general, tumors are poorly immunogenic; however, studies in our laboratory and others have shown that *Listeria* is a particularly good vector for TAA immunization [64,67,70–73]. A complete list of the antigens targeted by *Listeria* is shown in Table 17.2.

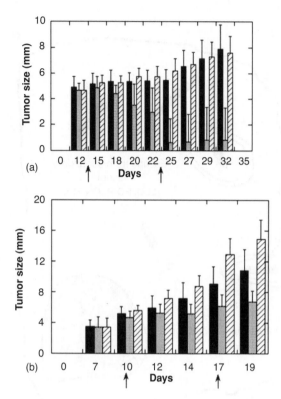

Figure 17.5 The first demonstration of the elimination of established tumors in mice by a *Listeria*-based immunotherapy. The tumor cell lines Renca (a renal carcinoma) and CT26 (a colorectal carcinoma), which had been transduced with influenza nucleoprotein (NP), were established in syngeneic mice. 5×10^5 tumor cells of either Renca-NP (a) or CT26-NP (b) were introduced subcutaneously to two groups of 30 mice. After measurable tumors had grown in the mice, in each group, 10 mice received a *Listeria monocytogenes* (Lm) recombinant that expressed and secreted NP fused to a truncated from of LLO, Lm-NP (darkly shaded bars), 10 mice received wild-type Listeria (lightly shaded bars), and 10 received saline (solid bars). The mice received immunizations on the days indicated by the arrows. Reproduced from Pan *et al.* [64] with permission from *Nature*.

Listeria-based immunotherapy for breast cancer

About 15–40% of all breast carcinomas overexpress the epidermal-like growth factor Her-2/neu. Thus, this protein can act as a TAA and as a target for immunotherapy [65,70,81,89–91]. Our laboratory initially targeted Her-2/neu by constructing five different *Listeria*-based constructs, each expressing a different region of the Her-2/neu molecule, three extracellular domains, and two intracellular domains [70]. Since *Listeria* has difficulty secreting large and hydrophobic molecules, each region was selected to avoid these problems. Each of the five *Listeria* constructs was able to impact tumor growth in a subcutaneous mouse model for breast cancer [70] and slow growth in an autochthonous model for breast cancer [89]. The use of *Listeria* as a shuttle vector revealed several immuno-subdominant epitopes not previously identified [70,90,91] and several of these epitopes would undergo immunoediting under immunologic pressure [89]. A more recent *Listeria* strain secreted a chimeric product composed of three immunodominant regions of three Her-2/neu fragments [81]. Vaccination with the Her-2/neu chimeric *Listeria* vaccine induced regression of established tumors and prevented lung metastasis in mouse models of breast cancer.

The use of *Listeria* to target tumor vasculature

Because of the instability of tumor cells and tumor antigen expression, a new strategy was undertaken to target the vasculature, which may be less susceptible to genetic mutation. The inhibition of tumor growth by attacking the tumor's vascular network was first pioneered by Folkman and colleagues [92]. Blood vessels in general are composed of two different cell types, the endothelial cells that interact directly with the blood stream, and the pericytes, a cell type responsible for orchestrating angiogenesis. Both cell types are crucial to vascular function. With this in mind, two different types of vaccines were constructed; one that would target the pericytes [85] and another that would target the endothelial cells [82].

One of the most important molecules in the formation of new blood vessels is the vascular endothelial growth factor receptor 2 (VEGFR2) or in the mouse, fetal liver kinase 1 (Flk-1). When tumors cells begin to grow and divide they can extract the necessary nutrients from the interstitial fluid via passive diffusion. However, once the tumor has reached a critical mass, 2–3 mm in diameter,

Table 17.2 Live *Listeria*-based anti-tumor vaccine efficacy in *in vivo* animal models of cancer.

Antigen	Cancer model	Vaccine type	Vaccine name	Strain	Ref.
E7, HPV-16	Cervical	Protein	Lm-LLO-E7	*prfA-*	[67]
		Protein	Lm-E7	Wild type	[67]
		Protein	Lm-PEST-E7	*prfA-*	[76]
		Protein	Lm-ActA-E7	*prfA-*	[75]
		Protein	rLm-E7	Wild type	[77]
		DNA	Lm-v1/Lm-v2 DNA vaccines	*dal-, dat-*	[78]
		Protein	Lm-dd-LO-E7	dal-, dat-	[79]
L1	Cervical	Protein	Lm-LLO-L1(1-258)	*prfA-*	[80]
		Protein	Lm-LLO-L1(238-474)	*prfA-*	[80]
E1, CRPV	Papilloma	Protein	E1-rLM	Wild type	[74]
Her2/neu	Breast	Protein	Lm-LLO-EC1	*prfA-*	[70]
		Protein	Lm-LLO-EC2	*prfA-*	[70]
		Protein	Lm-LLO-EC3	*prfA-*	[70]
		Protein	Lm-LLO-IC1	*prfA-*	[70]
		Protein	Lm-LLO-IC2	*prfA-*	[70]
		Protein	Lm-hHer-2/neu chimera	*prfA-*	[81]
Flk-1 (VEGFR2)	Breast	Protein	Lm-LLO-Flk- E1	*prfA-*	[82]
		Protein	Lm-LLO-Flk- E2	*prfA-*	[82]
		Protein	Lm-LLO-Flk- I1	*prfA-*	[82]
MAGE-b3	Breast	Protein	LM-LLO-Mage-b311-660	*prfA-*	[84]
TRP-2	Melanoma	Protein	Lm-TRP2	Wild type	[83]
HMWMAA		Protein	Lm-LLO-HMW-MAA-C	*prfA-*	[85]
GP70, AH1 epitope	Colon	Protein	actA-inlb-Ah1-A5	actA-, inlb-	[86]
PSA	Prostate	Protein	Lm-LLO-PSA	*prfA-*	[71]
		Protein	Lm-dal dat actA 142	*dal-, dat-, actA-*	[87]
Influenza nucleoprotein (NP)	Colon, renal	Protein	Lm-NP	Wild type	[72]
NP, LCMV	CNS	Protein	rLm-NP	Wild type	[73]
E. coli beta-galactosidase	Fibrosarcoma	Protein	Dmpl2GK20	*Delta mpl2*	[88]

a process known as "angiogenic switch" must occur, which requires the formation of new blood vessels. Flk-1 is strongly indicated as a therapeutic target [55,93], and has important roles in tumor growth, invasion, and metastasis [94].

Immunotherapeutic strategies that harness bacteria as a delivery mechanism for pro-angiogenic factors were first suggested by Reisfeld's group, who used DNA vaccines delivered orally by *Salmonella typhimurium* [55]. To construct *Listeria* vectors, we selected three polypeptide fragments of the VEGFR2 molecule and fused each to the microbial adjuvant LLO [82]. The Flk-1-expressing *Listeria* vaccines were able to cause tumor regression, Her-2/neu epitope spreading, reduce tumor microvascular density (MVD), and prevent the long-term growth of spontaneous tumors, all without significantly affecting normal tissue angiogenesis. In addition, tumors that escaped immune surveillance had acquired mutations in key regions of the Her-2/neu molecule responsible for both its recognition and targeting by anti-tumor CTLs [95]. The epitope-spreading phenomenon is further explained in Figure 17.6. Thus, targeting endothelial cells through Flk-1 could induce epitope spreading to an endogenous tumor protein and lead to tumor death. Destroying only endothelial cells has limitations, however, since tumors can survive with limited numbers of endothelial cells. However, tumor vasculature is critically dependent on other cells, called mural pericytes. Pericytes act as support cells for capillaries and support the normal function and integrity of vasculature. Pericyte loss is associated with loss of vessel integrity, leading

to eventual tissue starvation and hypoxia. Pericyte coverage of tumor vasculature is sparse, thus a further reduction in the numbers of these important cells could lead to the malfunctioning of mature blood vessels as the tumor grows in size.

As a blood vessel grows, pericytes arise from the vascular smooth muscles cells (vSMC). Pericytes express a specialized glycoprotein, high molecular weight melanoma-associated antigen (HMW-MAA), which interacts intimately with the extracellular matrix (ECM) and is responsible for binding vascular endothelial growth factor A (VEGF-A), matrix metalloproteinase (MMPs), and basic fibroblast growth factor (bFGF). Originally identified on melanoma, human HMW-MAA is a cell-surface, highly glycosylated, proteoglycan that is overexpressed on over 90% of benign nevi and melanoma lesions [96]. HMW-MAA is also known

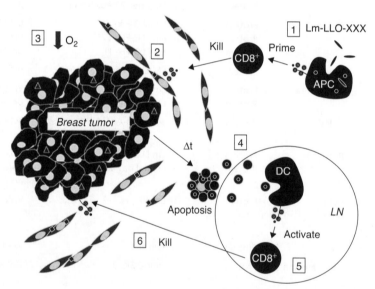

Figure 17.6 Targeting the vasculature using *Listeria*-based vaccines can overcome tolerance to an endogenous tumor protein and drive epitope-spreading to cryptic tumor epitopes. 1, An anti-angiogenesis *Lm* vaccine primes autoreactive CD8+ T cells to kill vascular cells expressing the cloned target ("XXX" may represent HMW-MAA or VEGFR2); 2, elicited CTLs attack and destroy the tumor vasculature; 3, destruction of key cells involved in maintaining the integrity of the tumor vasculature leads to increased tumor hypoxia and apoptosis; 4, apoptotic tumor cells are phagocytosed by resident DCs in the drain lymph nodes (LN) and

cross-present tumor proteins to naive CD8+ T cells; 5, due to the inflammatory milieu *Lm* induces, newly primed anti-tumor CTLs are generated and migrate back to the inflamed tumor site; 6, killing the tumor cells. Note this model requires that both targets express the appropriate antigen-expressing molecules, MHC I. Downregulation of MHC I may increase NK cell activity but immunosuppressive molecules and anti-NK proteins secreted by the tumor cells, like HLA-G, may prevent both mechanisms. However, the initial response against the vasculature should not be as easily mitigated.

as NG2 in the rat and AN2 in the mouse. Three different regions of the HMW-MAA molecule were cloned into *Listeria* fused to the truncated LLO molecule. Only one out of the three cloned molecules showed any efficacy, *Listeria*-LLO-HMW-MAA-C vaccine was able to slow the growth of transplanted B16F10 mouse melanoma cells in a subcutaneous model and eradicate primary breast tumors and lung metastases in a mouse model for breast cancer [85]. In addition, the vaccine induced a significant reduction in tumor volume, MVD, and pericyte coverage, which correlated with an increase in CD8+ cell infiltration into the tumor microenvironment. This vaccine failed to make a significant impact on pregnancy and wound healing in mice [85], indicating that it had few adverse effects.

Listeria as a vector for cDNA and mRNA delivery

Listeria monocytogenes has also been employed to deliver antigen-encoding cDNA by bactofection. Bactofection is a term used to describe the delivery of eukaryotic expression systems to mammalian cells by utilizing bacteria as a vector [97]. Bactofection is a relatively new technology that takes advantage of the ability of certain bacteria to be engulfed selectively by APCs. Once taken up by an APC, the bacterium lyses and delivers its tumor antigen-encoding cDNA to the cytosol. The delivered cDNA is then transcribed and the antigen expressed and presented to the immune system by the APC. The advantage of using intracellular bacteria to deliver cDNA in anti-tumor immune therapy, therefore, comes from selective delivery of cDNA to APCs for efficient processing of tumor antigens and effective co-stimulatory molecule production in response to the *Listeria* infection.

Bactofection by *Listeria monocytogenes* was initially developed by Goebel's group, utilizing an attenuated *Listeria* strain that expressed a suicide cassette upon entering the cytosol of an infected host cell [97,98]. The suicide cassette consists of a phage lysin under the regulation of the cytosol-specific *actA* promoter. Once *Listeria* escapes the confines of the phagosome and enters the cytosol, expression of the phage lysin under the control of the *actA* promoter leads to the death of the bacterium

and release of the cDNA plasmid to the cytosol. The cytosolic cDNA plasmid is then transferred to the nucleus instead of being degraded within the phagolysosome. Earlier bactofection vectors without a suicide cassette were still able to deliver cDNA that resulted in gene expression but with much lower efficiency. While initial optimization studies only involved the delivery of cDNA encoding for a reporter gene, eGFP, the *Listeria* bactofected cells were able to efficiently express and present the antigen, as evidenced by their ability to stimulate eGFP-specific CD8 T cells.

While bactofection of plasmid DNA by *Listeria monocytogenes* demonstrated effectiveness for *in vitro* CD8 T-cell stimulation, the results are less impressive in terms of *in vivo* effectiveness in a cervical cancer model [78]. In a direct comparison of *Listeria monocytogenes* strains that endogenously expressed and secreted the HPV-16 tumor antigen [67] with DNA delivery strains, the latter proved a great deal less effective in stimulating anti-tumor immune responses *in vivo* [78]. The decreased effectiveness of *Listeria*-delivered plasmid DNA vaccines was hypothesized to be due to the relatively late expression of the tumor antigen, because of the need for transcription and translation. In an effort to expedite the expression of the tumor antigen, delivery of translation-competent mRNA encoding for model tumor antigens by *Listeria* strains was pursued [99]. Much like the plasmid DNA delivery system, the mRNA strains contained a suicide cassette that would initiate the destruction of the *Listeria* vector upon entry of the bacterium into the cytosol. However, instead of releasing plasmid DNA upon lysis, the mRNA strains released T7 polymerase transcribed mRNA that contained an internal ribosome entry site (IRES) element rendering it translation-competent in the eukaryotic host cell. This allowed for earlier expression of the tumor antigen to coincide with the infection and, ultimately, this augmented *in vivo* anti-tumor immune responses in direct comparison to a plasmid DNA delivery strain. While the mRNA delivery system was more effective than the plasmid DNA delivery strain, it was still not as effective as the *Listeria* strains that endogenously expressed and secreted the tumor antigen as a protein [99].

Table 17.3 Median and mean survival of patients treated with Lm-LLO-E7 in the study reported and described in [100].

Dosage group	Patient no.	Study day 1	Date of death	Study day at death	Last date patient checked	Days alive as of January 1, 2011
1×10^9	01-001	Apr 4, 2006	Apr 6, 2007	367		
	01-002	Apr 26, 2006	Aug 22, 2006	118		
	01-003	May 10, 2006	Apr 22, 2007	347		
	01-004	Oct 5, 2006			January 1, 2011	1549
	04-001	Aug 28, 2006	Sep 13, 2007	381		
3.3×10^9	03-001	Dec 14, 2006	Nov 2, 2007	323		
	04-002	Oct 26, 2006	Apr 13, 2008	535		
	04-003	Nov 6, 2006	Oct 5, 2009	1064		
	04-004	Dec 14, 2006	Mar 11, 2007	87		
	04-005	Dec 14, 2006	Jan 19, 2007	36		
1×10^{10}	01-005	Feb 14, 2007	Aug 11, 2007	178		
	01-006	Jan 31, 2007	Aug 13, 2007	194		
	01-007	Feb 13, 2007			January 1, 2011	1418
	02-006[a]	Mar 15, 2007	Dec 11, 2007			
	04-006	Feb 15, 2007	Aug 10, 2008	542		
Median survival				347		
Mean survival				485		

Data courtesy of Dr Jon Rothman, Advaxis Inc.
[a] This patient was lost to follow-up. Her last contact date was on day 271.

Moving *Listeria*-based tumor immunotherapy into the clinic

The use of vaccine strains of *Listeria* to induce tumor regression have moved from the research laboratory to clinical trials, with treatment for cervical, breast, and prostate cancer in humans under development. Recently reported results of the first clinical phase I safety study of Lm-LLO-E7, a *Listeria* vaccine that secretes LLO-E7 fusion product [67], show that vaccinations were safe for use in patients with late-stage invasive carcinoma of the cervix [100]. All of the 15 patients enrolled experienced flu-like symptoms, which were alleviated by nonprescription symptomatic treatment. The study was not designed to evaluate efficacy, however more than half of the patients treated with the vaccine had stable disease and one patient was considered a partial responder. Although the Advaxis trial was not designed to evaluate efficacy, the median survival was 347 days for all the pa-

tients and almost 4 years for two patients at the close of the trial at the end of 2010. Table 17.3 shows survival data for patients who entered this study. These are remarkable results compared to historical controls since the median survival time of patients with previously treated metastatic, refractory, or recurrent cervical cancer is only 6–7 months [101]. This study showed for the first time that a live-attenuated *Listeria* immunotherapeutic is safe to be administered to late-stage invasive cancer patients and may provide some efficacy.

Discussion

Bacterial-based cancer immunotherapeutics have demonstrated great promise in preclinical settings and continue to make their way from the bench to the bedside. However, the development of bacterial vaccines for cancer treatment faces a number of technical and biological challenges. Bacteria are unable to carry out a variety of post-translational protein modifications observed in mammalian cells, limiting the pool of effector protein candidates that can serve as the basis of bacterial vaccine constructs. In addition, the expression of foreign antigens in bacteria can place a metabolic burden on the organism that can affect growth rate and select for plasmid loss in the case of plasmid-transformed bacteria or mutant bacteria that have shut down antigen expression [102]. Immune-based vaccines face challenges associated with host tolerance and tumor-associated self-antigens, which are poorly immunogenic and often heterogeneously expressed by genetically unstable, mutation-prone tumor cells. Tumors are also often characterized by immune suppressive microenvironments, limiting the responses of effector cells.

The use of live pathogen based vectors also raises concerns about safety in potentially immunocompromised hosts and efficacy in hosts that are immune incompetent. Attenuation of the virulence factors associated with each of the bacterial vectors under current investigation for potential treatments has enabled significant development of the most promising bacterial species. Recent research addresses concerns of bacterial-based vaccine efficacy in situations where there exists a level of immunity that has developed in response to prior exposures to relatively ubiquitous, wild-type versions of therapeutic pathogens found in nature [103]. Leong *et al.* found that mice with pre-existing cellular immunity to *L. monocytogenes* displayed attenuated CD8$^+$ T cell responses to recombinant strains of *Listeria* expressing a target antigen such as OVA, which were dependent on dose and time of exposure to wild-type *Listeria*, but this could be overcome by repeated immunizations [103].

Based upon our understanding of the similarities and the differences in the immune response to specific pathogens, investigators have addressed the notion that there exist qualitative differences in anti-tumor responses between live bacterial based vaccine vectors, including *Salmonella* and *Listeria* [104]. Specifically, immune responses generated by vaccination with *Listeria*-based vaccines were more effective at inducing tumor regression when compared to vaccination with a *Salmonella*-based vaccine. Vaccine efficacy was linked to favorable anti-tumor immune correlates, including faster antigen presentation by dendritic cells, greater homeostatic proliferation and homing, and the development of CD8$^+$ central memory T cells. In addition, it is now known that *Listeria* also has a propensity to invade and replicate in tumors and can directly cause tumor cell death through mitochondrial disruption mediated by activation of nicotinamide adenine dinucleotide phosphate (NADPH) oxidase, resulting in reactive oxygen species (ROS) production, and an increase in intracellular Ca^{2+} levels [105].

The uses of bacteria, within the context of cancer immunotherapy, are varied in their approach and effectiveness; however, research has revealed a potential place for each in the growing repertoire of therapeutic options for the treatment of cancer.

References

1 Pardoll D. Does the immune system see tumors as foreign or self? *Annu Rev Immunol* 2003;**21**: 807–39.
2 Sleator RD, Hill C. Patho-biotechnology: using bad bugs to do good things. *Curr Opin Biotechnol* 2006;**17**(2):211–16.
3 McCarthy EF. The toxins of William B. Coley and the treatment of bone and soft-tissue sarcomas. *Iowa Orthop J* 2006;**26**:154–8.
4 Groisman EA, Parra-Lopez C, Salcedo M, *et al.* Resistance to host antimicrobial peptides is necessary for *Salmonella* virulence. *Proc Natl Acad Sci U S A* 1992;**89**:11939–43.
5 Sturgill-Koszycki S, Schlesinger PH, Chakraborty P, *et al.* Lack of acidification in *Mycobacterium* phagosomes produced by exclusion of the vesicular proton-ATPase. *Science* 1994;**263**:678–81.
6 Buchmeier NA, Heffron F. Inhibition of macrophage phagosome-lysosome fusion by *Salmonella typhimurium*. *Infect Immun* 1991;**59**:2232–8.
7 Britton WJ, Roche PW, Winter N. Mechanisms of persistence of *mycobacteria*. *Trends Microbiol* 1994; **2**:284–8.
8 Alpuche-Aranda CM, Racoosin EL, Swanson JA, *et al. Salmonella* stimulate macrophage

macropinocytosis and persist within spacious phagosomes. *J Exp Med* 1994;**179**:601–8.

9 Portnoy DA, Chakraborty T, Goebel W, *et al*. Molecular determinants of *Listeria monocytogenes* pathogenesis. *Infect Immun* 1992;**60**:1263–7.

10 Southwick FS, Purich DL. *Listeria* and *Shigella* actin-based motility in host cells. *Trans Am Clin Climatol Assoc* 1998;**109**:160–73.

11 Biron CA, Gazzinelli RT. Effects of IL-12 on immune responses to microbial infections: a key mediator in regulating disease outcome. *Curr Opin Immunol* 1995;**7**(4):485–96.

12 Pamer, EG, Sijts AJ, Villanueva MS, *et al*. MHC class I antigen processing of *Listeria monocytogenes* proteins: implications for dominant and subdominant CTL responses. *Immunol Rev* 1997;**158**:129–36.

13 Wallecha A, Carroll KD, Maciag PC, *et al*. Multiple effector mechanisms induced by recombinant *Listeria monocytogenes* anti-cancer immunotherapeutics. *Adv Appl Microbiol* 2009;**66**:1–27.

14 Sizemore DR, Branstrom AA, Sadoff JC. Attenuated *Shigella* as a DNA delivery vehicle for DNA-mediated immunization. *Science* 1995;**270**:299–303.

15 Hess J, Miko D, Catic A, *et al*. *Mycobacterium bovis* Bacille Calmette-Guérin strains secreting listeriolysin of *Listeria monocytogenes*. *Proc Natl Acad Sci U S A* 1998;**95**(9):5299–304.

16 Grode L, Seiler P, Baumann S, *et al*. Increased vaccine efficacy against tuberculosis of recombinant *Mycobacterium bovis* bacille Calmette-Guérin mutants that secrete listeriolysin. *J Clin Invest* 2005;**115**(9): 2472–9.

17 Turner J, D'Souza CD, Pearl JE, *et al*. CD8⁻ and CD95/95L-dependent mechanisms of resistance in mice with chronic pulmonary tuberculosis. *Am J Respir Cell Mol Biol* 2001;**24**(2):203–9.

18 Colditz GA, Berkey CS, Mosteller F, *et al*. The efficacy of bacillus Calmette-Guérin vaccination of newborns and infants in the prevention of tuberculosis: meta-analyses of the published literature. *Pediatrics* 1995;**96**:29–35.

19 BCG vaccine. WHO position paper. *Wkly Epidemiol Rec* 2004;**79**:27–38.

20 Shelly MD, Kynaston H, Court J, *et al*. A systemic review of intravesical bacillus Calmette-Guérin plus transurethral resection vs transurethral resection alone in Ta and T1 bladder cancer. *BJU Int* 2001;**88**:209–16.

21 Bohle A. Recent knowledge on BCG's mechanism of action in the treatment of superficial bladder cancer. *Braz J Urol* 2000;**26**:488–502.

22 Hao M, Bao L, Gao L, *et al*. [Construction and screen of recombinant BCG strain expressing and secreting human interleukin12 protein]. *Sichuan Da Xue Xue Bao Yi Xue Ban* 2007;**38**(2):186–9 (in Chinese).

23 Liu HT, Sun XW, Zhang YN, *et al*. [Construction, expression and identification of recombinant bacillus Calmette-Guérin vaccine secreting human interferon alpha-2a]. *Zhonghua Yi Xue Za Zhi* 2006;**86**(34):2417–20 (in Chinese).

24 Ding GQ, Shen ZJ, Chen SW, *et al*. [Construction of recombinant bacillus Calmette-Guérin vaccine secreting human interferon-alpha 2b]. *Zhonghua Wai Ke Za Zhi* 2008;**46**(13):1022–6 (in Chinese).

25 Aldovini A, Young RA. Humoral and cell-mediated immune responses to live recombinant BCG-HIV vaccines. *Nature* 1991;**351**:479–82.

26 Chege GK, Thomas R, Shephard EG, *et al*. A prime-boost immunisation regimen using recombinant BCG and Pr55(gag) virus-like particle vaccines based on HIV type 1 subtype C successfully elicits Gag-specific responses in baboons. *Vaccine* 2009;**27**(35):4857–66.

27 Uno-Furuta S, Matsuo K, Tamaki S, *et al*. Immunization with recombinant Calmette-Guérin bacillus (BCG)-hepatitis C virus (HCV) elicits HCV-specific cytotoxic T lymphocytes in mice. *Vaccine* 2003;**21**(23):3149–56.

28 Kawahara M. Recombinant *Mycobacterium bovis* BCG vector system expressing SIV Gag protein stably and persistently induces antigen-specific humoral immune response concomitant with IFN gamma response, even at three years after immunization. *Clin Immunol* 2008;**129**(3):492–8.

29 He J, Shen D, O'Donnell MA, *et al*. Induction of MUC1-specific cellular immunity by a recombinant BCG expressing human MUC1 and secreting IL2. *Int J Oncol* 2002;**20**(6):1305–11.

30 Taylor-Papadimitriou J, Burchell J, Miles DW, *et al*. MUC1 and cancer. *Biochim Biophys Acta* 1999;**1455**(2–3):301–13.

31 Yuan S, Shi C, Han W, *et al*. Effective anti-tumor responses induced by recombinant bacillus Calmette-Guérin vaccines based on different tandem repeats of MUC1 and GM-CSF. *Eur J Cancer Prev* 2009;**18**(5):416–23.

32 Kweon MN. Shigellosis: the current status of vaccine development. *Curr Opin Infect Dis* 2008;**21**(3): 313–18.

33 Shata MT, Hone DM. Vaccination with a *Shigella* DNA vaccine vector induces antigen-specific CD8(+)

T cells and antiviral protective immunity. *J Virol* 2001;**75**(20):9665–70.

34 Fennelly GJ, Khan SA, Abadi MA, *et al.* Mucosal DNA vaccine immunization against measles with a highly attenuated *Shigella flexneri* vector. *J Immunol* 1999;**162**(3):1603–10.

35 Sizemore DR, Branstrom AA, Sadoff JC. Attenuated bacteria as a DNA delivery vehicle for DNA-mediated immunization. *Vaccine* 1997;**15**(8):804–7.

36 Chamekh M, Phalipon A, Quertainmont R, *et al.* Delivery of biologically active anti-inflammatory cytokines IL-10 and IL-1ra in vivo by the *Shigella* type III secretion apparatus. *J Immunol* 2008;**180**(6): 4292–8.

37 Pawelek JM, Low KB, Bermudes D. Bacteria as tumour-targeting vectors. *Lancet Oncol* 2003;**4**(9): 548–56.

38 Kasinskas RW, Forbes NS. *Salmonella typhimurium* lacking ribose chemoreceptors localize in tumor quiescence and induce apoptosis. *Cancer Res* 2007; **67**(7):3201–9.

39 Toso JF, Gill VJ, Hwu P, *et al.* Phase I study of the intravenous administration of attenuated *Salmonella typhimurium* to patients with metastatic melanoma. *J Clin Oncol* 2002;**20**(1):142–52.

40 Loeffler M, Le'Negrate G, Krajewska M, *et al.* Attenuated *Salmonella* engineered to produce human cytokine LIGHT inhibit tumor growth. *Proc Natl Acad Sci U S A* 2007;**104**(31):12879–83.

41 Loeffler M, Le'Negrate G, Krajewska M, *et al.* IL-18-producing *Salmonella* inhibit tumor growth. *Cancer Gene Ther* 2008;**15**(12):787–94.

42 Xiang R, Lode HN, Chao TH, *et al.* An autologous oral DNA vaccine protects against murine melanoma. *Proc Natl Acad Sci U S A* 2000;**97**(10):5492–7.

43 Xiang R, Silletti S, Lode HN, *et al.* Protective immunity against human carcinoembryonic antigen (CEA) induced by an oral DNA vaccine in CEA-transgenic mice. *Clin Cancer Res* 2001;**7**(3 Suppl):856s-64s.

44 Xiang R, Mizutani N, Luo Y, *et al.* A DNA vaccine targeting survivin combines apoptosis with suppression of angiogenesis in lung tumor eradication. *Cancer Res* 2005;**65**(2):553–61.

45 Nishikawa H, Sato E, Briones G, *et al. In vivo* antigen delivery by a *Salmonella typhimurium* type III secretion system for therapeutic cancer vaccines. *J Clin Invest* 2006;**116**(7):1946–54.

46 Low KB, Ittensohn M, Le T, *et al.* Lipid A mutant *Salmonella* with suppressed virulence and TNFalpha induction retain tumor-targeting in vivo. *Nat Biotechnol* 1999;**17**(1):37–41.

47 Luo X, Li Z, Lin S, *et al.* Antitumor effect of VNP20009, an attenuated *Salmonella*, in murine tumor models. *Oncol Res* 2001;**12**:501–8.

48 Chou CK, Hung JY, Liu JC, *et al.* An attenuated *Salmonella* oral DNA vaccine prevents the growth of hepatocellular carcinoma and colon cancer that express alpha-fetoprotein. *Cancer Gene Ther* 2006;**13**(8):746–52.

49 Revaz V, Benyacoub J, Kast WM, *et al.* Mucosal vaccination with a recombinant *Salmonella typhimurium* expressing human papillomavirus type 16 (HPV16) L1 virus-like particles (VLPs) or HPV16 VLPs purified from insect cells inhibits the growth of HPV16-expressing tumor cells in mice. *Virology* 2001;**279**(1):354–60.

50 Weth R, Christ O, Stevanovic S, *et al.* Gene delivery by attenuated *Salmonella typhimurium*: comparing the efficacy of helper versus cytotoxic T cell priming in tumor vaccination. *Cancer Gene Ther* 2001;**8**(8):599–611.

51 Xiang R, Primus FJ, Ruehlmann JM, *et al.* Dual-function DNA vaccine encoding carcinoembryonic antigen and CD40 ligand trimer induces T cell-mediated protective immunity against colon cancer in carcinoembryonic antigen-transgenic mice. *J Immunol* 2001;**167**(8):4560–65.

52 Niethammer AG, Wodrich H, Loeffler M, *et al.* Multidrug resistance-1 (MDR-1): a new target for T cell-based immunotherapy. *FASEB J* 2005;**19**(1): 158–9.

53 Loeffler M, Le'Negrate G, Krajewska M, *et al. Salmonella typhimurium* engineered to produce CCL21 inhibit tumor growth. *Cancer Immunol Immunother* 2009;**58**(5):769–75.

54 Lee SH, Mizutani N, Mizutani M, *et al.* Endoglin (CD105) is a target for an oral DNA vaccine against breast cancer. *Cancer Immunol Immunother* 2006;**55**(12):1565–74.

55 Niethammer AG, Xiang R, Becker JC, *et al.* A DNA vaccine against VEGF receptor 2 prevents effective angiogenesis and inhibits tumor growth. *Nat Med* 2002;**8**(12):1369–75.

56 Fensterle J, Bergmann B, Yone CL, *et al.* Cancer immunotherapy based on recombinant *Salmonella enterica* serovar Typhimurium *aroA* strains secreting prostate-specific antigen and cholera toxin subunit B. *Cancer Gene Ther* 2008;**15**(2):85–93.

57 Avogadri F, Martinoli C, Petrovska L, *et al.* Cancer immunotherapy based on killing of *Salmonella*-infected tumor cells. *Cancer Res* 2005;**65**(9): 3920–27.

58 Zhao M, Geller J, Ma H, *et al.* Monotherapy with a tumor-targeting mutant of *Salmonella typhimurium* cures orthotopic metastatic mouse models of human prostate cancer. *Proc Natl Acad Sci U S A* 2007;**104**(24):10170–74.

59 Zöller M, Christ O. Prophylactic tumor vaccination: comparison of effector mechanisms initiated by protein versus DNA vaccination. *J Immunol* 2001;**166**(5):3440–50.

60 Luo Y, Zhou H, Mizutani M, *et al.* Transcription factor Fos-related antigen 1 is an effective target for a breast cancer vaccine. *Proc Natl Acad Sci U S A* 2003;**100**(15):8850–55.

61 Cárdenas L, Clements JD. Oral immunization using live attenuated *Salmonella* spp. as carriers of foreign antigens. *Clin Microbiol Rev* 1992;**5**(3):328–42.

62 Old LJ. Cancer vaccines: an overview. *Cancer Immun* 2008;**8**(Suppl 1):1.

63 Schafer R, Portnoy DA, Brassell SA, *et al.* Induction of a cellular immune response to a foreign antigen by a recombinant *Listeria monocytogenes* vaccine. *J Immunol* 1992;**149**:53–9.

64 Pan ZK, Ikonomidis G, Lazenby A, *et al.* A recombinant *Listeria monocytogenes* vaccine expressing a model tumor antigen protects mice against lethal tumor cell challenge and causes regression of established tumors. *Nat Med* 1995;**1**(5):471–7.

65 Seavey MM, Verch T, Paterson Y. Anticancer vaccine strategies. In D Lie (Ed.) Handbook of *Listeria monocytogenes*. CRC Press, Boca Raton, FL, 2008, pp. 481–511.

66 Wood LM, Guirnalda PG, Seavey MM, *et al.* Cancer immunotherapy using *Listeria monocytogenes* and listerial virulence factors. *Immunol Res* 2008;**42**: 233–45.

67 Gunn GR, Zubair A, Peters C, *et al.* Two *Listeria monocytogenes* vaccine vectors that express different molecular forms of human papilloma virus-16 (HPV-16) E7 induce qualitatively different T cell immunity that correlates with their ability to induce regression of established tumors immortalized by HPV- 16. *J Immunol* 2001;**167**:6471–9.

68 Huang B, Zhao J, Shen S, *et al. Listeria monocytogenes* promotes tumor growth via tumor cell toll-like receptor 2 signaling. *Cancer Res* 2007;**67**:4346–52.

69 Kim SH, Castro F, Paterson Y, *et al.* High efficacy of a *Listeria*-based vaccine against metastatic breast cancer reveals a dual mode of action. *Cancer Res* 2009;**69**(14):5860–66.

70 Singh R, Dominiecki ME, Jaffee EM, *et al.* Fusion to listeriolysin O and delivery by *Listeria monocytogenes* enhances the immunogenicity of HER-2/neu and reveals subdominant epitopes in the FVB/N mouse. *J Immunol* 2005;**175**:3663–73.

71 Shahabi V, Reyes-Reyes M, Wallecha A, *et al.* Development of a *Listeria monocytogenes* based vaccine against prostate cancer. *Cancer Immunol Immunother* 2008;**57**(9):1301–13.

72 Pan ZK, Weiskirch LM, Paterson Y. Regression of established B16F10 melanoma with a recombinant *Listeria monocytogenes vaccine. Cancer Res* 1999;**59**:5264–9.

73 Liau LM, Jensen ER, Kremen TJ, *et al.* Tumor immunity within the central nervous system stimulated by recombinant *Listeria monocytogenes* vaccination. *Cancer Res* 2002;**62**(8):2287–93.

74 Jensen ER, Selvakumar R, Shen H, *et al.* Recombinant *Listeria monocytogenes* vaccination eliminates papillomavirus-induced tumors and prevents papilloma formation from viral DNA. *J Virol* 1997;**71**(11):8467–74.

75 Sewell DA, Douven D, Pan ZK, *et al.* Regression of HPV-positive tumors treated with a new *Listeria monocytogenes* vaccine. *Arch Otolaryngol Head Neck Surg* 2004;**130**(1):92–7.

76 Sewell DA, Shahabi V, Gunn GR, 3rd, *et al.* Recombinant *Listeria* vaccines containing PEST sequences are potent immune adjuvants for the tumor-associated antigen human papillomavirus-16 E7. *Cancer Res* 2004;**64**(24):8821–5.

77 Lin CW, Lee JY, Tsao YP, *et al.* Oral vaccination with recombinant *Listeria monocytogenes* expressing human papillomavirus type 16 E7 can cause tumor growth in mice to regress. *Int J Cancer* 2002;**102**(6): 629–37.

78 Souders NC, Verch T, Paterson Y. In vivo bactofection: *Listeria* can function as a DNA-cancer vaccine. *DNA Cell Biol* 2006;**25**(3):142–51.

79 Verch T, ZK Pan, Paterson Y. *Listeria monocytogenes*-based antibiotic resistance gene-free antigen delivery system applicable to other bacterial vectors and DNA vaccines. *Infect Immun* 2004;**72**(11): 6418–25.

80 Mustafa W, Maciag PC, Pan ZK, *et al. Listeria monocytogenes* delivery of HPV-16 major capsid protein L1 induces systemic and mucosal cell-mediated CD4$^+$ and CD8$^+$ T-cell responses after oral immunization. *Viral Immunol* 2009;**22**(3):195–204.

81 Seavey MM, Pan ZK, Maciag PC, *et al.* A novel human Her-2/neu chimeric molecule expressed by *Listeria monocytogenes* can elicit potent HLA-A2 restricted CD8-positive T cell responses and impact the

growth and spread of Her-2/neu-positive breast tumors. *Clin Cancer Res* 2009;**15**(3):924–32.

82 Seavey MM, Maciag PC, Al-Rawi N, *et al.* An antivascular endothelial growth factor receptor 2/fetal liver kinase-1 *Listeria monocytogenes* anti-angiogenesis cancer vaccine for the treatment of primary and metastatic Her-2/neu$^+$ breast tumors in a mouse model. *J Immunol* 2009;**182**(9):5537–46.

83 Kim SH, Castro F, Gonzalez D, *et al.* Mage-b vaccine delivered by recombinant *Listeria monocytogenes* is highly effective against breast cancer metastases. *Br J Cancer* 2008;**99**(5):741–9.

84 Bruhn KW, Craft N, Nguyen BD, *et al.* Characterization of anti-self CD8 T-cell responses stimulated by recombinant *Listeria monocytogenes* expressing the melanoma antigen TRP-2. *Vaccine* 2005;**23**(33):4263–72.

85 Maciag PC, Seavey MM, Pan ZK, *et al.* Cancer immunotherapy targeting the high molecular weight melanoma-associated antigen protein results in a broad antitumor response and reduction of pericytes in the tumor vasculature. *Cancer Res* 2008;**68**(19):8066–75.

86 Brockstedt DG, Giedlin MA, Leong ML, *et al.* *Listeria*-based cancer vaccines that segregate immunogenicity from toxicity. *Proc Natl Acad Sci U S A* 2004;**101**(38):13832–7.

87 Wallecha A, Maciag PC, Rivera S, *et al.* Construction and characterization of an attenuated *Listeria monocytogenes* strain for clinical use in cancer immunotherapy. *Clin Vaccine Immunol* 2009;**16**(1):96–103.

88 Paglia P, Arioli I, Frahm N, *et al.* The defined attenuated *Listeria monocytogenes* delta mp12 mutant is an effective oral vaccine carrier to trigger a long-lasting immune response against a mouse fibrosarcoma. *Eur J Immunol* 1997;**27**(6):1570–75.

89 Singh R, Paterson Y. Immunoediting sculpts tumor epitopes during immunotherapy. *Cancer Res* 2007;**67**:1887–92.

90 Ercolini AM, Machiels JP, Chen YC, *et al.* Identification and characterization of the immunodominant rat HER-2/neu MHC class I epitope presented by spontaneous mammary tumors from HER-2/neu-transgenic mice. *J Immunol* 2003;**170**:4273–80.

91 Singh R, Paterson Y. Vaccination strategy determines the emergence and dominance of CD8$^+$ T-cell epitopes in a FVB/N rat HER-2/neu mouse model of breast cancer. *Cancer Res* 2006;**66**:7748–57.

92 Folkman J. Tumor angiogenesis: therapeutic implications. *New Engl J Med* 1971;**285**:1182–6

93 Luo Y, Markowitz D, Xiang R, *et al.* FLK-1-based minigene vaccines induce T cell-mediated suppression of angiogenesis and tumor protective immunity in syngeneic BALB/c mice. *Vaccine* 2007;**25**: 1409–15.

94 Shibuya M. Vascular endothelial growth factor (VEGF)-receptor2: its biological functions, major signaling pathway, and specific ligand VEGF-E. *Endothelium* 2006;**13**:63–9.

95 Seavey MM, Paterson Y. Anti-angiogenesis immunotherapy induces epitope spreading to Her-2/neu resulting in tumor immunoediting. *Breast cancer (London)* 2009;**1**:19–30

96 Campoli MR, Chang CC, Kageshita T, *et al.* Human high molecular weight-melanoma-associated antigen (HMW-MAA): a melanoma cell surface chondroitin sulfate proteoglycan (MSCP) with biological and clinical significance. *Crit Rev Immunol* 2004;**24**:267–96.

97 Dietrich G, Bubert A, Gentschev I, *et al.* Delivery of antigen-encoding plasmid DNA into the cytosol of macrophages by attenuated suicide *Listeria monocytogenes*. *Nat Biotechnol* 1998;**16**(2):181–5.

98 Spreng S, Dietrich G, Niewiesk S, *et al.* Novel bacterial systems for the delivery of recombinant protein or DNA. *FEMS Immunol Med Microbiol* 2000;**27**(4):299–304.

99 Loeffler DI, Schoen CU, Goebel W, *et al.* Comparison of different live vaccine strategies in vivo for delivery of protein antigen or antigen-encoding DNA and mRNA by virulence-attenuated *Listeria monocytogenes*. *Infect Immun* 2006;**74**(7):3946–57.

100 Maciag PC, Radulovic S, Rothman J. The first clinical use of a live-attenuated *Listeria monocytogenes* vaccine: a phase I safety study of Lm-LLO-E7 in patients with advanced carcinoma of the cervix. *Vaccine* 2009;**27**(30):3975–83.

101 Moore DH, Tian C, Monk BJ, *et al.* Prognostic factors for response to cisplatin-based chemotherapy in advanced cervical carcinoma: a Gynecologic Oncology Group study. *Gynecol Oncol* 2010;**116**(1):44–9.

102 Galen JE, Pasetti MF, Sztein MB, *et al.* Attenuated *Salmonella* and *Shigella* as live vectors carrying either prokaryotic or eukaryotic expression systems. In MM Levine, JB Kaper, R Rappuoli, MA Liu, MF Good (Eds) *New Generation Vaccines*, 3rd edn. Marcel Dekker, New York, 2004, pp. 354–66.

103 Leong ML, Hampl J, Liu W, *et al.* Impact of preexisting vector-specific immunity on vaccine potency: characterization of *Listeria monocytogenes*-specific

humoral and cellular immunity in humans and modeling studies using recombinant vaccines in mice. *Infect Immun* 2009;**77**(9):3958–68.

104 Stark FC, Sad S, Krishnan L. Intracellular bacterial vectors that induce CD8(+) T cells with similar cytolytic abilities but disparate memory phenotypes provide contrasting tumor protection. *Cancer Res* 2009;**69**(10):4327–34.

105 Kim SH, Castro F, Paterson Y, *et al.* High efficacy of a *Listeria*-based vaccine against metastatic breast cancer reveals a dual mode of action. *Cancer Res* 2009;**69**(14):5860–66.

106 Paterson Y. The relationship between bacterial intracellular bacterial life-styles and immune responsiveness to bacterial delivered antigens. In Y Paterson (Ed.) *Intracellular Bacterial Vaccine Vectors: Immunology, Cell Biology, and Genetics.* John Wiley & Sons, Inc., New York, 1999.

107 Souders NC, Verch T, Paterson Y. Immunotherapeutic strategies against cancer using *Listeria monocytogenes* as a vector for tumor antigens. In RJ Orentas, BD Johnson, JW Hodge (Eds) *Cancer Vaccines and Tumor Immunity.* John Wiley & Sons, Hoboken, NJ, 2008, pp. 113–130.

CHAPTER 18

Nucleic Acid Vaccination

Britta Wahren[1] & Margaret A. Liu[2]
[1]Department of Virology, Karolinska Institutet and Swedish Institute for Infectious Disease Control, Stockholm, Sweden
[2]ProTherImmune, Lafayette, CA, USA

Background

A variety of novel technologies have been developed and evaluated in efforts to make vaccines against targets that have remained intractable to traditional approaches for making vaccines. While a number of the diseases are caused by infectious agents, immunologic approaches have extended from prophylaxis to immunotherapy for cancer, allergy, and autoimmune diseases. Many of the immune approaches focus on specific antigens, but the types of immune responses being generated range from the traditional ones aimed at killing a pathogen or stopping its replication, to more nuanced modulations of particular types of immune responses. This chapter will focus on the use of nucleic acids as vaccines against infectious diseases and cancer, and will describe the mechanisms involved, as well as potentials for therapy.

DNA vaccines were developed from the finding of plasmid DNA uptake by cells *in vivo*. Viruses have evolved structures and mechanisms to deliver their genetic material into cells. It was therefore thought that unformulated DNA would not be useful as a means to directly deliver genes into cells *in vivo*. Thus the observation by Felgner's group that bacterial plasmid DNA in saline resulted in the uptake of the DNA by muscle cells *in vivo* – with the subsequent transcription and translation of the encoded genes – came as a surprise [1].

DNA vaccines are the most developed form of nucleic acid vaccines, mostly as bacterial plasmids that code for antigens, and that have been modified in order to express in mammalian cells. The antigen or endogenous protein that is expressed in the person or animal is expressed from the plasmid rather than expressed by the pathogen itself. Thus there is no risk of infection from the pathogen from which the gene for the antigen is derived.

Because the antigen is synthesized *in situ* in the immunized host, cellular immune responses (including major histocompatibility complex (MHC) class I and class II restricted responses) as well as antibodies can be generated. Another attractive feature of DNA vaccines is that the technology for their creation and manufacture is amenable to the relatively rapid creation of new vaccines, with a manufacturing process that is quite similar for different entities since the same basic plasmid (with only different gene inserts) can be used. DNA vaccine technology thus offers advantages of both cost and speed. Given the continuing and increasing need for vaccines to be developed for pandemic diseases (such as influenza), the rapidity of development of a vaccine may be a critical feature.

For an influenza DNA vaccine, the advantage is not simply one of manufacturing, but also of making the initial vaccine construct. A plasmid encoding the desired genes of a newly arising pandemic strain can be quickly made, and moreover can be made without needing to work with the virus itself, since the desired genes can be directly sequenced, constructed, and inserted into the plasmid or a

Vaccinology: Principles and Practice, First Edition. Edited by W. John W. Morrow, Nadeem A. Sheikh, Clint S. Schmidt and D. Huw Davies.
© 2012 Blackwell Publishing Ltd. Published 2012 by Blackwell Publishing Ltd.

plasmid cassette already containing desirable additional genes.

The key issue for DNA vaccines has been that, despite the many potential advantages and applicability for a variety of diseases, their potency in humans has been disappointing. However, new technologies of delivery have resulted in improvements. Moreover, with the licensure of three DNA vaccines for veterinary applications (two for infectious diseases and one for cancer), the utility and feasibility of the technology has been demonstrated, providing hope that the appropriate modifications, delivery systems, and targets will be demonstrated to harness this technology (Figure 18.1).

The DNA plasmid itself also has immune effects that may potentiate the desired immune responses against an antigen. The vector backbone of the plasmid, because it is bacterial DNA with a different methylation pattern than mammalian DNA, stimulates the innate immune system (the topic of Chapter 2) via a Toll-like receptor (TLR) (Chapter 26), thus potentially enhancing the immunogenicity of the DNA vaccine [2]. Endogenous cytokines occur at the site of gene delivery, whether induced directly by the bacterial plasmid DNA or the RNA (as RNA has also been used to deliver genes encoding antigens), or as a result of the delivery technology, such as electroporation. These phenomena are desirable in vaccine attempts, but likely are counterproductive or even deleterious in gene therapy applications.

Efforts have focused on ways to increase the potency of DNA vaccines. The simplest strategy was to use larger doses of DNA. As data from early clinical trials demonstrated the safety of administering DNA vaccines to humans, increased doses of DNA have been used in clinical trials, increasing to as

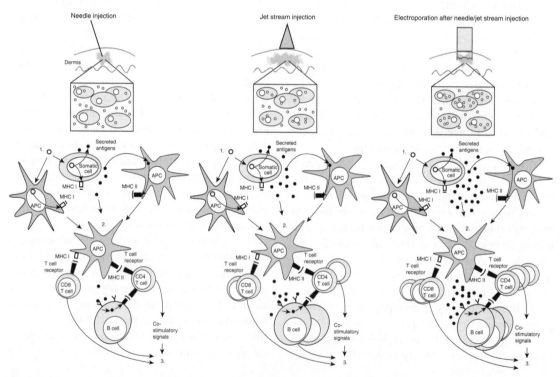

Figure 18.1 Schematic view of various modes of nucleic vaccine delivery. Needle delivery and jet spray delivery cause more plasmids to be distributed into cell supernatants than electroporation, which delivers plasmid DNA more effectively into cell cytoplasm and nuclei. Illustrated by David Hallengärd.

much as 1–8 milligram doses per vaccine [3]. Additional approaches have included means to increase the potency of the DNA vaccines themselves; alternate means of delivery, including with devices; prime-boost strategies; and the co-administration of immune-enhancing molecules.

Modifications of genes and gene expression

Pathogen diversity represents a challenge for vaccine construction. Several ways of representing common T-cell epitopes or neutralization-sensitive regions of a pathogen have been suggested. The most successful modification of microbe genes is the optimization for expression of the gene of interest. By taking into account the codons most common for expression in animal cells, most viral or bacterial genes can be modified to express their proteins in high amounts in mammalian cells (a process called "codon optimization"). This technology is now used universally to provide well-expressing nucleic acid vaccines.

Ligand linking of peptides of a certain optimal length to the cholera toxin B subunit strongly enhances immunogenicity of the peptide [4]. Such a point-directed boost may have its place in boosting desirable epitope reactivities induced by a DNA representing the whole gene of interest.

Conserved regions related to T-cell epitopes were included for HIV genes in the beads-on-a string concept. The epitopes were to be recognized by a high number of individuals with different HLA types and represented several viral subtypes [5]. This string-of-epitopes concept was tried in HIV vaccination, but did not give the expected high number of strong cytolytic T-cell responses, possibly due to interpeptide epitopes in the vaccines. Variants of these ideas include the shuffling and mosaic patterns to permit induction of a general response to many viral strains.

A recent finding is that hidden membrane epitopes give rise to strong neutralizing antibodies *in vitro*. Certain antibodies to HIV are rarely present in infected humans, perhaps due to lack of external exposure by parts of the transmembrane protein gp41, the MPER region [6]. A virus provided with an amino acid mutation within or close to the MPER region rendered a virus that is highly neutralization sensitive [7]. The mechanism is thought to be exposure of the epitope(s) close to the lipid membrane. It is possible that modification of a nucleotide vaccine may render the vaccine plasmid more immunogenic to induce the desired neutralizing antibodies. The capacity of these potential antibodies has, however, not been proven *in vivo*, since the access of such antibodies to their target *in vivo* is unclear. Passive immunization by an HIV anti-V3 antibody provided short-term viral antigen reduction in a small clinical trial [8] and passive immunization with anti-MPER antibodies a modest effect.

Mosaic and consensus envelope fragments

With a variable pathogen it is still possible to create recognizable epitopes for a large number of the proteins. Mosaic sequences derive from the optimal sequence of an epitope, and as many as possible should be included in a stretch of amino acid sequences [9]. Natural amino acid breakpoints should be protected in order not to create unnatural nonpathogen-related epitopes. The mosaic approach also takes into account the frequencies of the epitope in circulating viruses.

Cytotoxic T lymphocyte (CTL) epitopes are small and linear. Responses against conserved regions of a viral genome that overcome host gene limitations are being sought [9]. Multiple epitope responses were shown to occur in individuals with different HLA class I heterogeneities [10]. Mosaic antigens expand cellular breadth [11,12] but have not yet been put to the test of protection. B-cell epitopes are more variable, often nonlinear and conformation dependent. A typical example of this is the polio-neutralizing antibody. They cover amino acids protruding around a cleft formed by nucleocapsid molecules. The best mimic of such structures is the virus particle itself or a virus-like particle (VLP) [13], which are covered in detail in Chapter 13.

Many natural or fragment shuffled proteins have been tried [14]. Protection against *Mycoplasma pneumoniae* was obtained in a mouse model from a mixture of many DNA fragments [15] but this phenomenon has not been extensively used. A note of precaution is that innate immunity has a long duration after delivery of high and foreign DNA amounts, which might be taken as a pathogen-specific response.

The consensus sequences, like the ancestral sequences, are attempts to identify retroviruses of origin [16]. The ideas have also been used in attempts to obtain the most cross-reactive responses in as many individuals as possible. Nucleotide modifications are made in the envelope gene of HIV to insert in each position the amino acid that is either most frequent in many strains or has been calculated to be originally present early during evolution (Los Alamos databases). So far, such immunization attempts in primates have had varying successes to prove that they are more immunogenic than homologous or heterologous strain-specific amino acid sequences.

Cytokines as adjuvants

Cytokine administration has been one of the great successes of recombinant DNA technology. Recombinant cytokines have been used for the treatment of cancers and chronic viral infections. Administration of genes encoding these therapeutic proteins would enable the protein to be present for longer periods (compared to the short half-lives of a recombinant protein) and could avoid the toxicities due to the systemic administration of the recombinant protein if the gene were administered locally, such as directly into a tumor. Administration of genes encoding cytokines or co-stimulatory molecules has been evaluated preclinically and clinically. This has been done with the cytokine or cytokine gene in conjunction with or around the time of the DNA vaccine administration where the cytokine functions as an adjuvant [17].

Possible role of CpG motifs

While CpG motifs are more fully discussed in the chapter on Toll-like receptors (Chapter 26), a brief mention of them will be included here because of their putative role in the immunogenicity of DNA vaccines. DNA vaccines are of bacterial origin, and as such contain CpG motifs that stimulate Toll-like receptor 9 (TLR9) [18,19]. The presence of such motifs is thought to activate the innate immunity and thereby contribute to the adaptive immune responses generated against the DNA-encoded antigen, in part because the potency of a DNA vaccine was increased preclinically when noncoding plasmid was added to the DNA vaccine [20,21]. However, alteration of the backbone of plasmids to include more CpG motifs does not always increase the immunogenicity of the plasmid. More recent studies have cast additional doubt upon the importance of this interaction. For example, the immunogenicity of a DNA vaccine was similar in wild-type and TLR knockout mice [22], as was the potency for generation of CTL responses in TLR9-deficient or normal mice [23].

Prime-boost

In a variety of disease models and with several vaccine modalities, the observation has been made that plasmid DNA encoding an antigen, when given as a prime, followed by a boost of the same antigen either encoded by a different vector (such as an adenovector or vaccinia) or as a recombinant protein, results in a more potent immune response than either modality given alone. See Table 18.1 for a comparison of DNA vaccines with the two main viral vectors used independently and as a boost for the DNA.

Of note, the immune responses are most potent when the DNA vaccine is the priming agent. A variety of vectors used as the boost appear to be useful [24]. The immunologic mechanisms are not known in detail, but it is hypothesized that genes expressed in the DNA plasmid prime the immune response to the expressed protein without diversion by vector proteins. The vectorized immunogen then boosts the antigen-specific response and simultaneously induces a variety of cytokines, which aid induction of long-term memory.

Trials in nonhuman primates and humans are evaluating the novel and promising concept of using the DNA vaccine as a prime to be followed by immunization with viral vectors encoding the same

Table 18.1 Attributes of plasmid DNA vaccines compared to select vectors.

	Advantages	Disadvantages
Plasmid DNA	Simple design and construction Simple to modify Potent priming ability Stable	Needs more potency
Poxvectors	Carry large gene insert Large experience in humans	Vector immunity in vaccinated persons
Adenovirus vectors	Effective cellular uptake Effective expression	Vector immunity from prior exposure

antigen or a recombinant protein version of the antigen.

The prime-boost approach has advanced to the clinic for various diseases, including HIV and malaria. HIV DNA incorporated in a prime-boost schedule predicted the potent and broad immunogenicity subsequently found in humans [25]. Both prime and boost vaccination with subunits of the viral genes alone or introduced in a vector with heterogenous HIV gene inserts contributed to the striking and broad immunogenicity seen in the clinic [26,27].

Infectious diseases

The first demonstration that DNA vaccines could work preclinically *in vivo* was done using a simple plasmid of DNA coding for a protein from the influenza virus. That study showed that the DNA could result in the generation of both cytotoxic T lymphocytes and antibodies, and, more importantly, could protect from an otherwise lethal challenge with a strain of influenza different from the strain from which the gene had been cloned [28]. While the current influenza vaccine cannot protect against a virus of the same subtype that has drifted or shifted, the DNA vaccine protected against a challenge from a completely different subtype [28]. This raises hopes that DNA vaccines could provide a new means for making vaccines that would be broadly effective against a variety of strains, thereby helping to prevent the types of global epidemics such as the 1919 influenza pandemic that killed about 20 million people, or be a foundation

for a rapidly produced component against bird influenza (H5N1) or swine influenza (H1N1).

Also, antibodies against influenza could provide protection after DNA immunization [29]. Chen *et al.* have shown that DNA-encoded consensus H5 hemagglutinin can induce antibodies capable of inhibiting multiple subclades within H5N1 and providing various levels of protection in a murine challenge model [30].

The ability to protect animals in a cross-strain manner raised interest because it offered a potential means to design vaccines for mutating microbes such as HIV, influenza, and hepatitis C [31], whose multiple and/or evolving strains pose a tremendous challenge.

Interestingly, only a subunit of a microbe, when presented as a nucleic acid immunogen, may protect against serious disease. Two acute RNA viruses (rhabdo and filo) have been shown to confer protective capacity after vaccination with their DNA homologs. The single DNA of the G protein of rhabdovirus was early shown to protect mice, and recent expression analysis has shown that the antigen may act as an endogenous immune activator in specific species [32,33]. Envelope genes representing glycoproteins of Ebola virus strains from central Africa (Zaire and Sudan) together with the conserved nucleoprotein gene induced antibody in all healthy subjects, while one third of immunized persons obtained cytolytic T-cell reactivity [34].

Both cellular and humoral immune responses can be efficiently induced by the various nucleotide vaccines. The specific types or skewing of immune responses are determined or influenced by the dose, the number of immunizations, and the nature of the antigen (e.g., secreted, whether it forms VLPs, etc.). For example, hepatitis B virus DNA preferentially produces antibody responses [35], while DNA encoding proteins from the interior of retroviruses (e.g., HIV) and herpes virus can induce potent cellular responses [36].

Early phase clinical trials have been performed and are ongoing for DNA vaccines encoding antigens from pathogens, ranging from influenza and malaria to HIV [37]. While the studies have demonstrated the safety of the vaccines, immune responses were observed, but they were generally lower than anticipated. These included both antibodies and cellular immune responses [38,39]. Interesting observations included that certain HIV patients who had had long exposures to high levels of viral antigens (due to their high viral loads), yet who had not made cytolytic T-cell responses against a particular viral antigen, mounted cytolytic T-cell responses against epitopes of that protein following the DNA immunization [40]. This demonstrated that DNA differed from the virus in terms of the mechanism of generation of immune responses.

Cancer

DNA vaccines would be a means to make vaccines also against viruses that are related to the induction of tumors, such as papilloma virus [41], and hepatitis B and C viruses. The targets include a variety of antigens that are expressed uniquely or overexpressed on tumor cells, as well as proteins that play a role in the transformation of the cells from normal cells to cancerous ones. The latter include molecules such as carcinoembryonic antigen (CEA), which is expressed normally on fetal cells, or certain prostate antigens, which are present in higher amounts on tumor cells than on the normal prostate. Tyrosine kinase is another endogenous molecule that has been targeted in cancer cells. The challenge for such endogenous proteins has been both that tolerance needs to be broken, and then, once having broken tolerance, to determine whether the benefits of the immune response (killing tumor cells) will outweigh any deleterious effects against normal tissue. For targets such

as prostate antigens, for example prostate specific antigen (PSA), prostatic acid phosphatase (PAP), and prostate stem cell antigen (PSCA), this has been considered acceptable because the prostate, which is removed or ablated by the cancer therapy, is the only other site of expression. Electroporation with i.m. immunization of mice with DNA encoding PAP resulted in immune responses (i.e., tolerance was broken) [42].

For tyrosine kinase, it likewise has been possible to break tolerance against this enzyme and thus induce an immune response against the tumor melanoma, which is rich in such substances [43,44]. Patients with melanoma in stages 3–4 have received murine tyrosinase DNA followed by human tyrosinase DNA. Half of the patients developed cytolytic CD8$^+$ cells directed against a peptide. The median survival time was not yet reached, indicating a prolonged survival [44,45].

Targets that play a role in the cellular transformation include human papilloma virus proteins E6 and E7. Because of the role of E6 and E7 in cellular transformation, gene-based vaccines encode modified versions of the protein so as to deliver a protein that can induce immune responses but is not capable of cellular transformation. Other examples include survivin, which plays a role in apoptosis and angiogenesis [46]. In this study, mice were immunized with DNA encoding human survivin in order to facilitate the breaking of tolerance. Her-2/neu is a growth factor receptor whose presence is associated with aggressive breast cancer [47]. A monoclonal antibody directed against Her-2/neu has been quite useful in therapy of breast cancer, so efforts have been made to make DNA vaccines against this factor as well.

Allergy and autoimmune diseases

Because a hallmark of autoimmune diseases has been the presence of anti-DNA antibodies, a major safety concern initially for DNA vaccines was whether or not they would induce autoimmune diseases. To date, the clinical trials of DNA vaccines have not had significant safety issues. In contrast, a variety of DNA vaccines are being developed as therapies for autoimmune diseases such as diabetes, by changing the type of immune response against relevant antigens to being harmless rather than disease inducing. For example, DNA encoding proinsulin has been shown in a murine model of diabetes to decrease the number of animals that spontaneously develop the disease. This is thought to be mediated by a change in the type of T helper cells. The effect has recently been shown to depend upon factors such as the protocol of administration of the DNA, as well as the level and location of expression of the antigen [48].

One of the most interesting properties of a DNA vaccine is its property to not only induce predominantly Th1 responses but also to deviate the immune response away from pro-allergenic Th2 responses and certain classes of antibody production (notably IgE) [49]. Thus, allergic responses by IgE have been redirected by small doses of DNA encoding certain allergens in disease models of allergy and asthma [50]. A refinement of this general approach has been to direct the DNA vaccines to particular antigen-presenting cells for the generation of the Th1-type of immunity rather than simply depending upon the bias that occurs naturally with plasmid DNA vaccines (reviewed in [51]).

Licensed DNA vaccines

While DNA vaccines were effective in a variety of preclinical models of infectious diseases as prophylactic vaccines, clinical trials have generally resulted in disappointing immunogenicity. However, two vaccines and one immunotherapy have been licensed for veterinary applications [43,52,53]. These include a vaccine against West Nile virus in horses (Fort Dodge Laboratories), which induces antibodies more effectively than the killed virus vaccine in previous usage. A DNA vaccine for fish hematonecrosis virus is licensed for usage in salmon (Novartis Animal Health).

A DNA vaccine was approved in 2010 for the immunotherapy of melanoma in dogs. The vaccine for melanoma in dogs encodes molecules from the tyrosine kinase family. Immunization with foreign tyrosinase DNA improved survival and even cured dogs with progressing melanoma. In this case, the heterogenous (human) tyrosinase was able to break tolerance against the endogenous enzyme [43]. Antibodies appeared to be the major effector molecules occurring in parallel with tumor rejection.

The immunogenicity of DNA vaccine for horses leading to clinical licensure was surprising given that the failure to translate the broad efficacy of DNA vaccines in preclinical models into human potency was thought by many to be due to the larger mass of humans compared to small laboratory animals. One possible explanation is that the inherent immunogenicity of the antigen encoded by the DNA may determine whether the technology is useful for a given vaccine and disease. For example, the equine West Nile virus DNA vaccine encodes an extracellular particle that is a very potent immunogen [54]. Indeed, in a human trial of a DNA vaccine all the fully-immunized participants generated antibodies of titers high enough to be protective in horses [55]. Thus, as DNA vaccines are developed for human usage, it is important to marry the vaccine technology with the appropriately immunogenic antigens.

Delivery

Efforts have been directed at formulating the DNA in order to increase its cellular uptake, or to enable it to withstand extracellular degradation for longer. Encapsulating the DNA into or adhering the DNA onto microparticles or virus-like particles appears to increase the potency of DNA vaccines by either protecting the DNA from degradation or increasing its uptake by antigen-processing cells [56–58].

Different delivery devices or routes have also been employed in efforts to increase the potency of DNA vaccines, to stimulate, for instance, mucosal immune responses.

The initial demonstration of a DNA vaccine that could stimulate antibody responses employed a gene gun to shoot DNA-coated gold beads into the skin [59]. Such particle-mediated injection has been used in clinical trials to generate antibodies against hepatitis B surface antigen [60], or influenza using DNA encoding the antigen. Although the DNA immunizations resulted in lower titers and utilized more immunizations than the protein vaccine, they still showed the ability of DNA to clinically produce the desired immune response. In a further study, patients who had not responded well to the licensed recombinant protein hepatitis vaccine made antibodies following immunization with the DNA vaccine given by a gene gun [35].

DNA transfer by apoptotic cells appears to induce a receptor-independent immune response. The DNA, present in the apoptotic bodies from transfection by plasmids or by the infectious agent, is taken up by antigen-presenting cells and appears to induce good immune responses [61].

Devices other than traditional syringes are being tested to directly propel the DNA vaccine into the skin (for example, the Biojector or the coming Zetajet) [62, and Bioject.com] or the mucosa for the Syriject [63].

Another approach has been to couple the usual injection with subsequent *in vivo* electroporation (resulting in an increase in the amount of transfection of the DNA into cells (Figure 18.1)) [57,64]. The novel strategy of *in vivo* electroporation delivers DNA vaccines by either i.m. or i.d. routes. This technique has been used for a series of vaccines, with some entering human clinical trials [52,58]. Significant protection from severe disease can be offered by electroporation methodology in nonhuman primates [65].

Nevertheless, systematic studies regarding the impact of the route of vaccination of DNA vaccines delivered by *in vivo* electroporation on the type of immune responses in humans have not yet been performed.

Production

Nucleic acid vaccines have further potential advantages as a product, besides the immunologic and clinical issues. The manufacturing process is relatively generic compared to either small molecule drugs or other biologicals such as either recombinant proteins or live viral vaccines. DNA vaccines

are bacterial plasmids, with the differences generally being simply the gene insert and a promoter. The production process of growth in bacterial hosts and the subsequent purification of the plasmids are similar for different vaccines or therapies, and the plasmids are easier to purify than recombinant proteins. Moreover, DNA vaccines are more stable than live viruses. Current embodiments of DNA vaccines include formulations and delivery systems that may make them complicated as products, but the generic nature of the entity remains a compelling attribute.

References

1 Wolff JA, Malone RW, Williams P, *et al.* Direct gene transfer into mouse muscle in vivo. *Science* 1990;**247**(4949 Pt 1):1465–8.

2 Klinman DM, Xie H, Ivins BE. CpG oligonucleotides improve the protective immune response induced by the licensed anthrax vaccine. *Ann N Y Acad Sci* 2006;**1082**:137–50.

3 Moorthy VS, Imoukhuede EB, Milligan P, *et al.* A randomised, double-blind, controlled vaccine efficacy trial of DNA/MVA ME-TRAP against malaria infection in Gambian adults. *PLoS Med* 2004;**1**(2):e33.

4 Boberg A, Gaunitz S, Bråve A, Wahren B, Carlin N. Enhancement of epitope-specific cellular immune responses by immunization with HIV-1 peptides genetically conjugated to the B-subunit of recombinant cholera toxin. *Vaccine* 2008;**26**(40):5079–82.

5 McMichael A, Hanke T. The quest for an AIDS vaccine: is the CD8$^+$ T-cell approach feasible? *Nat Rev Immunol* 2002;**2**(4):283–91.

6 Hinz A, Schoehn G, Quendler H, *et al.* Characterization of a trimeric MPER containing HIV-1 gp41 antigen. *Virology* 2009;**390**(2):221–7.

7 Shen X, Dennison M, Gao F, *et al.* HIV-1 gp41 envelope MPER mutation altered epitope conformation in lipid and increased sensitivity to 2F5 and 4E10 neutralizing antibodies. *Retrovirology* 2009;**6**(Suppl 3): O16.

8 Hinkula J, Bratt G, Gilljam G, *et al.* Immunological and virological interactions in patients receiving passive immunotherapy with HIV-1 neutralizing monoclonal antibodies. *J Acquir Immune Defic Syndr* 1994;**7**(9):940–51.

9 Korber B, Gnanakaran G, Perkins S. New applications for mosaic antigen designs. Presented at AIDS Vaccine

2009, Symposium 6, Paris, October 19–22, Abstract S06–03. Available at www.hivvaccineenterprise.org/conference_archive/2009/Symposium-06.pdf. Accessed January 2012.

10 Zuniga R, Mothe B, Llano A, *et al*. HIV specific T cell responses and response patterns associated with viral control independent of classical non-progressor HLA class I alleles. *Retrovirology* 2009;**6**(Suppl 3):O3.

11 Barouch D, Korber B. HIV-1 mosaic antigens expand immune breadth and depth in rhesus monkeys. Presented at AIDS Vaccine 2009, Symposium 6, Paris, October 19–22, Abstract S06–04. Available at www.hivvaccineenterprise.org/conference_archive/2009/Symposium-06.pdf. Accessed January 2012.

12 Barouch DH, O'Brien KL, Simmons NL, *et al*. Mosaic HIV-1 vaccines expand the breadth and depth of cellular immune responses in rhesus monkeys. *Nat Med* 2010;**16**:319–23.

13 Buonaguro L, Devito C, Tornesello ML, *et al*. DNA-VLP prime-boost intra-nasal immunization induces cellular and humoral anti-HIV-1 systemic and mucosal immunity with cross-clade neutralizing activity. *Vaccine* 2007;**25**(32):5968–77.

14 Machesky LM, Johnston SA. MIM: a multifunctional scaffold protein. *J Mol Med* 2007;**85**(6):569–76.

15 Barry MA, Lai WC, Johnston SA. Protection against mycoplasma infection using expression-library immunization. *Nature* 1995;**377**:632–5.

16 Gao F, Scearce RM, Alam SM, *et al*. Cross-reactive monoclonal antibodies to multiple HIV-1 subtype and SIVcpz envelope glycoproteins. *Virology* 2009;**394**(1):91–8.

17 Chong SY, Egan MA, Kutzler MA, *et al*. Comparative ability of plasmid IL-12 and IL-15 to enhance cellular and humoral immune responses elicited by a SIVgag plasmid DNA vaccine and alter disease progression following SHIV(89.6P) challenge in rhesus macaques. *Vaccine* 2007;**25**(26):4967–82.

18 Klinman DM, Yamshchikov G, Ishigatsubo Y. Contribution of CpG motifs to the immunogenicity of DNA vaccines. *J Immunol* 1997;**158**:3635–9.

19 Hemmi H, Takeuchi O, Kawai T, *et al*. A Toll-like receptor recognizes bacterial DNA. *Nature* 2000;**408**:740–45.

20 Donnelly JJ, Friedman A, Martinez D, *et al*. Preclinical efficacy of a prototype DNA vaccine: enhanced protection against antigenic drift in influenza virus. *Nat Med* 1995;**1**:583–7.

21 Sato Y, Roman M, Tighe H, *et al*. Immunostimulatory DNA sequences necessary for effective intradermal gene immunization. *Science* 1996;**273**:352–4.

22 Babiuk S, Mookherjee N, Pontarollo R, *et al*. TLR9$^{-/-}$ and TLR9$^{+/+}$ mice display similar immune responses to a DNA vaccine. *Immunology* 2004;**113**:114–20.

23 Spies B, Hochrein H, Vabulas M, *et al*. Vaccination with plasmid DNA activates dendritic cells via Toll-like receptor 9 (TLR9) but functions in TLR9-deficient mice. *J Immunol* 2003;**171**:5908–12.

24 Bråve A, Ljungberg K, Wahren B, Liu MA. Vaccine delivery methods using viral vectors. *Mol Pharm* 2007;**4**(1):18–32.

25 Bråve A, Boberg A, Gudmundsdotter L, *et al*. A new multi-clade DNA prime/recombinant MVA boost vaccine induces broad and high levels of HIV-1-specific CD8(+) T-cell and humoral responses in mice. *Mol Ther* 2007;**15**(9):1724–33.

26 Sandström E, Nilsson C, Hejdeman B, *et al*. Broad immunogenicity of a multigene, multiclade HIV-1 DNA vaccine boosted with heterologous HIV-1 recombinant modified vaccinia virus Ankara. *J Infect Dis* 2008;**198**(10):1482–90.

27 Bakari M, Aboud S, Nilsson C, *et al*. A low dose of multigene, multiclade HIV DNA given intradermally induces strong and broad immune responses after boosting with heterologous HIV MVA. *Retrovirology* 2009;**6**(Suppl 3):P403.

28 Ulmer JB, Donnelly JJ, Parker SE, *et al*. Heterologous protection against influenza by injection of DNA encoding a viral protein. *Science* 1993;**259**(5102):1745–9.

29 Robinson HL, Hunt LA, Webster RG. Protection against a lethal influenza virus challenge by immunization with a hemagglutinin-expressing plasmid DNA. *Vaccine* 1993;**11**:957–60.

30 Chen M, Cheng T, Huang Y, *et al*. A consensus-hemagglutinin-based DNA vaccine that protects mice against divergent H5N1 influenza viruses. *Proc Natl Acad Sci USA* 2008;**105**(36):13538–43.

31 Ahlén G, Söderholm J, Tjelle T, *et al*. In vivo electroporation enhances the immunogenicity of hepatitis C virus nonstructural 3/4A DNA by increased local DNA uptake, protein expression, inflammation, and infiltration of CD3$^+$ T cells. *J Immunol* 2007;**179**(7):4741–53.

32 Purcell MK, Nichols KM, Winton JR, *et al*. Comprehensive gene expression profiling following DNA vaccination of rainbow trout against infectious hematopoietic necrosis virus. *Mol Immunol* 2006;**43**(13):2089–106.

33 Yasuike M, Kondo H, Hirono I, Aoki T. Difference in Japanese flounder, *Paralichthys olivaceus* gene expression profile following hirame rhabdovirus (HIRRV) G

and N protein DNA vaccination. *Fish Shellfish Immunol* 2007;**23**(3):531–41.

34 Sullivan NJ, Sanchez A, Rollin PE, Yang ZY, Nabel GJ. Development of a preventive vaccine for Ebola virus infection in primates. *Nature* 2000;**408**(6812): 605–9.

35 Rottinghaus ST, Poland GA, Jacobson RM, Barr LJ, Roy MJ. Hepatitis B DNA vaccine induces protective antibody responses in human non-responders to conventional vaccination. *Vaccine* 2003;**21**(31): 4604–8.

36 Liu MA, Wahren B, Karlsson Hedestam GB. DNA vaccines: recent developments and future possibilities. *Human Gene Therapy* 2006;**17**:1051–61.

37 Jaoko W, Karita E, Kayitenkore K, *et al.* Safety and immunogenicity study of multiclade HIV-1 adenoviral vector vaccine alone or as boost following a multiclade HIV-1 DNA vaccine in Africa. *PLoS One* 2010;**5**:e12873.

38 Calarota S, Bratt G, Nordlund S, *et al.* Cellular cytotoxic response induced by DNA vaccination in HIV-1-infected patients. *Lancet* 1998;**351**(9112):1320–25.

39 MacGregor RR, Boyer JD, Ugen KE, *et al.* First human trial of a DNA-based vaccine for treatment of human immunodeficiency virus type 1 infection: safety and host response. *J Infect Dis* 1998;**178**:92–100.

40 Gudmundsdotter L. HIV-1 immune responses induced by natural infection or immunisation, thesis, Karolinska Institute, Stockholm, 2009.

41 Donnelly JJ, Martinez D, Jansen KU, *et al.* Protection against papillomavirus with a polynucleotide vaccine. *J Infect Dis* 1996;**173**(2):314–20.

42 Low L, Mander A, McCann K, *et al.* DNA vaccination with electroporation induces increased antibody responses in patients with prostate cancer. *Hum Gene Ther* 2009;**20**(11):1269–78.

43 Bergman PJ, MA Camps-Palau, McKnight JA, *et al.* Development of a xenogeneic DNA vaccine program for canine malignant melanoma at the Animal Medical Center. *Vaccine* 2006;**24**(21):4582–5.

44 Wolchok JD, Yuan J, Houghton AN, *et al.* Safety and immunogenicity of tyrosinase DNA vaccines in patients with melanoma. *Mol Ther* 2007;**15**(11): 2044–50.

45 Bodles-Brakhop AM, Heller R, Draghia-Akli R. Electroporation for the delivery of DNA-based vaccines and immunotherapeutics: current clinical developments. *Mol Ther* 2009;**17**(4):585–92.

46 Lladser A, Ljungberg K, Tufvesson H, *et al.* (2009) Intradermal DNA electroporation induces survivin-specific CTLs, suppresses angiogenesis and confers protection against mouse melanoma. *Cancer Immunol Immunother* **59**(1):81–92.

47 De Giovanni C, Nicoletti G, Palladini A, *et al.* A multi-DNA preventive vaccine for p53/Neu-driven cancer syndrome. *Hum Gene Ther* 2009;**20**(5):453–64.

48 Solvason N, Lou Y, Peters W, *et al.* Improved efficacy of a tolerizing DNA vaccine for reversal of hyperglycemia through enhancement of gene expression and localization to intracellular sites. *J Immunol* 2008;**181**(12):8298–307.

49 Scheiblhofer S, Gabler M, Leitner WW, *et al.* Inhibition of type I allergic responses with nanogram doses of replicon-based DNA vaccines. *Allergy* 2006;**61**(7): 828–35.

50 Jarman ER, Lamb JR. Reversal of established CD4$^+$ type 2 T helper-mediated allergic airway inflammation and eosinophilia by therapeutic treatment with DNA vaccines limits progression towards chronic inflammation and remodelling. *Immunology* 2004; **112**(4):631–42.

51 Chua K, Kuo I, Huang CH. DNA vaccines for the prevention and treatment of allergy. *Curr Opin Allergy Clin Immunol* 2009;**9**(1):50–54.

52 Liu MA. Gene-based vaccines: Recent developments. *Curr Opin Mol Ther* 2010;**12**(1):86–93. Review.

53 Redding, L, Weiner DB. DNA vaccines in veterinary use. *Expert Rev Vaccines* 2009;**8**(9):1251–76.

54 Hall RA, Khromykh AA. West Nile virus vaccines. *Expert Opin Biol Ther* 2004;**4**:1295–305.

55 Martin JE, Pierson TC, Hubka S, *et al.* A West Nile virus DNA vaccine induces neutralizing antibody in healthy adults during a phase 1 clinical trial. *J Infect Dis* 2007;**196**:1732–40.

56 zur Megede J, Otten GR, Doe B, *et al.* Expression and immunogenicity of sequence-modified human immunodeficiency virus type 1 subtype B pol and gagpol DNA vaccines. *J Virol* 2003;**77**(11): 6197–207.

57 Otten GR, Schaefer M, Doe B, *et al.* Enhanced potency of plasmid DNA microparticle human immunodeficiency virus vaccines in rhesus macaques by using a priming-boosting regimen with recombinant proteins. *J Virol* 2005;**79**(13):8189–200.

58 Lu S, Wang S, Grimes-Serrano JM. Current progress of DNA vaccine studies in humans. *Expert Rev Vaccines* 2008;**7**(2):175–91.

59 Tang DC, DeVit M, Johnston SA, *et al.* Genetic immunization is a simple method for eliciting an immune response. *Nature* 1992;**356**(6365):152–4.

60 Roy MJ, Wu MS, Barr LJ, *et al.* Induction of antigen-specific CD8$^+$ T cells, T helper cells, and protective

levels of antibody in humans by particle-mediated administration of a hepatitis B virus DNA vaccine. *Vaccine* 2000;**19**(7–8):764–78.

61 Spetz AL, Sörensen AS, Walther-Jallow L, *et al.* Induction of HIV-1 specific immunity after vaccination with apoptotic HIV-1/murine leukemia virus-infected cells. *J Immunol* 2002;**169**(10):5771–9.

62 Trimble C, Lin CT, Hung CF, *et al.* Comparison of the CD8$^+$ T cell responses and antitumor effects generated by DNA vaccine administered through gene gun, biojector, and syringe. *Vaccine* 2003;**21**(25–26):4036–42.

63 Lundholm P, Leandersson AC, Christensson B, *et al.* DNA mucosal HIV vaccine in humans. *Virus Research* 2002;**82**(1–2):141–5.

64 Roos A, Eriksson F, Timmons JA, *et al.* Skin electroporation: effects on transgene expression, DNA persistence and local tissue environment. *PLoS One* 2009;**4**(9):e7226.

65 Luckay A, Sidhu MK, Kjeken R, *et al.* Effect of plasmid DNA vaccine design and in vivo electroporation on the resulting vaccine-specific immune responses in rhesus macaques. *J Virol* 2007;**81**(10):5257–69.

CHAPTER 19

Artificial Antigen-presenting Cells: Large Multivalent Immunogens

Matthew F. Mescher & Julie M. Curtsinger
Department of Laboratory Medicine & Pathology, Center for Immunology, University of Minnesota, Minneapolis, MN, USA

Introduction

Induction of long-lived cell-mediated immunity is a major goal of vaccine strategies, with establishment of protective CD8 T lymphocyte memory being a critical component of this immunity. Establishment of CD8 T cell memory is particularly important for pathogens where it has proven difficult to induce neutralizing antibodies, examples being HIV and tuberculosis, as well as for therapeutic vaccines that target cancers. Development of prophylactic and therapeutic vaccination strategies that lead to strong T-cell effector functions and memory has until recently been a largely empirical pursuit, with numerous antigen (Ag) delivery systems and adjuvants being tested. However, our understanding of the basis for T-cell activation has increased greatly in the past several years, and is providing information that is forming the basis for development of a variety of novel strategies for effectively activating T cells *in vivo* through immunization, as well as through *ex vivo* expansion for adoptive transfer therapies. One promising approach being pursued is the use of artificial antigen-presenting cells (APC), either engineered cell lines or inert supports that provide for presentation of Ag and other relevant ligands directly to the T cells. While engineered cells can have great utility for *ex vivo* expansion and adoptive therapy, artificial APCs made using inert supports have greater potential for use as vaccines on a large scale. Numerous such constructs are being developed and tested *in vitro*, and one approach, termed large multivalent immunogen (LMI), is being tested in clinical trials for cancer immunotherapy.

CD8 T-cell activation and memory development

Dendritic cells activate T cells

Dendritic cells (DC) play a central role in normal T-cell activation (Figure 19.1) [1,2]. They reside in peripheral and lymphoid tissues in an immature state, where they express relatively low levels of major histocompatibility complex (MHC) and co-stimulatory proteins but are actively phagocytic and continuously sample Ag from their environment. Upon activation, usually in response to ligation of Toll-like receptors (TLR) or other receptors that recognize products unique to pathogens, the DCs undergo a maturation process. Phagocytosis declines; Ag processing pathways are activated, leading to high levels of expression of MHC proteins displaying Ag-derived peptides; expression of co-stimulatory proteins and cytokines increases; and the DCs are stimulated to migrate to lymph nodes draining the peripheral site (Figure 19.1). Naïve T cells are localized to secondary lymphoid organs, and when they encounter Ag on a mature DC they are activated to undergo clonal expansion over two to three days. Assuming that the

Vaccinology: Principles and Practice, First Edition. Edited by W. John W. Morrow, Nadeem A. Sheikh, Clint S. Schmidt and D. Huw Davies.
© 2012 Blackwell Publishing Ltd. Published 2012 by Blackwell Publishing Ltd.

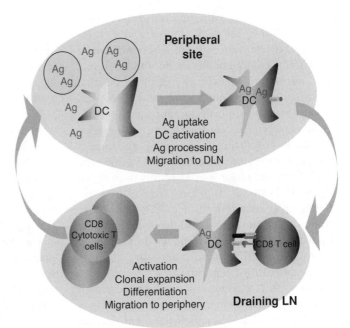

Figure 19.1 Dendritic cells (DC) carry Ag from peripheral sites to the draining lymph nodes (DLN), where they present it to T cells. The T cells respond by proliferating, differentiating to acquire effector functions, and migrating to peripheral sites to carry out their functions.

necessary signals are present, the T cells also differentiate to acquire effector functions and migratory capacity. They then exit the nodes and migrate to the peripheral site of Ag and inflammation, where they carry out their effector functions. Once Ag has been cleared, the majority of the T cells die, but about 5–10% remain as memory cells that reside in both peripheral and lymphoid tissue and are able to mount a rapid, protective response upon re-encounter of the specific Ag.

Conventional vaccines utilize this pathway by delivering the appropriate antigenic epitopes for presentation by DCs, along with an adjuvant to activate the DC. Although many vaccines are effective, in most cases they do not provide a level of protective memory that is comparable to that formed following infection and clearance of a live pathogen. Thus, infection with a live attenuated virus can provide superior protective memory, but applicability of this approach is limited. Development of effective conventional vaccines has been largely empirical, with numerous Ag and adjuvant formulations and dosing and timing regimens being tested to attempt to mimic the effective delivery of T-cell activating signals that are provided during

an infection. New insights into the nature of the critical T-cell activating signals, and their temporal requirements, are contributing to a more rational basis for the design of novel vaccines to optimize generation of effector and memory T cells.

Signals required for activation of naïve CD8 T cells for expansion, effector functions, and memory

Recognition by the T-cell receptor of an antigenic peptide bound to class I MHC protein provides the initial signals to activate cell division and differentiation. It has been appreciated for over twenty years that to be effective this must be accompanied by additional signals from non Ag-specific co-stimulatory receptors binding to their ligands on the APC (see Chapter 3). CD28 is the predominant co-stimulatory receptor, and binds to B7-1 and B7-2 ligands on the APC [3–6]. One consequence of CD28 signaling is increased production by the T cell of IL2, which can support proliferation and contribute to effector and memory development. More recently, it has been realized that, while necessary, the two signals provided by TCR and CD28 engagement are not sufficient to fully activate naïve CD8

T cells [7–9]. In fact, when the cells receive only these signals they proliferate but survival is compromised, effector functions are suboptimal, and a responsive memory population does not develop. Thus, tolerance is induced as a result of deletion and/or anergy induction. A productive CD8 T-cell response leading to full effector function and memory occurs when the cells also receive a third signal provided by an inflammatory cytokine, and there is considerable evidence in support of IL12 and type I IFNs being the major sources of this third signal (Figure 19.2) [8–10]. DCs can produce these cytokines upon activation through TLRs and other receptors [11], and upon CD40-dependent interaction with CD4 T helper cells, and are thus equipped to provide all three signals necessary to fully activate naïve CD8 T cells [11,12].

Naïve CD8 T cells not only need to receive all three signals, but the duration of the signaling is critical for a productive response. *In vivo* imaging studies have shown that an effective challenge with Ag and adjuvant results in the CD8 T cells undergoing prolonged interactions with DCs in the lymph node, lasting many hours to days [13,14]. In contrast, a tolerizing challenge with Ag in the absence of adjuvant results in only brief, transient interactions with the DC [13]. *In vitro* studies have provided additional evidence that prolonged signaling is necessary. Stimulation of naïve cells with Ag and B7-1 for as short a time as a few hours is sufficient to program them to undergo multiple rounds of cell division [15]. However, survival is compromised and effector functions do not develop; for optimum expansion and function, concomitant stimulation with Ag, B7-1, and IL12 for up to 60 hours is required [16].

The ability to form a memory population is programmed by the signals received during the first few days of activation, while expansion and differentiation are occurring [17], and the third signal provided by an inflammatory cytokine is also critical for this early memory programming [18]. Here too, the duration of signaling plays an important role in determining the magnitude and quality of the memory population that develops (unpublished results). Gaining a better understanding of how the cytokine milieu, including cytokines other than IL12 and type I IFNs, influences the magnitude and quality of CD8 memory populations, and how the duration of signaling influences these parameters, will be critical for developing more rational vaccine strategies for optimizing CD8 T cell-mediated protection. This will be particularly true for developing approaches that employ artificial APCs, where it should be possible to control much more precisely the strength, nature, and duration of the signals being delivered than is possible by simply providing a stimulus to endogenous DC.

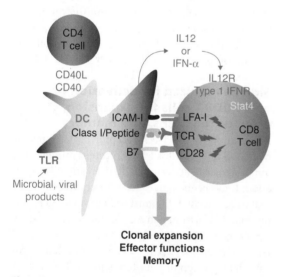

Figure 19.2 Activation of naïve CD8 T cells for optimal development of effector functions and formation of a memory population requires three signals. Signals from the TCR and a co-stimulatory receptor, usually CD28, are required to activate T cells, and are sufficient to stimulate proliferation. A third signal is required, however, to stimulate differentiation for function and memory, and can be provided by IL12 or type I IFN.

Activation of CD8 T cells for tumor immunotherapy

There is increasing evidence that many transformed cells may be eliminated by the immune system before they become detectable tumors or held in check for long periods of time by an ongoing immune response [19,20]. Thus, when overt tumors appear it is likely that they have altered in some way to circumvent the immune response. Nevertheless, in a great majority of cases tumors continue to express Ag that can be recognized by CD8 T cells. Furthermore, the technology now exists to identify these antigenic epitopes that result from mutation or overexpression of normal self-protein by the tumor, and large numbers of MHC class I-restricted Ags have been identified for both murine and human tumors. Despite this, developing strategies for delivering these as a tumor vaccine in a way that activates an effective tumor-specific response remains an elusive goal. Various approaches have shown some promise in murine models and clinical trials, but are not yet at a point of providing routine therapy.

There are numerous mechanisms that can limit T-cell responses to tumors, including low Ag expression, the presence of only low-affinity T cells due to the high-affinity cells having been tolerized through anergy induction or deletion, production of inhibitory factors such as TGF-β by the tumor, and active suppression by T regulatory cells [21]. These latter inhibitory mechanisms may act in part at the level of the T cell, but can also interfere with DC functions. Evidence from numerous models indicates that defective DC function may be a major barrier to activating tumor-specific T cells [21–25]. If so, this also presents a major barrier to conventional vaccine approaches, since attempting to activate responses by delivery of Ag and adjuvant relies on endogenous DC.

One approach for attempting to circumvent this problem has been that of isolating the patient's DC, loading them with Ag, and activating them *in vitro*, away from the suppressive environment, and reinfusing them into the patient to activate T-cell responses [26]. Similarly, there has been a great deal of interest in adoptive therapy using *in vitro* activated T cells from patients, and some limited but dramatic successes have been noted [27,28]. Nevertheless, adoptive therapy with a patient's *in vitro* activated DC or T cells remains a very custom and expensive approach, limiting the ability to treat large numbers of patients. An alternative for overcoming DC functional defects in cancers can potentially be provided by constructing artificial APCs that can bypass the reliance on endogenous DC and provide

all of the signals for activation directly to the T cell. With the exception of LMI, clinical application of artificial APCs has been limited to using them to stimulate the *in vitro* expansion of T cells prior to adoptive immunotherapy, as discussed in the next section.

Artificial APC for *ex vivo* activation and adoptive transfer of T cells

Adoptive transfer of *ex vivo* activated T cells has proven to be a promising approach to bypassing the regulatory mechanisms that limit *in vivo* activation of the cells. Stimulating a patient's specific T cells *in vitro* and expanding them to large numbers, followed by reinfusion, was first shown to have therapeutic potential in immunodeficient bone marrow transplant recipients who are at risk for cytomegalovirus (CMV) disease. Patients who received large numbers of CMV-specific T cells by adoptive transfer were protected from viremia and disease development [29], and this approach has been extended to other infectious diseases [30]. Infusion of *ex vivo* expanded tumor-specific T cells is also showing considerable promise in treating cancers [27,28].

In most of the studies done to examine adoptive immunotherapy, irradiated peripheral blood cells, lymphoblastoid cell lines, or autologous DCs have been used to present Ag or activating antibodies (anti-CD3, anti-CD28, etc.) to the T cells to stimulate activation and *ex vivo* expansion. As a better understanding of the requirements for effective T-cell activation has developed, this information has been used to engineer cell lines to produce artificial APCs that have more potent stimulatory activity. As an example, Maus *et al.* [31] engineered the human K562 cell line, which expresses ICAM and LFA-3 adhesion molecules but does not express class I MHC proteins, to be an effective artificial APC. Cells were transfected with Fcγ receptor (CD32), which allowed stimulatory antibodies such as anti-CD3 and anti-CD28 mAb to be displayed on the surface. The efficiency of stimulation was further increased when the cells were transfected with the ligand for 4-1BB (4-1BBL), a co-stimulatory receptor on T cells. These and other cell-based artificial APCs provide a more uniform and reproducible stimulus, and may circumvent some of the regulatory hurdles encountered when using poorly characterized cells that are of limited availability as APCs.

A further step toward a well-defined, uniform stimulus for activating T cells is the use of acellular particles displaying Ag and other ligands on the surface – that is, fully artificial APCs [32,33]. Such constructs were initially developed as a reductionist approach to defining the requirements for T-cell recognition and activation, where the nature and density of the ligands available for interaction with receptors on the T cell could be precisely defined and varied, and cytokines produced by the APC were not contributing to responses. Early work showed that liposomes having purified class I MHC proteins incorporated onto the surface had some activity in stimulating T-cell responses, but were suboptimal. More effective stimulation was achieved when the class I proteins were incorporated onto inert particles having about the same size as cells [34,35], as discussed in more detail in the following section. A variety of ligands could be incorporated onto the same particle to augment TCR-dependent signaling, including B7-1 and -2 ligands for the CD28 co-stimulatory receptor, and ICAM-1, the ligand for LFA-1 [36–38]. Alternatively, antibodies specific for receptors on the T cell could be immobilized on the particles. Particles of widely varying composition have been used to construct effective artificial APCs, including amorphous silica, latex, magnetic particles, and a variety of polymers, including biodegradable polymers [33]. It appears that the composition of the substrate is not critical as long as it allows formation of stable, cell-sized particles, and that ligands or Abs can be incorporated onto the surface through either adsorption or covalent attachment. There is a great deal of interest in using such artificial APC constructs for *ex vivo* expansion of T cells for adoptive therapy protocols because they provide a well-characterized, uniform, stable, easily modified, and potentially highly efficient stimulus, while avoiding the regulatory issues inherent in using cell-based

APCs. In addition, unlike engineered cellular APCs, there is the potential for using acellular APCs *in vivo* to stimulate T-cell responses. In contrast to particulate constructs designed to target Ag to DC, and activate the DC (see Chapters 13 and 24), acellular APC are designed to directly present Ag and co-stimulatory ligands to T cells. Silica microspheres of 5 μm diameter with Ag displayed on the surface, termed large multivalent immunogen, were the first acellular artificial APCs to be used to study *in vitro* activation of T cells [34]. LMI were also found to have T-cell stimulatory activity *in vivo*, and they are now being tested in clinical trials for tumor immunotherapy.

Artificial APC for *in vivo* T-cell activation: large multivalent immunogen

LMI development and preclinical studies

In early attempts to develop a reductionist approach for studying CD8 T-cell recognition using artificial APCs, we found that effective recognition of isolated class I MHC Ag only occurred if the Ag was displayed on a surface having cell-sized (or larger) dimensions [35]. Ag on the surface of 5 μm diameter microspheres was as effective as Ag-bearing cells in stimulating degranulation by cloned cytotoxic T lymphocyte (CTL) lines, but the response was substantially reduced when 3 μm beads were used, and no response occurred to Ag on 1 μm beads. Similar results were obtained in examining the stimulation of memory CD8 T cells to Ag. Thus, T cells discriminate between Ag having cell-sized dimensions versus Ag on somewhat smaller particles, and large numbers of small particles cannot overcome this size requirement. This suggests that sufficient receptor occupancy over a defined region of the cell surface is required for effective signal generation, perhaps related to the formation of the immunologic synapse.

At that time, there had been numerous reports of attempts to use various forms of tumor Ag to induce or enhance tumor-specific CTL responses for tumor therapy in murine models and in clinical trials. These were largely unsuccessful, but all used Ag in a form that did not meet the critical size requirement demonstrated by *in vitro* experiments. We therefore began experiments to examine the effects of Ag on the cell-sized beads, which we termed large multivalent immunogen, on *in vivo* CTL responses. Initially, we examined the effects of incorporating purified class I alloantigen onto LMI and injecting them into mice [39]. We were unable to detect any generation of a CTL response to the alloantigen; not surprising in retrospect, given the absence of co-stimulatory ligands and signal 3 cytokine. As a control for potential inhibitory effects, however, we also administered alloantigen on LMI to mice that were at the same time challenged by i.p. injection of allogeneic tumor. Mice challenged with allogeneic tumor generate a strong CTL response that is readily measured in a direct *ex vivo* ^{51}Cr release. Surprisingly, we found that the LMI dramatically augmented the CTL response to allogeneic tumor, with increases in lytic activity of 20- to 40-fold, while the same class I Ag incorporated into liposomes (<1 μm diameter) had no effect. Using LMI with purified H-2K^b, K^k, or D^d, and allogeneic EL-4 (H-2^b), P815 (H-2^d), and RDM-4 (H-2^k) tumors, we found that the augmenting effect was Ag-specific; LMI with syngeneic or third-party class I had no effect on response levels, and allo-LMI-augmented responses remained specific for the appropriate allogeneic target.

Prompted by these results, we also examined the effects of LMI on growth of syngeneic tumors and CTL responses to these tumors, in this case using plasma membranes isolated from the tumor cells as the Ag [39–41]. Isolation of plasma membranes results in bilayer membrane vesicles of heterogeneous sizes up to about 1 μm in diameter, and displaying class I MHC protein and other cell-surface proteins. These vesicles can be easily coated onto cell-size particles with a hydrophobic surface to prepare LMI. Using these, we found that administration of LMI at the time of challenge with syngeneic tumor resulted in a large reduction in tumor growth and generation of a detectable tumor-specific CTL response in the mice, while administering the same plasma membrane Ag in free form had no effect. Again, specificity of the LMI ef-

fect was shown using EL-4, P815, and RDM-4 tumors in their respective syngeneic hosts, demonstrating that only LMI prepared from the cognate tumor could mediate tumor growth reduction and CTL generation. Tumor growth was slowed in these experiments, but tumor was not eliminated.

Reduction of tumor growth did not require that the LMI be injected at the tumor site; similar efficacy was obtained whether the LMI were delivered s.c., i.v., or i.p. The effective dose range was between 0.1 and 10 × 10^6 beads/mouse, which is the approximate equivalent of Ag derived from the same number of tumor cells. LMI were found to be uniquely effective in mediating tumor growth reduction and CTL generation; irradiated tumor cells were ineffective, as was free plasma membrane Ag alone or in complete Freund's adjuvant. Finally, the composition of the bead used for preparing the LMI did not appear to influence the activity provided that the surface was sufficiently hydrophobic to allow adsorption of the membrane vesicles; 5 μm diameter beads composed of silica [39–41], latex [34], or polyanhydride polymer (unpublished results) were all found to be effective. Figure 19.3 shows T lymphocytes interacting with Ag on silica-based microspheres.

When we examined therapy of established, progressing tumors we found that treatment with LMI alone had only marginal effects on growth and survival, but found highly synergistic effects when LMI was combined with Cytoxan (Cy) treatment [40]. P815 mastocytoma grows as a solid tumor and spontaneously metastasizes within a few days to LN, spleen, and lungs, and kills the host in about 40 days. To examine LMI effects on established tumors, mice were inoculated with P815 s.c. and left untreated for 8 days, at which time all had visible, palpable tumors. Treatment with Cy alone transiently reduced tumor size, but the tumors began to grow progressively again within a few days and survival was only marginally extended. However, Cy followed 2 to 3 days later by a single injection of LMI resulted in prolonged reduction of growth and significant extension of survival, and in a large fraction of the mice tumor became undetectable and the mice survived indefinitely. When mice that had survived >150 days post-treatment were

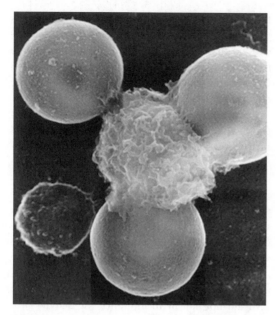

Figure 19.3 Scanning electron micrograph of a murine CD8$^+$ CTL interacting with three Ag-coated 5 μm diameter silica beads (LMI). Reproduced from Mitchell *et al.* [46] with permission from American Association of Cancer Research.

re-challenged with 10^7 P815 tumor cells (the 50% lethal dose of the line used in these experiments is 100 cells/mouse), survival of all of the mice was prolonged in comparison to a naïve control group, and about half survived indefinitely. Thus, mice "cured" in this way appear to have long-term memory.

Results similar to those with P815 were obtained in experiments examining treatment of two different fibrosarcomas (MCA-203 and MCA-207) in a lung metastasis model [40]. Treatment with LMI or Cy alone had marginal effects while combined treatment significantly extended survival, with some of the mice surviving indefinitely. As in the other models examined, LMI effects were specific in that LMI prepared using plasma membrane from a different tumor were ineffective. Again, LMI were uniquely effective in synergizing with Cy to result in prolonged control of tumor; irradiated tumor cells or free plasma membranes alone or with complete Freund's adjuvant were ineffective.

These experiments demonstrated that LMI could specifically augment tumor-specific CTL responses

to control of tumor growth, and could mediate significant therapeutic effects when used in combination with chemotherapy. Furthermore, Ag in this form appeared to be uniquely effective. CD8 T cells can directly recognize and respond to Ag on LMI *in vitro* [35], and the *in vivo* effects of LMI may also result from direct recognition. This would be consistent with the strong LMI-dependent augmentation of allogeneic CTL responses [39], where uptake and processing of the LMI would not lead to host re-presentation of the native alloantigen recognized by the CTL. It is possible that a mechanism exists for transfer of the intact alloantigen from the beads to the surface of host APC, although this seems unlikely. In the case of responses to syngeneic tumor Ag, LMI effects could result from either (or both) direct recognition of peptide/class I complexes on the membranes coating the LMI, or from uptake, processing, and re-presentation by host APC. Irrespective of the mechanism involved in LMI-mediated CTL augmentation, the unique therapeutic effects of Ag in this form warranted clinical testing of this approach.

Clinical trials using LMI immunotherapy

There have been numerous melanoma vaccine trials targeting CD8 T-cell responses, employing tumor cell lysates or peptide-epitopes as Ag, delivered in a variety of ways, including with adjuvants, DCs, or other forms of immune potentiation [42–44]. These trials have demonstrated that vaccination can increase the frequency of circulating melanoma-specific CD8 T cells in patients, yet objective responses evaluated according to Response Evaluation Criteria in Solid Tumors (RECIST) have been very rare. Some of these trials are promising when judged by criteria such as survival or time to progression, but the small numbers of patients in such trials make it difficult to judge their significance [45]. The initial clinical evaluation of LMI immunotherapy was carried out for melanoma.

Phase I trial of allogeneic LMI vaccine for melanoma

An initial phase I trial of LMI therapy for metastatic (stage IV) melanoma was conducted by Dr Malcolm

Mitchell at UC San Diego that demonstrated safety and suggested potential efficacy [46]. LMI were prepared by coating 5 μm silica beads with plasma membrane Ag purified from two melanoma cell lines grown *in vitro*, and patients were selected to be HLA-A2$^+$, an Ag expressed on one of the lines. A total of 15 patients were treated using 3 dose levels of LMI vaccine (10, 30, and 100 million beads) given monthly for 3 months without adjuvant. For each treatment, one-half of the dose was given intradermally and the other half s.c.; 8 of the 15 patients had a 2- to 10-fold increase in CTL precursor frequency above pretreatment baselines, usually by day 42. Precursor frequencies were assessed based on reactivity to the HLA-A2$^+$ melanoma cell line used to make the vaccine, and did not distinguish between alloreactive versus syngeneic tumor-specific CTL. Stable disease was seen in 5 patients at 12 weeks; one patient had a greater than 50% regression of a lung nodule but progression of disease to the brain; and another patient had partial remission of a 3 cm diameter solitary lung nodule. Most importantly, the vaccine was safe and well tolerated at all doses. Thus, injection of the artificial APC either intradermally or s.c. resulted in no significant detrimental effects either locally or systemically.

Autologous LMI vaccine for melanoma and renal carcinoma

Based on the phase I trial results [46], we initiated trials at the University of Minnesota Cancer Center to examine LMI therapy in stage IV metastatic melanoma and renal cell carcinoma (RCC) using plasma membrane from the surgically resected autologous tumors as the source of Ag for the LMI preparation. As for melanoma, there is considerable evidence to suggest that immune responses have the potential to be beneficial for RCC, and tumors can be obtained from many of these patients in sufficient quantity to isolate plasma membranes for LMI preparation.

The effects of Cy were examined in these trials because the murine studies had demonstrated synergistic effects of combining LMI and Cy [40]. In addition, low-dose IL2 was examined, based on the effects of IL2 found in murine tumor models. Upon acquisition of effector functions, activated CD8 T cells lose the ability to produce IL2 upon re-encounter with Ag, and cannot continue to expand in number, a state termed "activation-induced non-responsiveness" (AINR) [47]. However, the cells remain responsive to IL2, and if IL2 is provided they undergo further proliferation. Furthermore, within one to two days the cells regain the ability to produce IL2 and can then continue to proliferate in response to Ag without provision of additional exogenous IL2. Following an initial expansion in response to a syngeneic tumor, CTL that have become AINR can be reactivated to proliferate and continue to control tumor growth by administration of IL2 [48]. Similarly, CD8 T cells responding to lymphocytic choriomeningitis virus (LCMV) become anergic by day 8 [49], and administration of IL2 at this time leads to maintenance of higher numbers of cells [50]. AINR appears to act as a "helper-dependent check point" in the CD8 T cell response, with IL2 produced by the CD4 T helper cells giving "permission" to the CD8 cells to continue to expand. Thus, the absence of IL2-dependent help following the initial clonal expansion of the CD8 T cells can result in a form of tolerance, in that effector cells are present in insufficient numbers to clear the remaining Ag and cannot expand further. IL2 administration can have opposing effects on CD8 T cells responding to tumor; promoting expansion by reversing AINR but also inducing subsequent apoptotic death of the reactivated effector cells if given for a prolonged period [48], consistent with IL2 promoting activation-induced cell death (AICD) in activated T cells [51]. Based on these findings in murine models, one arm of the autologous melanoma and RCC LMI trials included administration of a short course of low-dose IL2 beginning 5 days after vaccination.

Thirty patients each for melanoma and renal carcinoma were randomized onto one of three treatment arms: (i) LMI alone (1 × 10^7), (ii) low-dose Cy (300 mg/m^2 i.v.) followed 8 days later by LMI, and (iii) Cy and LMI (day 8) followed in 5 days by a short course of low-dose IL2 (1.75 × 10^6 IU/m^2/day for 7 days). LMI were delivered by intradermal injection and treatments were given monthly while sufficient vaccine remained available, which depended upon the amount of tumor obtained from the patient. The median number of doses given was 2, and ranged from 1 to 8. No grade 4 toxicities were observed, and none of the patients discontinued protocol due to toxicity. The results of this autologous trial have recently been reported [52], and are briefly summarized here.

Tetramer analysis was done for six HLA-A2$^+$ melanoma patients using MART-1, gp100, and tyrosinase peptide epitopes (and EBV- and CMV-specific control tetramers). Three of the six patients showed an increase in frequency of binding of at least one of the melanoma-specific tetramers in the two post-vaccine samples examined, and two additional patients showed an increase in one of the two post-vaccine samples. Two patients had a partial clinical response, one RCC patient in group 3 and one melanoma patient in group 2. The latter had tumor shrinkage documented at 3, 8, and 12 months after LMI administration. In addition, two melanoma patients developed vitiligo during the course of treatment, both in group 1. Thus, the limited analysis that could be done for this autologous trial suggested that LMI therapy was increasing the numbers of tumor-specific CD8 T cells, at least in some patients.

Kaplan-Meier estimates for overall survival for the 30 RCC patients and 30 melanoma patients are shown in Figure 19.4, with superimposed survival curves taken from the literature for stage IV melanoma and RCC patients treated in various ways. For RCC, the median overall survival for the 30 LMI-treated patients was 46.2 months (95% CI: 30.3 – not assessable: upper bound not estimable due to small number of events). The superimposed curves show survival for 420 patients treated with IFN-α alone, IL2 alone, or the combination [53], and agree with other reports of 18-month median survival for patients receiving s.c. low-dose IL2 and IFN-α regimens [54,55].

For melanoma, median overall survival for all 30 LMI-treated patients was 20.4 months (95% CI: 8.0 – not assessable: upper bound not estimable due to small number of events). The superimposed survival curves are taken from a recent report of the analysis of the treatment history and survival of 212 metastatic melanoma pa-

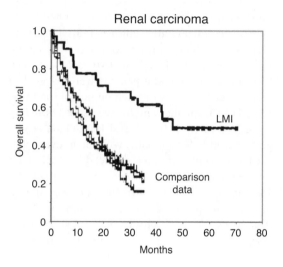

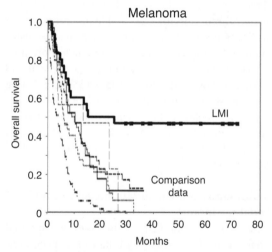

Figure 19.4 Kaplan-Meier estimates for overall survival of LMI-treated renal carcinoma ($n = 30$) and melanoma ($n = 30$) patients [52]. Comparison data for RCC is from Negrier *et al.* [53] for treatments with IL2 ($n = 140$), IFN-α ($n = 138$), and IL2/IFN-α ($n = 147$). Comparison data for melanoma is from Khan *et al.* [56] for untreated ($n = 70$) or treatments with DITC ($n = 40$), MDR ($n = 19$), biochemotherapy ($n = 57$), and Temozolamide/Thalidomide ($n = 21$).

tients treated at Moffitt Cancer Center from 1998 to 2003 [56], with treatments including chemotherapy and biochemotherapy (see legend to Figure 19.4). In the most recent trials by Rosenberg's group at the NIH [28] about 5×10^{10} *ex vivo* expanded tumor-infiltrating lymphocytes (TIL) were infused into melanoma patients following a non-myeloablative regimen that included Cy and fludarabine prior to infusion, and followed by administration of 7.2×10^5 IU/kg IL2 every 8 h for 2 to 3 days. Objective responses were seen in 21/43 patients (49%), and in 13/25 patients (52%) who also received 2 Gy total body irradiation. Three-year survival for patients with the chemotherapy regimen alone was 25%, versus 42% for patients who also received 2 Gy total body irradiation, while a group that received no lymphodepletion had 14% survival. While objective responses were much more frequent in this study than in our LMI trial, survival times were comparable. Comparison of survival for melanoma patients in the three LMI treatment groups showed that group 1 (LMI alone) had better overall survival than groups 2 and 3 ($p = 0.01$ and $p = 0.11$ versus groups 2 and 3, respectively). Although the small size of the groups (10 patients/group) clearly does not allow definitive conclusions, there is the impression that Cy may have interfered with an LMI effect, and that inclusion of IL2 partially reversed the interference.

While the results of these trials appear promising, there were significant limitations stemming from the use of autologous tumors as the source of Ag, including: (i) sufficient Ag could not be obtained from some patients for LMI preparation, and low Ag amounts limited the number of immunizations for others; (ii) the custom nature of autologous LMI therapy made the approach costly and of limited applicability; and (iii) immunomonitoring to assess responses to the therapy was limited by the lack of relevant tumor lines and identified class I epitopes. We have now begun a melanoma trial that circumvents these limitations by using a melanoma cell line as the source of Ag for preparation of the LMI, with enrollment limited to patients who share at least one class I MHC protein with the cell line. This will allow us to gain further information regarding the potential clinical efficacy of the LMI approach, allow a detailed assessment of immune responses in the patients, and make it possible to test a number of hypotheses regarding the status of melanoma-specific CD8 T cells in patients. Although it remains to be determined if LMI immunotherapy can have significant efficacy, the results of these trials clearly demonstrate that artificial APCs made using a solid support can safely be administered to patients.

Future directions

Studies of LMI in murine models have clearly shown that acellular artificial APCs can be used *in vivo* to significantly affect CD8 T-cell responses in an Ag-specific manner to promote tumor reduction. In addition, clinical trials using LMI have demonstrated that this approach is safe in humans, and suggested that tumor-specific immune responses may be affected. The effects of *in vivo* administration of Ag on LMI are summarized in Box 19.1. Numerous possibilities exist for refinement and optimization of the use of acellular APC for therapeutic vaccines, and potentially for prophylactic vaccines, and many of these are well along in development for *in vitro* applications.

The LMI used thus far for clinical trials were prepared using 5 μm diameter microspheres composed of amorphous silica. Following injection,

---

Box 19.1 Summary of the *in vivo* properties of Ag on LMI. The summary is based on results obtained in studies of murine models [35,39–41,57] and in clinical trials [46,52].

In vivo properties of Ag on LMI

- **Non-toxic when injected s.c. (mouse, human), i.d. (human), i.p. or i.v. (mouse)**

- **No detectable CTL response induced in absence of tumor**

- **Augments CTL responses to tumors**
  - Ag-specific: requires same Ag on LMI and tumor
  - Effector CTL are specific

- **Reduces growth of syngeneic tumor**

- **Injection at tumor site is not necessary for tumor reduction**
  - Intraperitoneal, subcutaneous and intravenous routes are effective

- **Physical form of Ag is critical**
  - Cell-size (5 μm diameter) support is optimal
  - No augmentation with Ag in membranes or adjuvant, or irradiated tumor cells)

these microspheres probably degrade over time at body temperature and pH, but use of biodegradable polymers would clearly be preferable. Many such polymers have been formulated that can be prepared as microspheres and have a chemistry compatible with attachment of membrane vesicles or proteins to the surface by adsorption or covalent attachment [33].

Murine studies have shown that purified class I MHC protein on LMI can mediate augmentation of allogeneic CTL responses [39], and that LMI bearing class I on the surface can be loaded with tumor-specific peptide and used to augment responses to syngeneic tumor [57]. Additional proteins can easily be co-immobilized on the microsphere surface, and this can contribute to enhanced *in vitro* activation of T cells [36–38]. Whether this approach will also enhance *in vivo* effects of LMI remains to be determined. Numerous T-cell epitopes expressed by human tumors have been identified and this, together with the ready availability of human recombinant MHC proteins, makes it feasible to design LMI targeted to specific tumors based on a patient's MHC haplotype.

While not as well defined, LMI made using plasma membranes from tumor cells [39,40,52] have the advantage that the entire spectrum of tumor-specific peptides should be displayed on the surface, potentially allowing recruitment into the response of more T cells than could be achieved using one or a few defined peptide epitopes. If allogeneic tumor cell lines that share at least one class I MHC protein with the patient prove to be effective, as is being tested in ongoing LMI trials, then a few cell lines would be sufficient for preparing LMI to treat the majority of patients. Here too, co-stimulatory ligands can readily be included by transfecting the tumor cell line so that the relevant protein is expressed on the cell surface, and thus on the LMI made from plasma membranes derived from the cell. We are employing this approach in the ongoing allogeneic melanoma trial by using a melanoma line that has been transfected with B7-1.

Finally, it may be possible to construct acellular APCs that fully mimic DCs by providing all of the signals needed to fully activate naïve CD8

T cells [9]. Thus, a biodegradable microsphere with encapsulated IL12 or type I IFN-α, and Ag and co-stimulatory ligands on the surface, could potentially provide all three signals needed for full activation of naïve CD8 T cells. It might also be possible to include IL2 in the microspheres so that it is released at the appropriate time (3 to 4 days) and in the appropriate amount following initial activation of the T cell to stimulate further expansion of the cells. In order to achieve the prolonged interaction with Ag that is necessary for CD8 T-cell activation, while providing the early cytokine signal, a microsphere that maintained surface presentation of Ag and co-stimulatory ligands while degrading to release the cytokines might be needed. Steenblock and Fahmy [58] have recently reported a significant step in the direction of such acellular APCs to mimic DCs. They prepared poly(lactide-co-glycolide) microparticles having anti-CD28 mAb and either anti-CD3 mAb or class I protein with bound peptide Ag attached to the surface, and having IL2 encapsulated in the biodegradable core, and demonstrated that these were highly effective in stimulating T-cell responses *in vitro*. In fact, provision of IL2 via the microparticles was more effective than exogenous addition of IL2 to the cultures. An acellular APC that fully reproduced the activation achieved by DCs would have potential for use not only for therapeutic vaccines, but also for prophylactic vaccines.

Acknowledgments

Research described was supported in part by grants RO1 CA82956 and RO1 AI34834 from the National Institutes of Health.

References

1 Heath WR, Carbone FR. Cross-presentation, dendritic cells, tolerance and immunity. *Annu Rev Immunol* 2001;**19**:47–64.

2 Steinman RM, Hemmi H. Dendritic cells: translating innate to adaptive immunity. *Curr Top Microbiol Immunol* 2006;**311**:17–58.

3 Allison JP. CD28-B7 interactions in T cell activation. *Curr Opin Immunol* 1994;**6**:414–19.

4 Jenkins M, Taylor P, Norton S, Urdahl K. CD28 delivers a costimulatory signal involved in antigen-specific IL-2 production by human T cells. *J Immunol* 1991;**147**:2461–6.

5 June CH, Bluestone JA, Nadler LM, Thompson CB. The B7 and CD28 receptor families. *Immunol Today* 1994;**15**:321–31.

6 Mueller D, Jenkins M, Schwartz R. Clonal expansion vs functional clonal inactivation. *Annu Rev Immunol* 1989;**7**:445–80.

7 Curtsinger JM, Lins DC, Mescher MF. Signal 3 determines tolerance versus full activation of naive CD8 T cells: dissociating proliferation and development of effector function. *J Exp Med* 2003;**197**:1141–51.

8 Curtsinger JM, Schmidt CS, Mondino A, *et al.* Inflammatory cytokines provide third signals for activation of naive CD4$^+$ and CD8$^+$ T cells. *J Immunol* 1999;**162**:3256–62.

9 Mescher MF, Curtsinger JM, Agarwal P, *et al.* Signals required for programming effector and memory development by CD8$^+$ T cells. *Immunol Rev* 2006; **211**:81–92.

10 Curtsinger JM, Valenzuela JO, Agarwal P, Lins D, Mescher MF. Type I IFNs provide a third signal to CD8 T cells to stimulate clonal expansion and differentiation. *J Immunol* 2005;**174**:4465–9.

11 Hochrein H, Shortman K, Vremec D, *et al.* Differential production of IL-12, IFN-alpha, and IFN-gamma by mouse dendritic cell subsets. *J Immunol* 2001;**166**:5448–55.

12 Cella M, Scheidegger D, Palmer-Lehmann K, *et al.* Ligation of CD40 on dendritic cells triggers production of high levels of interleukin-12 and enhances T cell stimulatory capacity: T-T help via APC activation. *J Exp Med* 1996;**184**:747–52.

13 Hugues S, Fetler L, Bonifaz L, *et al.* Distinct T cell dynamics in lymph nodes during the induction of tolerance and immunity. *Nature Immunol* 2004;**5**:1235–42.

14 Mempel TR, Henrickson SE, von Andrian UH. T-cell priming by dendritic cells in lymph nodes occurs in three distinct phases. *Nature* 2004;**427**:154–9.

15 van Stipdonk MJ, Lemmens EE, Schoenberger SP. Naive CTLs require a single brief period of antigenic stimulation for clonal expansion and differentiation. *Nat Immunol* 2001;**2**:423–9.

16 Curtsinger JM, Johnson CM, Mescher MF. CD8 T cell clonal expansion and development of effector function require prolonged exposure to antigen, costimulation, and signal 3 cytokine. *J Immunol* 2003;**171**:5165–71.

17 Kaech SM, Ahmed R. Memory CD8$^+$ T cell differentiation: initial antigen encounter triggers a developmental program in naive cells. *Nat Immunol* 2001; **2**:415–22.

18 Xiao Z, Casey KA, Jameson SC, Curtsinger JM, Mescher MF. Programming for CD8 T cell memory development requires IL-12 or type I IFN. *J Immunol* 2009;**182**:2786–94.

19 Bui JD, Schreiber RD. Cancer immunosurveillance, immunoediting and inflammation: independent or interdependent processes? *Curr Opin Immunol* 2007;**19**:203–8.

20 Dunn GP, Koebel CM, Schreiber RD. Interferons, immunity and cancer immunoediting. *Nat Rev Immunol* 2006;**6**:836–48.

21 Rabinovich GA, Gabrilovich D, Sotomayor EM. Immunosuppressive strategies that are mediated by tumor cells. *Annu Rev Immunol* 2007;**25**:267–96.

22 Gerner MY, Casey KA, Mescher MF. Defective MHC class II presentation by dendritic cells limits CD4 T cell help for antitumor CD8 T cell responses. *J Immunol* 2008;**181**:155–64.

23 Gerner MY, Mescher MF. Antigen processing and MHC-II presentation by dermal and tumor-infiltrating dendritic cells. *J Immunol* 2009;**182**:2726–37.

24 Perrot I, Blanchard D, Freymond N, *et al.* Dendritic cells infiltrating human non-small cell lung cancer are blocked at immature stage. *J Immunol* 2007;**178**:2763–9.

25 Vicari AP, Chiodoni C, Vaure C, *et al.* Reversal of tumor-induced dendritic cell paralysis by CpG immunostimulatory oligonucleotide and anti-interleukin 10 receptor antibody. *J Exp Med* 2002;**196**:541–9.

26 Nencioni A, Grünebach F, Schmidt SM, *et al.* The use of dendritic cells in cancer immunotherapy. *Crit Rev Oncol Hematol* 2008;**65**:191–9.

27 June CH. Adoptive T cell therapy for cancer in the clinic. *J Clin Invest* 2007;**117**:1466–76.

28 Rosenberg SA, Restifo NP, Yang JC, Morgan RA, Dudley ME. Adoptive cell transfer: a clinical path to effective cancer immunotherapy. *Nat Rev Cancer* 2008; **8**:299–308.

29 Walter EA, Greenberg PD, Gilbert MJ, *et al.* Reconstitution of cellular immunity against cytomegalovirus in recipients of allogeneic bone marrow by transfer of T-cell clones from the donor. *N Engl J Med* 1995;**333**:1038–44.

30 Ho WY, Yee C, Greenberg PD. Adoptive therapy with CD8$^+$ T cells: it may get by with a little help from its friends. *J Clin Invest* 2002;**110**:1415–17.

31 Maus MV, Thomas AK, Leonard DGB, *et al*. Ex vivo expansion of polyclonal and antigen-specific cytotoxic T lymphocytes by artificial APCs expressing ligands for the T-cell receptor, CD28 and 4-1BB. *Nat Biotechnol* 2002;**20**:143–8.

32 Oelke M, Krueger C, Giuntoli RL, 2nd, Schneck JP. Artificial antigen-presenting cells: artificial solutions for real diseases. *Trends Mol Med* 2005;**11**: 412–20.

33 Steenblock ER, Wrzesinski SH, Flavell RA, Fahmy TM. Antigen presentation on artificial acellular substrates: modular systems for flexible, adaptable immunotherapy. *Expert Opin Biol Ther* 2009;**9**:451–64.

34 Goldstein S, Mescher M. Cell-size, supported artificial membranes (pseudocytes): response of precursor cytotoxic T lymphocytes to class 1 proteins. *J Immunol* 1986;**137**:3383–92.

35 Mescher MF. Surface contact requirements for activation of cytotoxic T lymphocytes. *J Immunol* 1992;**149**:2402–5.

36 Deeths MJ, Mescher MF. B7-1-dependent costimulation results in qualitatively and quantitatively different responses in CD4$^+$ and CD8$^+$ T cells. *Eur J Immunol* 1997;**27**:598–608.

37 Deeths MJ, Mescher MF. ICAM-1 and B7-1 provide similar but distinct costimulation for CD8$^+$ T cells, while CD4$^+$ T cells are poorly costimulated by ICAM-1. *Eur J Immunol* 1999;**29**:45–53.

38 Tham EL, Jensen PL, Mescher MF. Activation of antigen-specific T cells by artificial cell constructs having immobilized multimeric peptide-class I complexes and recombinant B7-Fc proteins. *J Immunol Methods* 2001;**249**:111–19.

39 Rogers J, Mescher M. Augmentation of *in vivo* cytotoxic T lymphocyte activity and reduction of tumor growth by large multivalent immunogen. *J Immunol* 1992;**149**:269–76.

40 Mescher M, Rogers J. Immunotherapy of established murine tumors with large multivalent immunogen and cyclophosphamide. *J Immunother* 1996; **19**:102–12.

41 Mescher MF, Savelieva E. Stimulation of tumor-specific immunity using tumor cell plasma membrane antigen. *Methods* 1997;**12**:155–64.

42 Ribas A, Butterfield LH, Glaspy JA, Economou JS. Current developments in cancer vaccines and cellular immunotherapy. *J Clin Oncol* 2003;**21**:2415–32.

43 Slingluff CL, Chianese-Bullock KA, Bullock TN, *et al*. Immunity to melanoma antigens: from self-tolerance to immunotherapy. *Adv Immunol* 2006;**90**: 243–95.

44 Sondak VK, Sabel MS, Mulé JJ. Allogeneic and autologous melanoma vaccines: where have we been and where are we going? *Clin Cancer Res* 2006;**12** (7 Pt 2):2337s–41s.

45 Rosenberg SA, Yang JC, Restifo NP. Cancer immunotherapy: moving beyond current vaccines. 2004;**10**:909–15.

46 Mitchell MS, Kan-Mitchell J, Morrow PR, *et al*. Phase I trial of large multivalent immunogen derived from melanoma lysates in patients with disseminated melanoma. *Clin Cancer Res* 2004;**10**:76–83.

47 Deeths MJ, Kedl RM, Mescher MF. CD8$^+$ T cells become nonresponsive (anergic) following activation in the presence of costimulation. *J Immunol* 1999;**163**: 102–10.

48 Shrikant P, Mescher MF. Opposing effects of interleukin-2 in tumor immunotherapy: promoting CD8 T cell growth and inducing apoptosis. *J Immunol* 2002;**169**:1753–9.

49 Kaech SM, Hemby S, Kersh E, Ahmed R. Molecular and functional profiling of memory CD8 T cell differentiation. *Cell* 2002;**111**:837–51.

50 Blattman JN, Grayson JM, Wherry EJ, *et al*. Therapeutic use of IL-2 to enhance antiviral T-cell responses in vivo. *Nat Med* 2003;**9**:540–47.

51 Lenardo MJ. Interleukin-2 programs mouse alpha beta T lymphocytes for apoptosis. *Nature* 1991;**353**: 858–61.

52 Dudek AZ, Mescher MF, Okazaki I, *et al*. Autologous large multivalent immunogen vaccine (LMI) in patients with metastatic melanoma and renal cell carcinoma. *Am J Clin Oncol* 2008;**31**:173–81.

53 Negrier S, Escudier B, Lasset C, *et al*. Recombinant human interleukin-2, recombinant human interferon alfa-2a, or both in metastatic renal-cell carcinoma. *N Engl J Med* 1998;**338**:1272–8.

54 Figlin RA, Belldegrun A, Moldawer N, Zeffren J, deKernion J. Concomitant administration of recombinant human interleukin-2 and recombinant interferon alfa-2A: an active outpatient regimen in metastatic renal cell carcinoma. *J Clin Oncol* 1992;**10**: 414–21.

55 Yang JC, Sherry RM, Steinberg SM, *et al*. Randomized study of high-dose and low-dose interleukin-2 in patients with metastatic renal cancer. *J Clin Oncol* 2003;**21**:3127–32.

56 Khan MA, Andrews S, Ismail-Khan R, *et al.* Overall and progression-free survival in metastatic melanoma: analysis of a single-institution database. *Cancer Control* 2006;**13**:211–17.

57 Goldberg J, Shrikant P, Mescher MF. In vivo augmentation of tumor-specific CTL responses by class I/peptide antigen complexes on microspheres (large multivalent immunogen). *J Immunol* 2003; **170**:228–35.

58 Steenblock ER, Fahmy TM. A comprehensive platform for ex vivo T-cell expansion based on biodegradable polymeric artificial antigen-presenting cells. *Mol Ther* 2008;**16**:765–72.

PART 5

Delivery Systems

CHAPTER 20

Transcutaneous Immunization via Vaccine Patch Delivery System

Robert C. Seid, Jr & Gregory M. Glenn

Intercell USA, Inc., Gaithersburg, MD, USA

Introduction

Since the pioneering work of Glenn *et al.* [1,2], transcutaneous immunization (TCI) has been continually evolving as a noninvasive technique that capitalizes on the skin immune system. The skin offers an attractive site for vaccination due to the presence of a diverse population of resident antigen-presenting cells (APCs) and other immunocompetent cells. Most notable among the skin immune cells are the Langerhans cells (LCs), which reside in the viable epidermis, and are sufficiently networked to form a tight mesh to detect, capture, and process exogenous antigens that breach the stratum corneum (SC) barrier. Because of their specialized roles in antigen uptake and in transporting processed antigens to nearby skin-draining lymph nodes (LNs) to initiate immune responses, LCs appear to be the pivotal skin immune cells targeted by TCI.

To initiate adaptive immune responses to vaccine antigens via the skin, our laboratory has advanced two major platform applications of TCI (Figure 20.1). The first is the vaccine delivery patch (VDP), which involves a needle-free administration of antigen either alone or together with adjuvant, onto skin. The operating principle of the VDP involves passive diffusion of the antigen and/or adjuvant from the patch onto the skin and into the superficial layers of the skin. There, the LCs cap-

ture and process the antigen/adjuvant molecules and transport them to regional skin-draining LNs to induce antibody and cellular immune responses (see Chapter 3 for a review of antigen processing and presentation).

The second TCI platform is the vaccine enhancement patch (VEP), formerly known as the immunostimulant patch [3,4]. The VEP contains only the adjuvant and is used in combination with an injected vaccine (Figure 20.1). The VEP patch works similarly to the VDP. The adjuvant molecules passively diffuse out of the patch to reach the targeted epidermal LCs. Sensing the "danger signal," the LCs become activated and migrate to the same draining lymph node field as the injected vaccines. We have proposed that the adjuvant-activated LCs can exert bystander enhancing effects on the immune response to the vaccine antigen(s) injected in the same draining lymph node field [3–6].

Within the past decade, there has been a surge of interest in evaluating TCI as an alternative route of vaccine delivery. Table 20.1 gives a list of TCI studies published in scientific journals, and includes applications for bacterial [1,2,7–21], viral [3,4,22–39], and miscellaneous [40–42] diseases. While a vast majority of TCI studies have been performed and validated in animal models, several clinical studies have recently been published [9,12,15,27,38, 42]. Our aims for this chapter are (i) to provide current perspectives on skin immunology and TCI

Vaccinology: Principles and Practice, First Edition. Edited by W. John W. Morrow, Nadeem A. Sheikh, Clint S. Schmidt and D. Huw Davies.
© 2012 Blackwell Publishing Ltd. Published 2012 by Blackwell Publishing Ltd.

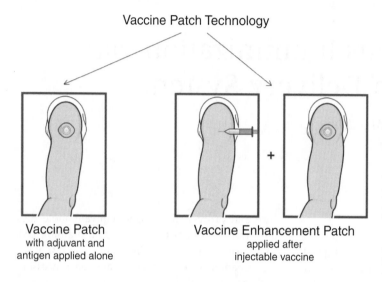

Vaccine Patch Technology

Vaccine Patch
with adjuvant and
antigen applied alone

Vaccine Enhancement Patch
applied after
injectable vaccine

Figure 20.1 Platform applications of vaccine patch technology. The vaccine patch (left) contains both antigen and adjuvant and is applied on the arm. The vaccine enhancement patch (right) contains only adjuvant and is applied on the arm receiving an injectable vaccine.

mechanism, (ii) to review lessons learned from TCI preclinical studies, (iii) to present key findings of recent TCI clinical studies, and (iv) to describe technical breakthroughs for a late-stage, integrated dry patch vaccine delivery system. In addition to TCI, there are other alternative needle-free routes for vaccine administration (see Chapter 4 for mucosal immunity and vaccine development and Chapter 21 for the use of Biojector® approaches for immunization).

Skin immunology system and TCI mechanism

The human skin consists of three layers – the SC (10–20 μm), the epidermis (50–100 μm), and the dermis (1–3 mm). The SC consists of dead or quiescent and flat keratinocytes (KCs) surrounded by a lipid mortar. The SC is the chief barrier to skin permeation by drugs and antigens. Underneath the SC is the epidermis, which is a continuously growing layer of viable KCs that constitute about 95% of epithelial cells. Populating the epidermis at about 1–3% of all epidermal cells are the LCs, which, because of their long dendrites, cover about 25% of the total skin surface area. Given their prominence in the epidermis, and their capacity to pick up antigen and carry it to skin-draining LNs, LCs

are considered to be the key APCs for TCI. Separated from the epidermis is the dermis, which contains connective tissues, blood vessels, lymphatics, nerve endings, hair follicles, and sweat glands. Also present is a second class of APCs, called the dermal dendritic cells (dDC), which are considered to play a pivotal role in the initiation of cutaneous immune response by intradermal (i.d.) immunization [43]. Other immunocompetent cells present in the epidermal and dermal layers are the KCs, macrophages, and T lymphocytes, as well as a low number of B cells and natural killer (NK) cells [44].

TCI generally utilizes passive diffusion of antigen from a skin patch to the resident, immature LCs in the epidermis. As immune sentinel cells, the LCs take up the antigens, become activated, and undergo a complex maturation process resulting in upregulation of major histocompatibility complex (MHC) class II proteins and co-stimulatory molecules [45–47]. During maturation, the LCs migrate from the epidermis to the regional skin-draining LNs where they present processed antigenic fragments to T and B cells to induce antigen-specific CD4+ and CD8+ T-cell production as well as systemic and mucosal immunity. The epidermal KCs also participate in the skin immune response to exogenous antigens. Bearing Toll-like receptors on their surfaces, the KCs become activated during

Table 20.1 TCI "proof-of-concept" studies within the past ten years.

Vaccines	TCI platform: VDP or VEP Wet or dry	Antigen(s)	Adjuvant(s)	Species tested	Pretreatment of shaved skin	Major finding(s)	Ref.
Bacterial							
Cholera	VDP Wet	Cholera toxin	Same as antigen	Mice	Vaccine solution on skin	Systemic and mucosal anti-CT IgG and IgA induced; protection against lethal mucosal toxin challenge	[1]
Diphtheria	VDP Wet	Diphtheria toxoid	CT	Mice	Vaccine solution on skin	Anti-DT Ab responses comparable to i.m. and i.n. routes	[2]
Tetanus	VDP Wet	Tetanus fragment C and tetanus toxoid	CT	Mice	Vaccine solution on skin	Anti-TetC and anti-TTx Ab induced; protection against systemic toxin challenge	[11]
	VDP Wet	TTxd	LTR72 and other LT mutants	Mice	Hydration followed by vaccine solution on skin	Enhanced anti-TT Ab responses; passive protection in mice	[19]
	VDP Wet	TetC and TTxd	None	Mice	Skin treated with depilatory cream followed by hydration	TetC more potent than TTx in inducing toxin neutralizing Abs; T-cell responses elicited	[20]
	VDP Wet	TTx	None	Mice	Wet TTx patch on unshaved ear for prolonged time	Non-adjuvanted TCI induced serum anti-TTx Ab comparable to adjuvanted TCI; protection provided against TT challenge	[16]

(Continued)

Table 20.1 TCI "proof-of-concept" studies within the past ten years. (*Continued*)

Vaccines	TCI platform: VDP or VEP Wet or dry	Antigen(s)	Adjuvant(s)	Species tested	Pretreatment of shaved skin	Major finding(s)	Ref.
Haemophilus influenza type b	VDP Wet	PRP-CRM$_{197}$ glycoconjugate	CT and LT mutants	Rats	Hydration followed by vaccine solution on skin	High-titer Abs induced to PRP; passive protection in infant rats	[14]
Bacillus anthracis	VDP Wet	rPA	LT	Mice, rabbits	Hydration followed by skin abrasion	Toxin neutralizing anti-rPA Ab induced; protection against aerosolized *B. anthracis* in mice	[13]
	VDP Wet	rPA	LT	Mice	Hydration followed by skin abrasion	Higher toxin-neutralizing Ab titer than i.m.; partial protection against lethal i.n. dose of *B. anthracis* spores	[17]
Chlamydia muridarum	VDP Wet	Chlamydia major outer membrane proteins	CT + CpG	Mice	Hydration followed by vaccine solution on skin	Serum IgG and mucosal IgG and IgA induced to MOMP; enhanced clearance of organisms following intravaginal challenge	[7]
Vibrio cholerae	VDP Wet	Toxin-coregulated pilin A (TcpA)	CT	Mice	Tape-stripping	Prominent serum anti-TcpA IgG and IgA produced; protective immunity induced in pups born to TCI immunized mothers in infant mouse challenge model	[18]

Disease	Formulation	Antigen	Adjuvant	Species	Delivery	Results	Ref.
ETEC	VDP Wet	CS6 (colonization factor)	LT	Humans	Hydration via semiocclusive "wet" patch	Serum anti-CS6 IgG and IgA induced; anti-CS6 ASCs induced	[12]
	VDP Wet	LT	Same as antigen	Humans	Skin abrasion followed by "wet" patch	Robust serum anti-LT IgG and IgA induced; anti-LT mucosal responses induced; mitigation of ETEC diseases following high-dose challenge of virulent ETEC strain	[15]
	VDP Dry	LT	Same	Humans	Skin abrasion	Similar immune responses and mitigation of diarrheal illnesses as noted above; dry patch LT conferred 75% and 84% efficacy against moderate-to-severe and severe diarrhea, respectively	[9]
Enterohemorrhagic E. coli	VDP Wet	Shiga toxin subunit B (StxB1B)	LT	Rabbits	Skin abrasion	Significant levels of serum anti-StxB1 IgG and toxin neutralization titers induced. Weight gain and reduced histopathology observed for TCI group challenged with virulent Stx1 strain	[21]
Clostridium difficile	VDP Wet	C. difficile toxin A	CT	Mice	Skin abrasion	Serum anti-CDA IgG and IgA and mucosal IgA induced; serum neutralization of toxin A activity demonstrated	[10]

(Continued)

Table 20.1 TCI "proof-of-concept" studies within the past ten years. (*Continued*)

Vaccines	TCI platform: VDP or VEP Wet or dry	Antigen(s)	Adjuvant(s)	Species tested	Pretreatment of shaved skin	Major finding(s)	Ref.
Yersinia pestis	VDP Wet	F1 and V protein subunits	CT	Mice	Hydration followed by vaccine solution on skin	Significant levels of anti-F1 and V Ab induced; cell-mediated response elicited; protection in mice against challenge with virulent strain observed	[8]
Viral							
Herpes simplex virus, type 1	VDP Wet	Whole inactivated virus and HSV-1 antigens	CT	Mice	Vaccine solution on skin	Serum and mucosal anti-HSV Ab induced; cell-mediated immune response protected mice against live virus epidermal challenge	[26]
Respiratory syncytial virus	VDP Wet	G proteins: G2Na and G5	CT	Mice	Vaccine solution on skin	Serum anti-G2Na IgG1 Ab induced; protection against RSV infection in lung and nasal tract	[31]
Seasonal influenza virus	VDP Wet	Inactivated whole flu virus	CT	Mice	Tape-stripping	Anti-influenza HI Ab and cellular immune responses induced; protection against i.n. virus challenge	[37]
	VDP Dry	Inactivated whole flu virus	LT	Guinea pigs	Skin abrasion	Robust serum anti-influenza HAI Ab titers induced; dry and wet TIV patches were equally potent	[29]

	VEP Wet	Flu vaccine (injected)	LT	Mice	Skin abrasion	LT patch increased anti-flu serum IgG, HAI Ab titers, mucosal Ab and T-cell responses	[3,4]
	VEP Wet	Seasonal flu vaccine (injected)	LT	Humans	Skin abrasion	Improved HAI Abs induced in elderly compared to control group without VEP	[28]
	VEP Wet	DNA encoding hemagglutinin (injected)	LT	Mice	Skin abrasion	Anti-HA Ab enhanced; T-cell responses amplified	[34]
	VDP Wet	Influenza vaccine	None	Humans	Glue + tape-stripping	Influenza-specific CD4 and CD8 T-cell responses induced by TCI; only CD4 induced by i.m.	[38]
Human immunodeficeny virus	VDP Wet	Synthetic TAT protein	CT	Mice	Vaccine solution on skin	Serum and mucosal anti-Tat IgG and IgA induced; anti-TAT Ab neutralized Tat activity; cellular immune responses also induced	[35]
	VDP Wet	HIV peptide	CT + CpG	Mice	Skin abrasion	Robust systemic and mucosal CTLs induced; protection in mice against intrarectal challenge with HIV-recombinant vaccinia virus observed	[23]

(Continued)

Table 20.1 TCI "proof-of-concept" studies within the past ten years. (*Continued*)

Vaccines	TCI platform: VDP or VEP Wet or dry	Antigen(s)	Adjuvant(s)	Species tested	Pretreatment of shaved skin	Major finding(s)	Ref.
Foot-and-mouth disease virus	VDP Wet	VP1 synthetic peptide-BSA conjugate	CT+CpG	Mice	Vaccine solution on skin	Potent neutralizing anti-FMDV antibodies induced	[22]
Human papilloma, type 16 virus	VDP Wet	HPV-16 E7 peptide	CT + CpG	Mice	Cold wax depilation and hydration	Strong E-7-specific CTL response induced; protection in mice against tumor growth after challenge with HPV E-7 tumor cells	[25]
Measles virus	VDP Wet	Live-attenuated measles vaccine	None	Humans	Tape-stripping	MV-specific salivary IgA induced; increase rate of MV-specific IFN-γ production observed	[27]
Rabbit hemorrhagic virus	VDP Wet	Virus-like particles	CT + CpG	Mice	Vaccine solution on skin	Systemic anti-RHDV IgG1 and mucosal IgA induced in vagina; cell-mediated Th1 responses also induced	[39]
Pandemic influenza	VDP Wet	rH5 HA protein	CpG	Mice	Thermal ablation	HAI Ab induced; protection in mice against lethal H5N1 virus challenge	[30]

Application	Format	Antigen	Adjuvant	Additive	Model	Skin preparation	Outcome	Ref
VEP	Wet	rH5 HA protein, injected intradermally	LT		Mice	Skin abrasion	Significant dose sparing achieved for rH5 HA protein with VEP	[32]
VEP	Dry	H5N1 inactivated virus	LT		Humans	Skin abrasion	Enhanced HAI response observed with a single 45 μg LT VEP	[72][a]
Hepatitis B virus	VDP Wet	Hepatitis B surface antigen on elastic liposomes		None	Mice	Vaccine solution on skin	Robust systemic and mucosal anti-HBsAg induced; higher IgA titers for TCI versus i.m.	[33]
JEV	VDP Wet	Plasmid DNA encoding JEV envelope proteins on liposomes		None	Mice	Depilation cream	Significant immune protection in mice against lethal doses of JEV challenges	[24]
Miscellaneous								
Melanoma cancer	VDP Wet	Synthetic peptide expressing CTL epitope		Imiquimod	Mice	Tape-stripping	Strong CTLs induced; significant delay of tumor growth in a mice melanoma model system	[40]
	VDP Wet	Melanoma-associated peptides		None	Humans	Glue-stripping	CTL and IFN-γ induced; reduction in lesion size and suppression of tumor growth	[42]
Alzheimer's disease	VDP Wet	Aβ		CT	Mice	Hydration followed by vaccine solution on skin	High-titer Aβ IgG1 Ab and Aβ splenocytes induced; significant reduction of cerebral amyloidosis without side effects	[41]

[a]See section below, "Recent clinical applications with LT dry patches"

Aβ, β-amyloid peptide; Ab, antibodies; ASC, antibody-secreting cell; CDA, *Clostridium difficile* toxin A; CpG, CpG oligodeoxynucleotide; CT, cholera toxin; CTL, cytotoxic lymphocytes; Dry, vaccine applied in dry patch type format; DTxd, diphtheria toxoid; ETEC, enterotoxic *E. coli*; FMDV, foot-and-mouth virus; HA, hemagglutinin protein; HAI, hemagglutinin inhibition; HBsAg, hepatitis B surface antigen; HSV-1, herpes simplex type 1 virus; JEV, Japanese encephalitis virus; i.m., intramuscular; i.n., intranasal; LT, heat-labile *E. coli* enterotoxin; LTR72, nontoxic derivative of heat-labile enterotoxin; MOMP, major outer membrane protein; PRP-CRM$_{197}$ polyribosyl ribitol phosphate-cross-reacting material$_{197}$ glycoconjugate vaccine; rH5 HA, recombinant H5 hemagglutinin; rPA, recombinant protective antigen of *B. anthracis*; RHDV, rabbit hemorrhagic virus; RSV, respiratory syncytial virus; TcpA, toxin-coregulated pilin A; TetC, tetanus fragment C; TTxd, tetanus toxoid; VDP, vaccine delivery patch; VEP, vaccine enhancement patch; VP, vaccine patch; Wet, vaccine applied in wet patch type format.

exposure to "danger signals" of a microbial antigen [48,49]. When activated, the KCs secrete proinflammatory cytokines (i.e., IL1 and TNF-α), which can modulate antigen uptake and processing by the LCs and promote their maturation and migration to the skin-draining LNs [50–52].

In the absence of "danger" signals, epidermal homeostasis is maintained by both KCs and immature LCs. The former secrete constituent levels of IL10 and TGF-β cytokines, which maintain the immature LCs in a resting state. Under noninflammatory conditions, the immature LCs express low levels of MHC class I/II and co-stimulatory molecules, and can capture and process self-antigens and innocuous antigens (i.e., skin bacterial commensals). It has been proposed that immature LCs can transport the self-antigens or harmless antigens to the skin-draining LNs to establish CD4 and CD8 T-cell tolerance via induction of regulatory T cells [53]; thus autoimmunity to self-antigens as well as inappropriate inflammatory response to bacterial commensals are prevented.

Dermal DCs can also take up antigens, migrate to the draining LNs, and orchestrate antigen-specific immune responses. Most interestingly, the dermis has been recently found to contain a novel subpopulation of dermal DCs, known as the langerin+ dDCs, which are phenotypically similar to LCs in terms of maturation and co-stimulatory molecules. Situated in the upper dermis, these langerin+ dDCs can capture, process, and transport antigens to regional skin-draining LNs [54–56]. Even though the LCs are the first APCs to contact antigens at the skin surface and, thus, are presumed to play the key role for TCI, the relative contribution of other skin immune cells to the induction of innate and adaptive immune responses via skin are beginning to be elucidated. Given that LCs are just one of many subsets of DCs in the skin immune system, and the possibility that an antigen may be able to approach the LCs in the epidermis and the langerin+ dDCs in the upper dermis, the paradigm for TCI may need refinement. In any case, there is a consensus that the skin is replete with a repertoire of immunocompetent cells that potentially could be exploited to optimize the efficacy of various skin immunization approaches, including transcutaneous, epidermal, and intradermal vaccinations.

General TCI principles learned from preclinical studies

As indicated in Table 20.1, numerous TCI experiments have been conducted in animals to demonstrate that skin-delivered antigens can induce both humoral and cellular immunity. Most studies were performed by applying the antigen and/or adjuvant in a "wet" patch format. The term "wet" patch is used broadly here to represent any of these scenarios: (i) placing a gauze pad, previously soaked in antigen/adjuvant solution, onto the skin; (ii) placing a dry gauze pad on the skin and pipetting an antigen/adjuvant solution onto it; or (iii) applying an antigen/adjuvant solution directly onto the skin, allowing time for skin absorption, and then covering the vaccination site with a semi-occlusive patch. Based on numerous preclinical studies, some common principles of TCI have emerged:

• TCI can be practicable with large size macromolecules. TCI should be differentiated from transdermal delivery, which is restricted to small molecules up to 500 Da. TCI has been successfully demonstrated with a diversity of antigens, ranging from small synthetic peptides to high molecular weight subunit proteins, and to large, complex macromolecular assemblies, such as split and whole inactivated viruses (Table 20.1).

• Skin pretreatment to disrupt the SC, the principal barrier to delivery, can enhance antigen penetration to the epidermis, thereby augmenting the adaptive immune responses (Table 20.1). Various physical techniques (e.g., abrasion with emery paper, tape-stripping, ultrasound [57], electroporation [58], ballistic particle-based guns [59], etc.), chemical methods (e.g., water hydration [1,5]), use of penetration enhancers such as anionic surfactants [60], and vesicular carrier systems [61,62] have been used to alter the SC barrier to increase antigen delivery.

• The use of an adjuvant can augment the immune response in TCI applications. The most common adjuvants used are the bacterial ADP-ribosylating exotoxins, cholera toxin (CT) from *Vibrio cholera*, and heat-labile enterotoxin (LT) from *E. coli*. Their use would be prohibited for the i.m., s.c., i.n., or oral routes; however, these potent adjuvants can be safely used in the context of skin immunization [1,5,6,11]. Also, pre-existing anti-CT or anti-LT antibodies do not appear to negatively affect their adjuvant properties upon repeated use for TCI.

Some studies have revealed that TCI is possible without adjuvant [27,33,38,42]. Evidently, in these studies, the SC physical disruption process itself, such as tape-stripping, can prompt surrounding KCs to secrete proinflammatory cytokines for LC activation. Interestingly, one preclinical study showed that even prolonged contact of the antigen with the skin could induce adequate levels of anti-TTx antibodies to provide protection against TT challenge [16].

• Other types of adjuvants, such as CpG and imiquimod, have been used as topical adjuvants to augment or modulate the immune response. CpG in combination with CT or LT has been shown to modulate a Th2- to a Th1-type response to co-administered antigens [63–65]. The small molecule imiquimod, when applied on the skin, triggers release of inflammatory cytokines needed by LCs for antigen uptake and processing and their mobilization to the LNs [66]. Interestingly, no SC disruption was required when imiquimod was used as an adjuvant for a TCI study in mice involving a peptide antigen [67].

• TCI is an effective vaccine route for peptide antigens. In contrast, peptides are not effective immunogens via traditional vaccination routes. Peptide immunization via TCI can induce strong antigen-specific CD4 [63,68] or even cytotoxic CD8 T-cell responses [23,42]. In an insightful study, topical application of an HIV peptide antigen with LT or CT was shown to induce robust HIV gp160 CTL responses in the spleen and gut [23]. The TCI protocol protected mice against a mucosal challenge with a recombinant viral carrier expressing the HIV gp160 construct. The study provided evidence that activated skin dendritic cells, carrying the HIV peptide antigen, migrated not only to regional skin-draining LNs, but also to immune-inductive sites of secondary lymphoid organs.

Clinical studies involving TCI using early-stage, "wet" patch format

In this section, we provide synopses of five clinical studies performed with antigens or adjuvants delivered via "wet" patch format. The first three studies were performed by delivering vaccines onto human skin in which the SC had been disrupted by glue and/or tape-stripping. Most interestingly, these studies were performed without adjuvants. The fourth and fifth studies used LT as an adjuvant (VEP), and as an antigen (VDP), respectively, onto skin that was lightly abraded with EKG-grade emery paper. A later section describes two clinical studies involving LT delivered in a "dry" patch format.

Measles-virus vaccine patch

In a phase I clinical trial, a vaccine patch containing a live attenuated measles vaccine (MV) induced higher levels of MV-specific salivary IgA in human volunteers, whereas no increase in mucosal IgA was seen for the s.c. group [27]. The study demonstrated that homing of MV-specific IgA B cells to a remote mucosal site (i.e., salivary glands) distinct from the skin immunization site had occurred. In addition, there was a rise in the frequency of MV-specific IFN-γ producing cells for the TCI group. Interestingly, humoral MV-neutralizing was induced by the s.c. route, but not by TCI. The discrepancy in the humoral response is not clear, but it should be noted that no adjuvant was used with the MV vaccine patch.

Flu vaccine patch

Vogt *et al.* demonstrated differences in the quality of cellular immune responses in humans vaccinated by TCI versus i.m. routes with a seasonal influenza vaccine [38]. The "wet" flu patch induced both effector CD4 and CD8 T-cell responses, while the i.m. route induced stronger Th1 CD4 but no CD8 T-cell responses. Their clinical data also showed that i.m. delivery is more efficient than TCI in inducing hemagglutination inhibition assay (HAI) antibody titers; however, no significant differences in the geometric mean HAI titers were observed between the two groups. Again, it should be emphasized that no adjuvant was used in conjunction with the "wet" flu vaccine patch.

Melanoma vaccine patch

In a pilot study involving patients with advanced melanoma, skin immunization was conducted with small, synthetic, melanoma-associated antigenic peptides [42]. Following application of peptides onto glue barrier-disrupted skin, potent CTL responses were induced, as evidenced by CD8 effector cells appearing in the blood with strong cytolytic activity. Importantly, tumor regression and suppression of further tumor development in four of seven patients with advanced melanoma were obtained. The clinical findings validate preclinical studies showing that topically administered peptides containing cytotoxic T-cell peptide epitopes can induce effective anti-tumor immunity [40].

Vaccine enhancement patch for flu vaccine for elderly

A "wet" VEP containing LT was tested in elderly adults (over 65 years) vaccinated with an injectable commercial influenza vaccine [28]. The VEP improved the elderly seroconversion rates by 23%, 18%, and 12% for the H1N1, H3N2, and B strains, respectively, as compared to an elderly control group receiving the i.m. vaccination alone. The stimulation of a greater immune response offered by VEP suggests the potential to overcome current limitations in vaccine potency of commercial seasonal flu vaccines for the elderly population.

Vaccine patch for travelers' diarrhea

In a phase 1 challenge study, McKenzie *et al.* demonstrated that a wet LT patch induced strong systemic and mucosal anti-LT immune responses that were higher than a control group following challenge with a virulent LT-expressing enterotoxic *E. coli* ETEC strain [15]. Moreover, fecal anti-LT IgG and IgA as well as LT-specific IgG and IgA antibody-secreting cells (ASCs) in the peripheral blood were higher after a single patch dose than after challenge with the ETEC strain. The VDP mitigated ETEC disease in the inpatient challenge setting. For example, TCI vaccinees had significantly lower rates of

stooling, reduced stool weights, longer time to onset of diseases, and decreased need for IV therapy. Since this phase I study, a "dry" LT patch, representing an improved version of the "wet" LT patch, has been recently tested in a double blind, placebo-controlled field trial [9] (see below, "Recent clinical applications with LT dry patches").

Technical advances: dry vaccine patch delivery system

Simple, easy-to-use skin preparation system

As a pretreatment for immunization via a patch, a simple skin preparation system (SPS) has been developed by our laboratory to disrupt the SC in a controlled, single-step manner with little, if any, discomfort [69]. The SPS is a disposable hand-held device (Figure 20.2, left) containing an aperture over which an abrasive strip is pulled. Over the aperture is a small push-button dome that provides controlled pressure during contact of the abrasive surface with the skin. As the strip is pulled out, about 25% of the SC covering the skin is gently disrupted. The SPS device is intended to be packaged together with the dry VDP or VEP as an integrated vaccine patch delivery system (Figure 20.2) with the potential for self-administration.

Use of the SPS increases transepidermal water loss (TEWL) from the disrupted SC area. TEWL has been correlated to the degree of SC disruption as well as to enhanced immune responses in human volunteers [69]. The TEWL is trapped by the patch's occlusive backing, and is essential for patch hydration. This patch reconstitution process, occurring *in situ* on the skin, enhances antigen delivery since the early solubilization stage of the patch formulation results in saturated concentrations of antigen/adjuvant on the skin surface. This higher concentration gradient provides the thermodynamic driving force to deliver more antigen/adjuvant into the epidermis.

The SPS device has been described in a human volunteer study [69] and used in several human clinical studies involving LT used as a dry VDP and as a dry VEP (see the following section). These

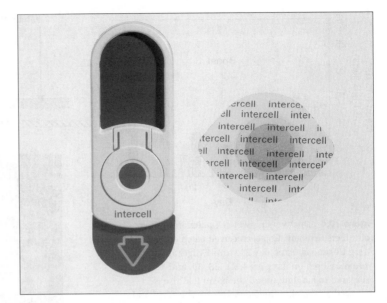

Figure 20.2 An integrated vaccine patch delivery system. On the left is the Skin Preparation System device used to gently disrupt the stratum corneum. On the right is a representation of a dry vaccine patch or vaccine enhancement patch that is applied to the pretreated skin.

studies indicated that the SPS system was simple to use, well tolerated, and able to provide a controlled method of SC disruption to achieve good immune responses.

Patch formulation science: high-throughput screening method

A "dry" patch offers certain advantages over a "wet" patch – ease of use, improved stability, better delivery, and commercial viability. We have developed a rapid high-throughput microplate screening method to identify optimal combinations of excipients for formulating and stabilizing biologics in a dry format. Briefly, prototype formulations containing certain proprietary combinations of excipients are added into 96-well microplates and dried to a solid state. Following short-term storage at 37°C, the dried antigens are reconstituted with appropriate diluents and assessed for stability via routine chemical and biological assays. More importantly, prior to sample reconstitution, the dried formulations are visually inspected for crystal appearance under a microscope. Since crystallization is known to destabilize proteins, dried formulations exhibiting crystals can be eliminated from further consideration (Figure 20.3). This microscopic

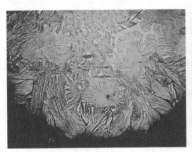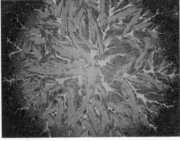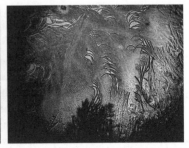

Figure 20.3 Crystallization occurring in dried solid blend formulations. Crystals were visually observed under a light microscope during the high-throughput 96-well microplate screening process. Thus, these three prototype blend formulations were rapidly removed from further consideration.

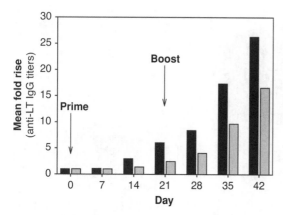

Figure 20.4 "Dry" versus "wet" LT patch in human volunteers. Human subjects received patch containing 50 μg LT on day 0 and day 21. Anti-LT IgG antibodies were measured on days 7, 14, 21, 28, 35, and 42 and compared to baseline titers. The mean fold rise is indicated by the black and gray bars for the "dry" and "wet" patches, respectively.

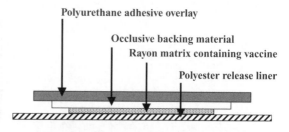

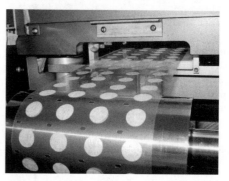

Figure 20.5 Dry patch design and production. The dry rayon/cellulose patch (vaccine patch or vaccine enhancement patch) is assembled between the occlusive backing and release liner (top). After peeling off the release liner, the adhesive overlay is used to adhere the dry patch onto the skin. A pilot patch manufacturing process is shown and is inherently scalable to meet mass production (bottom).

evaluation has enabled us to determine optimal combinations of stabilizing excipients for final patch products in a rather short time: months rather than years.

As proof that a dry patch formulation can deliver more effectively than a wet patch, we conducted a head-to-head comparison of a "dry" versus "wet" LT patch in human volunteers. As shown in Figure 20.4, the dry patch produced significantly higher fold rises (ratio over background) of anti-LT IgG than the corresponding wet patch (at equal LT dose) at all time points from day 14 onward.

Disc matrix-assisted drying and patch assembly

Our laboratory has developed an efficient drying process to efficiently transform liquid patch formulations to dry dosage forms. Essentially, small volumes of the formulations are dispensed onto a nonwoven, rayon/cellulose disc matrix. The open and large surface area of the matrix serves as a scaffold to allow rapid water evaporation. Under mild drying conditions, bulk water is efficiently removed and the blend formulation is readily dried into a solid formulation that coats the

nonwoven fibers. Following the drying process, the formulation-dosed disc is assembled as a vaccine patch (Figure 20.5). Essentially, the rayon/cellulose disc, heat-tacked on an occlusive film backing, is sandwiched between a polyurethane adhesive tape and a polyester release liner. The patch assembly is then placed in a foil pouch, sealed under nitrogen, and stored at 2–8 °C. The disc-matrix-assisted drying process and patch assembly steps are inherently scalable, and can be developed as a low-cost operation capable of producing patches at high volumes to meet mass vaccination campaign needs.

Stability of antigens in dry patches

In previous reports, we have shown that proprietary dry patch formulations, developed for the heat-labile enterotoxin *E. coli* LT as well as for an inactivated trivalent influenza vaccine (TIV), impart excellent long-term stability for these two dry patches stored under ambient conditions (e.g., >9 months for LT; >12 months for TIV) [29, 32]. Based on thermocycling experiments, we also demonstrated that both the dry LT and TIV patches can withstand extreme temperature excursions that may be encountered during shipping and distribution.

As another example that a dry and thermostable product can be generated by our patch formulation technologies, we provide the 6-month stability profiles of the recombinant protective antigen (rPA) of *Bacillus anthracis* stored at 40 °C. Figure 20.6 shows the rPA content, as determined by SEC-HPLC, for four different dry patch formulations containing 25 μg of rPA at 40 °C. Patch A represents an rPA formulation typically used for lyophilized biologics. Patches B, C, and D represent three leading "excipient stabilizing" formulations identified by our high-throughput microplate screening technology. As shown in Figure 20.6, the rPAs in the Patch B, C, and D formulations were stable for 6 months at 40 °C. On the other hand, Patch A was stable for approximately two weeks. It is clear that the proprietary combinations of excipients used for the Patch B, C, and D formulations offered enhanced stability for rPA.

Taken together, the stability studies demonstrate that dry formulated patches can be developed with excellent thermostable characteristics that can al-

low cold-chain-free distribution, ambient storage, and field use.

Recent clinical applications with LT dry patches

Dry vaccine patch for travelers' diarrhea

As mentioned earlier, a phase I challenge study demonstrated that a wet LT patch could ameliorate the severity of ETEC illness [15]. The phase I data suggested that the vaccine effect could be amplified in the field, where the ingested ETEC dose could be 1–3 orders less than used in the challenge study.

In the follow-up field study, a dry VDP containing 37.5 μg LT was used in a randomized, double blind, placebo-controlled field trial [9]. Altogether, 170 healthy US travelers (aged 18–64 years) to Guatemala and Mexico were vaccinated twice, two weeks apart, with the LT VDP or a dry placebo patch in a 1:2 ratio. Volunteers were pretreated on the arms with the single-use, disposable SPS device prior to patch application. The LT VDP led to high levels of protective efficacy against clinically significant diarrhea. For instance, the number of cases of moderate or severe diarrheal disease from any cause was significantly greater in placebo recipients than in vaccinees (Table 20.2). Moderate diarrhea was graded as 4–5 loose stools in a 24-hour period, whereas severe diarrhea was defined as ≥6 loose

Figure 20.6 Stability of dry rPA patches (25 μg dose) at 40 °C. SEC-HPLC was used to monitor rPA content (*y*-axis) over time in months (*x*-axis). A lower 75% recommended specification limit is indicated by the dotted line.

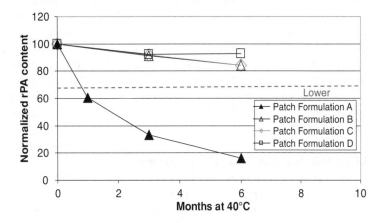

Table 20.2 Incidence and severity of diarrhea in US travelers to Guatemala and Mexico

Diarrhea severity[a]	LT patch (n = 59)	Placebo (n = 111)	p	Protective efficacy (95% CI)
Individuals with diarrhea of any cause	9	24	0.32	29% (−13 to 72)
Moderate to severe	3	23	0.007	75% (948 to 103)
Severe	1	12	0.033	84% (54 to 115)
Individuals with ETEC diarrhea	3	11	0.28	49% (−8 to 105)
Moderate to severe	2	11	0.13	66% (19 to 112)
Severe	1	5	0.34	62% (−11 to 136)

[a]Moderate diarrhea was considered as 4–5 loose stools in a 24-hour period, whereas severe diarrhea was graded as ≥6 loose stools per 24-hour period. Altogether, 170 US travelers were vaccinated twice, two weeks apart, with a dry LT vaccine patch or a dry placebo patch in a 1 to 1.88 ratio.
Reproduced from Frech *et al.* [9] with permission from Elsevier.

stools per 24-hour period. Overall, the LT VDP conferred 75% vaccine efficacy against moderate to severe diarrhea and 85% efficacy against severe diarrhea from any cause. Moreover, the few vaccinees who developed diarrhea had a short and relatively mild illness (0.45 day) versus the placebo groups (2.1 days).

Based on the expected 10–20% incidence of LT-secreting ETEC in these countries, the protective data suggest that the anti-LT immune responses extended protection beyond LT-secreting ETEC. This broad protective effect is in concert with two field studies using oral vaccines containing cholera toxin B-subunit (CTB) [70,71]. In these CTB-based vaccine trials, cross-protection against *Salmonella*, mixed *Salmonella*/ETEC infections [71], and *Campylobacter* [70] was observed. Together, the data suggest that the LT patch may be able to confer protection against other pathogens that cause travelers' diarrhea, in addition to LT-producing ETEC. We suggest that anti-LT antibodies block the conditioning of the gut wall for enhanced enteric pathogenicity caused by other intestinal disease-causing microorganisms. This hypothesis warrants further study.

LT as VEP for injected H5N1 vaccine

A dry patch containing 50 μg LT was recently used as a VEP to improve the immune response rates in subjects who received an injected A/H5N1 pandemic influenza vaccine candidate [72]. In this study, 500 adults received two injections of a re-assortant A/Vietnam/1194/2004 A/H5N1 (5 μg, 15 μg, and 45 μg) or a placebo 21 days apart. The VEP was placed over the injection site at days 0 and 21 or at day 21 only and compared to vaccine alone. In subjects receiving LT patches, the injection site was prepared using the SPS system to disrupt the SC.

A summary of the HAI titers is provided in Table 20.3. Clearly, at day 21, for all A/H5N1 dose levels, the groups receiving patches (i.e., groups 3, 6, and 9) manifested higher anti-H5N1 HAI geometric mean titers, higher fold rises, and higher rates of seroconversion and seroprotection than the corresponding non-adjuvanted groups (groups 1 and 2 combined, groups 4 and 5 combined, and groups 7 and 8 combined). However, the most significant finding in this study was the induction of high levels of seroprotection (HAI titer ≥40) in 73% of subjects receiving the patch, a 24% improvement over the vaccine alone. Table 20.3 suggests that the VEP, given only at the second dose (groups 2, 5, and 8), resulted in only a modest but not significant enhancement. On the other hand, with the two-VEP regimen, pairwise comparisons of A/H5N1 alone and A/H5N1 + VE-P showed higher HAI titers and geometric mean fold-rise (GMFR) at all three HA doses, with significance achieved in the 45 μg HA + VEP group (HAI 226 versus 94, $p < 0.05$; GMFR

Table 20.3 Summary of HAI responses in three H5N1 dose groups.[a]

	CHMP criteria	5 µg IM			15 µg IM			45 µg IM		
		Group 1 −/−	Group 2 −/+	Group 3 +/+	Group 4 −/−	Group 5 −/+	Group 6 +/+	Group 7 −/−	Group 8 −/+	Group 9 +/+
N = Day 21			92	43		93	45		86	48
GMT			11	15[b]		18	25		49	86[b]
GMFR	>2.5		1.8	2.6[b]		3.2	4.9[b]		8.9	12.5
% SC	>40%		7	14[b]		20	36[b]		49	67[b]
% SP	>70%		13	16		24	36[b]		49	73[b]
N = Day 42		48	44	43	48	45	45	43	43	48
GMT		21	29	25	37	37	44	94	90	226
GMFR	>2.5	3.5	4.0	4.2	6.2	6.7	8.6	16.9	17.0	33.1[b]
% SC	>40%	23	32	33	46	53	47	79	84	94[b]
% SP	>70%	27	39	37	50	58	49	79	84	94

[a]All groups were vaccinated twice with the injectable H5N1 vaccine on day 0 and day 21. Groups 1, 4, and 7 did not receive LT VEP. Groups 2, 5, and 8 received the LT VEP on day 21. Groups 3, 6, and 9 received the LT VEP on day 0 and day 21. The HAI responses are indicated by geometric mean titer (GMT), geometric mean fold rise (GMFR), % seroconversion (SC), and % seroprotection (SP) for day 21 and day 42.
[b]Significantly higher than injection dose alone.
−/−: Day 0 and day 21 no patch.
−/+: Day 21 patch only.
+/+: Day 0 and day 21 patch.

33.1 versus 16.9, $p < 0.05$, at day 42) along with a 94% versus 79% seroprotection rate. The combination of an injected A/H5N1 and VEP was also found to be safe and well tolerated. A single 45 µg HA dose + VEP meeting European CHMP criteria [73] for pandemic influenza vaccine licensure would be a highly desirable modality for pandemic preparedness. Research to date has indicated that H5N1 influenza vaccine candidates are inherently poor immunogens. So far, the only approved vaccine in the United States for the H5N1 influenza virus has required two 90 µg doses to generate a protective level in about 45% of vaccinated individuals. By comparison, a VEP coupled with a single dose of A/H5N1 can generate an immune response that exceeds the protective levels of the licensed vaccine, thus potentially eliminating the need for a second round of vaccination and reducing the amount of H5N1 vaccine by fourfold. Thus, a single-dose regimen is inherently dose sparing and will improve the logistics and feasibility of a successful mass immunization campaign.

Commentary and future direction

In recent years, various protocols of TCI have been translated from preclinical into clinical applications. For example, three early-stage clinical studies have demonstrated that vaccine antigens, such as a live-attenuated measles [27], a trivalent inactivated influenza vaccine [38], and melanoma-associated peptides [42], could be successfully delivered across tape-stripped skin to induce immune responses. In these studies, the vaccines were applied in a "wet" patch format, and, interestingly, without adjuvants. The studies reveal that TCI could be potentially useful where cellular and mucosal immune responses are critical for control of viral diseases and cancer.

With respect to small- to larger-scale clinical studies, our laboratory has transitioned from using a "wet' to a "dry" patch form of LT. Recently, we have used LT as an antigen in a dry VDP to protect travelers from infectious diarrhea, and as an adjuvant in a dry VEP for human volunteers receiving an injected pandemic vaccine candidate. For both clinical studies, an improved late-stage SPS device was also used to gently disrupt the SC prior to patch application. We found that the LT VDP conferred clinically significant protective efficacy and disease amelioration in travelers going to Guatemala and Mexico [9]. In the VEP study, the dry LT VEP improved the immune response rates in humans receiving an injected pandemic influenza vaccine [72]. This latter study verified that the LT-activated LCs can migrate to the same draining lymph node field as the injected vaccine and greatly enhanced the immune response to the injected vaccine.

Our formulation patch technologies have enabled us to produce dry vaccine patches with superior thermostable characteristics, suggesting the possibility of cold-chain-free shipping and distribution. In clinical settings, the dry VP or VEP along with the SPS device has proven to be an effective single-use skin patch delivery system offering advantages in terms of safety, convenience, compliance, and the potential for self-administration.

The experience gained by us and others from recent clinical studies will surely lead to development of other vaccines delivered topically to the skin. We foresee new skin patch vaccines with novel antigens or reformulation of current vaccines used in routine immunization. As for future direction, we feel that further development of TCI will be forthcoming in the following areas:

• In-depth understanding of skin immunology. There are still many questions about which skin dendritic cells are responsible for inducing adaptive immunity following skin immunization. Most studies have assumed that epidermal LCs are the major APC players. Recent experiments have shown that dDCs can mediate skin immune responses [74]. Further studies are needed to elucidate the precise role played by the various skin immunocompetent cells in the epidermal and dermal layers.

• Formulation optimization for TCI delivery. We anticipate more novel and improved formulations will be developed to enhance antigen delivery across the skin. For example, chemical enhancers can be used as additives to make the SC barrier more permeable. Physiochemical factors, such as particle size, zeta potential, and pH of the delivered antigen(s) at the skin surface will also be systematically evaluated in the development of new and improved formulations.

Acknowledgments

We thank Dr Vladimir Frolov for providing the stability profiles of the dry formulated patches of the recombinant protective antigen of *Bacillus anthracis*. We also thank Wanda Hardy for excellent editorial assistance.

References

1 Glenn GM, Scharton-Kersten T, Alving CR. Advances in vaccine delivery: transcutaneous immunisation. *Exp Opin Invest Drugs* 1999;**8**(6):797–805.

2 Glenn GM, Scharton-Kersten T, Vassell R, *et al.* Transcutaneous immunization with cholera toxin protects mice against lethal mucosal toxin challenge. *J Immunol* 1998;**161**(7):3211–14.

3 Guebre-Xabier M, Hammond SA, Ellingsworth LR, Glenn GM. Immunostimulant patch enhances immune responses to influenza vaccine in aged mice. *J Virol* 2004;**78**(14):7610–18.

4 Guebre-Xabier M, Hammond SA, Epperson DE, *et al.* Immunostimulant patch containing heat labile enterotoxin from *E. coli* enhances immune responses to injected influenza vaccine through activation of skin dendritic cells. *J Virol* 2003;**77**(9):5218–25.

5 Glenn GM, Kenney RT. Transcutaneous immunization. In MM Levine, JB Kaper, R Rappuoli, M Liu, M Good (Eds) *New Generation Vaccines*, 3rd edn. Marcel Dekker, New York, 2004, pp. 401–12.

6 Glenn GM, Kenney RT, Ellingsworth LR, *et al.* Transcutaneous immunization and immunostimulant strategies: capitalizing on the immunocompetence of the skin. *Expert Rev Vaccines* 2003;**2**(2):253–67.

7 Berry LJ, Hickey DK, Skelding KA, *et al.* Transcutaneous immunization with combined cholera toxin and CpG adjuvant protects against *Chlamydia muridarum* genital tract infection. *Infect Immun* 2004; **72**(2):1019–28.

8 Eyles JE, Elvin SJ, Westwood A, *et al.* Immunisation against plague by transcutaneous and intradermal application of subunit antigens. *Vaccine* 2004; **22**(31–2):4365–73.

9 Frech SA, DuPont HL, Bourgeois AL, *et al.* Use of a patch containing heat-labile toxin from *Escherichia*

coli against travellers' diarrhoea: a phase II, randomized, double-blind, placebo-controlled field trial. *Lancet* 2008;**371**(9629):2019–25.

10 Ghose C, Kalsy A, Shiekh A, *et al.* Transcutaneous immunization with *Clostridium difficile* toxoid A induces systemic and mucosal immune responses and toxin A neutralizing antibodies in mice. *Infect Immun* 2007;**75**(6):2826–32.

11 Glenn GM, Scharton-Kersten T, Vassell R, Matyas GR, Alving CR. Transcutaneous immunization with bacterial ADP-ribosylating exotoxins as antigens and adjuvants. *Infect Immun* 1999;**67**(3):1100–106.

12 Güereña-Burgueño F, Hall ER, Taylor DN, *et al.* Safety and immunogenicity of a prototype enterotoxigenic *Escherichia coli* vaccine administered transcutaneously. *Infect Immun* 2002;**70**(4):1874–80.

13 Kenney R, Yu J, Guebre-Xabier M, *et al.* Induction of protective immunity against lethal anthrax challenge with a patch. *J Infect Dis* 2004;**190**:774–82.

14 Mawas F, Peyre M, Beignon AS, *et al.* Successful induction of protective antibody responses against *Haemophilus influenzae* type b and diphtheria after transcutaneous immunization with the glycoconjugate polyribosyl ribitol phosphate-cross-reacting material 197 vaccine. *J Infect Dis* 2004;**190**(6):1177–82.

15 McKenzie R, Bourgeois AL, Frech SA, *et al.* Transcutaneous immunization with the heat-labile toxin (LT) of enterotoxigenic *Escherichia coli* (ETEC): protective efficacy in a double-blind, placebo-controlled challenge study. *Vaccine* 2007;**25**(18):3684–91.

16 Naito S, Maeyama J, Mizukami T, *et al.* Transcutaneous immunization by merely prolonging the duration of antigen presence on the skin of mice induces a potent antigen-specific antibody response even in the absence of an adjuvant. *Vaccine* 2007;**25**(52):8762–70.

17 Peachman KK, Rao M, Alving CR, *et al.* Correlation between lethal toxin-neutralizing antibody titers and protection from intranasal challenge with *Bacillus anthracis* Ames strain spores in mice after transcutaneous immunization with recombinant anthrax protective antigen. *Infect Immun* 2006;**74**(1):794–7.

18 Rollenhagen JE, Kalsy A, Cerda F, *et al.* Transcutaneous immunization with toxin-coregulated pilin A induces protective immunity against *Vibrio cholerae* O1 El Tor challenge in mice. *Infect Immun* 2006;**74**(10):5834–9.

19 Tierney R, Beignon AS, Rappuoli R, *et al.* Transcutaneous immunization with tetanus toxoid and mutants of *Escherichia coli* heat-labile enterotoxin as adjuvants elicits strong protective antibody responses. *J Infect Dis* 2003;**188**(5):753–8.

20 Johnston L, Mawas F, Tierney R, *et al.* Transcutaneous delivery of tetanus toxin Hc fragment induces superior tetanus toxin neutralizing antibody response compared to tetanus toxoid. *Hum Vaccin* 2009;**5**(4):230–36.

21 Zhu C, Yu J, Yang Z, Davis K, *et al.* Protection against Shiga toxin-producing *Escherichia coli* infection by transcutaneous immunization with Shiga toxin subunit B. *Clin Vaccine Immunol* 2008;**15**(2):359–66.

22 Beignon AS, Brown F, Eftekhari P, *et al.* A peptide vaccine administered transcutaneously together with cholera toxin elicits potent neutralising anti-FMDV antibody responses. *Vet Immunol Immunopathol* 2005;**104**(3–4):273–80.

23 Belyakov IM, Hammond SA, Ahlers JD, Glenn GM, Berzofsky JA. Transcutaneous immunization induces mucosal CTLs and protective immunity by migration of primed skin dendritic cells. *J Clin Invest* 2004;**113**:998–1007.

24 Cheng JY, Huang HN, Tseng WC, *et al.* Transcutaneous immunization by lipoplex-patch based DNA vaccines is effective vaccination against Japanese encephalitis virus infection. *J Control Release* 2009;**135**(3):242–9.

25 Dell K, Koesters R, Gissmann L. Transcutaneous immunization in mice: induction of T-helper and cytotoxic T lymphocyte responses and protection against human papillomavirus-induced tumors. *Int J Cancer* 2005;**118**(2):364–72.

26 El-Ghorr AA, Williams RM, Heap C, Norval M. Transcutaneous immunisation with herpes simplex virus stimulates immunity in mice. *FEMS Immunol Med Microbiol* 2000;**29**(4):255–61.

27 Etchart N, Hennino A, Friede M, *et al.* Safety and efficacy of transcutaneous vaccination using a patch with the live-attenuated measles vaccine in humans. *Vaccine* 2007;**25**(39–40):6891–9.

28 Frech SA, Kenney RT, Spyr CA, *et al.* Improved immune responses to influenza vaccination in the elderly using an immunostimulant patch. *Vaccine* 2005;**23**(7):946–50.

29 Frolov VG, Seid RC, Jr, Odutayo O, *et al.* Transcutaneous delivery and thermostability of a dry trivalent inactivated influenza vaccine patch. *Influenza Other Respi Viruses* 2008;**2**(2):53–60.

30 Garg S, Hoelscher M, Belser JA, *et al.* Needle-free skin patch delivery of a pandemic influenza vaccine protects mice from lethal viral challenge. *Clin Vaccine Immunol* 2007;**14**:926–8.

31 Godefroy S, Goestch L, Plotnicky-Gilquin H, *et al.* Immunization onto shaved skin with a bacterial

enterotoxin adjuvant protects mice against respiratory syncytial virus (RSV). *Vaccine* 2003;**21**(15):1665–71.

32 Look JL, Butler B, Al-Khalili M, *et al.* The adjuvant patch: a universal dose sparing approach for pandemic and conventional vaccines. *BioPharm Int* 2007; **20**(Suppl Aug 2007):34–45.

33 Mishra D, Dubey V, Asthana A, Saraf DK, Jain NK. Elastic liposomes mediated transcutaneous immunization against hepatitis B. *Vaccine* 2006;**24**(22): 4847–55.

34 Mkrtichyan M, Ghochikyan A, Movsesyan N, *et al.* Immunostimulant adjuvant patch enhances humoral and cellular immune responses to DNA immunization. *DNA Cell Biol* 2007;**27**(1):19–24.

35 Partidos CD, Moreau E, Chaloin O, *et al.* A synthetic HIV-1 Tat protein breaches the skin barrier and elicits Tat-neutralizing antibodies and cellular immunity. *Eur J Immunol* 2004;**34**(12):3723–31.

36 Seid RC, Jr, Glenn GM. Advances in transcutaneous vaccine delivery. In MM Levine (Ed.) *New Generation Vaccines*, 4th edn. Taylor & Francis, New York, 2009, ch. 40.

37 Skountzou I, Quan FS, Jacob J, Compans RW, Kang SM. Transcutaneous immunization with inactivated influenza virus induces protective immune responses. *Vaccine* 2006;**24**(35–36):6110–19.

38 Vogt A, Mahe B, Costagliola D, *et al.* Transcutaneous anti-influenza vaccination promotes both CD4 and CD8 T cell immune responses in humans. *J Immunol* 2008;**180**(3):1482–9.

39 Young SL, Wilson M, Wilson S, *et al.* Transcutaneous vaccination with virus-like particles. *Vaccine* 2006; **24**(26):5406–12.

40 Itoh T, Celis E. Transcutaneous immunization with cytotoxic T-cell peptide epitopes provides effective antitumor immunity in mice. *J Immunother* 2005; **28**(5):430–37.

41 Nikolic WV, Bai Y, Obregon D, *et al.* Transcutaneous beta-amyloid immunization reduces cerebral beta-amyloid deposits without T cell infiltration and microhemorrhage. *PNAS* 2007;**104**(7):2507–12

42 Yagi H, Hashizume H, Horibe T, *et al.* Induction of therapeutically relevant cytotoxic T lymphocytes in humans by percutaneous peptide immunization. *Cancer Res* 2006;**66**(20):10136–44.

43 Nicolas JF, Guy B. Intradermal, epidermal and transcutaneous vaccination: from immunology to clinical practice. *Expert Rev Vaccines* 2008;**7**(8):1201–14.

44 Bos JD, Das PK, Kapsenberg ML. Skin immune system (SIS). In JD Bos (Ed.) *Skin Immune System (SIS): Cutaneous Immunology and Clinical Immunoderma-* *tology*, 2nd edn. CRC Press, Boca Raton, FL, 1997, ch. 1.

45 Banchereau J, Steinman RM. Dendritic cells and the control of immunity. *Nature* 1998;**392**(6673):245–52.

46 Partidos CD, Muller S. Decision-making at the surface of the intact or barrier disrupted skin: potential applications for vaccination or therapy. *Cell Mol Life Sci* 2005;**63**(13):1418–24.

47 Steinman RM, Banchereau J. Taking dendritic cells into medicine. *Nature* 2007;**449**(7161):419–26.

48 Kollisch G, Kalali BN, Voelcker V, *et al.* Various members of the Toll-like receptor family contribute to the innate immune response of human epidermal keratinocytes. *Immunology* 2005;**114**(4):531–41.

49 Lebre MC, van der Aar AM, van Baarsen L, *et al.* Human keratinocytes express functional Toll-like receptor 3, 4, 5, and 9. *J Invest Dermatol* 2007;**127**(2): 331–41.

50 Steinhoff M, Brzoska T, Luger TA. Keratinocytes in epidermal immune responses. *Curr Opin Allergy Clin Immunol* 2001;**1**(5):469–76.

51 Stoitzner P, Zanella M, Ortner U, *et al.* Migration of Langerhans cells and dermal dendritic cells in skin organ cultures: augmentation by TNF-alpha and IL-1beta. *J Leukoc Biol* 1999;**66**(3):462–70.

52 Wang B, Amerio P, Sauder DN. Role of cytokines in epidermal Langerhans cell migration. *J Leukoc Biol* 1999;**66**(1):33–9.

53 Yamazaki S, Iyoda T, Tarbell K, *et al.* Direct expansion of functional CD25$^+$ CD4$^+$ regulatory T cells by antigen-processing dendritic cells. *J Exp Med* 2003; **198**(2):235–47.

54 Bursch LS, Wang L, Igyarto B, *et al.* Identification of a novel population of langerin$^+$ dendritic cells. *J Exp Med* 2007;**204**(13):3147–56.

55 Ginhoux F, Collin MP, Bogunovic M, *et al.* Blood-derived dermal langerin$^+$ dendritic cells survey the skin in the steady state. *J Exp Med* 2007;**204**(13): 3133–46.

56 Poulin LF, Henri S, de Bovis B, *et al.* The dermis contains langerin$^+$ dendritic cells that develop and function independently of epidermal Langerhans cells. *J Exp Med* 2007;**204**(13):3119–31.

57 Tezel A, Paliwal S, Shen Z, Mitragotri S. Low-frequency ultrasound as a transcutaneous immunization adjuvant. *Vaccine* 2005;**23**(29):3800–807.

58 Misra A, Ganga S, Upadhyay P. Needle-free, non-adjuvanted skin immunization by electroporation-enhanced transdermal delivery of diphtheria toxoid and a candidate peptide vaccine against hepatitis B virus. *Vaccine* 1999;**18**(5–6):517–23.

59 Chen D, Maa YF, Haynes JR. Needle-free epidermal powder immunization. *Expert Rev Vaccines* 2002;**1**(3): 265–76.

60 Huang CM, Wang CC, Kawai M, Barnes S, Elmets CA. Surfactant sodium lauryl sulfate enhances skin vaccination: molecular characterization via a novel technique using ultrafiltration capillaries and mass spectrometric proteomics. *Mol Cell Proteomics* 2006;**5**(3): 523–32.

61 Mahor S, Gupta PN, Rawat A, Vyas SP. A needle-free approach for topical immunization: antigen delivery via vesicular carrier system(s). *Curr Med Chem* 2007;**14**(27):2898–910.

62 Mishra V, Mahor S, Rawat A, *et al.* Development of novel fusogenic vesosomes for transcutaneous immunization. *Vaccine* 2006;**24**(27–8):5559–70.

63 Beignon AS, Briand JP, Muller S, Partidos CD. Immunization onto bare skin with synthetic peptides: immunomodulation with a CpG-containing oligodeoxynucleotide and effective priming of influenza virus-specific CD4$^+$ T cells. *Immunology* 2002; **105**(2):204–12.

64 Partidos CD, Beignon AS, Briand JP, Muller S. Modulation of immune responses with transcutaneously deliverable adjuvants. *Vaccine* 2004;**22**(19):2385–90.

65 von Hunolstein C, Mariotti S, Teloni R, *et al.* The adjuvant effect of synthetic oligodeoxynucleotide containing CpG motif converts the anti-*Haemophilus influenzae* type b glycoconjugates into efficient anti-polysaccharide and anti-carrier polyvalent vaccines. *Vaccine* 2001;**19**(23–4):3058–66.

66 Rechtsteiner G, Warger T, Osterloh P, Schild H, Radsak MP. Priming of CTL by transcutaneous peptide immunization with imiquimod. *J Immunol* 2005; **174**(5):2476–80.

67 Warger T, Schild H, Rechtsteiner G. Initiation of adaptive immune responses by transcutaneous immunization. *Immunol Lett* 2007;**109**(1):13–20.

68 Partidos CD, Beignon AS, Brown F, *et al.* Applying peptide antigens onto bare skin: induction of humoral and cellular immune responses and potential for vaccination. *J Control Release* 2002;**85**(1–3):27–34.

69 Frerichs DM, Frech SA, Flyer DC, Yu J, Glenn GM. Controlled, single-step, stratum corneum disruption as a pretreatment for immunization via a patch. *Vaccine* 2008;**26**(22):2782–7.

70 Bourgeois AL, Halpern J, Grahek S, et al. Vaccination of travelers to Guatemala (GU) and Mexico (MX) with an oral killed vaccine (OKV) for enterotoxigenic *E. coli* (ETEC): impact of vaccine "take" on risk of ETEC disease and infection with enteric pathogens. 4th International Conference on Vaccines for Enteric Diseases (VED 2007), April 25–27, 2007, Lisbon, Portugal.

71 Peltola H, Siitonen A, Kyronseppa H, *et al.* Prevention of travellers' diarrhoea by oral B-subunit/whole-cell cholera vaccine. *Lancet* 1991;**338**(8778):1285–9.

72 Glenn GM, Thomas DN, Poffenberger KL, *et al.* Safety and immunogenicity of an influenza vaccine A/H5N1 (A/Vietnam/1194/2004) when coadministered with a heat-labile enterotoxin (LT) adjuvant patch. *Vaccine* 2009;**27**(Suppl 6):G60–66.

73 Guideline on dossier structure and content for pandemic influenza vaccine marketing authorisation application (Revision) 2008, EMEA/CPMP/VEG/4717/03-Rev. 1.

74 Kaplan DH, Kissenpfennig A, Clausen BE. Insights into Langerhans cell function from Langerhans cell ablation models. *Eur J Immunol* 200;**38**(9):2369–76.

CHAPTER 21

Needle-free Jet Injection for Vaccine Administration

Brian R. Sloat[1], Hoi K. Tran[2], & Zhengrong Cui[1]

[1]Pharmaceutics Division, College of Pharmacy, University of Texas-Austin, Austin, TX, USA
[2]Department of Pharmaceutical Sciences, College of Pharmacy, Oregon State University, Corvallis, OR, USA

Introduction

Vaccination has historically been accomplished by needle and syringe injection to the subcutaneous, intramuscular, or intradermal spaces. While vaccination by needle and syringe injection has led to advances in the control of several infectious diseases, the use of needles and syringes comes with the risk of accidental needle-sticks and patient fear and discomfort [1]. Needle-based injection also requires trained medical professionals, creates large volumes of medical waste, has the potential to lead to cross-contamination, and is prohibitively expensive in developing countries [2–7]. Thus, the advent of technological innovation has led to new devices that deliver vaccines across the skin without the use of needles. The key advantages of needle-free injection of vaccines may include improved safety for the medical professional, patients, and the community; decreased pain at the injection site; greater patient comfort and compliance; faster and easier vaccination; and low cost [7–9].

As the largest organ and an easily accessible site for vaccine delivery, the human skin poses the greatest challenge in vaccine delivery [10]. The three layers of the skin can be recognized as the epidermis, dermis, and subcutis. The epidermis is composed of five layers, which are from outside to inside: stratum corneum, stratum lucidum, stratum granulosum, stratum spinosum, and stra-

tum basal cell layer. The outer three layers primarily consist of dead cells that form a highly effective barrier, which plays a crucial role in shielding the body from the external environment. This protective layer is believed to hinder the passage of molecules larger than 500 Da [11]. The inner two layers of the epidermis, particularly the stratum basale, contain keratinocytes, Langerhans cells (LCs), which are epidermal dendritic cells (DCs), and melanocytes. Skin-associated lymphoid tissue, blood vessels, and additional immune cells (DCs, macrophages, lymphocytes, and granulocytes) are located in the dermal skin layer. The connective tissues of the skin are filled with a jelly-like interstitium harboring immune cells, which allow for fast cellular migration in the case of inflammation [12].

Professional antigen-presenting cells (APCs), most notably the DCs, are activated at the site of injection, take up and process antigens, and migrate to the local draining lymph nodes, where they mediate the activation of B or T cells [13]. The population of DCs involved in an immunization event belong to one of three distinct categories, the epidermis-resident LCs, dermis-resident DCs [14], and DCs that infiltrate the skin in response to inflammatory events [15–17]. Mast cells are also important skin-resident immune cells. Not only do they play a role in initiating the migration of LCs, but they are required for the full induction of a cytotoxic T lymphocyte (CTL) response.

Vaccinology: Principles and Practice, First Edition. Edited by W. John W. Morrow, Nadeem A. Sheikh, Clint S. Schmidt and D. Huw Davies.
© 2012 Blackwell Publishing Ltd. Published 2012 by Blackwell Publishing Ltd.

Table 21.1 A comparison of needle and syringe injection and needle-free jet injection for vaccine administration.

	Needle and syringe	Liquid jet injection		Solid jet injection
		MUNJIs	DCJIs	
Use of needles	Yes	Needle-free	Needle-free	Needle-free
Single or multiple use	Disposable or multiple use	Multiple use	Disposable	Multiple use
Vaccine formulation	Liquid	Liquid	Liquid	Solid powder
Target tissue	i.d., s.c., i.m.	s.c., i.m., i.d. (i.d. needs improvement)		Excellent i.d.
Immune responses	Good	Equivalent or stronger than the responses induced by needle and syringe injection		
Safety and patient issues	Fear and discomfort caused by needles	Cross-contamination potential	Safe and well received	Safe and well tolerated in clinical trials
Cost of vaccination	Medium to high	Low	High	Unknown

MUNJI, multiple use nozzle jet injector; DCJI, disposable cartridge jet injector; i.d., intradermal;, i.m., intramuscular; s.c., subcutaneous.

Keratinocytes respond to physical trauma and secrete interleukin (IL)-10, IL-12, type I interferons, and several other chemokines [18–23]. Keratinocytes also influence epidermal and dermal DCs and may play a role in mediating the activation and migration of skin-derived APCs to secondary lymphoid organs and the induction of an adaptive immune response.

Over the past decades, a number of minimally invasive transdermal delivery devices using an active mechanism for skin permeation have entered the market or are under clinical development. The most notable of these devices can be divided into two categories: liquid jet injectors and solid jet injectors. Both types of injectors deliver a vaccine across the skin by using an added driving force for vaccine transport and by transiently disrupting the skin barrier. The injectors rely on compressed springs or gases to propel the vaccine to a velocity sufficient for skin penetration in the absence of needles. The devices and application parameters can be adjusted to an individual's skin properties, such as the varying skin thickness among regions of the body, as well as a person's sex and age [24]. The rapid injection and interchangeable nozzle design of these injectors are ideal for rapid, mass immunization, in addition to routine clinical usage [1,7,8]. Further, when the jet injection de-

vices are optimized, their simplicity of use and reduced costs may make them cost-effective for vaccination in developing countries. Herein, we briefly describe the design, application, and efficacy of liquid jet and solid jet injectors for vaccine delivery. For comparison, Table 21.1 summarizes the similarities and differences between needle and syringe injection and needle-free jet injections.

Liquid jet injectors

Devices and mechanism

Arnold Sutermeister is credited with developing the first liquid jet injector in the US. He noticed the accidental injection of diesel oil into the hands of workers when small leaks occurred in high-pressure lines [25]. Liquid jet injectors utilize a high-speed jet to penetrate the skin to deliver vaccine in a liquid form without the use of needles. The design of commercial liquid jet injectors consists of a piston adjacent to a vaccine-loaded compartment and a nozzle with an orifice diameter ranging between 150 and 300 μm, all attached to a power source – either compressed gas or a spring mechanism [1]. When the device is activated, the power source pushes the piston, which impacts the vaccine-loaded compartment. A rapid increase in pressures forces the vaccine in liquid through the nozzle orifice with a velocity ranging between 100 and 200 m/s [8,26]. The diameter of the liquid jet approximately equals the diameter of the nozzle orifice, but increases with distance traveled. When entering the skin, the formation of a hole is speculated to occur by a combination of skin erosion and fractionation and is completed within the first few hundred ms [24]. As the jet progresses deeper into the skin, the velocity decreases until it does not have sufficient energy to continue hole formation, completing the penetration stage where the maximum injection depth is defined. A stagnation event follows where the fluid begins to build up at the maximum injection depth. Finally, a fluid dispersion event takes place, where the fluid is absorbed by the penetrated tissue surfaces [24,27–29].

The diameter of the nozzle orifice and velocity of the liquid jet determine the depth of penetration and the shape of liquid dispersion. The dispersion of the fluid appears to be approximately hemispherical in shape, which tends to be governed by the jet power. An increase in penetration depth is reported to occur by increasing the jet velocity, the diameter of the nozzle orifice, or the energy output of the power source. Increasing the diameter of the nozzle orifice was reported to increase the size of the dispersion within the skin, and increasing the output of the power source also changed the shape of the dispersed liquid within the tissue [8].

Two main classes of liquid jet injectors have been developed: single-dose jet injectors, which are also known as disposable cartridge jet injectors (DCJIs), and multiple-use nozzle jet injectors (MUNJIs). MUNJIs do not contain any disposable parts and were developed for rapid mass immunization. However, due to reports linking the use of such devices to the spread of hepatitis B viruses in the 1980s, their use was abandoned. The cause of the outbreak was believed to arise from cross-contamination due to splash-back of the interstitial fluid from the skin onto the nozzle [30]. The focus of most research using liquid jet injectors has since focused only on DCJIs. There are currently more than two dozens DCJIs on the market or under development. Devices with FDA approval include the Biojector® 2000 (Bioject Medical Technologies,

Inc., Portland, OR), the Injex™ (Equidyne Systems, Inc., Tustin, CA), and the Lectrajet® (D'Antonio Consultants International, Inc., East Syracuse, NY), which has the potential capacity to deliver more than 600 doses of vaccine per hour by using auto-disposable vaccine cartridges.

Applications

Liquid jet injectors have been used to administer several different vaccines to humans. Mass immunization programs for the administration of traditional measles, small pox, influenza, polio, cholera, and hepatitis B vaccines have all made use of MUNJIs [31]. Patients would be immunized using the same nozzle and vaccine reservoir. Generally, liquid jet injection was found to be equivalent or better than needle and syringe injection [31,32]. One study aimed at comparing the immune response generated by using the Biojector® 2000 or traditional needle and syringe injection of a type A hepatitis vaccine showed that the anti-HAV immune response induced by the Biojector® 2000 was significantly greater than that induced by injection using needles and syringes [33]. Each human subject received two immunizations on months 0 and 6 in the deltoid muscle, and the resultant immune response was measured 15 and 30 days, and 7 months after the first immunization. Subjects who received the vaccine via the Biojector® 2000 developed significantly greater anti-HAV antibody titers than those receiving the injection using needles and syringes on all measured days [33]. It was reasoned that needle-based intramuscular injection deposits the vaccine within the muscle where it is absorbed and circulated, whereas injection by Biojector® 2000 disperses the vaccine more widely into the injected tissue [34]. The greater dispersion within the tissue is believed to be responsible for the observed inflammation after administration, which may mean greater contact of the vaccine with immune-competent inflammatory cells and earlier development of stronger immune response [34]. Similar results were also observed in another human study administering a type A hepatitis vaccine using the Imule® liquid jet injector [35]. However, in a study by Mathei *et al.* administration of a hepatitis B vaccine (recombinant HBsAg purified from yeast and adjuvanted with aluminum) using the Biojector® 2000 induced slightly lower anti-HBsAg antibody titers than needle and syringe injection [36].

In general, any vaccine that is administered by needles and syringes can also be injected using a liquid jet injector because extra reformulation work is usually not needed. Therefore, it is not surprising that liquid jet injectors have also been used to administer plasmid DNA for genetic immunization [37–49] (see Chapter 18). Davis *et al.* reported that a needle-free jet injection using Biojector® was able to deliver plasmid DNA encoding HBsAg into the normal muscle in rats and rabbits such that a substantial immune response was induced [50]. The Biojector® injection induced a 4-fold greater antibody production 8 weeks after injection as compared to injection with needles and syringes. Liquid jet injection of DNA vaccine has also been employed in nonhuman primates and clinical trials. For example, Raviprakash *et al.* administered a dengue-1 DNA vaccine to *Aotus* monkeys using Biojector® or needle and syringes [39]. Vaccination using the Biojector® resulted in a higher antibody response than using the needles and syringes. A plague reduction neutralization test revealed a mean dengue antibody titer of 161 at 6 months in the needle-injected group, while the Biojector® group had a value almost twice as much [39]. Titers among animals injected using the Biojector® were also more uniform and consistent, remaining at a stabilized level from months 6 through 11, possibly providing the animals with long-term protection from virus challenge [39]. Many clinical trials using the Biojector® 2000 to administer DNA vaccines have been completed or are active (clinicaltrials.gov). For example, the Biojector® 2000 was used to intramuscularly inject an influenza DNA vaccine in a phase I clinical trial recently completed by Vical, Inc. (San Diego, CA). The trivalent vaccine contained a plasmid encoding the hemagglutinin (HA) surface protein from the H5N1 influenza virus strain A/Vietnam/1203/4 and separate plasmids encoding the consensus sequences of two highly conserved influenza virus proteins, the nucleoprotein (NP) and the ion channel protein

(M2). After two injections on days 0 and 21, by day 56, at least 50% and up to 67% of the evaluable subjects were responders in the cohorts receiving the DNA vaccine, but there were no responders in the placebo cohort (IBC Life Sciences Next Generation Vaccines conference, National Harbor, MD, July 17–18, 2008).

Finally, besides vaccine administration, liquid jet injectors have been primarily used for the administration of drugs. The most notable macromolecules include growth hormones, insulin, interferon, and erythropoietin [25,51–70]. For example, the control of blood glucose level was found to be as effective when insulin was administered by liquid jet injection as by traditional needle and syringe injections [60,67,68]; however, a faster onset of plasma insulin was observed after administration by jet injection [69,70]. Liquid jet injectors have also been used to deliver small drug molecules such as lidocaine, midazolam, and ketamine [71–75]. MUNJIs have been used to administer drugs for the treatment of plantar warts, hypertrophic scars, and leishmaniasis [76–81].

Safety and limitations

Due to the increased risk of cross-contamination, the World Health Organization recommends that MUNJIs should not be used for immunization until all of their safety issues are resolved. However, the Centers for Disease Control and Prevention recommend the use of MUNJIs for rapid and mass immunization when the risks of using them are outweighed by the risk of the disease. Efforts have been made to minimize the risks of cross-contamination from MUNJIs. For example, a new device was designed to use a disposable nozzle cap to reduce the risk of transmission of infections via splash-back [31]. The device features an interlock design to prevent the use of the injector without the protective cap. Studies carried out with this device showed no risk of contamination [82]. Further, detailed protocols for cleaning the MUNJIs between uses have been proposed to minimize the risk of contamination, but their effectiveness remains undetermined [83].

Children and adults are routinely immunized using DCJIs as the physician deems appropriate.

However, the acceptability of DCJIs for immunization has been mixed due to the variability of reactions at the injection site. Some reports claimed no difference in pain when compared to that experienced after needle and syringe injection [84], while other studies reported that DCJIs caused higher levels of pain [32], as well as soreness, redness, and swelling at the injection site [33,36], bleeding, and the formation of hematomas [59]. In contrast, some reports stated the absence of any local reactions at the injection site altogether [85]. The variability of adverse reactions at the injection site caused by liquid jet injection is thought to arise from the large dosing volume (tens to hundreds of microliters) and nozzle orifice diameter [1] and the device's inability to respond to the large variations of the mechanical properties of the skin [26]. To overcome these problems, novel pulsed microjet injectors are being developed, which offer control over the depth of penetration into the skin and minimize the injection volume. Using a small jet diameter (50–100 μm) and nano-volume (2–15 nl) of liquid limited the penetration depth, whereas the high velocity (>100 m/s) of the microjet allowed entry into the skin [8].

Solid jet injectors

Devices and mechanism

Much of the development of solid jet injectors was performed by Klein *et al.*, who transfected plant cells with DNA and RNA nucleic acid–coated tungsten particles [86]. Since then, solid jet injectors have been developed to deliver vaccines or drugs in a powder form into the superficial layers of the skin. Powder jet injector and biolistic injector, as well as gene gun, are additional terms for solid jet injectors.

Solid jet injectors are comprised of a compartment to hold the drug powder formulation, a nozzle that directs the flow of the powder, and a power source in the form of compressed gas [87]. The drug compartment is between a pair of diaphragms a few microns thick. When the injector is activated, compressed gas from the power source expands, ruptures the diaphragms, and carries the particu-

lates or powders into the skin. Through the force of momentum, the drug particles penetrate the stratum corneum and continue through this superficial layer of skin, with a significant percentage of them reaching the viable epidermis for the desired therapeutic effect [8]. A variation of this mechanism uses a light gas gun, which uses an accelerating piston to generate particle velocity. Upon activation, the piston accelerates, carrying the particles, and decelerates, causing the particles to leave the surface of the piston. The particles are ejected from the injector and penetrate the targeted tissue surface.

Successful delivery of drug across the stratum corneum relies on several parameters: particle density (ρ), particle radius (r), and impact velocity (v). A composite parameter, called the particle impact parameter (PIP), is defined as the product of the particle density, radius, and velocity (PIP = ρrv), and represents the momentum per unit cross-sectional area of the particle. The depth of penetration and the fraction of particles penetrating the stratum corneum were found to be directly proportional to the PIP. When PIP is fixed, increasing the particle radius corresponds to a decrease in particle velocity at constant density, resulting in a decrease in penetration depth. With a given set of parameters, varying the gas pressure allows for control over particle velocity.

Applications

In theory, all types of vaccines that can be formulated into a powder form or a particulate form can be delivered using a solid jet injector, such as the PowderJect injector, although in reality solid jet injection has been used very intensively for DNA vaccine delivery. Typically, plasmid DNA encoding antigen(s) of interest is coated onto gold or tungsten particles and delivered into the epidermal layer of the skin using the injector. Vaccination by solid jet injection of DNA-coated gold particles differs from intramuscular and intradermal injection in that the jet injection results in the direct delivery of the vaccine intracellularly into viable cells in the skin [88]. DNA can be delivered into both professional and nonprofessional APCs of the epidermis [89,90]. The enhanced immune response is likely due to the deposition of DNA into cells

[88,90] and the immune competence of the epidermal skin layer [91,92]. Vaccination of mice using plasmid DNA encoding antigens specific to hepatitis B, rabies, HIV, and influenza using solid jet injectors has demonstrated the induction of both humoral and cellular immune responses [93–106], while preventing the induction of long-term IgE antibody production [107]. Further, injection of mice with tumor-specific antigen-encoding plasmid DNA on gold particles or entrapped in polymeric particles was shown to afford the mice protection against a tumor challenge [108–112]. For example, Trimble *et al.* evaluated the immunologic and antitumor responses generated by the pNGVL4a-Sig/E7 (detox)/HSP70, a plasmid encoding human papillomavirus type 16 E7 protein linked to a *Mycobacterium tuberculosis* heat shock protein 70 [49]. The plasmid was administered to mice by three different routes: intramuscular injection by needles and syringes, liquid jet injection using Biojector®, or solid jet injection using gene gun. Following two injections of the plasmid, mice vaccinated using the gene gun exhibited significantly higher numbers of E7-specific IFNγ^+ CD8$^+$ T cell precursors with only 2 μg of DNA per injection (50 μg of DNA for the Biojector® and i.m. needle and syringe injection). Further, these mice exhibited the lowest number of pulmonary nodules and lowest pulmonary weight following a hematogenous spread TC-1 tumor model challenge, as compared with the naïve, needle and syringe, or Biojector® vaccinated mice [49]. However, other factors such as the antigen of interest, the plasmid DNA *per se*, the dosing schedule, and the genetic background of the animals may even play a dominant role in determining the type of immune responses induced by a particular DNA vaccine [113].

Similar results were also obtained in preclinical studies using large animal models such as swine and nonhuman primates [114–122]. Fuller *et al.* published a comprehensive review in this aspect [123]. Antigens specific to a great variety of pathogens have been used, which included HIV, SIV, HSIV, hepatitis B, encephalitis, Ebola, Andes virus, dengue, measles, rabies, influenza, small pox, and foot and mouth disease. In general, solid jet injection of plasmid DNA vaccine into monkeys or

pigs was able to induce specific neutralizing antibody, CD8$^+$ T-cell responses, which in some cases afforded the animals protection against pathogen challenges. Administration of DNA vaccines to humans by needles and syringes proved to be disappointing due to the irregular and relatively poor immune responses elicited as compared with that in small animal models [124,125]. One of the focuses on improving the efficacy of DNA vaccines in humans is the delivery methods, and solid jet injectors have shown promise through the induction of robust cytotoxic T-cell and antibody responses [126–131]. In fact, solid jet injection of DNA coated on gold particles using only 1–4 μg of DNA was shown to consistently induce both humoral and cellular immune responses in all or most subjects without adjuvants or boosting with other vaccine formulations [123].

Solid jet injector has also been used to deliver non-DNA vaccines, including peptide, protein, and inactivated viruses [100,101,113]. The vaccines were formulated into a powder form with sugar excipients (e.g., trehalose) to generate particles or granules of 20–70 μm, or a particulate form by precipitating the protein or peptide antigens onto gold particles of 1–3 μm. For example, Chen *et al.* formulated the commercial human influenza vaccine used for the 1998–1999 vaccination season with trehalose into dried powder of 20–53 μm, which was then used to immunize mice using the PowderJect device or using needles and syringes for intramuscular or subcutaneous injections [96]. The PowderJect injector was found to be superior. After a single immunization, the PowderJect injector elicited a serum IgG titer to influenza virus that was significantly higher than that induced by either intramuscular injection ($p < 0.05$) or subcutaneous injection ($p < 0.01$). Comparison of the sera after a single boosting showed that the antibody titer elicited by the PowderJect injector was approximately 4–8-fold higher than that induced by intramuscular or subcutaneous needle-based injection ($p < 0.01$). Importantly, it is known that nonreplicating vaccines administered by intramuscular injection using needles and syringes elicit predominantly humoral responses and not CTL responses. Because the PowderJect injector can deliver protein and peptide antigens precipitated on gold particles intracellularly into viable epidermal cells, including LCs, Chen *et al.* reported that epidermal powder immunization using the PowderJect to deliver protein (HBsAg) or peptide (TYQRTRALV of influenza virus NP) antigens precipitated on 1.5–2.5 μm gold particles to the epidermis elicited CTL responses to the nonreplicating protein and peptide [101]. When proteins and peptides are formulated into a powder form with sugar excipients, the size and physical properties of the sugar particles preclude intracellular delivery. Therefore, the immune responses induced were predominantly humoral responses, but adjuvants such as the CpG DNA oligos can be co-formulated with the protein antigens to modify the resultant immune responses [113]. For example, using diphtheria toxoid (DT) as the antigen, which was formulated into a dry powder using trehalose as an excipient, with or without CpG DNA oligos as an adjuvant, Chen *et al.* showed that the serum anti-DT IgG titer following the PowderJect injection was augmented by 250-fold when DT was co-delivered with a CpG DNA oligo [100]. Moreover, PowderJect injection of the DT powder alone induced an IgG1-biased response, whereas co-delivery of CpG oligo adjuvant with the DT led to an increased production of anti-DT IgG2a antibodies [100].

Safety and limitations

Unlike liquid jet injection, which has been used worldwide to deliver millions of doses of vaccines, solid jet injection is still limited to clinical trial use. Therefore, the safety data for solid jet injection in humans are not as comprehensive as those for liquid jet injection. Several human clinical trials using solid jet injectors to deliver DNA vaccines have been performed [126,127,129–131]. Generally, it seems that solid jet injection is safe and well tolerated in humans. Subjects report painless delivery of the vaccine at the time of administration. However, symptoms after administration included mild erythema, hyperpigmentation, skin flaking, and discoloration at the injection site. Burning, tingling, or tightening of the skin have also been reported, although symptoms typically subside within a month [127,130]. However, mild discoloration was re-

ported to persist in a few injection sites for up to 180 days [127,130].

Raju *et al.* found that DNA-coated particles delivered via solid jet injectors resulted in cell death, and, based on their findings, a particle density less than 2 microparticles per 1000 μm² would minimize cell death [132].

Conclusion

The long-standing needles and syringes have proven to be effective in delivering vaccines across human skin, but there are limits to the range of products available for use, as well as safety concerns. The development of needle-free injection devices in recent decades is aimed at filling in gaps where traditional methods have been lacking. It has been said that the stigma of sharp needles and the pain associated with shots can be avoided with needle-free injectors; these may be personal preferences that vary from one person to another. Studies have demonstrated that needle-free devices are useful in eliciting greater humoral and cellular immune responses compared to traditional needles and syringes, but there are also studies that conclude otherwise. There are many factors preventing needle-free devices from becoming mainstream, not least the cost of disposable devices. The future of needle-free injection devices holds many promises as well as room for improvement. With increasing focus and gaining popularity in clinical studies, perhaps the day of seeing this new injection method becoming common will not be too far away. Nevertheless, needles and syringes will not likely become obsolete anytime in the near future.

References

1 Mitragotri S. Current status and future prospects of needle-free liquid jet injectors. *Nat Rev Drug Discov* 2006;**5**:543–8.
2 Jacobson RM, Swan A, Adegbenro A, *et al.* Making vaccines more acceptable – methods to prevent and minimize pain and other common adverse events associated with vaccines. *Vaccine* 2001;**19**:2418–27.

3 Nir Y, Paz A, Sabo E, *et al.* Fear of injections in young adults: prevalence and associations. *Am J Trop Med Hyg* 2003;**68**:341–4.

4 Dicko M, Oni AQ, Ganivet S, *et al.* Safety of immunization injections in Africa: not simply a problem of logistics. *Bull World Health Organ* 2000;**78**: 163–9.

5 Miller MA, Pisani E. The cost of unsafe injections. *Bull World Health Organ* 1999;**77**:808–11.

6 Simonsen L, Kane A, Lloyd J, *et al.* Unsafe injections in the developing world and transmission of bloodborne pathogens: a review. *Bull World Health Organ* 1999;**77**:789–800.

7 Giudice EL, Campbell JD. Needle-free vaccine delivery. *Adv Drug Deliv Rev* 2006;**58**:68–89.

8 Arora A, Prausnitz MR, Mitragotri S. Micro-scale devices for transdermal drug delivery. *Int J Pharm* 2008;**364**:227–36.

9 Ekwueme DU, Weniger BG, Chen RT. Model-based estimates of risks of disease transmission and economic costs of seven injection devices in sub-Saharan Africa. *Bull World Health Organ* 2002;**80**: 859–70.

10 Scheuplein RJ, Blank IH. Permeability of the skin. *Physiol Rev* 1971;**51**:702–47.

11 Bos JD, Meinardi MM. The 500 Dalton rule for the skin penetration of chemical compounds and drugs. *Exp Dermatol* 2000;**9**:165–9.

12 Warger T, Schild H, Rechtsteiner G. Initiation of adaptive immune responses by transcutaneous immunization. *Immunol Lett* 2007;**109**:13–20.

13 Banchereau J, Steinman RM. Dendritic cells and the control of immunity. *Nature* 1998;**392**:245–52.

14 Valladeau J, Saeland S. Cutaneous dendritic cells. *Semin Immunol* 2005;**17**:273–83.

15 Palamara F, Meindl S, Holcmann M, *et al.* Identification and characterization of pDC-like cells in normal mouse skin and melanomas treated with imiquimod. *J Immunol* 2004;**173**:3051–61.

16 Urosevic M, Dummer R, Conrad C, *et al.* Disease-independent skin recruitment and activation of plasmacytoid predendritic cells following imiquimod treatment. *J Natl Cancer Inst* 2005;**97**: 1143–53.

17 Wollenberg A, Wagner M, Gunther S, *et al.* Plasmacytoid dendritic cells: a new cutaneous dendritic cell subset with distinct role in inflammatory skin diseases. *J Invest Dermatol* 2002;**119**: 1096–102.

18 Grone A. Keratinocytes and cytokines. *Vet Immunol Immunopathol* 2002;**88**:1–12.

19 Kollisch G, Kalali BN, Voelcker V, *et al.* Various members of the Toll-like receptor family contribute to the innate immune response of human epidermal keratinocytes. *Immunology* 2005;**114**:531–41.

20 Kono T, Kondo S, Pastore S, *et al.* Effects of a novel topical immunomodulator, imiquimod, on keratinocyte cytokine gene expression. *Lymphokine Cytokine Res* 1994;**13**:71–6.

21 Lebre MC, van der Aar AM, van Baarsen L, *et al.* Human keratinocytes express functional Toll-like receptor 3, 4, 5, and 9. *J Invest Dermatol* 2007; **127**:331–41.

22 Mempel M, Voelcker V, Kollisch G, *et al.* Toll-like receptor expression in human keratinocytes: nuclear factor kappaB controlled gene activation by *Staphylococcus aureus* is toll-like receptor 2 but not toll-like receptor 4 or platelet activating factor receptor dependent. *J Invest Dermatol* 2003;**121**: 1389–96.

23 Uchi H, Terao H, Koga T, *et al.* Cytokines and chemokines in the epidermis. *J Dermatol Sci* 2000;**24** (Suppl 1):S29–38.

24 Baxter J, Mitragotri S. Jet-induced skin puncture and its impact on needle-free jet injections: experimental studies and a predictive model. *J Control Release* 2005;**106**:361–73.

25 Bremseth DL, Pass F. Delivery of insulin by jet injection: recent observations. *Diabetes Technol Ther* 2001;**3**:225–32.

26 Schramm J, Mitragotri S. Transdermal drug delivery by jet injectors: energetics of jet formation and penetration. *Pharm Res* 2002;**19**:1673–9.

27 Schramm-Baxter J, Katrencik J, Mitragotri S. Jet injection into polyacrylamide gels: investigation of jet injection mechanics. *J Biomech* 2004;**37**:1181–8.

28 Schramm-Baxter J, Mitragotri S. Needle-free jet injections: dependence of jet penetration and dispersion in the skin on jet power. *J Control Release* 2004;**97**:527–35.

29 Schramm-Baxter JR, Mitragotri S. Investigations of needle-free jet injections. *Conf Proc IEEE Eng Med Biol Soc* 2004;**5**:3543–6.

30 Canter J, Mackey K, Good LS, *et al.* An outbreak of hepatitis B associated with jet injections in a weight reduction clinic. *Arch Intern Med* 1990;**150**:1923–7.

31 Weniger BG. Jet injection of vaccines: overview and challenges for mass vaccination with jet injections (JIs). Presented at Innovative Administration Systems for Vaccines, Rockville, MD, Dec 18–19, 2003.

32 Jackson LA, Austin G, Chen RT, *et al.* Safety and immunogenicity of varying dosages of trivalent

inactivated influenza vaccine administered by needle-free jet injectors. *Vaccine* 2001;**19**:4703–9.

33 Williams J, Fox-Leyva L, Christensen C, *et al.* Hepatitis A vaccine administration: comparison between jet-injector and needle injection. *Vaccine* 2000;**18**:1939–43.

34 Lemon SM, Scott RM, Bancroft WH. Subcutaneous administration of inactivated hepatitis B vaccine by automatic jet injection. *J Med Virol* 1983;**12**:129–36.

35 Parent du Chatelet I, Lang J, Schlumberger M, *et al.* Clinical immunogenicity and tolerance studies of liquid vaccines delivered by jet-injector and a new single-use cartridge (Imule): comparison with standard syringe injection. Imule Investigators Group. *Vaccine* 1997;**15**:449–58.

36 Mathei C, Van Damme P, Meheus A. Hepatitis B vaccine administration: comparison between jet-gun and syringe and needle. *Vaccine* 1997;**15**:402–4.

37 Manam S, Ledwith BJ, Barnum AB, *et al.* Plasmid DNA vaccines: tissue distribution and effects of DNA sequence, adjuvants and delivery method on integration into host DNA. *Intervirology* 2000;**43**:273–81.

38 Mumper RJ, Cui Z. Genetic immunization by jet injection of targeted pDNA-coated nanoparticles. *Methods* 2003;**31**:255–62.

39 Raviprakash K, Ewing D, Simmons M, *et al.* Needle-free Biojector injection of a dengue virus type 1 DNA vaccine with human immunostimulatory sequences and the GM-CSF gene increases immunogenicity and protection from virus challenge in *Aotus* monkeys. *Virology* 2003;**315**:345–52.

40 Aguiar JC, Hedstrom RC, Rogers WO, *et al.* Enhancement of the immune response in rabbits to a malaria DNA vaccine by immunization with a needle-free jet device. *Vaccine* 2001;**20**:275–80.

41 Brave A, Ljungberg K, Boberg A, *et al.* Multigene/multisubtype HIV-1 vaccine induces potent cellular and humoral immune responses by needle-free intradermal delivery. *Mol Ther* 2005;**12**:1197–205.

42 Choi AH, Smiley K, Basu M, *et al.* Protection of mice against rotavirus challenge following intradermal DNA immunization by Biojector needle-free injection. *Vaccine* 2007;**25**:3215–18.

43 Cui Z, Baizer L, Mumper RJ. Intradermal immunization with novel plasmid DNA-coated nanoparticles via a needle-free injection device. *J Biotechnol* 2003;**102**:105–15.

44 Gramzinski RA, Millan CL, Obaldia N, *et al.* Immune response to a hepatitis B DNA vaccine in *Aotus* monkeys: a comparison of vaccine formula-tion, route, and method of administration. *Mol Med* 1998;**4**:109–18.

45 Larmour CJ, Chadwick RG. Effects of a commercial orthodontic debonding agent upon the surface microhardness of two orthodontic bonding resins. *J Dent* 1995;**23**:37–40.

46 Meseda CA, Stout RR, Weir JP. Evaluation of a needle-free delivery platform for prime-boost immunization with DNA and modified vaccinia virus Ankara vectors expressing herpes simplex virus 2 glycoprotein D. *Viral Immunol* 2006;**19**:250–59.

47 Rao SS, Gomez P, Mascola JR, *et al.* Comparative evaluation of three different intramuscular delivery methods for DNA immunization in a nonhuman primate animal model. *Vaccine* 2006;**24**:367–73.

48 Smith BF, Baker HJ, Curiel DT, *et al.* Humoral and cellular immune responses of dogs immunized with a nucleic acid vaccine encoding human carcinoembryonic antigen. *Gene Ther* 1998;**5**:865–8.

49 Trimble C, Lin CT, Hung CF, *et al.* Comparison of the CD8$^+$ T cell responses and antitumor effects generated by DNA vaccine administered through gene gun, biojector, and syringe. *Vaccine* 2003;**21**:4036–42.

50 Davis HL, Michel ML, Mancini M, *et al.* Direct gene transfer in skeletal muscle: plasmid DNA-based immunization against the hepatitis B virus surface antigen. *Vaccine* 1994;**12**:1503–9.

51 Bareille P, MacSwiney M, Albanese A, *et al.* Growth hormone treatment without a needle using the Preci-Jet 50 transjector. *Arch Dis Child* 1997;**76**:65–7.

52 Brodell RT, Bredle DL. The treatment of palmar and plantar warts using natural alpha interferon and a needleless injector. *Dermatol Surg* 1995;**21**:213–18.

53 Dorr HG, Zabransky S, Keller E, *et al.* Are needle-free injections a useful alternative for growth hormone therapy in children? Safety and pharmacokinetics of growth hormone delivered by a new needle-free injection device compared to a fine gauge needle. *J Pediatr Endocrinol Metab* 2003;**16**:383–92.

54 Mitragotri S. Immunization without needles. *Nat Rev Immunol* 2005;**5**:905–16.

55 Suzuki T, Takahashi I, Takada G. Daily subcutaneous erythropoietin by jet injection in pediatric dialysis patients. *Nephron* 1995;**69**:347.

56 Chang CH, Rickes EL, Marsilio F, *et al.* Activity of a novel nonpeptidyl growth hormone secretagogue, L-700,653, in swine. *Endocrinology* 1995;**136**:1065–71.

57 Chiasson JL, Ducros F, Poliquin-Hamet M, *et al.* Continuous subcutaneous insulin infusion (Mill-Hill

Infuser) versus multiple injections (Medi-Jector) in the treatment of insulin-dependent diabetes mellitus and the effect of metabolic control on microangiopathy. *Diabetes Care* 1984;**7**:331–7.

58 Houtzagers CM, Berntzen PA, van der Stap H, *et al.* Absorption kinetics of short- and intermediate-acting insulins after jet injection with Medi-Jector II. *Diabetes Care* 1988;**11**:739–42.

59 Houtzagers CM, Visser AP, Berntzen PA, *et al.* The Medi-Jector II: efficacy and acceptability in insulin-dependent diabetic patients with and without needle phobia. *Diabet Med* 1988;**5**:135–8.

60 Katoulis EC, Drosinos EK, Dimitriadis GK, *et al.* Efficacy of a new needleless insulin delivery system monitoring of blood glucose fluctuations and free insulin levels. *Int J Artif Organs* 1989;**12**:333–8.

61 Lalezari JP, Saag M, Walworth C, *et al.* An open-label safety study of enfuvirtide injection with a needle-free injection device or needle/syringe: the Biojector 2000 Open-label Safety Study (BOSS). *AIDS Res Hum Retroviruses* 2008;**24**:805–13.

62 Malone JI, Lowitt S, Grove NP, *et al.* Comparison of insulin levels after injection by jet stream and disposable insulin syringe. *Diabetes Care* 1986;**9**:637–40.

63 Oberye J, Mannaerts B, Huisman J, *et al.* Local tolerance, pharmacokinetics, and dynamics of ganirelix (Orgalutran) administration by Medi-Jector compared to conventional needle injections. *Hum Reprod* 2000;**15**:245–9.

64 Solnica A, Oh C, Cho MM, *et al.* Patient satisfaction and clinical outcome after injecting gonadotropins with use of a needle-free carbon dioxide injection system for controlled ovarian hyperstimulation for in vitro fertilization. *Fertil Steril* 2009;**92**(4): 1369–71.

65 True AL, Chiu YY, Demasi RA, *et al.* Pharmacokinetic bioequivalence of enfuvirtide using a needle-free device versus standard needle administration. *Pharmacotherapy* 2006;**26**:1679–86.

66 Verrips GH, Hirasing RA, Fekkes M, *et al.* Psychological responses to the needle-free Medi-Jector or the multidose Disetronic injection pen in human growth hormone therapy. *Acta Paediatr* 1998;**87**:154–8.

67 Lindmayer I, Menassa K, Lambert J, *et al.* Development of new jet injector for insulin therapy. *Diabetes Care* 1986;**9**:294–7.

68 Weller C, Linder M. Jet injection of insulin vs the syringe-and-needle method. *JAMA* 1966;**195**:844–7.

69 Kerum G, Profozic V, Granic M, *et al.* Blood glucose and free insulin levels after the administration of insulin by conventional syringe or jet injector in insulin treated type 2 diabetics. *Horm Metab Res* 1987;**19**:422–5.

70 Pehling GB, Gerich JE. Comparison of plasma insulin profiles after subcutaneous administration of insulin by jet spray and conventional needle injection in patients with insulin-dependent diabetes mellitus. *Mayo Clin Proc* 1984;**59**:751–4.

71 Cooper JA, Bromley LM, Baranowski AP, *et al.* Evaluation of a needle-free injection system for local anaesthesia prior to venous cannulation. *Anaesthesia* 2000;**55**:247–50.

72 Domino EF, Zsigmoid EK, Kovacs V, *et al.* A new route, jet injection for anesthetic induction in children: IV. Midazolam plasma levels. *Int J Clin Pharmacol Ther* 1998;**36**:458–62.

73 Domino EF, Zsigmond EK, Kovacs V, *et al.* A new route, jet injection for anesthetic induction in children: III. Ketamine pharmacokinetic studies. *Int J Clin Pharmacol Ther* 1997;**35**:527–30.

74 Florentine BD, Frankel K, Raza A, *et al.* Local anesthesia for fine-needle aspiration biopsy of palpable breast masses: the effectiveness of a jet injection system. *Diagn Cytopathol* 1997;**17**:472–6.

75 Bennett J, Nichols F, Rosenblum M, *et al.* Subcutaneous administration of midazolam: a comparison of the Bioject jet injector with the conventional syringe and needle. *J Oral Maxillofac Surg* 1998;**56**: 1249–54.

76 Agius E, Mooney JM, Bezzina AC, *et al.* Dermojet delivery of bleomycin for the treatment of recalcitrant plantar warts. *J Dermatolog Treat* 2006;**17**:112–16.

77 Bogenrieder T, Lehn N, Landthaler M, *et al.* Treatment of Old World cutaneous leishmaniasis with intralesionally injected meglumine antimoniate using a Dermojet device. *Dermatology* 2003;**206**:269–72.

78 Gibson JR, Harvey SG, Kemmett D, *et al.* Treatment of common and plantar viral warts with human lymphoblastoid interferon-alpha – pilot studies with intralesional, intramuscular and Dermojet injections. *Br J Dermatol* 1986;**115**(Suppl 31):76–9.

79 Saray Y, Gulec AT. Treatment of keloids and hypertrophic scars with Dermojet injections of bleomycin: a preliminary study. *Int J Dermatol* 2005;**44**:777–84.

80 Vadoud-Seyedi J. Treatment of plantar hyperhidrosis with botulinum toxin type A. *Int J Dermatol* 2004;**43**:969–71.

81 Vadoud-Seyedi J, Simonart T, Heenen M. Treatment of plantar hyperhidrosis with Dermojet injections of botulinum toxin. *Dermatology* 2000;**201**:179.

82 Dimache G, Croitoru M, Balteanu M, *et al.* A clinical, epidemiological and laboratory study on

avoiding the risk of transmitting viral hepatitis during vaccinations with the Dermojet protected by an anticontaminant disposable device. *Vaccine* 1997;**15**:1010–13.

83 Weintraub AM, Ponce de Leon MP. Potential for cross-contamination from use of a needleless injector. *Am J Infect Control* 1998;**26**:442–5.

84 Sarno MJ, Blase E, Galindo N, *et al.* Clinical immunogenicity of measles, mumps and rubella vaccine delivered by the Injex jet injector: comparison with standard syringe injection. *Pediatr Infect Dis J* 2000;**19**:839–42.

85 Resman Z, Metelko Z, Skrabalo Z. The application of insulin using the jet injector DG-77. *Acta Diabetol Lat* 1985;**22**:119–25.

86 Klein RM, Wolf ED, Wu R, *et al.* High-velocity microprojectiles for delivering nucleic acids into living cells. 1987. *Biotechnology* 1992;**24**:384–6.

87 Mulholland WJ, Kendall MA, White N, *et al.* Characterization of powdered epidermal vaccine delivery with multiphoton microscopy. *Phys Med Biol* 2004;**49**:5043–58.

88 Yang NS, Burkholder J, Roberts B, *et al.* In vivo and in vitro gene transfer to mammalian somatic cells by particle bombardment. *Proc Natl Acad Sci U S A* 1990;**87**:9568–72.

89 Condon C, Watkins SC, Celluzzi CM, *et al.* DNA-based immunization by in vivo transfection of dendritic cells. *Nat Med* 1996;**2**:1122–8.

90 Eisenbraun MD, Fuller DH, Haynes JR. Examination of parameters affecting the elicitation of humoral immune responses by particle bombardment-mediated genetic immunization. *DNA Cell Biol* 1993;**12**:791–7.

91 Falo LD, Jr. Targeting the skin for genetic immunization. *Proc Assoc Am Physicians* 1999;**111**:211–19.

92 Tuting T, Storkus WJ, Falo LD, Jr. DNA immunization targeting the skin: molecular control of adaptive immunity. *J Invest Dermatol* 1998;**111**:183–8.

93 Chen D, Burger M, Chu Q, *et al.* Epidermal powder immunization: cellular and molecular mechanisms for enhancing vaccine immunogenicity. *Virus Res* 2004;**103**:147–53.

94 Chen D, Endres R, Maa YF, *et al.* Epidermal powder immunization of mice and monkeys with an influenza vaccine. *Vaccine* 2003;**21**:2830–36.

95 Chen D, Endres RL, Erickson CA, *et al.* Epidermal powder immunization using non-toxic bacterial enterotoxin adjuvants with influenza vaccine augments protective immunity. *Vaccine* 2002;**20**:2671–9.

96 Chen D, Endres RL, Erickson CA, *et al.* Epidermal immunization by a needle-free powder delivery technology: immunogenicity of influenza vaccine and protection in mice. *Nat Med* 2000;**6**:1187–90.

97 Chen D, Erickson CA, Endres RL, *et al.* Adjuvantation of epidermal powder immunization. *Vaccine* 2001;**19**:2908–17.

98 Chen D, Maa YF, Haynes JR. Needle-free epidermal powder immunization. *Expert Rev Vaccines* 2002;**1**:265–76.

99 Chen D, Payne LG. Targeting epidermal Langerhans cells by epidermal powder immunization. *Cell Res* 2002;**12**:97–104.

100 Chen D, Periwal SB, Larrivee K, *et al.* Serum and mucosal immune responses to an inactivated influenza virus vaccine induced by epidermal powder immunization. *J Virol* 2001;**75**:7956–65.

101 Chen D, Weis KF, Chu Q, *et al.* Epidermal powder immunization induces both cytotoxic T-lymphocyte and antibody responses to protein antigens of influenza and hepatitis B viruses. *J Virol* 2001;**75**:11630–40.

102 Chen D, Zuleger C, Chu Q, *et al.* Epidermal powder immunization with a recombinant HIV gp120 targets Langerhans cells and induces enhanced immune responses. *AIDS Res Hum Retroviruses* 2002;**18**:715–22.

103 Dean HJ, Chen D. Epidermal powder immunization against influenza. *Vaccine* 2004;**23**:681–6.

104 Lodmell DL, Ray NB, Ulrich JT, *et al.* DNA vaccination of mice against rabies virus: effects of the route of vaccination and the adjuvant monophosphoryl lipid A (MPL). *Vaccine* 2000;**18**:1059–66.

105 Osorio JE, Zuleger CL, Burger M, *et al.* Immune responses to hepatitis B surface antigen following epidermal powder immunization. *Immunol Cell Biol* 2003;**81**:52–8.

106 Brave A, Hallengard D, Malm M, *et al.* Combining DNA technologies and different modes of immunization for induction of humoral and cellular anti-HIV-1 immune responses. *Vaccine* 2009;**27**:184–6.

107 Ludwig-Portugall I, Montermann E, Kremer A, *et al.* Prevention of long-term IgE antibody production by gene gun-mediated DNA vaccination. *J Allergy Clin Immunol* 2004;**114**:951–7.

108 Frelin L, Alheim M, Chen A, *et al.* Low dose and gene gun immunization with a hepatitis C virus nonstructural (NS) 3 DNA-based vaccine containing NS4A inhibit NS3/4A-expressing tumors in vivo. *Gene Ther* 2003;**10**:686–99.

109 Han R, Cladel NM, Reed CA, *et al.* DNA vaccination prevents and/or delays carcinoma development of papillomavirus-induced skin papillomas on rabbits. *J Virol* 2000;**74**:9712–16.

110 Han R, Cladel NM, Reed CA, *et al.* Protection of rabbits from viral challenge by gene gun-based intracutaneous vaccination with a combination of cottontail rabbit papillomavirus E1, E2, E6, and E7 genes. *J Virol* 1999;**73**:7039–43.

111 Han R, Peng X, Reed CA, *et al.* Gene gun-mediated intracutaneous vaccination with papillomavirus E7 gene delays cancer development of papillomavirus-induced skin papillomas on rabbits. *Cancer Detect Prev* 2002;**26**:458–67.

112 Han R, Reed CA, Cladel NM, *et al.* Immunization of rabbits with cottontail rabbit papillomavirus E1 and E2 genes: protective immunity induced by gene gun-mediated intracutaneous delivery but not by intramuscular injection. *Vaccine* 2000;**18**:2937–44.

113 Dean HJ, Fuller D, Osorio JE. Powder and particle-mediated approaches for delivery of DNA and protein vaccines into the epidermis. *Comp Immunol Microbiol Infect Dis* 2003;**26**:373–88.

114 Kamili S, Spelbring J, Carson D, *et al.* Protective efficacy of hepatitis E virus DNA vaccine administered by gene gun in the cynomolgus macaque model of infection. *J Infect Dis* 2004;**189**:258–64.

115 Lodmell DL, Ray NB, Parnell MJ, *et al.* DNA immunization protects nonhuman primates against rabies virus. *Nat Med* 1998;**4**:949–52.

116 McCluskie MJ, Brazolot Millan CL, Gramzinski RA, *et al.* Route and method of delivery of DNA vaccine influence immune responses in mice and non-human primates. *Mol Med* 1999;**5**:287–300.

117 Polack FP, Lee SH, Permar S, *et al.* Successful DNA immunization against measles: neutralizing antibody against either the hemagglutinin or fusion glycoprotein protects rhesus macaques without evidence of atypical measles. *Nat Med* 2000;**6**:776–81.

118 Macklin MD, McCabe D, McGregor MW, *et al.* Immunization of pigs with a particle-mediated DNA vaccine to influenza A virus protects against challenge with homologous virus. *J Virol* 1998;**72**: 1491–6.

119 Barfoed AM, Kristensen B, Dannemann-Jensen T, *et al.* Influence of routes and administration parameters on antibody response of pigs following DNA vaccination. *Vaccine* 2004;**22**:1395–1405.

120 Barfoed AM, Blixenkrone-Møller M, Jensen MH, *et al.* DNA vaccination of pigs with open reading frame 1–7 of PRRS virus. *Vaccine* 2004;**22**:3628–41.

121 Rompato G, Ling E, Chen Z, *et al.* Positive inductive effect of IL-2 on virus-specific cellular responses elicited by a PRRSV-ORF7 DNA vaccine in swine. *Vet Immunol Immunopathol* 2006;**109**:151–60.

122 Beard C, Ward G, Rieder E, *et al.* Development of DNA vaccines for foot-and-mouth disease, evaluation of vaccines encoding replicating and non-replicating nucleic acids in swine. *J Biotechnol* 1999; **73**:243–9.

123 Fuller DH, Loudon P, Schmaljohn C. Preclinical and clinical progress of particle-mediated DNA vaccines for infectious diseases. *Methods* 2006;**40**:86–97.

124 Liu MA, Ulmer JB. Human clinical trials of plasmid DNA vaccines. *Adv Genet* 2005;**55**:25–40.

125 Cui Z. DNA vaccine. *Adv Genet* 2005;**54**:257–89.

126 Roy MJ, Wu MS, Barr LJ, *et al.* Induction of antigen-specific CD8$^+$ T cells, T helper cells, and protective levels of antibody in humans by particle-mediated administration of a hepatitis B virus DNA vaccine. *Vaccine* 2000;**19**:764–78.

127 Roberts LK, Barr LJ, Fuller DH, *et al.* Clinical safety and efficacy of a powdered hepatitis B nucleic acid vaccine delivered to the epidermis by a commercial prototype device. *Vaccine* 2005;**23**:4867–78.

128 Rottinghaus ST, Poland GA, Jacobson RM, *et al.* Hepatitis B DNA vaccine induces protective antibody responses in human non-responders to conventional vaccination. *Vaccine* 2003;**21**:4604–8.

129 Tacket CO, Roy MJ, Widera G, *et al.* Phase 1 safety and immune response studies of a DNA vaccine encoding hepatitis B surface antigen delivered by a gene delivery device. *Vaccine* 1999;**17**: 2826–9.

130 Drape RJ, Macklin MD, Barr LJ, *et al.* Epidermal DNA vaccine for influenza is immunogenic in humans. *Vaccine* 2006;**24**:4475–81.

131 McConkey SJ, Reece WH, Moorthy VS, *et al.* Enhanced T-cell immunogenicity of plasmid DNA vaccines boosted by recombinant modified vaccinia virus Ankara in humans. *Nat Med* 2003;**9**: 729–35.

132 Raju PA, McSloy N, Truong NK, *et al.* Assessment of epidermal cell viability by near infrared multiphoton microscopy following ballistic delivery of gold micro-particles. *Vaccine* 2006;**24**:4644–7.

CHAPTER 22

Oral Vaccines: An Old Need and Some New Possibilities

Amit A. Lugade, Kalathil Suresh, & Yasmin Thanavala
Department of Immunology, Roswell Park Cancer Institute, Buffalo, NY, USA

Introduction

The mucosal immune system provides the first line of defense for epithelial surfaces that are in continuous contact with the environment. It is comprised of specialized cells that patrol the various tissues in order to ensure that immediate responses are generated against invading pathogens and other foreign antigens. Reducing the potential pathogenic burden upon infection and limiting the proinflammatory tissue damage in response to infection are critical to maintaining a functional mucosal barrier. The immune system in the intestine has developed mechanisms to prevent pathogen colonization as the first line of defense to complement adaptive immune responses. These include the expression of mucosal secretions, such as antimicrobial peptides and gastric acids that create an inhospitable environment for noncommensal microorganisms. In addition, epithelial cells in the mucosa express cilia to deter pathogen attachment and physically expel the agent from the host's body. When this first line of defense is insufficient for protection, the mucosal immune system has also evolved pathways to respond to pathogens while simultaneously preventing unnecessary and potentially detrimental responses to dietary antigens. To maintain the homeostasis at mucosal surfaces, the immune system has developed two strategies: (i) physical exclusion of pathogens by the presence of secreted IgA to limit epithelial contact and invasion by microorganisms, and (ii) immunosuppressive mechanisms to prevent damage against innocuous antigens mediated by an overexuberant proinflammatory responses [1]. The second mechanism, referred to as "oral tolerance," depends largely on the development of regulatory T cells [2]. Because of this tolerance mechanism, we do not normally respond to dietary antigens. Several investigators are developing methods to exploit this feature of oral tolerance in the gut to treat autoimmune diseases such as Crohn's and celiac, where disregulated mucosal tolerance leads to the activation of immune responses against the host's own tissue [3,4] (for further details, see Chapter 4).

In order to mount appropriate responses against pathogens and avoid generating responses against dietary antigens, the intestinal mucosa is organized as a complex network of anatomical structures and immune cells to effectively protect this surface [5,6]. The immune network in mucosal tissues, termed mucosal-associated lymphoid tissue (MALT), is organized with distinct features depending on the tissue in which it is located. These include the gut-associated lymphoid tissue (GALT), which is also composed of enterocytes and mucus-secreting goblet cells in addition to the immune cells [7]. The GALT is ideally situated at

Vaccinology: Principles and Practice, First Edition. Edited by W. John W. Morrow, Nadeem A. Sheikh, Clint S. Schmidt and D. Huw Davies.
© 2012 Blackwell Publishing Ltd. Published 2012 by Blackwell Publishing Ltd.

the interface at which orally administered, dietary, pathogen-associated, or vaccine antigens make the first contact with the host's epithelium. Enterocytes and goblet cells make up the outermost layer of the GALT, which is distinct from the epithelial layer located directly below, termed the lamina propria. Within the small intestine, the lamina propria forms finger-like projections with the surrounding epithelial layer into structures known as intestinal villi and crypts of Lieberkühn, involved in absorption of nutrients from ingested food. Lymphocytes in the GALT are organized into lymphoid follicles and are surrounded by an epithelial layer containing a specialized cell known as the M cell. Unlike the surrounding epithelial cells, M cells have the unique ability to endocytose antigen from the lumen of the intestine and deliver the antigen via transcytosis to the dendritic cells (DCs) in the lymphoid follicles [8]. The high efficiency of antigen sampling by the M cells is attributed to their lack of apical microvilli and the presence of microfolds. Antigen delivered by M cells to DCs or directly endocytosed by a subset of lamina propria DCs, which extend their dendrites into the lumen, is processed and is then able to stimulate specific T cells. Activated CD4$^+$ T cells within these lymphoid follicles and Peyer's patches are then capable of providing help to B cells for the production of antibodies, specifically secretory IgA, which is critical for mucosal protection [9].

The propensity of tolerance induction via antigen introduction in mucosal tissue, especially in the oral and nasal tissue, is an important hurdle for mucosal vaccine development. The factors that induce oral tolerance, such as amount of antigen and frequency of dosing, are also critical for the generation of effective immune responses following vaccination. To overcome this limitation and elicit protective immune responses, mucosal adjuvants and delivery systems, including transgenic plants, have been developed in order to utilize the oral route of immunization [10]. There are currently four licensed vaccines against important childhood diseases that are administered orally: polio (Sabin), cholera, typhoid, and rotavirus.

Polio vaccine

Infection with the polio virus occurs in the intestinal mucosa, and the oral live attenuated vaccine induces antibodies that prevent virus attachment to the intestinal epithelium, and thus infection and transmission. As one of the first approved mucosal vaccines, the live attenuated oral polio vaccine (OPV) developed by Albert Sabin generated protective immune responses similar to the injectable inactivated polio vaccine (IPV) developed earlier by Jonas Salk [11]. Both are trivalent vaccines that elicit antibody responses against the three serotypes of the polio virus. The OPV produces a higher titer of virus-specific IgG in the serum compared to the IPV; however, the main advantage of the OPV is the induction of mucosal IgA, which the IPV is incapable of eliciting [12–14]. As infection with the virus occurs primarily in the intestinal mucosa, the OPV offers the benefit of local mucosal immunity, which cannot be achieved by the IPV. Thus, while the IPV is considered to be a safe vaccine as it prevents polio virus infection, one of the disadvantages is its inability to induce mucosal immune responses [15]. Developing nations continue to use the OPV because it induces effective immunity at a lower cost of administration than the injectable IPV, which requires sterile needles and trained health care staff to administer the injection and carefully dispose of the needles [13]. However, despite the advantages of the OPV in terms of efficacy and administration, the oral polio vaccine does have the disadvantage that it has the ability to revert to a form that can cause neurovirulence and paralysis (vaccine-associated paralytic poliomyelitis) [16]. The rate of vaccine-associated poliomyelitis is rare, being approximately one case in 750,000 administered doses. Outbreaks of paralytic polio caused by the vaccine have been reported every year since 2000 [17]. Since the widespread use of the polio vaccine, the rate of poliomyelitis has declined dramatically in most industrialized nations; since 2000, the OPV has not been used in the USA or in the UK. In order to achieve global eradication of polio, the OPV will require improvements in its safety. An effective mucosal adjuvant will also be a necessity in order to elicit robust polio-specific immunity in both mucosal and systemic tissue.

Cholera vaccine

Diarrheal diseases represent a major global health problem and are attributable for approximately 2.2 million deaths annually, of which a great proportion occur in children under 5 years of age in developing nations. Half of the cases of diarrhea are caused by pathogenic bacteria that produce enterotoxins, and infection with *Vibrio cholerae* is one of the most severe enteropathies. The global burden of cholera still remains substantial in the developing world, which lacks access to clean, safe drinking water and good sanitation [18]. An injectable vaccine containing inactivated *V. cholerae* was used to prevent cholera until the end of the 20th century. Although it is still available, the injectable vaccine is now not prescribed as frequently due to adverse side reactions and induction of short-lived immune responses [19]. To overcome the limitations of the injectable vaccine, two oral cholera vaccines were developed. One of the newer vaccines, licensed under the name Orochol, is a recombinant live attenuated vaccine generated by modifying the cholera toxin (CT) gene. The *V. cholerae* Inaba strain 569B used in the vaccine no longer expresses the toxic A subunit [20]. The nontoxic but immunogenic B subunit (CTB) is left intact and provides adjuvant activity for immunization with the vaccine. The vaccine strain CVD 103 HgR is given as a single oral dose and prevented cholera in adults living in industrialized nations [21,22]. However, when the vaccine was tested in Thailand and Indonesia no significant protection was observed, leading to a cessation in production of this vaccine [23,24]. The second licensed oral vaccine (Dukoral) utilizes an inactivated *V. cholerae* strain (O1) combined with recombinant CTB. Volunteers given three oral doses of Dukoral generated both mucosal IgA in the intestinal tract and serum IgG [25]. A clinical trial conducted in Bangladesh demonstrated that protective responses were observed in children aged 2–5 years and in adults with 63% efficacy [26,27]. An important analysis

from the clinical trial in Bangladesh was the tangible proof of herd immunity, a process in which vaccination of a portion of the population (or herd) provides protection to nonvaccinated individuals. This effect occurred in areas in which vaccine coverage was achieved in 50% of individuals, thus fewer cases of cholera were observed in nonvaccinated individuals who lived in close proximity to vaccinated individuals [27]. Herd immunity from cholera vaccination has the advantage of reducing the cholera burden for regions in which the disease is endemic with the use of fewer vaccine doses. The vaccine was also shown to produce short-term protection against severe cholera in regions of sub-Saharan Africa with high prevalence of HIV [28]. An added benefit of this oral vaccine was the elicitation of cross-protective responses against enterotoxigenic *Escherichia coli* (ETEC) [29]. This pathogen expresses the heat-labile enterotoxin (LT), which is highly homologous to CT [30], thus leading to cross-protection against another pathogen that is also responsible for diarrheal diseases in developing nations.

Typhoid vaccine

Typhoid fever is caused by *Salmonella enterica* serovar Typhi and the prevalence of this disease is highest in children aged 5–19 years in developing nations. Two types of vaccines are currently available, an injectable vaccine comprised of the Vi polysaccharide and an oral vaccine comprised of a live attenuated Ty21a strain (Vivotif) [31,32]. The injectable vaccine induces protective responses against the O antigen of the polysaccharide, found in the outer membrane of the bacteria. A single dose of the parenteral vaccine provided 70% protection over three years in South African children, but was not as efficacious in infants, resulting in lower titers of antigen-specific antibodies [33]. The oral vaccine was initially administered as three doses and provided 67% protection over three years due to the induction of both serum IgG and mucosal IgA [34,35]. Chemical mutagenesis of the *S. enterica* Typhi strain Ty21a resulted in an attenuated vaccine but the possibility remains for the strain to revert to virulence, although revertants have yet to be isolated [36,37]. Unfortunately, the oral version of the vaccine requires three to four oral doses for optimal protection [38]. A version of the oral vaccine that elicits protection from a single dose is therefore highly desirable. The original oral vaccine strain was shown to be deficient in the expression of the Vi polysaccharide; however, a new strain that constitutively expresses the Vi polysaccharide is currently under testing [39,40]. The newer live attenuated vaccine strain CVD 909 (HolaVax-Typhoid) is in phase II testing and has shown no difference in the rates of diarrhea after vaccination among volunteers receiving low and high doses of vaccine [39]. Serum anti-polysaccharide antibodies and T-cells responses against the Typhi antigen were observed in volunteers given the oral CVD 909 vaccine, thereby providing encouraging data for the success of an oral vaccine against typhoid fever.

Rotavirus vaccine

Rotavirus is the causative agent of acute gastroenteritis in children younger than 5 years of age. Two surface proteins on the virion capsid, VP4 and VP7, are the main targets for neutralizing antibodies against virus serotypes P and G, respectively [41,42]. Five combinations of the P and G serotypes account for roughly 90% of all human infective rotavirus strains – G1P8, G2P4, G3P8, G4P8, and G9P8 – thereby specifying the targets required for a successful vaccine [41]. Analysis of vaccine recipients has shown that levels of rotavirus-specific serum IgA in general are associated with intestinal levels of antigen-specific IgA [43,44]. Thus, the induction of intestinal IgA is likely the most important indicator of protection against rotavirus gastroenteritis. The first licensed oral vaccine against rotaviruses was a live attenuated tetravalent vaccine composed of rhesus and human rotavirus strains, named RotaShield. The treatment schedule for RotaShield was three doses, the first given at 8 weeks of age, and follow-up oral boosters at 8-week intervals [45]. The vaccine was efficacious at preventing diarrhea and rotavirus infection, but was withdrawn from the market in 1999 due to the perceived risk of vaccine-associated intussusception, or bowel obstruction, in one of every 10,000–32,000 vaccinated infants. To replace RotaShield, there are two new licensed vaccines, RotaTeq (licensed in 2006) and Rotarix (licensed in 2008), both of which are live attenuated rotavirus given orally. The Rotarix vaccine is comprised of a tissue culture-adapted rotavirus strain of serotype G1P8. This strain was chosen as the only serotype to be included in the vaccine as G1P8 is the predominant strain for infections worldwide, and neutralizing antibodies against G1P8 are to some extent broadly cross-reactive with other strains. This version of the vaccine is given as two oral doses, at 2 and 4 months of age. A phase III trial of the vaccine in infants showed great efficacy at preventing gastroenteritis without an increased risk of intussusception [46]. In contrast, RotaTeq is composed of five reassortant rotavirus strains derived from a bovine strain engineered to express P and G serotypes of human origin. RotaTeq is administered as three oral doses at 2, 4, and 6 months of age. A phase III trial of RotaTeq in infants was also efficacious in preventing rotavirus gastroenteritis; and the risk of intussusception was similar between vaccine and placebo recipients [47].

Plant-derived vaccines: current status and challenges ahead

Plants are emerging as an attractive platform for vaccine antigen expression and are superior to other approaches in several aspects. Plant virus based transient expression system are suitable for rapid engineering, scaling up, and low-cost effective production in bulk quantities within a short span of time to meet contingencies of natural outbreaks, and accidental or intended release of biothreats such as *Bacillus anthracis* and *Yersinia pestis*. Plant-derived vaccines can be relatively inexpensively processed for oral delivery, obviating the need for time consuming and expensive fermentation, purification, cold storage, and transportation. Plant-generated therapeutic proteins, as in other eukaryotic systems, are subject to post-translational modifications, including proper folding and disulfide bond formation in chloroplasts or endoplasmic reticulum [48,49]. However, therapeutic proteins are not glycosylated in chloroplasts; this only occurs when targeted to the endoplasmic reticulum. Although an enormous number of proteins have been expressed in plants, transgene silencing is one of the formidable challenges to be addressed in nuclear transgenic plants. Limited studies have been carried out on purification and characterization of proteins and contaminants, and stability of the protein after harvest, processing, and storage. As in the case of recombinant proteins developed in other system, plant-derived therapeutic proteins have to circumvent regulatory hurdles in order for them to be administered orally. Over the past two decades, vaccine antigens expressed via the plant nuclear genome have elicited robust immune responses and have conferred protection upon oral delivery [50,51], but no transgenic plant-based vaccine for human use has yet moved beyond a phase I clinical trial.

Stably integrated nuclear transgene

The earliest reported study that used plants for the recombinant expression of vaccine antigens was performed using stable transformation of the nuclear genome of tobacco (*Nicotiana tobacum*) [52]. The nuclear transgene methodology facilitated by *Agrobacterium*-mediated gene delivery was easy and it dominated the field for several years. This approach has several advantages, including the ability to scale up large quantity of vaccine antigens from seed stock with a possibility to express in fruits and edible plant products, enabling the oral delivery of minimally processed antigens. However, stably integrated nuclear antigens had very low levels of expression, which varied from plant to plant or generation, which could be attributed to gene silencing or position effect [53]. Oral delivery of antigens elicited specific antibody responses in mice as well as in clinical trials. Antigens derived from enteric pathogens such as Norwalk virus capsid protein (NVCP), rotavirus capsid protein, and the cholera toxin B subunit (CTB) and *E. coli* heat-labile enterotoxin B subunit (LTB) have been generated in nuclear transgenic plants, and oral administration

of these proteins in mice has been shown to protect against cholera toxin challenges [54,55]. Several other antigens from non-enteric pathogens, such as the F protein of respiratory syncytial virus [56] and hepatitis B surface antigen (HBsAg) [57], also stimulate antigen-specific antibodies after oral delivery. The requirement of adjuvants for such stimulation was inevitable, as in the case of HBsAg fed to mice in transgenic potato tubers, along with CT, a potent mucosal adjuvant, to stimulate significant levels of anti-HBsAg antibodies [58]. Interestingly, the same transgenic HBsAg-expressing potato tubers fed to humans without adjuvant as a booster dose provoked serum anti-HBs immunoglobulin in a significant majority of the volunteers. Potatoes and other plant organs except seeds have a limited shelf life and freeze-drying can compromise the efficacy of the vaccine as compared to fresh potato due to oxidation of phenolic compounds in the potato tissue during freeze drying [59].

Chloroplast-derived vaccine antigens

Chloroplast-derived therapeutic antigens are generated by homologous recombination of foreign antigens into chloroplasts. The major advantages of chloroplast transgenic lines are high expression levels of the transgene in transformed plants without gene silencing effects, and minimal risk of gene contamination via pollen from genetically modified plants to other related crops or weeds through maternal inheritance of transgene [60]. Expression of vaccine antigens in leaves, which facilitates their harvest before the development of any reproductive structures, is yet another strategy for containment. Chloroplast expression systems have been exploited to produce several functional vaccine antigens against bacterial, viral, and protozoan pathogens. One major disadvantage of the system is that many therapeutic proteins are expressed in tobacco leaves and the leaf of this plant is not suitable for human consumption. Addictiveness of nicotine rules out the feasibility of oral delivery of therapeutic proteins expressed in tobacco leaves. The levels of transgene expression and regeneration in lettuce chloroplast are comparable to tobacco and this system is being optimized to develop several therapeutic proteins such as proinsulin [61,62]. Chloroplast-derived therapeutic proteins, delivered orally via plant cells, are protected from degradation in the stomach, presumably because of the encapsulation of antigen by plant cell wall. The translocation of the therapeutic protein from the gut lumen to circulation is facilitated by fusing with CTB, which can bind to the epithelial receptor GM1 [63]. Oral or subcutaneous administration of chloroplast-derived bacterial antigen has been shown to confer protection in mice challenged with CT, through elaboration of both IgA and IgG1 antibody [49]. Vaccine antigen against tetanus also conferred complete protection against pathogen challenge. An anthrax vaccine expressed in transgenic tobacco chloroplast is devoid of extraneous bacterial contaminant responsible for side effects and has been shown to protect mice immunized subcutaneously from lethal doses of toxin challenges [64]. Oral delivery of plague F1 antigen expressed in chloroplasts has been shown to be protective against a large dose of aerosolized *Yersinia pestis* plague challenge [65]. Canine parvovirus (CPV) antigen was the first viral antigen capable of eliciting protective immune responses when expressed in chloroplasts in mice. Human papilloma virus 16 capsid L1, expressed in chloroplasts, displayed conformation-specific epitope and on intraperitoneal administration in mice elicited neutralizing antibody responses. Protozoan antigens, such as *Entamoeba histolytica* antigen, LecA, and malaria vaccine candidates AMA1 and MSP1 fused with CTB, expressed in tobacco chloroplasts or lettuce leaves, produced antigen-specific anybody titers in mice immunized orally or subcutaneously [49,66]. Autoantigens, including human proinsulin, fused with CTB were expressed in chloroplasts, and immunization of mice elicited Th2-type responses with elaboration of immunosuppressive cytokines IL4 and IL10 in pancreas, resulting in oral tolerance with concomitant reduction in the infiltrating lymphocytes (insulitis) into the pancreas [62]. Several other human proteins, such as human serum albumin, IFN-γ, IFN-α-2b, and human α1 antitrypsin, have also been expressed in chloroplasts, and the biological properties of these blood proteins were validated in functional assays. Proper functionality

of these proteins revealed that the requisite post-translational modifications such as disulfide bonding were carried out in chloroplasts [67].

A major advantage of plant-derived vaccines and biopharmaceuticals is that there is no need for expensive fermentation and purification systems and other expenses associated with cold storage, transportation, and sterile delivery. Even though stable nuclear expression systems have been developed over the past decades and are available in a large number of crops, with the ability to facilitate tissue-specific expression and inducible expression, expression levels are often inadequate for commercial development. Chloroplast expression systems offer a higher level of expression of vaccine antigens against a broad spectrum of pathogens such as bacterial, viral, and protozoan pathogens, and biopharmaceuticals. However, glycosylated proteins cannot be expressed in chloroplast systems in their glycosylated form. Viral expression systems produce therapeutic proteins rapidly; however, they are not suitable for oral delivery. Therefore, expenses associated with purification, storage, and sterile delivery will be major challenges in viral system. Research in viral expression systems has made great strides in recent years, with the development of passive antibody against non-Hodgkin's lymphoma for clinical trials, development of anti-HIV peptides, and testing of F1-V plague vaccine in monkeys. Transient expression systems may be ideally suited for pandemic responses such as H1N1 influenza strains. The ultimate success of plant-derived vaccines will depend on the commercially viable targets for transitioning through clinical trials.

Plant-based vaccine trials

Transgenic plants have several advantages for oral vaccine delivery over the customary parenteral vaccinations. Newer iterations of plant-based vaccines have minimal requirement for cold storage, during either transportation or storage. The obvious need for sterile needles and syringes, and trained health care workers to use and dispose of these items properly, is also of nominal concern with oral delivery of plant-derived vaccines. An increased emphasis on vaccine safety has also been a critical driving force behind the development of subunit vaccines. Although plant-based vaccines have been in development for almost 20 years, only one plant-derived vaccine has reached licensure. In 2006, Dow Agroscience (IN, USA) received regulatory approval from the US Department of Agriculture Center for Veterinary Biologics for a plant-made vaccine targeting a viral disease in poultry [68]. Our group will begin conducting a phase I/II dose escalation trial of safety and immunogenicity with HBsAg-transgenic potatoes in July 2012. Inadequate expression levels of vaccine antigens within the transgenic plant have been improved upon through new techniques such as stable transformation of the nuclear genome and homologous recombination into chloroplasts. To date, the leaves and fruits of transgenic plants have been utilized for oral vaccine delivery in phase I clinical trials. Although a large number of candidate antigens from human pathogens have been introduced into many transgenic plant models [69], only a few prototype antigens have been tested in humans. These include enterotoxigenic *E. coli*, Norwalk virus, and hepatitis B virus.

Enterotoxigenic *Escherichia coli*

The plant-based vaccine against ETEC utilizes the highly immunogenic heat-labile enterotoxin B subunit of *E. coli*. The LT toxin consists of an enzymatically active A subunit associated with five LTB subunits. LTB is responsible for bacterial adherence to epithelial cell via binding to GM1 ganglioside; therefore, antibodies against LTB induced by vaccination prevent toxin binding to the epithelia and the resulting infection and diarrheal disease. This vaccine antigen was first successfully introduced into tobacco and potato plants by Haq and colleagues in 1995 [70]. LTB expressed in the plant self-assembled into the pentameric structures observed in the bacteria and was capable of binding to GM1 ganglioside *in vitro*. Preclinical studies in mice fed multiple doses of LTB-expressing potato tubers demonstrated that LTB-specific serum IgG and mucosal IgA could be generated [71]. In fact, these LTB-specific titers were higher in potato-fed mice than in mice immunized with bacterial-derived LTB. Vaccinated mice challenged with the fully toxinogenic LT were slightly protected and had a significant reduction in intestinal fluid accumulation in the patent mouse assay, thereby providing proof for the potential of this plant-based vaccine.

A phase I clinical trial using the LTB-expressing potato tuber was conducted by Tacket and colleagues based on the encouraging responses observed in mice given the vaccine [72]. Raw transgenic potatoes and control potatoes were given to healthy volunteers in three separate 100 g doses. Each dose of transgenic potato contained approximately 0.4–1.1 mg of LTB. All volunteers developed LTB-specific antibody secreting cells, which were detectable in blood, following the complete course of transgenic potato consumption. In addition, a significant majority of volunteers who received the transgenic potatoes developed at least four-fold increases in LT-specific serum IgG, which also showed evidence of LT neutralization in a functional assay. In addition, half of the volunteers developed LT-specific IgA detectable in stool samples; thus representing the first proof of principle that a transgenic plant vaccine could be immunogenic in humans. LTB has also been introduced into transgenic corn, as this vaccine plant model is inexpensive to produce and scale up. In fact, expressed genes are highly concentrated in the corn germ at levels up to 10 mg/g. In 2002, Streatfield and colleagues reported that defatted corn germ meal from the LTB-expressing transgenic corn was well tolerated in mice and induced antigen-specific serum IgG and fecal IgA [73]. The transgenic corn germ meal given to healthy volunteers in a phase I clinical trial as three 2 g doses resulted in the generation of LT-specific serum IgG and IgA after the last dose of transgenic vaccine [74]. Four of nine volunteers displayed increases in antigen-specific IgA detected in stool samples. Work from these groups has shown that systemic and mucosal immune responses can be generated following ingestion of either whole fruit or plant extract.

Norwalk virus

Norwalk virus (NV) is a member of the *Caliciviridae* enteric virus family, which is an important etiological agent of gastroenteritis. The major capsid protein (NVCP) self-assembles into virus-like particles (VLP) when it is expressed in cloned insect cells. The naked VLPs of the capsid protein are highly immunogenic when administered orally, and this result has prompted the development of a transgenic potato that expresses NVCP as a source for increased antigen production [75]. Plant-derived NVCP also assemble into particles that are structurally identical to the VLPs generated from insect cells. Mice that were fed these transgenic potatoes developed serum IgG and fecal IgA responses, providing the necessary proof to proceed with testing in human volunteers.

In the phase I clinical trial, volunteers received either two or three doses of transgenic potato or three doses of control potato [76]. Each dose consisted of 150 g of raw potato tuber and the transgenic potato contained approximately 500 μg of NVCP, only half of which was assembled into VLPs. Volunteers from both of the transgenic potato fed groups developed IgA secreting cells that were detectable in the blood after ingestion of the first dose. Only 4 of the 20 volunteers developed anti-NVCP serum IgG responses and stool IgA was detected in 6 volunteers who ingested the transgenic potatoes. Current work is focused on improving the expression and VLP assembly of NVCP in the potato tuber in order to enhance immunogenicity.

Hepatitis B virus

Hepatitis B virus (HBV) is the causative agent of chronic hepatitis, cirrhosis, and hepatocellular carcinoma. Although HBV is primarily a sexually transmitted disease, a chronic carrier mother can also transmit the virus to the baby due to viral exposure at the time of birth. The current parenteral vaccine is comprised of a yeast-derived recombinant form of HBV surface antigen (HBsAg) adsorbed to alum as an adjuvant. HBsAg plays an important role in viral infection and induction of anti-HBs antibodies is protective. This vaccine antigen was first introduced into tobacco plants by Mason and colleagues, and was shown to self-assemble into VLPs in the plant tissue with similar characteristics to the particles made by HBV and the yeast-derived vaccine antigen [52]. Tobacco leaf extracts

were utilized to generate purified HBsAg and subsequently fed to mice to test the immunogenicity of tobacco-derived HBsAg particles. Levels of serum anti-HBs antibodies elicited to the tobacco-derived HBsAg were found to be similar to those in mice immunized with the yeast-derived HBsAg, thus establishing that plant-derived vaccine antigens had equivalent immunologic properties to non-plant-derived vaccine antigens [77]. Preclinical studies in mice were extended to measuring the immunogenicity of HBsAg-expressing potato tubers [78]. Mice that were fed three times with 5 g of transgenic potato tubers expressing 8 μg of HBsAg along with 10 μg of CT mucosal adjuvant developed a primary response and a strong and sustained secondary response when boosted with recombinant HBsAg. These studies also established the ability of transgenic plant vaccines to provide a booster response in mice immunized with a suboptimal dose of parenteral vaccine.

A randomized, placebo-controlled, double blind phase I clinical trial was conducted to test the efficacy of HBsAg-expressing potato tubers to boost serum anti-HBs levels in volunteers who had previously received the parenteral vaccine 1–15 years earlier [57]. Study subjects consumed two or three doses of raw transgenic tubers or three doses of control potatoes. Volunteers who ingested the transgenic tubers developed serum anti-HBs titers that were significantly higher than their own baseline controls. Overall, 63% of volunteers who consumed the three doses of transgenic HBsAg-expressing tubers showed marked increases in antibody titers compared with their own titers at the start of the study (up to 33-fold after two doses and 56-fold after three doses). In this trial, no adjuvant was utilized. Thus, remarkably, HBsAg, an antigen from a non-enteric pathogen (HBV), stimulated antibody responses when delivered to humans by ingestion of transgenic potatoes. This has prompted the development of an additional phase II clinical trial to test whether high titers and increased numbers of responders can be achieved by oral administration of transgenic potatoes in conjunction with a mucosal adjuvant. Lettuce leaves expressing HBsAg have also been tested in three human volunteers who had not been previously immunized

[79]. Two of the three volunteers made anti-HBs response greater than 10 mIU/mL but the responses were not sustained.

Although plant-made vaccines will likely not supplant other vaccine technologies, they offer the promise of serving as an alternative and economical system that will find its most promising application in underdeveloped nations.

Acknowledgments

The work in the Thanavala laboratory was supported by grants from the National Institutes of Health AI42836, R44 HL083553 and a World Health Organization Vaccines and Other Biologicals Grant (15/181/416).

References

1 Mowat AM, Parker LA, Beacock-Sharp H, *et al.* Oral tolerance: overview and historical perspectives. *Ann N Y Acad Sci* 2004;**1029**:1–8.

2 Ishikawa H, Tanaka K, Maeda Y, *et al.* Effect of intestinal microbiota on the induction of regulatory CD25$^+$ CD4$^+$ T cells. *Clin Exp Immunol* 2008;**153**: 127–35.

3 Meresse B, Ripoche J, Heyman M, *et al.* Celiac disease: from oral tolerance to intestinal inflammation, autoimmunity and lymphomagenesis. *Mucosal Immunol* 2009;**2**:8–23.

4 Hyun JG, Barrett TA. Oral tolerance therapy in inflammatory bowel disease. *Am J Gastroenterol* 2006; **101**:569–71.

5 Garside P, Millington O, Smith KM. The anatomy of mucosal immune responses. *Ann N Y Acad Sci* 2004; **1029**:9–15.

6 Nagler-Anderson C. Man the barrier! Strategic defences in the intestinal mucosa. *Nat Rev Immunol* 2001; **1**:59–67.

7 Kunisawa J, Fukuyama S, Kiyono H. Mucosa-associated lymphoid tissues in the aerodigestive tract: their shared and divergent traits and their importance to the orchestration of the mucosal immune system. *Curr Mol Med* 2005;**5**:557–72.

8 Corr SC, Gahan CC, Hill C. M-cells: origin, morphology and role in mucosal immunity and microbial pathogenesis. *FEMS Immunol Med Microbiol* 2008;**52**:2–12.

9 Makala LH, Suzuki N, Nagasawa H. Peyer's patches: organized lymphoid structures for the induction of mucosal immune responses in the intestine. *Pathobiology* 2002;**70**:55–68.

10 Ogra PL, Faden H, Welliver RC. Vaccination strategies for mucosal immune responses. *Clin Microbiol Rev* 2001;**14**:430–45.

11 Ehrenfeld E, Modlin J, Chumakov K. Future of polio vaccines. *Expert Rev Vaccines* 2009;**8**:899–905.

12 Dowdle WR, De GE, Kew OM, *et al.* Polio eradication: the OPV paradox. *Rev Med Virol* 2003;**13**:277–91.

13 Falleiros-Carvalho LH, Weckx LY. Universal use of inactivated polio vaccine. *J Pediatr (Rio J)* 2006;**82**: S75–S82.

14 Zaman S, Carlsson B, Jalil F, *et al.* Comparison of serum and salivary antibodies in children vaccinated with oral live or parenteral inactivated poliovirus vaccines of different antigen concentrations. *Acta Paediatr Scand* 1991;**80**:1166–73.

15 Ivanov A, Dragunsky E, Ivanova O, *et al.* Determination of poliovirus-specific IgA in saliva by ELISA tests. *J Virol Methods* 2005;**126**:45–52.

16 Laassri M, Lottenbach K, Belshe R, *et al.* Analysis of reversions in the 5'-untranslated region of attenuated poliovirus after sequential administration of inactivated and oral poliovirus vaccines. *J Infect Dis* 2006;**193**:1344–9.

17 Jackson ST, Mullings AM, Booth TF, *et al.* Molecular analysis and implications of neurovirulent circulating vaccine-derived poliovirus in Jamaica. A case report and review of literature. *West Indian Med J* 2008;**57**:511–14.

18 Sack DA, Sack RB, Nair GB, *et al.* Cholera. *Lancet* 2004; **363**:223–33.

19 Mosley WH, Aziz KM, Mizanur-Rahman AS, *et al.* Report of the 1966–67 cholera vaccine trial in rural East Pakistan. *Bull World Health Organ* 1972;**47**:229–38.

20 Levine MM, Kaper JB, Herrington D, *et al.* Safety, immunogenicity, and efficacy of recombinant live oral cholera vaccines, CVD 103 and CVD 103-HgR. *Lancet* 1988;**2**:467–70.

21 Cryz SJ, Levine MM, Kaper JB, *et al.* Randomized double-blind placebo controlled trial to evaluate the safety and immunogenicity of the live oral cholera vaccine strain CVD 103-HgR in Swiss adults. *Vaccine* 1990;**8**:577–80.

22 Kotloff KL, Wasserman SS, O'Donnell S, *et al.* Safety and immunogenicity in North Americans of a single dose of live oral cholera vaccine CVD 103-HgR: results of a randomized, placebo-controlled, double-blind crossover trial. *Infect Immun* 1992;**60**:4430–32.

23 Su-Arehawaratana P, Singharaj P, Taylor DN, *et al.* Safety and immunogenicity of different immunization regimens of CVD 103-HgR live oral cholera vaccine in soldiers and civilians in Thailand. *J Infect Dis* 1992;**165**:1042–8.

24 Richie EE, Punjabi NH, Sidharta YY, *et al.* Efficacy trial of single-dose live oral cholera vaccine CVD 103-HgR in North Jakarta, Indonesia, a cholera-endemic area. *Vaccine* 2000;**18**:2399–410.

25 Shamsuzzaman S, Ahmed T, Mannoor K, *et al.* Robust gut associated vaccine-specific antibody-secreting cell responses are detected at the mucosal surface of Bangladeshi subjects after immunization with an oral killed bivalent *V. cholerae* O1/O139 whole cell cholera vaccine: comparison with other mucosal and systemic responses. *Vaccine* 2009;**27**:1386–92.

26 Clemens JD, Sack DA, Harris JR, *et al.* Field trial of oral cholera vaccines in Bangladesh: results from three-year follow-up. *Lancet* 1990;**335**:270–73.

27 Ali M, Emch M, Von SL, *et al.* Herd immunity conferred by killed oral cholera vaccines in Bangladesh: a reanalysis. *Lancet* 2005;**366**:44–9.

28 Lucas ME, Deen JL, Von SL, *et al.* Effectiveness of mass oral cholera vaccination in Beira, Mozambique. *N Engl J Med* 2005;**352**:757–67.

29 Clemens JD, Sack DA, Harris JR, *et al.* Cross-protection by B subunit-whole cell cholera vaccine against diarrhea associated with heat-labile toxin-producing enterotoxigenic *Escherichia coli*: results of a large-scale field trial. *J Infect Dis* 1988;**158**:372–7.

30 Dallas WS, Falkow S. Amino acid sequence homology between cholera toxin and *Escherichia coli* heat-labile toxin. *Nature* 1980;**288**:499–501.

31 Plotkin SA, Bouveret-Le CN. A new typhoid vaccine composed of the Vi capsular polysaccharide. *Arch Intern Med* 1995;**155**:2293–9.

32 Fraser A, Goldberg E, Acosta CJ, *et al.* Vaccines for preventing typhoid fever. *Cochrane Database Syst Rev* 2007 Jul **18**(3):CD001261.

33 Klugman KP, Koornhof HJ, Robbins JB, *et al.* Immunogenicity, efficacy and serological correlate of protection of *Salmonella typhi* Vi capsular polysaccharide vaccine three years after immunization. *Vaccine* 1996;**14**:435–8.

34 Levine MM, Ferreccio C, Abrego P, *et al.* Duration of efficacy of Ty21a, attenuated *Salmonella typhi* live oral vaccine. *Vaccine* 1999;**17**(Suppl 2):S22–S27.

35 Salerno-Goncalves R, Pasetti MF, Sztein MB. Characterization of CD8(+) effector T cell responses in volunteers immunized with *Salmonella enterica* serovar Typhi strain Ty21a typhoid vaccine. *J Immunol* 2002;**169**:2196–203.

36 McKenna AJ, Bygraves JA, Maiden MC, *et al.* Attenuated typhoid vaccine *Salmonella typhi* Ty21a: fingerprinting and quality control. *Microbiology* 1995;**141** (Pt 8):1993–2002.

37 Garmory HS, Brown KA, Titball RW. Salmonella vaccines for use in humans: present and future perspectives. *FEMS Microbiol Rev* 2002;**26**:339–53.

38 World Health Organization. Typhoid vaccines: WHO position paper. *Wkly Epidemiol Rec* 2008;**83**:49–59.

39 Tacket CO, Pasetti MF, Sztein MB, *et al.* Immune responses to an oral typhoid vaccine strain that is modified to constitutively express Vi capsular polysaccharide. *J Infect Dis* 2004;**190**:565–70.

40 Wang JY, Noriega FR, Galen JE, *et al.* Constitutive expression of the Vi polysaccharide capsular antigen in attenuated *Salmonella enterica* serovar Typhi oral vaccine strain CVD 909. *Infect Immun* 2000;**68**:4647–52.

41 Santos N, Hoshino Y. Global distribution of rotavirus serotypes/genotypes and its implication for the development and implementation of an effective rotavirus vaccine. *Rev Med Virol* 2005;**15**:29–56.

42 Pesavento JB, Crawford SE, Estes MK, *et al.* Rotavirus proteins: structure and assembly. *Curr Top Microbiol Immunol* 2006;**309**:189–219.

43 Franco MA, Angel J, Greenberg HB. Immunity and correlates of protection for rotavirus vaccines. *Vaccine* 2006;**24**:2718–31.

44 Velazquez FR, Matson DO, Guerrero ML, *et al.* Serum antibody as a marker of protection against natural rotavirus infection and disease. *J Infect Dis* 2000;**182**:1602–9.

45 Matson DO. RotaShield: the ill-fated rhesus-human reassortant rotavirus vaccine. *Pediatr Ann* 2006;**35**:44–50.

46 Ruiz-Palacios GM, Perez-Schael I, Velazquez FR, *et al.* Safety and efficacy of an attenuated vaccine against severe rotavirus gastroenteritis. *N Engl J Med* 2006;**354**:11–22.

47 Vesikari T, Matson DO, Dennehy P, *et al.* Safety and efficacy of a pentavalent human-bovine (WC3) reassortant rotavirus vaccine. *N Engl J Med* 2006;**354**:23–33.

48 Moravec T, Schmidt MA, Herman EM, *et al.* Production of *Escherichia coli* heat labile toxin (LT) B subunit in soybean seed and analysis of its immunogenicity as an oral vaccine. *Vaccine* 2007;**25**:1647–57.

49 Voodi-Semiromi A, Samson N, Daniell H. The green vaccine: a global strategy to combat infectious and autoimmune diseases. *Hum Vaccin* 2009;**5**:488–93.

50 Aviezer D, Brill-Almon E, Shaaltiel Y, *et al.* A plant-derived recombinant human glucocerebrosidase enzyme – a preclinical and phase I investigation. *PLoS One* 2009;**4**:e4792.

51 Yusibov V, Rabindran S. Recent progress in the development of plant derived vaccines. *Expert Rev Vaccines* 2008;**7**:1173–83.

52 Mason HS, Lam DM, Arntzen CJ. Expression of hepatitis B surface antigen in transgenic plants. *Proc Natl Acad Sci U S A* 1992;**89**:11745–9.

53 Voinnet O, Rivas S, Mestre P, *et al.* An enhanced transient expression system in plants based on suppression of gene silencing by the p19 protein of tomato bushy stunt virus. *Plant J* 2003;**33**:949–56.

54 Nochi T, Yuki Y, Matsumura A, *et al.* A novel M cell-specific carbohydrate-targeted mucosal vaccine effectively induces antigen-specific immune responses. *J Exp Med* 2007;**204**:2789–96.

55 Rosales-Mendoza S, Puche-Solis AG, Soria-Guerra RE, *et al.* Expression of an *Escherichia coli* antigenic fusion protein comprising the heat labile toxin B subunit and the heat stable toxin, and its assembly as a functional oligomer in transplastomic tobacco plants. *Plant J* 2009;**57**:45–54.

56 Sandhu JS, Krasnyanski SF, Domier LL, *et al.* Oral immunization of mice with transgenic tomato fruit expressing respiratory syncytial virus-F protein induces a systemic immune response. *Transgenic Res* 2000;**9**:127–35.

57 Thanavala Y, Mahoney M, Pal S, *et al.* Immunogenicity in humans of an edible vaccine for hepatitis B. *Proc Natl Acad Sci U S A* 2005;**102**:3378–82.

58 Kong Q, Richter L, Yang YF, *et al.* Oral immunization with hepatitis B surface antigen expressed in transgenic plants. *Proc Natl Acad Sci U S A* 2001;**98**:11539–44.

59 Zhang X, Buehner NA, Hutson AM, *et al.* Tomato is a highly effective vehicle for expression and oral immunization with Norwalk virus capsid protein. *Plant Biotechnol J* 2006;**4**:419–32.

60 Daniell H. Transgene containment by maternal inheritance: effective or elusive? *Proc Natl Acad Sci U S A* 2007;**104**:6879–80.

61 Lelivelt CL, McCabe MS, Newell CA, *et al.* Stable plastid transformation in lettuce (*Lactuca sativa* L.). *Plant Mol Biol* 2005;**58**:763–74.

62 Ruhlman T, Ahangari R, Devine A, *et al.* Expression of cholera toxin B-proinsulin fusion protein in lettuce and tobacco chloroplasts – oral administration protects against development of insulitis in non-obese diabetic mice. *Plant Biotechnol J* 2007;**5**:495–510.

63 Limaye A, Koya V, Samsam M, *et al.* Receptor-mediated oral delivery of a bioencapsulated green fluorescent protein expressed in transgenic chloroplasts into the mouse circulatory system. *FASEB J* 2006;**20**:959–61.

64 Watson J, Koya V, Leppla SH, *et al.* Expression of *Bacillus anthracis* protective antigen in transgenic chloroplasts of tobacco, a non-food/feed crop. *Vaccine* 2004;**22**:4374–84.

65 Arlen PA, Singleton M, Adamovicz JJ, *et al.* Effective plague vaccination via oral delivery of plant cells expressing F1-V antigens in chloroplasts. *Infect Immun* 2008;**76**:3640–50.

66 Chebolu S, Daniell H. Stable expression of Gal/GalNAc lectin of *Entamoeba histolytica* in transgenic chloroplasts and immunogenicity in mice towards vaccine development for amoebiasis. *Plant Biotechnol J* 2007;**5**:230–39.

67 Staub JM, Garcia B, Graves J, *et al.* High-yield production of a human therapeutic protein in tobacco chloroplasts. *Nat Biotechnol* 2000;**18**:333–8.

68 Agriculture.com. First vaccine made in plant cells receives regulatory approval. Available at www.agriculture.com/news/business/First-vaccine-made-in-plant-cells-receives-regulatory-approval_5-ar165. Accessed Feb 2012.

69 Tiwari S, Verma PC, Singh PK, *et al.* Plants as bioreactors for the production of vaccine antigens. *Biotechnol Adv* 2009;**27**:449–67.

70 Haq TA, Mason HS, Clements JD, *et al.* Oral immunization with a recombinant bacterial antigen produced in transgenic plants. *Science* 1995;**268**:714–16.

71 Mason HS, Haq TA, Clements JD, *et al.* Edible vaccine protects mice against *Escherichia coli* heat-labile enterotoxin (LT): potatoes expressing a synthetic LT-B gene. *Vaccine* 1998;**16**:1336–43.

72 Tacket CO, Mason HS, Losonsky G, *et al.* Immunogenicity in humans of a recombinant bacterial antigen delivered in a transgenic potato. *Nat Med* 1998;**4**:607–9.

73 Lamphear BJ, Streatfield SJ, Jilka JM, *et al.* Delivery of subunit vaccines in maize seed. *J Control Release* 2002;**85**:169–80.

74 Tacket CO, Pasetti MF, Edelman R, *et al.* Immunogenicity of recombinant LT-B delivered orally to humans in transgenic corn. *Vaccine* 2004;**22**:4385–9.

75 Mason HS, Ball JM, Shi JJ, *et al.* Expression of Norwalk virus capsid protein in transgenic tobacco and potato and its oral immunogenicity in mice. *Proc Natl Acad Sci U S A* 1996;**93**:5335–40.

76 Tacket CO, Mason HS, Losonsky G, *et al.* Human immune responses to a novel Norwalk virus vaccine delivered in transgenic potatoes. *J Infect Dis* 2000;**182**:302–5.

77 Thanavala Y, Yang YF, Lyons P, *et al.* Immunogenicity of transgenic plant-derived hepatitis B surface antigen. *Proc Natl Acad Sci U S A* 1995;**92**:3358–61.

78 Richter LJ, Thanavala Y, Arntzen CJ, *et al.* Production of hepatitis B surface antigen in transgenic plants for oral immunization. *Nat Biotechnol* 2000;**18**:1167–71.

79 Kapusta J, Modelska A, Pniewski T, *et al.* Oral immunization of human with transgenic lettuce expressing hepatitis B surface antigen. *Adv Exp Med Biol* 2001;**495**:299–303.

CHAPTER 23

Adjuvants: From Serendipity to Rational Discovery

Derek T. O'Hagan[1] & Andreas Wack[2]
[1]Novartis Vaccines and Diagnostics, Inc., Cambridge, MA, USA
[2]Division of Immunoregulation, National Institute for Medical Research, London, UK

What are adjuvants and why do we need them?

One of the consequences of most self-limiting infections is the induction of antigen (Ag)-specific immunologic memory leading to long-term protection from a second infection by the same pathogen. Simply put, the aim of vaccination is to achieve the same goal but to avoid disease in the process. The logical consequence of this was that the original development of vaccines was based on attenuated, fixed, and split pathogens, similar enough to the natural pathogen to induce specific immunity, but disabled enough to avoid disease and tissue damage. While many of these vaccines were and still are very successful, this approach is limited in some cases either by insufficient immunogenicity or unacceptable reactogenicity profiles of the vaccine antigens [1]. Therefore, most future vaccines will be based on highly purified soluble recombinant protein antigens, which by their nature tend to be poorly immunogenic. This is the first and foremost reason why adjuvants will be needed in future-generation vaccines. Moreover, adjuvants offer important advantages, including the induction of greater breadth of the antibody response, to cover pathogen diversity; the induction of potent functional antibody responses, to ensure pathogen killing or neutralization; and the in-

duction of more effective T-cell responses, for direct and indirect pathogen killing. In addition, adjuvants may be necessary to achieve more pragmatic effects, including antigen dose reduction and overcoming antigen competition in combination vaccines. Last but not least, the target groups of vaccination are often at-risk populations such as infants, the elderly, and immunocompromised individuals, groups that share reduced immune responses due to immaturity of their immune system, immunosenescence, or pre-existing medical conditions.

The earliest definition of a vaccine adjuvant describes it as a component that is added to vaccine antigens to make them more immunogenic [2]. Therefore, the term "vaccine adjuvant" is based on function, not on what substances they actually are, which reflects the mostly empirical, if not serendipitous, nature of adjuvant discovery. As a consequence, a very heterogeneous assortment of substances is used under this name, and new adjuvants are regularly described in the literature. Moreover, as the signaling pathways involved in immune activation are becoming better defined, many more "new" adjuvants will emerge, or be rediscovered. Attempts have been made to classify adjuvants, including the distinction between "delivery systems," which means that their predominant mechanism of action was thought to be delivery of antigens to immune cells, and "immune potentiators," which

Vaccinology: Principles and Practice, First Edition. Edited by W. John W. Morrow, Nadeem A. Sheikh, Clint S. Schmidt and D. Huw Davies.
© 2012 Blackwell Publishing Ltd. Published 2012 by Blackwell Publishing Ltd.

exert direct effects on immune cells, leading to their activation [3]. However, in this classification system, delivery systems that were thought to be inert have to be shifted to the alternative category once an ability to directly activate immune cells is ascribed to them, and this has happened regularly in recent years [4–7]. Here we use a classification based on the idea of different adjuvant generations, which takes into account the heterogeneity of the substances used and of the mechanisms they employ. This offers an opportunity to find commonality among the diverse approaches under evaluation, while not being prone to regular reassessments. For a long time, there was very little progress in understanding the mechanism of action of adjuvants, but there has been a recent renaissance in this area. Knowledge of the effects of adjuvants on the immune system is a rapidly expanding and evolving field, with many notable recent observations.

The canonical member of the first generation of vaccine adjuvants is represented by insoluble aluminum salts, generically called alum (Table 23.1), which was originally identified in the 1920s [8] and is now used in licensed vaccines all over the world [9] (Figure 23.1). Emulsion adjuvants were first introduced only a decade later by Freund [10] and also belong to the first generation of adjuvants. A second emulsion adjuvant that is a success is the MF59 oil in water emulsion, which has been licensed for more than a decade in a significant number (>20) of countries [11]. Emulsions were originally thought to work similarly to alum, since they released antigen over an extended time period from the entrapped water in heavy mineral oils [12]. An additional adjuvant technology that has gained approval is virosomes, which, like MF59, has been licensed as a component of an influenza vaccine [13]. Hence, the most successful generation 1 adjuvants are linked by their physical structure and dimensions; they are particulate dispersions (alum aggregates or emulsion droplets), to which antigen may be bound or associated. Moreover, they were originally designed to extend the duration of antigen persistence at the injection site. It was also thought to be important that the adjuvant induced a degree of local inflammation, to help recruit antigen-presenting cells. More practical considerations underpinning the success of these adjuvant technologies include their ability to be scaled and reproducibly manufactured, within parameters that can be easily quantified. To optimize their chances of success, adjuvants should ideally be comprised of cheap and easily obtainable components that are not inherently variable and should be biodegradable, or at least biocompatible and well tolerated. Although it might be argued that only alum has really achieved broad success as an adjuvant, since it is used in a range of vaccines produced by different manufacturers, preclinical data show that MF59 is a more potent adjuvant for a broad range of vaccines than alum [14]. Moreover, additional manufacturers are also bringing forward adjuvant technologies similar to MF59, although sometimes additional components are added, which are claimed to be immune potentiating [15,16]. In addition, several alternative particulate carriers were also evaluated as adjuvants in the 1970s, including polymeric nanoparticles [17] and liposomes [18]. Like alum, these alternative approaches had the appropriate dimensions to promote uptake into immune cells and they were able to adsorb or encapsulate antigen to enhance persistency and improve delivery. Based on their particulate structure and dimensions, nanoparticles (or microparticles) and liposomes also belong to the first generation of adjuvants.

Generation 2 adjuvants were initiated in the 1970s, following the discovery of synthetic components that activated the immune system, including muramyl dipeptide (MDP). MDP was originally identified as the smallest water-soluble component of mycobacterial cell wall with adjuvant activity [19]. It was quickly realized, however, that components extracted from microorganisms would not be optimally effective as single components, so they were coupled to, or linked to, the existing generation 1 adjuvants, including liposomes [20]. Even before MDP had been identified, synthetic double-stranded RNA had been added to an emulsion adjuvant to improve its potency for influenza vaccines [21]. Hence, generation 2 adjuvants, which comprise more than one adjuvant component, have been around for more than 40 years (Table 23.1).

Table 23.1 Examples of first- and second-generation adjuvant formulations tested in humans.

Name	Company	Class	Indications	Stage
Generation 1 adjuvants				
Alum	Various	Mineral salt	Various	Licensed
MF59	Novartis	O/W emulsion	Influenza (Fluad)/ pandemic influenza	Licensed (EU)
Liposomes	Crucell	Lipid vesicles	HAV, influenza	Licensed (EU)
Montanide	Various	W/O emulsion	Malaria, cancer	Phase III
PLG	Novartis	Polymeric microparticle	DNA vaccine (HIV)	Phase I
Flagellin	Vaxinnate	Flagellin linked to antigen	Influenza	Phase I
QS21	Antigenics	Saponin	Various	Phase I
Generation 2 combination adjuvants				
AS01	GSK	MPL + liposomes + QS21	Malaria, TB	Phase II
AS02	GSK	MPL + O/W emulsion + QS21	Malaria	Phase II
AS03	GSK	O/W emulsion + α-tocopherol	Pandemic influenza (Pandemrix)	Licensed (EU)
AS04	GSK	MPL + alum	HBV (Fendrix), HPV (Cervarix)	Licensed (EU)
RC-529	Dynavax	Synthetic MPL + alum	HBV	Phase II
Iscom	CSL, Isconova	Saponins + cholesterol + phospholipids	Various	Phase I
IC31	Intercell	Peptide + oligonucleotides	TB	Phase I
CpG 7909	Coley/Pfizer Novartis	Oligonucleotide + alum, oligonucleotide + MF59	HBV, malaria, HCV	
ISS	Dynavax	Oligonucleotide alum	HBV	Phase II
MF59 + MTP-PE	Chiron/Novartis	Lipidated MDP + O/W emulsion	HIV, influenza	Phase I

O/W, oil in water; W/O water in oil; MPL, monophosphoryl lipid A; MDP, muramyl dipeptide.

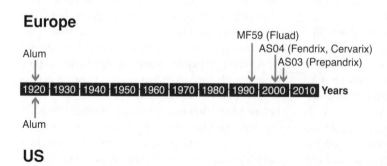

Figure 23.1 Chronology of the introduction of adjuvants for use in humans. Alum was licensed in both Europe and the US in the 1920s and was for a long time the only adjuvant approved for human use. Progress has accelerated but continues to be slow.

Only now, however, are generation 2 adjuvants reaching licensure in approved vaccine products. An example for this is alum/monophosphoryl lipid A (MPL) (trade name ASO4 by GlaxoSmithKline), which has been licensed in a significant number of countries as a component of a vaccine against human papilloma virus [22] and for an improved vaccine against hepatitis B virus [23]. In addition, there are a number of alternative generation 2 adjuvants in various phases of development (Table 23.1). Unfortunately, there is already a long and largely unsuccessful history of previous attempts to include immune potentiators in vaccines. Hence, the decision on which immune potentiator to include in second-generation adjuvant formulations will continue to be a difficult one, until more success is achieved and the path to success becomes clearer. Moreover, given this challenging environment, a key early question in any vaccine development program is to consider the need for a more potent adjuvant. Clearly, the path to vaccine licensure will be significantly longer if a second-generation adjuvant is required to enable vaccine efficacy. It will be important to show that the second-generation adjuvant is necessary to achieve the desired response and that it shows a clear and consistent benefit over first-generation alternatives, to justify inclusion. The challenges to including a second-generation adjuvant in a vaccine product are very demanding from a regulatory perspective, and this needs to be fully appreciated by the group developing the vaccine candidate. To summarize, adjuvant development is a slow and laborious process and approval of new adjuvants in licensed products has been and will remain a very challenging endeavor.

Safety safety safety

As pointed out above, the approval of new adjuvants is complex, and safety issues, rather than effectiveness, can be considered the limiting step in successful adjuvant development [24]. Safety issues represent a complex and evolving challenge and need to be considered as an informed risk/benefit analysis. Some "safety" issues are immediate, but these may really be issues of tolerability, which may or may not reflect a longer-term issue. Nevertheless, if an adjuvant induces a significant degree of local reactions, then almost certainly the adjuvant would be considered unsuitable for further development. The "acceptability" of the tolerability profile needs, however, to be defined in the context of the vaccine target indication, taking into consideration the incidence of infection and the severity of the disease. In a simple illustration, the acceptable tolerability profile for an adjuvant to be used in a therapeutic cancer vaccine would be very different from that of a prophylactic vaccine to be used in infants. Hence, important questions in adjuvant selection include: What is the indication? Who are the target population? and What is the acceptable balance of risk to benefit in this population? The tolerance for even a perception of "risk" for a vaccine to be used in large numbers of healthy children is understandably very low.

An additional problem for current candidates is the origin of some of the materials being used as immune potentiators. The adjuvants often comprise natural products with inherent variability, some of which have proven impossible to synthesize. Sometimes, the extraction of sufficient quantities of fully characterized and reproducible material becomes an issue, as does the expense involved. Synthetic analogs of some of the natural compounds are, however, now becoming available [25]. Moreover, some new-generation adjuvants are highly amenable to rapid, efficient, and inexpensive synthetic approaches [3].

Mechanisms of adjuvanticity: the target cells

Immunologists widely agree that dendritic cells (DCs) represent the crucial relay between the initial phase of innate immune activation and the slower but more Ag-specific adaptive immune activation that eventually confers immune memory, the desired outcome of vaccination. The reason for the prominent role of DCs is their unique ability to migrate into the T-cell areas of lymph nodes, to present processed antigen to naïve T cells, to activate ("prime") them, and thereby to trigger the adaptive arm of the immune response [26]. While this "DC-centric" view of the immune response is certainly supported by a wealth of published data, it has led to the assumption that adjuvants function by directly activating DCs, and many adjuvant discovery programs are based on this assumption. For first-generation adjuvants such as alum and MF59, the available data on DC activation was contradictory for years, and recent publications show that an important, if not the crucial, effect of these adjuvants is to induce recruitment of innate immune cells into the site of application, thereby generating an environment of increased immunostimulation, with the ultimate outcome of DC activation [4–6]. This means that, eventually, DCs are more activated when vaccine Ag is given together with adjuvant rather than without it, but the actual target cells of these adjuvants are not DCs and their direct effect is upstream of DC activation.

In the case of MF59, it became clear that vast amounts of chemoattractants are produced by direct activation of purified human granulocytes, monocytes, or monocyte-derived macrophages, but not by DCs purified from blood or by monocyte-derived DCs. The results obtained for alum were broadly similar, showing that monocytes were the direct target cells of intraperitoneally applied alum, but DCs were crucial further downstream to generate the increased immune response [6]. The immune cells that are recruited into the injection site of conventional vaccines include neutrophils, eosinophils, and others, suggesting an ancillary role in inducing adaptive immune responses. While for some of these cell types, it remains to be determined whether their appearance is a collateral consequence of adjuvant use, for some adjuvants, a potential contribution to adjuvant function appears more likely. A number of recent publications propose a role for neutrophils in presentation and cross-presentation, suggesting that they take over the part of antigen-presenting cells from DCs [27, 28]. An important alternative mechanism is more indirect: It has been shown that DCs are activated through interaction with neutrophils, and this appears to depend on cell-surface receptor DC-SIGN interaction with Mac-1 [29] or CEACAM [29,30],

and on the production of TNF-α by neutrophils. Alternatively, since neutrophils are among the first and most numerous cells to be recruited into the injection site, and at the same time are producers of copious amounts of cytokines, their role may simply be that of an early source of chemoattractants to enhance cell recruitment in a positive feedback loop [4,31].

A mouse study has shown that alum induces the migration to the spleen of $Gr1^+$ myeloid cells, which have been implicated in priming and expansion of antigen-specific B cells [32]. More recently, it has been demonstrated that this $Gr1^+$ cell population responsible for B-cell priming in the spleen is represented by eosinophils [33], thus adding these cells to the growing list of innate cells with accessory function in adjuvanticity. A role for basophils in enhancing memory responses was also shown, as a cytokine source for both T and B cells after boosting with soluble antigen [34]. The proposed mechanism is that antibodies formed in the primary response are pre-bound to basophil Fc receptors, and that a secondary antigen administration activates basophils, leading to a wave of cytokines such as IL6 and IL4, which act as natural adjuvants for T and B cells, thus enhancing cognate interaction. The interesting possibility that mast cells contribute to the induction of adaptive immune response was raised by a study showing that the compound c48/80, a commonly used mast-cell activator, acts as an adjuvant [35]. It was shown that the adjuvanticity of c48/80 depends on the mast cell–dependent activation of DCs, which triggers an efficient migration of DCs to lymph nodes.

Other cell types that have long been shown to be able to enhance and modulate adaptive immune responses are natural killer (NK) cells, by the early, rapid, and strong production of cytokines [36], and invariant natural killer T (iNKT) cells through stimulation of their semi-invariant T-cell receptor (TCR) by CD1d-presented glycosphingolipid antigens. Therefore, such lipids can be used as adjuvants, and the adjuvant properties of the prototype compound, α-galactosylceramide (αGalCer) have been demonstrated in many animal models in which this iNKT agonist was able to enhance both T and B cell specific responses to the co-administered antigen [37–39]. In addition, activation of iNKT cells by αGalCer used as adjuvant for vaccination against influenza was shown to promote survival of memory cytotoxic T lymphocytes (CTL) [40]. It is as yet unclear whether the mechanism of αGalCer adjuvanticity is by direct iNKT help to B cells [41,42], or through a more indirect effect involving the licensing of DCs that present both CD1d-αGalCer and MHC II-antigen peptide on their surface [43]. To summarize, many of the innate immune cell populations are now directly implicated in adjuvanticity, although their precise contribution to the adjuvant effects is in many cases upstream of DC activation, and this is currently under intense study.

For Toll-like receptor agonists (see below) used as adjuvants, the same considerations as described above need to be made, taking into account cells both upstream and downstream of DCs: many innate immune cells apart from monocytes and DCs – for instance, neutrophils and basophils – express a wide range of TLRs, and the effects of their TLR-mediated activation are not known. Therefore, it may be that at least some of the effects of this adjuvant group (immune potentiators) are not directly on DCs, but on other innate cells as discussed above. In addition, some subsets of T cells and most B cells express a number of different TLRs, and adjuvanticity may be due to the synergy of simultaneous stimulation through their Ag receptors and their TLRs. For B cells, this view emerges from studies in mice where either B cells or DCs were unresponsive to TLR signaling. In some cases, enhanced antibody responses depended more on the TLR responsiveness of B cells than of the DCs [44,45] (see also Chapter 26).

In conclusion, from a cellular point of view, both first- and second-generation adjuvants appear to have complex mechanisms of action and more than one target is directly or indirectly involved (Figure 23.2). These mechanistic questions are not merely esoteric considerations, but are very important to understand better how first- and second-generation adjuvants work, and why they sometimes work too well or not enough. Moreover, these questions are important to expand the scope of agents that might work as adjuvants and

to be able to design improved versions for third-generation adjuvants.

Mechanisms of adjuvanticity: the target molecules

The target cells for many of the first-generation adjuvants were not identified until recently, and the often-described "depot" effect implied that there may be no such thing as a specific target cell. This is rapidly beginning to change, but clearly identified molecular targets are still lacking for some common adjuvants. For alum, the inflammasome was recently shown to mediate the activation of immune cells, leading to the activation of caspase 1, a protease that is required for maturation of several proinflammatory cytokines, including IL1β [46]. A number of *in vitro* studies have confirmed that alum activates the inflammasome in concert with TLR agonists such as lipopolysaccharide (LPS), but *in vivo* studies addressing the requirement of inflammasome components for alum adjuvanticity have provided conflicting results [45–48]. While the precise molecular mechanism remains unclear, alum appears to employ a mechanism similar to that of silica, asbestos, and other crystal-like substances that are phagocytosed, probably involving the release of cathepsins from unstable phagosomes into the cytosol [49]. Uric acid, a crystalline substance released from dying cells, is also able to activate inflammasomes, and was shown to be a mediator of alum adjuvanticity, suggesting another more indirect link between alum and the inflammasome [6]. Another "antigen delivery system," polylactide-co-glycolide (PLG) microparticles, was also shown to activate the inflammasome *in vitro* [7]. However, the molecular target of MF59 and other emulsion adjuvants is as yet unclear (see also Chapter 24).

In contrast to first-generation adjuvants, most of the immune potentiators that are components of second-generation adjuvants have a more defined molecular target and a fairly clear signaling pathway mediating activation. The targets are in most cases pattern recognition receptors (PRRs), part of an ancient system of pathogen recognition by distinct molecular patterns specific for

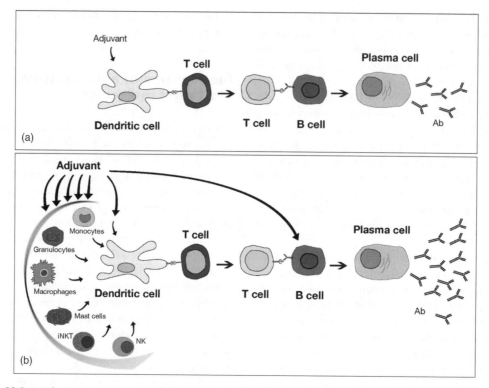

Figure 23.2 (a) The intervention point of adjuvants was originally thought to be predominantly the dendritic cell. (b) Recent evidence indicates that many types of innate immune cells can be activated upstream of DC activation, and that B cells can receive direct signals as well.

microbes, but not for the host organism (pathogen-associated molecular patterns, PAMPs) [50]. In fact, the majority of immune potentiators under evaluation today are microbial products, including flagellin, MDP, derivatives of LPS such as MPL, or mimics of bacterial or viral DNA or RNA such as methylated cytidine-guanine (CpG) motifs and polyinosinic:polycytidylic acid (poly I:C) oligonucleotides. All of these adjuvant molecules target a specific subset of PRRs called Toll-like receptors (TLRs), which are found on the surface or in the endosomal lumen of many immune cells and enable these cells to recognize extracellular or phagocytosed microorganisms [51]. Most TLR agonists increase the immunogenicity of co-administered antigens in preclinical models [52], and some of them have been successfully tested as vaccine adjuvants in human clinical trials: For example, CpG

oligonucleotides have been evaluated in combination with a number of antigens [53], and MPL is a component of a licensed vaccine product [54] (Table 23.2). Other PRR classes such as non-obese diabetic (NOD) -like receptors (NLRs), of which the NALP inflammasome components are members, and RIG-I-like helicases (RLHs) are found in the cytosol and activate immune cells and other cells when their ligands of microbial origin accumulate intracellularly, for instance in the case of viral infection of these cells. In conclusion, PRRs such as those included in inflammasomes and TLRs have been identified as targets of known adjuvants, and more adjuvants will be discovered through target-based screens. In contrast, first-generation adjuvants such as alum and Freund's incomplete adjuvant were shown to be TLR-independent [55, 56], leaving space for improvement by combining

Table 23.2 Toll like receptor (TLR) as vaccine adjuvant target (immune potentiators).

TLR	Localization	Natural elicitor	Elicitor	Vaccine target
TLR1–2	Plasma membrane	Cell wall components of Gram-positive bacteria, fungi	Triacyl lipopeptides (PAM3CSK4)	Preclinical
TLR2–6	Plasma membrane	Cell wall components of Gram-positive bacteria, fungi	Diacyl lipoptides (PAM2CSK4), MALP2, peptidoglycan	Preclinical
TLR3	Endosome	Viral RNA	dsRNA (Poly I:C)	Preclinical
TLR4	Plasma membrane	Cell wall components of Gram-negative bacteria, viral proteins	LPS (MPL, synthetic MPL)	MPL approved in EU for HBV and HPV vaccines in EU (GSK)
TLR5	Plasma membrane	Bacterial Flagellae	Flagellin	Preclinical
TLR7	Endosome	Viral RNA	ssRNA, imiquimod	Preclinical
TLR8	Endosome	Viral RNA	ssRNA, resiquimod	Preclinical
TLR9	Endosome	Bacterial and viral DNA	DNA, CpG oligonucleotides	CpG oligonucleotides in clinical trials for Antrax and melanoma vaccines
TLR10	Plasma membrane	Unknown	Unknown	

different components into potent combination adjuvants to trigger a variety of different activation pathways [57].

Outlook: what will the adjuvants of the future look like?

Accumulated lessons and setbacks have, hopefully, given us some insight on which to base our predictions of what a generation 3 adjuvant will look like. In essence, we propose that a delivery system should be used to ensure co-delivery of antigens and immune potentiators to the key immune cells. Moreover, the delivery system should ensure that the delivery of the immune potentiator is specific to the cells of interest and not more generalized, and good examples for this already exist [58]. The immune potentiator should be localized at the injection site, to minimize the impact on more diverse immune cells. As outlined above, TLRs and other PRRs are expressed on a diverse range of cells and are not specialized only to immune cells. Therefore, for reasons of safety, the delivery of potent immune potentiators needs to be controlled and focused. The objective will be to deliver the right molecule or molecules to the right site, for the right amount of time, but we still know very little about what is really required, particularly in relation to the temporal issues. Nevertheless, we believe that the technology for delivery is in place, although the immunology is still far behind and we have much to learn. We propose that delivery can be achieved using biodegradable microparticles, which have already been successfully scaled up for manufacturing, and have already been commercialized for drug delivery.

The adjuvant effect of linking antigens to synthetic microparticles was first described quite some time ago [59] and nondegradable particles have been used extensively since [60]. The development of biodegradable polymers to form the microparticles allowed this area to advance significantly. Microparticles prepared from biodegradable polymers were initially evaluated for systemic [61] and oral [62] vaccine delivery at the end of the 1980s. A subsequent development was the use of the more common biodegradable polymer, poly(lactide co-glycolide) (PLG), for vaccine delivery [63]. Since this polymer had already been used for the development of several drug delivery systems, it was an attractive approach. Although there were some significant challenges in the early stages of this technology, mostly due to the degradation of entrapped antigens [64], an important advance was the use of preformed microparticles for the delivery of adsorbed antigen [65,66]. The use of preformed microparticles allowed PLGs to be used more like the established alum adjuvant, but with the advantages of a biodegradable polymer with the potential to co-deliver additional adjuvant components. Second-generation microparticles are able to co-deliver adjuvants, which can be adsorbed [67] or entrapped [68]. Although microparticles worked better for traditional vaccines, if they were combined with alum [69], this eliminated some of the advantages of the technology. A similar path has also been followed for nanoparticles, which were originally described as adjuvants in the 1970s [17], but have more recently been described using the PLG polymer [70]. Nanoparticles, however, do not yet appear to have advantages in terms of potency over microparticles [71], but they may have other advantages, including ease of manufacture [70]. Although both microparticles and nanoparticles are capable of modifying the release of entrapped agents, it is not yet clear what is the desirable release profile for immune potentiators. This is likely to be a productive area of research.

As discussed briefly earlier, new-generation adjuvants include small-molecule immune potentiators (SMIPs), which have many inherent advantages over microbial-derived compounds. Small molecules can be synthesized easily and inexpensively and can be optimized to be highly specific for the preferred target, while avoiding undesired toxic effects. In addition, their potency may be modified relatively easily, as can their pharmacokinetic and pharmacodynamic properties to avoid systemic exposure. Moreover, synthetic drugs can be modified by appropriate linkers to enable easier for-

mulation and delivery. Despite these many potential advantages, so far only a few small molecules, mainly belonging to the imidazoquinoline class and targeting TLR7 and 8, have been used as vaccine adjuvants. The future development of new classes of SMIPs targeting selective PRRs such as TLRs, NLRs, or RLHs is, however, very promising. The development of new SMIPs, highly specific for their target, will also allow the investigation of which PRR is the best target for a given class of pathogens. For example, one intracellular RNA sensor such as TLR3, 7, 8, or RIG-I could be the optimal target for vaccination against RNA viruses, while a plasma membrane microbial sensors such as TLR2 or 4 may be the optimal PRR to target in order to achieve protective immunity to extracellular bacteria.

Conclusions

This chapter should make it clear that vaccine adjuvants are difficult to develop. Moreover, with increasing regulatory concerns in relation to safety, it is not going to get any easier. In this context, it is important to consider how we can enhance our chances of success. Unnecessary complexity must be avoided. A simple and scaleable formulation needs to be identified early, preferably using readily available and inexpensive materials, which have an established safety profile, ideally in an existing medical product. In interactions with regulators, it will be necessary to show a clear and compelling need for the inclusion of all active components in the formulation, particularly those that are added for an adjuvant effect. The impact of a second adjuvant component must be clear and easily quantifiable, preferably improving clinical protection, or enhancing an immune correlate of protective immunity. Although the approval of vaccines containing novel adjuvants will continue to be challenging, we believe that the path is becoming somewhat clearer, if not less challenging, but more clarity is urgently sought. Overall, we believe that the MF59 adjuvant will attain additional success in the near future, gaining further approvals, since it has a well-established safety profile and a clear case for contributing to the potency of influenza vaccines, particularly in the pre-pandemic arena. In this setting, it seems appropriate to ask "If not now, when?"' It is, however, the regulatory agencies that will make decisions about vaccine approval.

As discussed, ASO4-containing vaccines have recently gained significant regulatory approvals, but it is difficult to predict how quickly approval will be gained in the US. Although the use of immune potentiators, including TLR agonists, in second-generation adjuvants holds huge promise, clinically this area is in its infancy. Immune manipulation using TLR agonists and other innate activators is a poorly understood area, with many unanswered questions, which raise a number of concerns. Much of the work performed so far has been empirical and observational, mostly highlighting that one plus one may equal more than two. To make serious advances, we need to apply the tools of drug discovery, delivery, and evaluation to the field of vaccine adjuvants. We need to focus on the optimal molecules to deliver and enable them to selectively activate the appropriate targets, to induce only the desired protective immune responses. Advances in biomarkers can be applied through the use of translational medicine to better understand and quantify the immune activation achieved, while also evaluating more thoroughly the safety profile. The extent to which translational medicine can contribute to safety evaluation of adjuvants, through the judicious application of novel biomarkers, needs to be determined, but is an important area of research.

The safety issues surrounding adjuvants have been with us for quite some time and were discussed knowledgeably back in 1980 [72]. Most of the concerns raised almost 30 years ago still remain valid today, although perhaps we now know a little more about how the adjuvants work. Even back in 1980, it was highlighted that there were concerns that potent immune stimulators could potentially trigger autoimmune diseases, since this had been seen with Freund's adjuvants in animal models. More recently, this has also been discussed in the literature as a concern for TLR agonists [73]. Unfortunately, this will remain a challenging issue, particularly since the available animal models are unlikely to be predictive. The models are

not helped by the TLR differences between species, along with immunologic differences, which further limit their likely predictability. The development of improved preclinical models to better predict the safety of vaccine adjuvants is obviously an area requiring further research. Encouragingly, although infections have been associated with triggering autoimmune disease, vaccination has not been directly linked with autoimmune disease [74]. Moreover, with significant experience worldwide, autoimmune disease does not seem to be a problem for generation 1 adjuvants, including alum and MF59. The use of alum as a vaccine adjuvant was re-evaluated at an international workshop in 2002 and it was concluded that alum had an excellent safety record, with a low incidence of adverse events [75]. However, the safety and acceptability of generation 2 adjuvants, including TLR agonists, will need to be established in the clinic, with extensive monitoring of patients likely to be necessary in early stages of clinical evaluation.

References

1 Rappuoli R. Bridging the knowledge gaps in vaccine design. *Nat Biotechnol* 2007;**25**(12):1361–6.

2 Ramon G. Procédés pour accroitre la production des antitoxines. *Ann Inst Pasteur* 1926;**40**: 1–10.

3 O'Hagan DT, Valiante NM. Recent advances in the discovery and delivery of vaccine adjuvants. *Nat Rev Drug Discov* 2003;**2**(9):727–35.

4 Seubert A, Monaci E, Pizza M, O'Hagan DT, Wack A. The adjuvants aluminum hydroxide and MF59 induce monocyte and granulocyte chemoattractants and enhance monocyte differentiation toward dendritic cells. *J Immunol* 2008;**180**(8):5402–12.

5 Mosca F, Tritto E, Muzzi A, *et al*. Molecular and cellular signatures of human vaccine adjuvants. *Proc Natl Acad Sci U S A* 2008;**105**(30):10501–6.

6 Kool M, Soullie T, van Nimwegen M, *et al*. Alum adjuvant boosts adaptive immunity by inducing uric acid and activating inflammatory dendritic cells. *J Exp Med* 2008;**205**(4):869–82.

7 Sharp FA, Ruane D, Claass B, *et al*. Uptake of particulate vaccine adjuvants by dendritic cells activates the NALP3 inflammasome. *Proc Natl Acad Sci U S A* 2009;**106**(3):870–75.

8 Glenny AT, Pope CG, Waddington H, Wallace U. The antigenic value of toxoid precipitated by potassium alum. *J Pathol Bacteriol* 1926;**29**(29):31–40.

9 Clements CJ, Griffiths E. The global impact of vaccines containing aluminium adjuvants. *Vaccine* 2002;**20**(Suppl 3):S24–33.

10 Freund J, Casals J, Hosmer EP. Sensitization and antibody formation after injection of tubercle bacilli and paraffin oil. *Proc Soc Exp Biol Med* 1937;**37**: 509–13.

11 O'Hagan DT. MF59 is a safe and potent vaccine adjuvant that enhances protection against influenza virus infection. *Expert Rev Vaccines* 2007;**6**(5):699–710.

12 Herbert WJ. The mode of action of mineral-oil emulsion adjuvants on antibody production in mice. *Immunology* 1968;**14**(3):301–18.

13 Metcalfe IC, Gluck R. Virosomes for vaccine delivery. In V Schijns, DT O'Hagan (Eds) *Immunopotentiators in Modern Vaccines*. Elsevier, London, 2006, pp. 179–89.

14 Singh M, Ugozzoli M, Kazzaz J, *et al.* A preliminary evaluation of alternative adjuvants to alum using a range of established and new generation vaccine antigens. *Vaccine* 2006;**24**(10):1680–86.

15 Leroux-Roels I, Borkowski A, Vanwolleghem T, *et al.* Antigen sparing and cross-reactive immunity with an adjuvanted rH5N1 prototype pandemic influenza vaccine: a randomised controlled trial. *Lancet* 2007;**370**(9587):580–89.

16 Levie K, Leroux-Roels I, Hoppenbrouwers K, *et al.* An adjuvanted, low-dose, pandemic influenza A (H5N1) vaccine candidate is safe, immunogenic, and induces cross-reactive immune responses in healthy adults. *J Infect Dis* 2008;**198**(5):642–9.

17 Kreuter J, Mauler R, Gruschkau H, Speiser PP. The use of new polymethylmethacrylate adjuvants for split influenza vaccines. *Exp Cell Biol* 1976;**44**(1): 12–19.

18 Allison AG, Gregoriadis G. Liposomes as immunological adjuvants. *Nature* 1974;**252**(5480):252.

19 Webster RG, Glezen WP, Hannoun C, Laver WG. Potentiation of the immune response to influenza virus subunit vaccines. *J Immunol* 1977;**119**(6):2073–7.

20 Siddiqui WA, Taylor DW, Kan SC, *et al.* Vaccination of experimental monkeys against *Plasmodium falciparum*: a possible safe adjuvant. *Science* 1978;**201**(4362): 1237–9.

21 Woodhour AF, Friedman A, Tytell AA, Hilleman MR. Hyperpotentiation by synthetic double-stranded RNA of antibody responses to influenza virus vaccine in adjuvant 65. *Proc Soc Exp Biol Med* 1969;**131**(3): 809–17.

22 Harper DM, Franco EL, Wheeler CM, *et al.* Sustained efficacy up to 4.5 years of a bivalent L1 virus-like particle vaccine against human papillomavirus types 16 and 18: follow-up from a randomised control trial. *Lancet* 2006;**367**(9518):1247–55.

23 Boland G, Beran J, Lievens M, *et al.* Safety and immunogenicity profile of an experimental hepatitis B vaccine adjuvanted with AS04. *Vaccine* 2004;**23**(3): 316–20.

24 Vogel FR, Powell MF. A compendium of vaccine adjuvants and excipients. In MF Powell, MJ Newman (Eds) *Vaccine Design: The Subunit and Adjuvant Approach*. Plenum Press, New York, 1995, pp. 141–228.

25 Ishizaka ST, Hawkins LD. E6020: a synthetic Toll-like receptor 4 agonist as a vaccine adjuvant. *Expert Rev Vaccines* 2007;**6**(5):773–84.

26 Pulendran B, Ahmed R. Translating innate immunity into immunological memory: implications for vaccine development. *Cell* 2006;**124**(4):849–63.

27 Beauvillain C, Delneste Y, Scotet M, *et al.* Neutrophils efficiently cross-prime naive T cells in vivo. *Blood* 2007;**110**(8):2965–73.

28 Culshaw S, Millington OR, Brewer JM, McInnes IB. Murine neutrophils present class II restricted antigen. *Immunol Lett* 2008;**118**(1):49–54.

29 van Gisbergen KP, Ludwig IS, Geijtenbeek TB, van Kooyk Y. Interactions of DC-SIGN with Mac-1 and CEACAM1 regulate contact between dendritic cells and neutrophils. *FEBS Lett* 2005;**579**(27):6159–68.

30 Bogoevska V, Horst A, Klampe B, *et al.* CEACAM1, an adhesion molecule of human granulocytes, is fucosylated by fucosyltransferase IX and interacts with DC-SIGN of dendritic cells via Lewis x residues. *Glycobiology* 2006;**16**(3):197–209.

31 Nathan C. Neutrophils and immunity: challenges and opportunities. *Nat Rev Immunol* 2006;**6**(3):173–82.

32 Jordan MB, Mills DM, Kappler J, Marrack P, Cambier JC. Promotion of B cell immune responses via an alum-induced myeloid cell population. *Science* 2004;**304**(5678):1808–10.

33 Wang HB, Weller PF. Pivotal advance: eosinophils mediate early alum adjuvant-elicited B cell priming and IgM production. *J Leukoc Biol* 2008;**83**(4):817–21.

34 Denzel A, Maus UA, Rodriguez Gomez M, *et al.* Basophils enhance immunological memory responses. *Nat Immunol* 2008;**9**(7):733–42.

35 McLachlan JB, Shelburne CP, Hart JP, *et al.* Mast cell activators: a new class of highly effective vaccine adjuvants. *Nat Med* 2008;**14**(5):536–41.

36 Martin-Fontecha A, Thomsen LL, Brett S, *et al.* Induced recruitment of NK cells to lymph nodes

provides IFN-gamma for T(H)1 priming. *Nat Immunol* 2004;**5**(12):1260–65.

37 Fujii S, Shimizu K, Smith C, Bonifaz L, Steinman RM. Activation of natural killer T cells by alpha-galactosylceramide rapidly induces the full maturation of dendritic cells in vivo and thereby acts as an adjuvant for combined CD4 and CD8 T cell immunity to a coadministered protein. *J Exp Med* 2003;**198**(2): 267–79.

38 Nieda M, Okai M, Tazbirkova A, *et al.* Therapeutic activation of Valpha24$^+$Vbeta11$^+$ NKT cells in human subjects results in highly coordinated secondary activation of acquired and innate immunity. *Blood* 2004;**103**(2):383–9.

39 Cerundolo V, Silk JD, Masri SH, Salio M. Harnessing invariant NKT cells in vaccination strategies. *Nat Rev Immunol* 2009;**9**(1):28–38.

40 Guillonneau C, Mintern JD, Hubert FX, *et al.* Combined NKT cell activation and influenza virus vaccination boosts memory CTL generation and protective immunity. *Proc Natl Acad Sci U S A* 2009;**106**(9): 3330–35.

41 Galli G, Nuti S, Tavarini S, *et al.* Innate immune responses support adaptive immunity: NKT cells induce B cell activation. *Vaccine* 2003;**21**(Suppl 2):S48–54.

42 Galli G, Pittoni P, Tonti E, *et al.* Invariant NKT cells sustain specific B cell responses and memory. *Proc Natl Acad Sci U S A* 2007;**104**(10):3984–9.

43 Tonti E, Galli G, Malzone C, *et al.* NKT-cell help to B lymphocytes can occur independently of cognate interaction. *Blood* 2009;**113**(2):370–76.

44 Delgado MF, Coviello S, Monsalvo AC, *et al.* Lack of antibody affinity maturation due to poor Toll-like receptor stimulation leads to enhanced respiratory syncytial virus disease. *Nat Med* 2009;**15**(1):34–41.

45 Pasare C, Medzhitov R. Control of B-cell responses by Toll-like receptors. *Nature* 2005;**438**(7066):364–8.

46 Petrilli V, Dostert C, Muruve DA, Tschopp J. The inflammasome: a danger sensing complex triggering innate immunity. *Curr Opin Immunol* 2007;**19**(6): 615–22.

47 Eisenbarth SC, Colegio OR, O'Connor W, Sutterwala FS, Flavell RA. Crucial role for the Nalp3 inflammasome in the immunostimulatory properties of aluminium adjuvants. *Nature* 2008;**453**(7198):1122–16.

48 Franchi L, Nunez G. The Nlrp3 inflammasome is critical for aluminium hydroxide-mediated IL-1beta secretion but dispensable for adjuvant activity. *Eur J Immunol* 2008;**38**(8):2085–9.

49 Hornung V, Bauernfeind F, Halle A, *et al.* Silica crystals and aluminum salts activate the NALP3 inflam-

masome through phagosomal destabilization. *Nat Immunol* 2008;**9**(8):847–56.

50 Akira S, Uematsu S, Takeuchi O. Pathogen recognition and innate immunity. *Cell* 2006;**124**(4):783–801.

51 Kawai T, Akira S. Pathogen recognition with Toll-like receptors. *Curr Opin Immunol* 2005;**17**(4):338–44.

52 van Duin D, Medzhitov R, Shaw AC. Triggering TLR signaling in vaccination. *Trends Immunol* 2006;**27**(1): 49–55.

53 Krieg AM. Therapeutic potential of Toll-like receptor 9 activation. *Nat Rev Drug Discov* 2006;**5**(6):471–84.

54 Garçon N, Chomez P, Van Mechelen M. Glaxo-SmithKline adjuvant systems in vaccines: concepts, achievements and perspectives. *Expert Rev Vaccines* 2007;**6**(5):723–39.

55 Gavin AL, Hoebe K, Duong B, *et al.* Adjuvant-enhanced antibody responses in the absence of toll-like receptor signaling. *Science* 2006;**314**(5807): 1936–8.

56 Nemazee D, Gavin A, Hoebe K, Beutler B. Toll-like receptors and antibody responses. *Nature* 2006;**441**:E4.

57 Wack A, Baudner BC, Hilbert AK, *et al.* Combination adjuvants for the induction of potent, long-lasting antibody and T-cell responses to influenza vaccine in mice. *Vaccine* 2008;**26**(4):552–61.

58 Eckl-Dorna J, Batista FD. BCR-mediated uptake of antigen linked to TLR9 ligand stimulates B-cell proliferation and antigen-specific plasma cell formation. *Blood* 2009;**113**(17):3969–77.

59 Litwin SD, Singer JM. The adjuvant action of latex particulate carriers. *J Immunol* 1965;**95**(6):1147–52.

60 Raychaudhuri S, Rock KL. Fully mobilizing host defense: building better vaccines. *Nat Biotechnol* 1998; **16**(11):1025–31.

61 Artursson P, Martensson IL, Sjoholm I. Biodegradable microspheres. III: some immunological properties of polyacryl starch microparticles. *J Pharm Sci* 1986;**75**(7):697–701.

62 O'Hagan DT, Palin K, Davis SS, Artursson P, Sjoholm I. Microparticles as potentially orally active immunological adjuvants. *Vaccine* 1989;**7**(5):421–4.

63 O'Hagan DT, Rahman D, McGee JP, *et al.* Biodegradable microparticles as controlled release antigen delivery systems. *Immunology* 1991;**73**(2):239–42.

64 Gupta RK, Singh M, O'Hagan DT. Poly(lactide-co-glycolide) microparticles for the development of single-dose controlled-release vaccines. *Adv Drug Deliv Rev* 1998;**32**(3):225–46.

65 Kazzaz J, Neidleman J, Singh M, Ott G, O'Hagan DT. Novel anionic microparticles are a potent adjuvant for the induction of cytotoxic T lymphocytes against

recombinant p55 gag from HIV-1. *J Control Release* 2000;**67**(2–3): 347–56.

66 Singh M, Kazzaz J, Chesko J, *et al.* Anionic microparticles are a potent delivery system for recombinant antigens from *Neisseria meningitidis* serotype B. *J Pharm Sci* 2004;**93**(2):273–82.

67 Singh M, Ott G, Kazzaz J, *et al.* Cationic microparticles are an effective delivery system for immune stimulatory cpG DNA. *Pharm Res* 2001;**18**(10):1476–9.

68 Kazzaz J, Singh M, Ugozzoli M, *et al.* Encapsulation of the immune potentiators MPL and RC529 in PLG microparticles enhances their potency. *J Control Release* 2006;**110**(3):566–73.

69 Singh M, Li XM, Wang H, *et al.* Immunogenicity and protection in small-animal models with controlled-release tetanus toxoid microparticles as a single-dose vaccine. *Infect Immun* 1997;**65**(5):1716–21.

70 Wendorf J, Singh M, Chesko J, *et al.* A practical approach to the use of nanoparticles for vaccine delivery. *J Pharm Sci* 2006;**95**(12):2738–50.

71 Wendorf J, Chesko J, Kazzaz J, *et al.* A comparison of anionic nanoparticles and microparticles as vaccine delivery systems. *Hum Vaccin* 2008;**4**(1):44–9.

72 Edelman R. Vaccine adjuvants. *Rev Infect Dis* 1980; **2**(3):370–83.

73 Marshak-Rothstein A. Toll-like receptors in systemic autoimmune disease. *Nat Rev Immunol* 2006;**6**(11): 823–35.

74 Wraith DC, Goldman M, Lambert PH. Vaccination and autoimmune disease: what is the evidence? *Lancet* 2003;**362**(9396):1659–66.

75 Eickhoff TC, Myers M. Workshop summary. Aluminum in vaccines. *Vaccine* 2002;**20**(Suppl 3): S1–4.

CHAPTER 24

Immunostimulatory Properties of Biodegradable Microparticles

Fiona A. Sharp[1] *& Ed C. Lavelle*[2]

[1] Fahmy Research Group, Department of Biomedical Engineering, School of Engineering and Applied Science, Yale University, New Haven, CT, USA

[2] Adjuvant Research Group, School of Biochemistry and Immunology, Trinity Biomedical Sciences Institute, Trinity College, Dublin, Ireland

Introduction

The development of vaccines has progressed significantly since the days of Edward Jenner and Louis Pasteur. Due to increased safety concerns and advances in molecular biology and immunology, we have moved away from the use of whole organism based vaccines and toward recombinant subunit vaccines. These subunit vaccines generally have an improved safety profile but the price paid for this is reduced immunogenicity. In order to enhance the efficacy of subunit vaccines, adjuvants are added. Adjuvants were originally defined as "substances used in combination with a specific antigen that produce more immunity than the antigen alone" [1]. Gaston Ramon tested a diverse range of substances, including tapioca, inorganic salts, oil, and pyogenic bacteria with diphtheria toxoid. He demonstrated that they all had the ability to enhance antibody responses toward the toxin [1]. Following on from Ramon's observations, Alexander Glenny later showed that the combination of diphtheria toxoid and aluminum potassium sulfate, or "potash alum," induced enhanced antibody responses compared with the toxoid alone [2]. Today aluminum compounds remain the most widely used adjuvants.

The inclusion of adjuvants can have several positive effects on the efficacy of vaccines, including increased stimulation of cell-mediated immunity and the promotion of mucosal immunity. In addition, adjuvants can reduce the amount of antigen necessary to induce protective responses and enable the use of combination vaccines by preventing antigen competition. Furthermore, adjuvants can increase the efficacy of vaccines in newborns with underdeveloped immune systems or in elderly and immune-compromised individuals. In all cases, safety is a prime concern, and the balance between efficacy and reactogenicity is a key determinant in the choice of vaccine adjuvant. There are many examples of highly potent adjuvants that are too toxic for clinical application. Local reactions such as pain, inflammation, and necrosis have been reported but these symptoms are often short-lived and self-limiting. The ideal adjuvant should satisfy a number of criteria; it should be biocompatible, biodegradable, promote long-lasting protective immune responses, and remain stable before administration [3]. In addition, adjuvants should be well defined both chemically and physically, allowing for reproducibility from a manufacturing point of view as well as quality control.

Current adjuvants may be broadly classified into immunostimulatory and particulate adjuvants (Table 24.1). Immunostimulatory adjuvants act as agonists of pathogen recognition receptors (PRR), which are a large family of innate germline

Vaccinology: Principles and Practice, First Edition. Edited by W. John W. Morrow, Nadeem A. Sheikh, Clint S. Schmidt and D. Huw Davies.
© 2012 Blackwell Publishing Ltd. Published 2012 by Blackwell Publishing Ltd.

Table 24.1 Examples of immunostimulatory and particulate vaccine adjuvants in current use both experimentally and in clinical trials.

Particulate vaccine adjuvants	Immunostimulatory adjuvants
Mineral salts	*TLR agonists*
Alhydrogel (alum)	MPL
Aluminum phosphate (potash)	Flagellin
Calcium phosphate	Imiquimods
Imject (aluminum and magnesium hydroxide)	CpG
Lipid-based systems	*NLR agonists*
MF59	CFA (MDP)
Montanides	Alhydrogel (alum)[a]
CFA	PLG microparticles[a]
IFA	QS21[a]
Virosomes	ISCOMs[a]
Liposomes	
ISCOMs	
Nano- and microparticles	*CLR agonists*
Biodegradable polymers (PLGA)	Trehalose dimycolate (cord factor)
Proteosomes	Yeast β-glucans
	Zymosan
Polysaccharides	*Bacterial toxoids*
Chitosan	Cholera toxin
	Escherichia coli, heat-labile enterotoxin derivatives

CFA, complete Freund's adjuvant; IFA, incomplete Freund's adjuvant; MDP, *N*-acetyl muramyl-L-alanyl-D-isoglutamine; PLG, poly (lactide-coglycolide).
[a]All shown to activate NLRP3 in combination with a TLR agonist.

encoded receptors with the ability to recognize conserved sequences commonly expressed on invading microorganisms. PRR equip cells of the immune system with the ability to distinguish "infectious non-self" from "non-infectious self" [4]. These innate receptors can be further subdivided into several families based on their structure, including Toll-like receptors (TLR), NOD-like receptors (NLR), RIG-like receptors (RLR), and C-type lectin receptors (CLR) [5]. Activation of these receptors triggers intracellular signaling cascades, which ultimately results in the expression of inflammatory effector molecules, such as cytokines, reactive oxygen species (ROS), and co-stimulatory molecules. A growing number of agonists for these innate sensors are under investigation as adjuvants for both injectable and mucosal vaccines. In contrast to immunostimulatory adjuvants, particulate vaccine adjuvants are not thought to directly activate PRR but act as delivery systems targeting the antigen to antigen-presenting cells (APCs), which have the ability to activate the adaptive arm of the immune system (Table 24.1).

It is becoming increasingly clear that in addition to fulfilling a "delivery" role, many particulate vaccine adjuvants also exert powerful immunostimulatory effects. As well as generating more potent adjuvant systems, many immunostimulatory adjuvants are currently being incorporated into particulate systems to enhance their delivery and efficacy. The main focus of this chapter will, however, be on the nature and mode of action of particulate adjuvants and their application in preclinical studies and clinical trial vaccines.

Particulate vaccine adjuvants

Mineral salts

Aluminum-containing adjuvants have been contributing to the efficacy of vaccines for almost a century. The adjuvant properties of these compounds were first discovered by Glenny in the 1920s. A precipitate of diphtheria toxoid and aluminum potassium sulphate (potash alum) was produced and the precipitated vaccine induced greater protective immunity than the toxoid alone [2]. Several other aluminum salts have also been shown to possess adjuvant properties, including aluminum potassium phosphate (Adju-phos), aluminum hydroxide (Alhydrogel or alum), and a combination of aluminum hydroxide and magnesium hydroxide (Imject Alum). The most commonly used aluminum salt adjuvants are Adju-phos and Alhydrogel due to the ease of manufacturing and reproducibility. Although it is not completely correct, Adju-phos and Aldydrogel are commonly referred to as alum. Aluminum-containing adjuvants have proved to be highly effective and are licensed for use in multiple vaccines, including diptheria-pertussis-tetanus, diptheria-tetanus, diptheria-tetanus combined with hepatitis B vaccine, *Haemophilus influenzae* B and inactivated polio virus, and human papilloma virus (HPV) [6].

However, despite this and their acceptable safety profile, aluminum-containing adjuvants are poor inducers of cell-mediated immunity, making them unsuitable for use in vaccines against diseases such as tuberculosis, malaria, and HIV, which require long-lasting antibody responses along with potent cell-mediated immunity, based on CD4$^+$ and CD8$^+$ T-cell responses [7].

Lipid-based particulates

Emulsions

The use of emulsions in vaccines to boost immune responses can be traced back to work by Le Moignic and Pinoy in 1916, who used the first oil emulsion, water and Vaseline, with inactivated *Salmonella typhimurium* [8].

Less than ten years later, Ramon demonstrated that starch oil increased antibody responses to diphtheria toxoid [9]. In the 1930s, Freund developed paraffin oil–based emulsions with or without heat-killed *Mycobacteria*, producing Freund's complete (FCA) and incomplete (FIA) adjuvants, respectively [10]. Freund's adjuvant is an example of a water-in-oil (W/O) emulsion, which is made up of antigen-containing water droplets in a continuous oil phase. Oil-in-water (O/W) emulsions are composed of antigen in a water phase with oil droplets in the solution, and double emulsions can be produced with water droplets trapped within larger oil droplets, dispersed in a water phase (W/O/W) [11].

Herbert showed that oil-in-water emulsions have the ability to retain an antigen at the site of injection, allowing prolonged exposure to the immune system [12]. O/W emulsions have shown the best safety profile, while W/O emulsions have proven too toxic for human use, even though they are more efficient at enhancing immune responses [11]. Syntax adjuvant formulation (SAF) is an O/W emulsion developed in the 1980s as a replacement for Freund's adjuvant. SAF contains the biodegradable oil squalene, but was too toxic for clinical use due to the presence of muramyl dipeptide and induced severe local reactogenicity in an HIV clinical trial [7,13]. Subsequent work led to the development of a safer emulsion adjuvant known as MF59, a micro-fluidized O/W emulsion comprising squalene oil with Tween 80 and Span 85 as surfactants but with no additional immunostimulators [14]. MF59 has been shown to be an effective adjuvant with an acceptable safety profile. A large number of subjects have been immunized with MF59 and the adjuvant was well tolerated and was safe in newborns and the elderly. FLUAD™ is an MF59-adjuvanted influenza vaccine currently licensed for use in the elderly by 12 European health authorities and in some non-EU countries, with at least 45 million doses administered to date [15].

The Montanides are a series of W/O emulsions that are currently being developed for use as vaccine adjuvants in response to safety concerns with IFA [16,17]. Montanides ISA 51 and ISA 720 are both biodegradable emulsions that use mannide-mono-oleate as an emulsifier. They are currently being tested in clinical trials for vaccines against malaria and cancer [3].

Immune-stimulating complexes

In 1971 immune-stimulating complexes (ISCOMs) were first visualized by electron microscopy in a preparation of virus particles treated with saponin [18]. However, it was not until 1984 that Morein *et al.* first described the formation of these saponin-containing complexes with viral membrane proteins [19]. Negative stain transmission electron microscopy shows these well-defined particles as spherical, cage-like structures of approximately 40 nm in diameter [20]. Their formation occurs spontaneously upon mixing cholesterol, *Quillaja saponaria* saponins, and phospholipids. It is the interaction of the cholesterol and saponins

it can range from days to weeks and possibly years. The optimal size range for vaccination is likely to depend on the application but it has been proposed that microparticles of 1–3 μm are optimal in some settings [46]. However, it is likely that in addition to the magnitude, the type of immune response induced may be dictated to some degree by particle size, the size of the PLG particles should be taken into careful consideration and tailored for the specific indication.

Antigens can be encapsulated within PLG using a technique known as microencapsulation. During this process, antigens can be exposed to various potentially damaging conditions such as low pH, high shear, and organic solvents [49,50]. This and the susceptibility of encapsulated antigen to acid-mediated hydrolysis encouraged scientists to develop alternative means of associating antigens with microparticles [51,52]. Kazzaz *et al.* described the preparation of charged microparticles, using sodium dodecyl sulphate (SDS) to produce anionic PLG, which were easier to adsorb proteins onto [53]. Factors such as protein charge and hydrophobicity affect antigen adsorption and the optimal adsorption conditions are protein specific [54]. Cationic particles were developed, using sodium dioctyl sulfosuccinate as the particle stabilizer, by the same group, and these have been optimized for the delivery of DNA vaccines [55]. Along with the ability of PLG microparticles to promote antibody responses, studies in rodents have demonstrated that PLG microparticles also promote cell-mediated immunity [56,57]. T cells isolated from mice immunized either parenterally or orally with PLG and OVA demonstrated cytolytic activity when restimulated *ex vivo* [56,57]. In addition, both oral and nasal delivery of PLG microparticles have been shown to elicit strong mucosal and systemic responses [47,48,56,58]. Others have also demonstrated that manipulation of PLG microparticles, such as coating with poly(ethelyne glycol) (PEG) or chitosan, enhances movement of the microparticles across the mucosa due to neutralization of their negative charge [59,60]. Cationic PLG particles have been tested in nonhuman primates as a delivery system for a hepatitis C vaccine and successfully induced seroconversion in all animals tested [54].

One of the main issues for the use of PLG particles as vaccine delivery systems is the ability to manufacture these particulates in a consistent manner on a large scale, sufficient to meet the demands required for global vaccination. However, PLG microspheres have already been FDA approved for the delivery of commercially available anti-cancer treatments, such as Lupron, demonstrating that these particles can be manufactured on a large scale. Furthermore, the development of PLG particles with surface modifications, such as cationic and anionic particles, allows for adsorption of antigen on the particle surface, removing the need for complex formulation and conjugation steps. In addition, the adjuvant effect of particulates may rely more on properties such as size [61] and shape than the specific chemical composition, therefore the constituents of the particles themselves could be modified in order to enhance both adjuvanticity and ease of manufacturing. However, given the strong safety record associated with PLGA copolymers and the fact that PLGA-based particles have previously been FDA approved for human use, these represent a most attractive adjuvant system for use in vaccines. Vaccines for clinical use must be terminally sterilized or produced under aseptic conditions, the former being the more commonly used technique. Indeed, it has been demonstrated that γ-irradiation can be used to terminally sterilize PLG microparticles following lyophilization with no negative effects on the adjuvant activities of these particles [62].

Combination vaccine adjuvants

Increased understanding of the activation of the innate immune system and the relationship between innate and adaptive immunity has allowed for engineering of the next generation of vaccine adjuvants. This is necessary in order to aid the development of vaccines to target diseases for which there are currently no effective vaccines available, including HIV and malaria. These attributes will include the ability to promote the development of more heterologous antibodies, thus allowing for increased cross-reactivity among different strains of the same microorganism; the induction of more effective T-cell responses; and the induction of more potent functional antibody responses to allow for pathogen killing or neutralization [3]. In addition, future adjuvants will be expected to allow for more practical applications, such as a reduction in antigen dose.

One of the first combination adjuvants tested was FCA. Although the adjuvant is too toxic for human use, it is one of the original combination adjuvants consisting of a particulate delivery system (oil in water emulsion) and dead mycobacteria, the immunostimulatory component. Prime examples of the next generation of adjuvants, most of which are combination adjuvants, are the adjuvant systems (AS) developed by GSK. These include AS01, AS02, AS03, and AS04. AS01 is a liposomal formulation containing MPL, which has been shown to promote strong cell-mediated responses and is currently being tested in GSK's malaria vaccine candidate [66]. Another combination vaccine adjuvant, known as AS02, is a combination of MPL and QS21 in an O/W emulsion and has been shown to induce both strong humoral and cell-mediated responses [7]. In addition, the GSK RTS/S malaria vaccine combined with AS02 provided 65% protection against first-time infections in infants. However, in earlier trials in children (1–4 years), the vaccine was only effective in 35% of candidates [66]. GSK's H1N1 vaccine, Pandemrix™, is adjuvanted with AS03, which is composed of α-tocopherol, a synthetic form of vitamin E, in an O/W-based emulsion [67]. Another GSK adjuvant system, AS04, is composed of the TLR4 agonist MPL and the particulate vaccine adjuvant alum. A recent study has shown that this combination of MPL and alum induces the local secretion of cytokines, including IL6, TNF-α, and the chemokines CCL2 and CCL3 [68]. This enhancement of proinflammatory mediators occurred rapidly and was short lived, with maximal levels detected between 6 and 24 h following injection of adjuvants. In addition, the numbers of DCs and inflammatory monocytes infiltrating local lymph nodes were increased when mice received MPL and alum in comparison to alum alone [68]. AS04 is one of the first new-generation vaccines to be approved for use in a

vaccine against HPV (Cervarix) by the FDA [69]. Cervarix contains two types of VLP, HPV 16 and 18 [70]. Adding further complexity to the design of adjuvants, GSK has also developed AS15, which consists of AS01 (liposomal-based MPL) and CpG. AS15 is currently being tested as an adjuvant for therapeutic cancer vaccines [71]. These new adjuvant systems have been proven to have a high safety profile, with over 1.4 million people receiving AS04 and an estimated 29 million people in Europe receiving the AS03-adjuvanted GSK influenza vaccine [72,73].

In addition to GSK, others have also reported the successful use of combination adjuvant systems. For example, immunization (i.m.) with a *Neisseria meningitides* serogroup B antigen encapsulated in PLG microparticles containing CpG induced stronger antibody responses than antigen mixed with soluble CpG or encapsulated in PLG microparticles without CpG [74]. Another study reported enhanced mucosal antigen-specific IgA responses when a group B streptococcus antigen (GBS) was co-encapsulated with CpG in PLG [75]. Furthermore, the adjuvant was shown to enhance immune responses when administered by several routes of immunization, including oral, vaginal, nasal, intramuscular, and intraperitoneal [75].

A liposome-based vaccine containing MPL known as Stimuvax® has been developed for the treatment of non-small-cell lung cancer [76]. This vaccine has moved on to phase III trials and Stimuvax® has also been tested for the treatment of breast cancers and multiple myelomas. However, one of the patients involved in the multiple myeloma trial developed encephalitis, resulting in the FDA putting all trials involving Stimuvax® on hold for the foreseeable future [77,78].

IC31® is a two-component adjuvant system developed by Intercell. It consists of KLK, an antimicrobial peptide, and a TLR9-activating oligodeoxynucleotide, ODN1a. Studies have demonstrated that IC31 promotes the formation of a depot at the injection site via KLK. In addition, IC31 has been shown to activate APC and strongly enhance both humoral and cell-mediated responses, with a bias toward Th1-type responses [79–81]. Furthermore, IC31 has been shown to enhance immune responses to several influenza antigens in aged mice, suggesting that it may be a prime candidate for use in influenza vaccines for the elderly [81]. This novel adjuvant is currently being tested in vaccines against tuberculosis and influenza. Reports so far suggest that IC31 is well tolerated in subjects, with no serious adverse events observed [82].

These examples of combination adjuvants are but the tip of the iceberg in terms of current activity in this area. The potency of a number of these systems provides great encouragement that this approach can generate new and improved vaccines, particularly in cases where strong cell-mediated immunity is a prerequisite.

How do particulate vaccine adjuvants work?

Particulate vaccine adjuvants were originally proposed to act as delivery systems. Alexander T. Glenny's early studies into alum suggested that antigen completely adsorbed to the particulate, which led to the idea that particulates act as an "antigen depot" at the site of injection [2]. For decades this depot theory has been used to explain the efficacy of particulate adjuvants and is so widely accepted that the regulatory guidelines outlined by the WHO state that the antigens must be adsorbed to the aluminum-containing adjuvants [83]. However, a recent renaissance of interest in particulate vaccine adjuvants has provided a strong body of evidence which suggests that particulates act as more than delivery agents and can exert stimulatory effects on the immune system, suggesting a more complicated mode of action.

Previous studies into particulates have demonstrated that particle-associated antigens are more readily phagocytosed by APC, thereby enhancing antigen presentation [48,84]. This enhanced phagocytosis by APC also promotes trafficking of antigen to secondary lymphoid organs, thereby promoting induction of cell-mediated immunity [85]. The degree of phagocytosis depends on particle size, and both this and intracellular trafficking can be decisive factors in determining the type of

response that is induced [61,86]. As well as promoting antigen uptake by APCs, microparticles allow multimeric presentation of antigens, which is required for optimal B-cell activation [87].

It was proposed 60 years ago that antigen adsorption was not a prerequisite for functionality of particulate vaccine adjuvants. Specifically, it was shown that removal of the antigen-adjuvant nodule from the injection site had no effect on the level of antibodies produced [88]. In addition, biodistribution studies have shown that the majority of antigen is rapidly cleared from the injection site following immunization, suggesting that particulates do not retain antigen within the local injection site [89]. However, it may be valuable to revisit these studies now that improved technologies are available to track antigens and adjuvants. The key events in innate immune system activation are likely to occur in the first few hours after injection so it may not be surprising that the adjuvant can be removed after these decisive events have taken place. Additionally, the adjuvant may be taken up and transported to lymph nodes rapidly after injection, where it may act for some time.

Adding further evidence against the "depot theory," more recent findings have highlighted the immunostimulatory effects of particulate adjuvants on the immune system. For example, injection of alum or MF59 is sufficient to increase the local production of proinflammatory mediators, including IL1β, CC-chemokine ligand 2 (CCL-2), CCL-11 or eotaxin, and IL5, as well as the recruitment of neutrophils and inflammatory monocytes [90–92]. Others have also demonstrated that injection of particulate adjuvants promotes the local release of the endogenous danger signal, uric acid [90]. The release of uric acid has the ability to promote the recruitment of inflammatory DCs, which play a central role in the enhancement of CD4$^+$ T-cell-mediated responses [90]. With regard to PRR, alum-mediated humoral immune responses have been shown to occur independently of TLR signaling [93,94]. Several groups have demonstrated the ability of alum to enhance secretion of IL1β by both primary murine DC and human monocytes [61,95–99]. Further studies have subsequently identified the NLR, NLRP3, as being the key

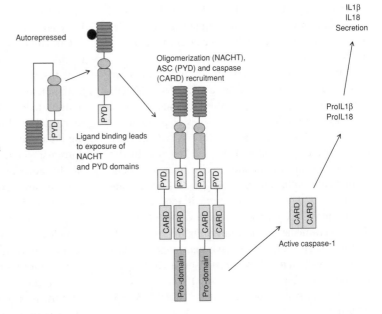

Figure 24.1 Current theories suggest that NLR proteins are present in an autorepressed state in the cytoplasm in a conformation that conceals the NACHT/NOD and effector domains, preventing any interaction with other proteins. Once the NLRP protein is activated a conformational change is induced, exposing the PYD/CARD domains. This leads to recruitment of ASC and, subsequently, caspase-1 activation, which then goes on to convert proIL1β into active IL1β and proIL18 into active IL18 [101].

mediator of alum-driven IL1β and IL18 secretion [61,95–99]. NLRP3 is a cytosolic NLR that forms part of a multiprotein complex with the ability to activate caspase-1, subsequently resulting in the processing of proIL1β into its biologically active form (Figure 24.1) [100,101]. We have recently demonstrated that PLG microparticles can also promote NLRP3 inflammasome activation and the secretion of IL1β (Figure 24.2a) and IL18 secretion [61]. Thus the ability to promote NLRP3 inflammasome

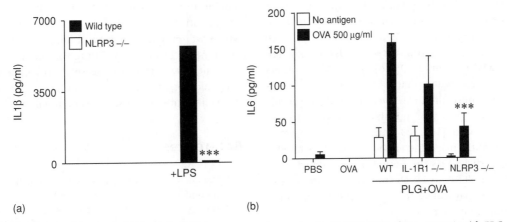

(a)

(b)

Figure 24.2 (a) PLG-mediated enhancement of pro-inflammatory cytokines is NLRP-3 dependent [61]. BMDC (6.25×10^5 cells/mL) from WT C57BL/6 mice and NLRP3$^{-/-}$ mice were pre-incubated with medium or PLG alone for 1 h before medium or LPS was added to the cells. After 24 h, supernatants were removed from the cells and analyzed for IL1β by ELISA. Particles + LPS WT C57BL/6 versus particles + LPS NLRP3$^{-/-}$ mice, ***p < 0.001. (b) WT, IL1R1$^{-/-}$ and NLRP3$^{-/-}$ C57BL/6 were immunized with PBS, OVA alone, or OVA with PLG subcutaneously on day 0 and day 14. After 21 days the mice were sacrificed and spleens were removed. Cells isolated from spleens were restimulated with OVA. After 3 days, supernatants were removed and analyzed for IL6 by ELISA. OVA WT mice versus OVA IL1R1$^{-/-}$ mice or OVA NLRP3$^{-/-}$ mice, ***p < 0.001. Reproduced from [61] with permission from PNAS.

activation appears to be shared by a wide range of particulates and is a clear example that these "delivery systems" can activate specific components of innate immune signaling pathways.

While the ability of particulates, including alum and PLG microparticles, to activate the NLRP3 inflammasome *in vitro* is well established, the role of NLRP3 in the adjuvant activities of particulates *in vivo* remains controversial. Several studies have demonstrated that NLRP3 plays a key role in the recruitment of inflammatory cells, including neutrophils and inflammatory DCs [95,96], to the site of injection. Furthermore, there is evidence that NLPR3 plays a role in alum and PLG microparticle-driven cell-mediated immunity (Figure 24.2b) [61, 95,96,98]. Several groups have demonstrated that particulate-driven cellular responses, including secretion of antigen-specific IL5 and IL6 in secondary lymphoid organs, is dependent on NLRP3 [61,95, 96,98].

However, since these particulates alone are poor inducers of Th1 and Th17 responses, the role of NLRP3 in the case of combination adjuvants that are more effective promoters of such responses should be investigated.

With respect to the role of NLRP3 in the promotion of antibody responses by adjuvants, there are several conflicting studies. Some groups have demonstrated that NLRP3-deficient mice produce significantly less antigen-specific IgG1 and IgE than wild-type mice [95,96]. In contrast, others have demonstrated that NLRP3- and caspase-1-deficient mice produce levels of antigen-specific IgG, IgG1, IgG2, and IgE that are comparable to wild-type mice [102,103]. Additionally, the induction of antigen-specific antibody responses by PLG microparticles was unaffected in mice deficient in IL1R1 or NLRP3 [61]. Overall, the requirement of NLRP3 for particulate-mediated humoral immunity remains controversial.

The identification of the ability of particulates to activate NLRP3 has been a major milestone in demonstrating that particulate adjuvants can trigger specific innate sensing pathways. However, the discrepancies between *in vivo* studies to date regarding the requirement of NLRP3 for the adjuvant effects of particulates suggests that other currently unidentified pathways are also activated by particulate adjuvants.

Our increased understanding of the requirements for modulating innate and adaptive immunity fused with advances in the design and formulation of biomaterials, such as PLG micro- and nanoparticles, offers great hope for development of specifically tailored vaccine formulations. This has the potential to overcome one of the major limitations associated with currently available particulate vaccine adjuvants, their limited capacity to promote cell-mediated immunity. PLG particles may be tailored to facilitate greater activation of cellular immune responses in several ways. For example, the particles can be engineered on the nanoscale in order to increase their access to the lymphatics, therefore promoting their interaction with lymph node resident cells including CD8$^+$ DCs, which are proficient in cross-presentation. In addition, the particle surface can be modified to present antigen in a multimeric form, which will enhance the activation of B cells. PRR agonists, such as CpG, may be conjugated to the surface of PLG particles, promoting the ability of these particles to promote the secretion of key cytokines such as IL12 and activate specialized cells, including plasmacytoid DCs. These surface modifications can include the attachment of targeting antibodies, for example targeting DC-SIGN, which will enhance delivery of antigen to professional APCs. In summary, future vaccines based on PLG microparticles will increasingly resemble artificial microorganisms that can induce targeted protective immune responses with minimal toxicity.

References

1 Ramon G. Sur la toxine et sur l'anatoxine diphtheriques. *Ann Inst Pasteur* 1924;**38**:1–10.

2 Glenny A, Pope CG, Waddington H, Wallace U. Immunological notes XVII–XXIV. *J Pathol* 1926;**29**: 31–40.

3 O'Hagan DT, De Gregorio E. The path to a successful vaccine adjuvant – "the long and winding road". *Drug Discov Today* 2009;**14**:541–51.

4 Janeway CA, Jr. Approaching the asymptote? Evolution and revolution in immunology. *Cold Spring Harb Symp Quant Biol* 1989;**54**(Pt 1):1–13.

5 Baccala R, Gonzalez-Quintial R, Lawson BR, *et al.* Sensors of the innate immune system: their mode of action. *Nat Rev Rheumatol* 2009;**5**:448–56.

6 Clements CJ, Griffiths E. The global impact of vaccines containing aluminium adjuvants. *Vaccine* 2002;**20**(Suppl 3):S24–33.

7 Reed SG, *et al.* New horizons in adjuvants for vaccine development. *Trends Immunol* 2009;**30**:23–32.

8 Le Moignic, Pinoy. Les vaccines en emulsion dans les corps gras ou "lipo-vaccins". *C R Seances Soc Biol Fil* 1916;**79**:201–3.

9 Ramon G. Procedes pour accroître la production des antitoxins. *Ann Inst Pasteur* 1926;**40**:1–10.

10 Freund J, Casals J, Hosmer EP. Sensitization and antibody formation after injection of tubercle bacilli and paraffin oil. *Proc Soc Exp Biol* 1937;**37**:509–13.

11 Jansen T, Hofmans MP, Theelen MJ, Manders F, Schijns VE. Structure- and oil type-based efficacy of emulsion adjuvants. *Vaccine* 2006;**24**:5400–405.

12 Herbert WJ. The mode of action of mineral-oil emulsion adjuvants on antibody production in mice. *Immunology* 1968;**14**:301–18.

13 Allison AC, Byars NE. An adjuvant formulation that selectively elicits the formation of antibodies of protective isotypes and of cell-mediated immunity. *J Immunol Methods* 1986;**95**:157–68.

14 Ott G, Barchfeld GL, Van Nest G. Enhancement of humoral response against human influenza vaccine with the simple submicron oil/water emulsion adjuvant MF59. *Vaccine* 1995;**13**:1557–62.

15 O'Hagan DT. MF59 is a safe and potent vaccine adjuvant that enhances protection against influenza virus infection. *Expert Rev Vaccines* 2007;**6**(5):699–710.

16 Aucouturier J, Ascarateil S, Dupuis L. The use of oil adjuvants in therapeutic vaccines. *Vaccine* 2006;**24**(Suppl 2):S2-44–5.

17 Scalzo AA, Elliott SL, Cox J, *et al.* Induction of protective cytotoxic T cells to murine cytomegalovirus by using a nonapeptide and a human-compatible adjuvant (Montanide ISA 720). *J Virol* 1995;**69**:1306–9.

18 Horzinek M, Mussgay M. Studies on the substructure of togaviruses. I. Effect of urea, deoxycholate, and saponin on the Sindbis virion. *Arch Gesamte Virusforsch* 1971;**33**:296–305.

19 Morein B, Sundquist B, Höglund S, Dalsgaard K, Osterhaus A. Iscom, a novel structure for antigenic presentation of membrane proteins from enveloped viruses. *Nature* 1984;**308**:457–60.

20 Sanders MT, Brown LE, Deliyannis G, Pearse MJ. ISCOM-based vaccines: the second decade. *Immunol Cell Biol* 2005;**83**:119–28.

21 Kersten GF, Teerlink T, Derks HJ, *et al.* Incorporation of the major outer membrane protein of *Neisseria gonorrhoeae* in saponin-lipid complexes (iscoms): chemical analysis, some structural features, and comparison of their immunogenicity with three other antigen delivery systems. *Infect Immun* 1988;**56**:432–8.

22 Lovgren K, Morein B. The requirement of lipids for the formation of immunostimulating complexes (iscoms). *Biotechnol Appl Biochem* 1988;**10**:161–72.

23 Pearse MJ, Drane D. ISCOMATRIX adjuvant for antigen delivery. *Adv Drug Deliv Rev* 2005;**57**:465–74.

24 Frazer IH, Quinn M, Nicklin JL, *et al.* Phase 1 study of HPV16-specific immunotherapy with E6E7 fusion protein and ISCOMATRIX adjuvant in women with cervical intraepithelial neoplasia. *Vaccine* 2004;**23**:172–81.

25 Davis ID, Chen W, Jackson H, *et al.* Recombinant NY-ESO-1 protein with ISCOMATRIX adjuvant induces broad integrated antibody and CD4(+) and CD8(+) T cell responses in humans. *Proc Natl Acad Sci U S A* 2004;**101**:10697–702.

26 Bangham AD, Standish MM, Miller N. Cation permeability of phospholipid model membranes: effect of narcotics. *Nature* 1965;**208**:1295–7.

27 Li S, Nickels J, Palmer AF. Liposome-encapsulated actin-hemoglobin (LEAcHb) artificial blood substitutes. *Biomaterials* 2005;**26**:3759–69.

28 Gregoriadis G, Allison AC. Entrapment of proteins in liposomes prevents allergic reactions in pre-immunised mice. *FEBS Lett* 1974;**45**:71–4.

29 Gabizon AA. Selective tumor localization and improved therapeutic index of anthracyclines encapsulated in long-circulating liposomes. *Cancer Res* 1992;**52**:891–6.

30 Maruyama K, Okuizumi S, Ishida O, *et al.* Phosphatidyl polyglycerols prolong liposome circulation in vivo. *Int J Pharm* 1994;**111**:103–7.

31 Foged C, Arigita C, Sundblad A, *et al.* Interaction of dendritic cells with antigen-containing liposomes: effect of bilayer composition. *Vaccine* 2004;**22**:1903–13.

32 Chen H, Torchilin V, Langer R. Lectin-bearing polymerized liposomes as potential oral vaccine carriers. *Pharm Res* 1996;**13**:1378–83.

33 Scheerlinck JP, Greenwood DL. Virus-sized vaccine delivery systems. *Drug Discov Today* 2008;**13**:882–7.

34 Wilschut J. Influenza vaccines: the virosome concept. *Immunol Lett* 2009;**122**:118–21.

35 Glück R, Moser C, Metcalfe IC. Influenza virosomes as an efficient system for adjuvanted vaccine delivery. *Expert Opin Biol Ther* 2004;**4**:1139–45.

36 Grgacic EV, Anderson DA. Virus-like particles: passport to immune recognition. *Methods* 2006;**40**: 60–65.

37 Huckriede A, Bungener L, Stegmann T, *et al.* The virosome concept for influenza vaccines. *Vaccine* 2005;**23**(Suppl 1):S26–38.

38 Peek LJ, Middaugh CR, Berkland C. Nanotechnology in vaccine delivery. *Adv Drug Deliv Rev* 2008; **60**:915–28.

39 Villa LL, Costa RL, Petta CA, *et al.* Prophylactic quadrivalent human papillomavirus (types 6, 11, 16, and 18) L1 virus-like particle vaccine in young women: a randomised double-blind placebo-controlled multicentre phase II efficacy trial. *Lancet Oncol* 2005;**6**:271–8.

40 Harper DM, Franco EL, Wheeler C, *et al.* Efficacy of a bivalent L1 virus-like particle vaccine in prevention of infection with human papillomavirus types 16 and 18 in young women: a randomised controlled trial. *Lancet* 2004;**364**:1757–65.

41 Harper DM, Franco EL, Wheeler CM, *et al.* Sustained efficacy up to 4.5 years of a bivalent L1 virus-like particle vaccine against human papillomavirus types 16 and 18: follow-up from a randomised control trial. *Lancet* 2006;**367**:1247–55.

42 Bosch FX, de Sanjosé S. Human papillomavirus and cervical cancer – burden and assessment of causality. *J Natl Cancer Inst Monogr* 2003(31):3–13, ch. 1.

43 Tissot AC, Renhofa R, Schmitz N, *et al.* Versatile virus-like particle carrier for epitope based vaccines. *PLoS One* 2010;**5**:e9809.

44 O'Hagan DT. Microparticles and polymers for the mucosal delivery of vaccines. *Adv Drug Deliv Rev* 1998;**34**:305–20.

45 Singh M, Chakrapani A, O'Hagan D. Nanoparticles and microparticles as vaccine-delivery systems. *Expert Rev Vaccines* 2007;**6**:797–808.

46 O'Hagan DT, Singh M. Microparticles as vaccine adjuvants and delivery systems. *Expert Rev Vaccines* 2003;**2**:269–83.

47 Challacombe SJ, Rahman D, Jeffery H, Davis SS, O'Hagan DT. Enhanced secretory IgA and systemic IgG antibody responses after oral immunization with biodegradable microparticles containing antigen. *Immunology* 1992;**76**:164–8.

48 Eldridge JH, Staas JK, Chen D, *et al.* New advances in vaccine delivery systems. *Semin Hematol* 1993;**30**:16–24; discussion 25.

49 Shenderova A, Burke TG, Schwendeman SP. The acidic microclimate in poly(lactide-co-glycolide) microspheres stabilizes camptothecins. *Pharm Res* 1999;**16**:241–8.

50 Singh M, Ugozzoli M, Kazzaz J, *et al.* A preliminary evaluation of alternative adjuvants to alum using a range of established and new generation vaccine antigens. *Vaccine* 2006;**24**:1680–86.

51 Lavelle EC, Yeh MK, Coombes AG, Davis SS. The stability and immunogenicity of a protein antigen encapsulated in biodegradable microparticles based on blends of lactide polymers and polyethylene glycol. *Vaccine* 1999;**17**:512–29.

52 Takahata H, Lavelle EC, Coombes AG, Davis SS. The distribution of protein associated with poly(DL-lactide co-glycolide) microparticles and its degradation in simulated body fluids. *J Control Release* 1998;**50**:237–46.

53 Kazzaz J, Neidleman J, Singh M, Ott G, O'Hagan DT. Novel anionic microparticles are a potent adjuvant for the induction of cytotoxic T lymphocytes against recombinant p55 gag from HIV-1. *J Control Release* 2000;**67**:347–56.

54 Singh M, Chesko J, Kazzaz J, *et al.* Adsorption of a novel recombinant glycoprotein from HIV (Env gp120dV2 SF162) to anionic PLG microparticles retains the structural integrity of the protein, whereas encapsulation in PLG microparticles does not. *Pharm Res* 2004;**21**:2148–52.

55 Singh M, Briones M, Ott G, O'Hagan D. Cationic microparticles: a potent delivery system for DNA vaccines. *Proc Natl Acad Sci U S A* 2000;**97**:811–16.

56 Maloy KJ, Donachie AM, O'Hagan DT, Mowat AM. Induction of mucosal and systemic immune responses by immunization with ovalbumin entrapped in poly(lactide-co-glycolide) microparticles. *Immunology* 1994;**81**:661–7.

57 Nixon DF, Hioe C, Chen PD, *et al.* Synthetic peptides entrapped in microparticles can elicit cytotoxic T cell activity. *Vaccine* 1996;**14**:1523–30.

58 Moldoveanu Z, Novak M, Huang WQ, *et al.* Oral immunization with influenza virus in biodegradable microspheres. *J Infect Dis* 1993;**167**:84–90.

59 Vila A, Sánchez A, Tobío M, Calvo P, Alonso MJ. Design of biodegradable particles for protein delivery. *J Control Release* 2002;**78**:15–24.

60 Wang YY, Lai SK, Suk JS, *et al.* Addressing the PEG mucoadhesivity paradox to engineer nanoparticles

that "slip" through the human mucus barrier. *Angew Chem Int Ed Engl* 2008;**47**:9726–9.

61 Sharp FA, Ruane D, Claass B, *et al.* Uptake of particulate vaccine adjuvants by dendritic cells activates the NALP3 inflammasome. *Proc Natl Acad Sci U S A* 2009;**106**:870–75.

62 Jain S, Malyala P, Pallaoro M, *et al.* A two-stage strategy for sterilization of poly(lactide-co-glycolide) particles by gamma-irradiation does not impair their potency for vaccine delivery. *J Pharm Sci* 2011;**100**:646–54.

63 Coombes AG, Lavelle EC, Davis SS. Biodegradable lamellar particles of poly(lactide) induce sustained immune responses to a single dose of adsorbed protein. *Vaccine* 1999;**17**:2410–22.

64 Conway MA, Madrigal-Estebas L, McClean S, Brayden DJ, Mills KH. Protection against *Bordetella pertussis* infection following parenteral or oral immunization with antigens entrapped in biodegradable particles: effect of formulation and route of immunization on induction of Th1 and Th2 cells. *Vaccine* 2001;**19**:1940–50.

65 Delgado A, Lavelle EC, Hartshorne M, Davis SS. PLG microparticles stabilised using enteric coating polymers as oral vaccine delivery systems. *Vaccine* 1999;**17**:2927–38.

66 GSK. Two new studies in the New England Journal of Medicine show malaria vaccine candidate advancing in Africa. Dec 8, 2008. Available at www.gsk.com/media/pressreleases/2008/2008_us_pressrelease_10168.htm. Accessed Feb 2012.

67 GSK. New data for GlaxoSmithKline's pre-pandemic H5N1 influenza vaccine, Prepandrix™, show administration flexibility for pandemic planning, Sep 16, 2008. Available at www.gsk.com/media/pressreleases/2008/2008_pressrelease_10106.htm. Accessed Feb 2012.

68 Didierlaurent AM, Morel S, Lockman L, *et al.* AS04, an aluminum salt- and TLR4 agonist-based adjuvant system, induces a transient localized innate immune response leading to enhanced adaptive immunity. *J Immunol* 2009;**183**:6186–97.

69 GSK. FDA approves Cervarix, GlaxoSmithKline's cervical cancer vaccine, Oct 16, 2009. Available at www.gsk.com/media/pressreleases/2009/2009_pressrelease_10112.htm. Accessed Feb 2012.

70 Schiller JT, Castellsagué X, Villa LL, Hildesheim A. An update of prophylactic human papillomavirus L1 virus-like particle vaccine clinical trial results. *Vaccine* 2008;**26**(Suppl 10):K53–61.

71 GSK/Duke University. Study to assess dHER2+AS15 cancer vaccine given in combination with Lapatinib to patients with metastatic breast cancer. Available at clinicaltrials.gov/ct2/show/NCT00952692. Accessed Feb 2012.

72 Verstraeten T, Descamps D, David MP, *et al.* Analysis of adverse events of potential autoimmune aetiology in a large integrated safety database of AS04 adjuvanted vaccines. *Vaccine* 2008;**26**:6630–38.

73 GSK. Adjuvants briefing paper, Apr 2010. Available at www.gsk.com/policies/adjuvants.pdf. Accessed Feb 2012.

74 Malyala P, Chesko J, Ugozzoli M, *et al.* The potency of the adjuvant, CpG oligos, is enhanced by encapsulation in PLG microparticles. *J Pharm Sci* 2007;**3**:1155–64.

75 Hunter SK, Andracki ME, Krieg AM. Biodegradable microspheres containing group B Streptococcus vaccine: immune response in mice. *Am J Obstet Gynecol* 2001;**185**:1174–9.

76 Palmer M, Parker J, Modi S, *et al.* Phase I study of the BLP25 (MUC1 peptide) liposomal vaccine for active specific immunotherapy in stage IIIB/IV non-small-cell lung cancer. *Clin Lung Cancer* 2001;**3**:49–57; discussion 58.

77 Merck. Merck Initiates Phase III Study of Stimuvax in Breast Cancer, Jun 22, 2009. Available at www.merckgroup.com/en/media/extNewsDetail.html?newsId=53CE16569ABA8129C12575DA004270D7&newsType=1. Accessed Feb 2012.

78 Merck. Merck KGaA: Stimuvax Clinical Program Temporarily Suspended, Mar 23, 2010. Available at www.merckgroup.com/en/media/extNewsDetail.html?newsId=E01571A622782EADC12576EE00702854&newsType=1. Accessed Feb 2012.

79 Agger EM, Rosenkrands I, Olsen AW, *et al.* Protective immunity to tuberculosis with Ag85B-ESAT-6 in a synthetic cationic adjuvant system IC31. *Vaccine* 2006;**24**:5452–60.

80 Schellack C, Prinz K, Egyed A, *et al.* IC31, a novel adjuvant signaling via TLR9, induces potent cellular and humoral immune responses. *Vaccine* 2006;**24**:5461–72.

81 Riedl K, Riedl R, von Gabain A, Nagy E, Lingnau K. The novel adjuvant IC31 strongly improves influenza vaccine-specific cellular and humoral immune responses in young adult and aged mice. *Vaccine* 2008;**26**:3461–8.

82 Intercell. Adjuvant IC31®. Available at www.intercell.com/main/forvaccperts/technologies/adjuvant-ic31r./ Accessed Feb 2012.

83 WHO. Immunological adjuvants. WHO technical report series no. 595. WHO, Geneva:1976, pp. 6–8.

84 O'Hagan DT, Jeffery H, Davis SS. Long-term antibody responses in mice following subcutaneous immunization with ovalbumin entrapped in biodegradable microparticles. *Vaccine* 1993;**11**:965–9.

85 Watson DL, Watson NA, Fossum C, Lövgren K, Morein B. Interactions between immune-stimulating complexes (ISCOMs) and peritoneal mononuclear leucocytes. *Microbiol Immunol* 1992;**36**:199–203.

86 Fifis T, Gamvrellis A, Crimeen-Irwin B, *et al.* Size-dependent immunogenicity: therapeutic and protective properties of nano-vaccines against tumors. *J Immunol* 2004;**173**:3148–54.

87 Bachmann MF, Zinkernagel RM. Neutralizing antiviral B cell responses. *Annu Rev Immunol* 1997;**15**:235–70.

88 Holt LB. *Developments in Diptheria Prophylaxis.* Heinemann, London, 1950.

89 Gupta RK, Chang AC, Griffin P, Rivera R, Siber GR. In vivo distribution of radioactivity in mice after injection of biodegradable polymer microspheres containing 14C-labeled tetanus toxoid. *Vaccine* 1996;**14**:1412–16.

90 Kool M, Soullié T, van Nimwegen M, *et al.* Alum adjuvant boosts adaptive immunity by inducing uric acid and activating inflammatory dendritic cells. *J Exp Med* 2008;**205**(4):869–82.

91 McKee AS, MacLeod M, White J, *et al.* Gr1+IL-4-producing innate cells are induced in response to Th2 stimuli and suppress Th1-dependent antibody responses. *Int Immunol* 2008;**20**:659–69.

92 Seubert A, Monaci E, Pizza M, O'Hagan DT, Wack A. The adjuvants aluminum hydroxide and MF59 induce monocyte and granulocyte chemoattractants and enhance monocyte differentiation toward dendritic cells. *J Immunol* 2008;**180**:5402–12.

93 Gavin AL, Hoebe K, Duong B, *et al.* Adjuvant-enhanced antibody responses in the absence of toll-like receptor signaling. *Science* 2006;**314**:1936–8.

94 Schnare M, Barton GM, Holt AC, *et al.* Toll-like receptors control activation of adaptive immune responses. *Nat Immunol* 2001;**2**:947–50.

95 Eisenbarth SC, Colegio OR, O'Connor W, Sutterwala FS, Flavell RA. Crucial role for the Nalp3 inflammasome in the immunostimulatory properties of aluminium adjuvants. *Nature* 2008;**453**:1122–6.

96 Kool M, Pétrilli V, De Smedt T, *et al.* Alum adjuvant stimulates inflammatory dendritic cells through activation of the NALP3 inflammasome. *J Immunol* 2008;**181**:3755–9.

97 Li H, Nookala S, Re F. Aluminum hydroxide adjuvants activate caspase-1 and induce IL-1beta and IL-18 release. *J Immunol* 2007;**178**:5271–6.

98 Li H, Willingham SB, Ting JP, Re F. Inflammasome activation by alum and alum's adjuvant effect are mediated by NLRP3. *J Immunol* 2008;**181**:17–21.

99 Sokolovska A, Hem SL, HogenEsch H. Activation of dendritic cells and induction of CD4(+) T cell differentiation by aluminum-containing adjuvants. *Vaccine* 2007;**25**:4575–85.

100 Martinon F, Burns K, Tschopp J. The inflammasome: a molecular platform triggering activation of inflammatory caspases and processing of proIL-beta. *Mol Cell* 2002;**10**:417–26.

101 Pétrilli V, Dostert C, Muruve DA, Tschopp J. The inflammasome: a danger sensing complex triggering innate immunity. *Curr Opin Immunol* 2007;**19**:615–22.

102 Franchi L, Nune G. The Nlrp3 inflammasome is critical for aluminium hydroxide-mediated IL-1beta secretion but dispensable for adjuvant activity. *Eur J Immunol* 2008;**38**:2085–89.

103 McKee AS, Munks MW, MacLeod MK, *et al.* Alum induces innate immune responses through macrophage and mast cell sensors, but these sensors are not required for alum to act as an adjuvant for specific immunity. *J Immunol* 2009;**183**:4403–14.

CHAPTER 25

Co-administration of Co-stimulatory Moieties

Carolina Arancibia-Cárcamo[1] & Yvette Latchman[2]
[1]Translational Gastroenterology Unit, Nuffield Department of Clinical Medicine, University of Oxford, Oxford, UK
[2]The Puget Sound Blood Center, Seattle, WA, USA

Introduction

Vaccine development requires the understanding of how the immune system recognizes antigens and the sequential pathways that are activated during an immune response. One of the key targets of vaccination is the activation of antigen-specific T cells and the generation of subsequent memory T cells.

T cells acquire specificity through their T-cell receptor (TCR) by recognizing their cognate peptide bound to major histocompatibility complex (MHC) molecules expressed on antigen-presenting cells (APC). The notion that optimal activation of T cells required secondary signals independent of TCR signaling was first postulated by Lafferty and Cunningham to clarify their functional observation that naïve T cells were not activated by antigen alone (reviewed in [1]). From this data they proposed a two-signal hypothesis whereby naïve T cells were activated through the TCR (signal 1) and an inducible molecule with co-stimulatory activity (signal 2) [1]. Further studies by Jenkins *et al.* demonstrated that a lack of signal 2 resulted in T-cell anergy or unresponsiveness to successive antigen challenge [1]. The generation of monoclonal antibodies to the human T-cell surface molecules and cloning led to the discovery of the best-characterized co-stimulatory molecule, CD28. Human and murine studies showed that cross-

linking of CD28 together with anti-CD3 induced full activation of naïve T cells, thereby confirming the two-signal theory. By the early 1990s, CD80 and CD86, members of the B7 family, were found to be the ligands for CD28. However, the discovery of cytotoxic T lymphocyte antigen 4 (CTLA4) as a homolog of CD28 highlighted the complexity of T-cell co-stimulation as it was shown to provide an inhibitory signal. The implication of this finding was that co-stimulators could either stimulate and sustain T-cell responses or negatively regulate T-cell responses [2]. Thus, anergy induction or tolerance occurred through an active process of engaging negative receptors. Over the past ten years there has been an expansion of the CD28 co-stimulatory family with various potential targets for use in conjunction with established vaccination protocols (Table 25.1). Some of these pathways will be discussed further in this chapter. The uniqueness and overlapping functions of diverse co-stimulators – that is, targeting naïve versus effector T cells or effectors versus regulatory T cells (Tregs) – adds to their intricacy in determining the best option for therapeutic benefit. Interestingly, clinical trials using anti-CTLA4 antibody as a component of a cancer vaccine has opened up the field of co-stimulation for therapeutic use in enhancing or blocking immune responses. As well as the CD28 superfamily, the tumor necrosis

Vaccinology: Principles and Practice, First Edition. Edited by W. John W. Morrow, Nadeem A. Sheikh, Clint S. Schmidt and D. Huw Davies.
© 2012 Blackwell Publishing Ltd. Published 2012 by Blackwell Publishing Ltd.

Table 25.1 CD28 superfamily members.

Receptor	Expression	Signaling	Ligand	Expression	Clinical use
Positive co-stimulatory pathways					
CD28	Human/mouse: Constitutively expressed on most T cells, NK cells, and plasma cells Mouse (only T cells)	YMNM motif phosphatidylinositol-3-kinase (PI3K) Grb2	CD80 CD86	Human/mouse: Upregulated on APC Human/mouse: Constitutively and upregulated on APC Upregulated T cells (mouse)	CTLA4Ig (abatacept) Approved for RA patients failing anti-TNF-α therapy Phase I/II IBD, lupus nephritis, and diabetes
ICOS (CD278)	Human/mouse: Upregulated on T cells	YMFM motif PI3K	ICOSL (CD275)	Human/mouse: Upregulated on APC, fibroblasts, endothelial cells and renal epithelial cells (human)	
Negative regulatory pathways					
CTLA4 (CD152)	Human/mouse: Upregulated on T cells (constitutively expressed on Tregs)	YVKM motif SHP-2 PP2A	CD80 CD86	As above	Anti-CTLA4 (ipilimumab, tremelimumab) Phase I–III melanoma, ovarian cancer, lung cancer, prostate cancer, leukemia, and myelodysplastic syndromes
PD1 (CD279)	Human/mouse: Upregulated on T cells, B cells, monocytes, and NKT cells (mouse)	Imunoreceptor tyrosine-based inhibitory motif (ITIM) Imunoreceptor tyrosine-based switch motif (ITSM) SHP-2 (ITSM) SHP-1 (ITSM)	PD-L1[a] (CD274) PD-L2 (CD273)	Human/mouse: Constitutively expressed on T, B cells, and DC NKT cells (mouse), non-lymphoid organs and upregulated by activation. Human/mouse: Upregulated by activation on DC, monocytes and B1 B cells and some non-lymphoid organs	Anti-PD1 (MDX-1105/ONO-4538, CT-011) Anti-PD-L1 (MDX-1105) Phase I solid tumors

(Continued)

Table 25.1 CD28 superfamily members. (*Continued*)

Receptor	Expression	Signaling	Ligand	Expression	Clinical use
BTLA (CD272)	Human/mouse: Constitutively expressed on B cells and downregulated on activation Upregulated on DC, myeloid, and T cells	ITIM SHP-2 SHP-1	HVEM	Human/mouse: Constitutively expressed on T cells, B cells, DC, NK, and myeloid cells. Liver, kidney, and lung (mouse)	
Unknown			B7-H4	Human/mouse: Upregulated on APC, T cells, NK cells, tumor cells (mouse)	
Unknown			BTNL2	Human/mouse: B cells and intestinal epithelial cells	
TREM-like transcript 2 (mouse only)	Constitutively expressed on B cell, CD8+ T cells and upregulated on CD4+ T cells	Unknown	B7-H3 (CD276)[b]	Human/mouse: Upregulated on APC, T cells, NK cells Constitutively expressed on fibroblasts and tumor cells (human)	

[a]PD-L1 also interacts with CD80 to give a negative signal.
[b]Reported to have positive co-stimulatory and negative regulatory activity.

factor (TNF) and CD2/signaling lymphocyte activation molecule (SLAM) superfamilies can provide important second signals for the activation of T cells. However, due to the extensive research on all three pathways it would not be feasible to discuss all these and their relevance to vaccine development. In this chapter, we will discuss recent advances on co-stimulation through the CD28 superfamily and the potential for their use as monotherapies or combination therapies in vaccines against cancer, viruses, and autoimmune diseases.

Negative regulatory members of the CD28 superfamily

Cytotoxic T lymphocyte-associated molecule 4 (CTLA4, CD152)

Within the CD28 superfamily, the counterbalance of positive and negative signals can be clearly demonstrated by the engagement of CD80 (B7-1) and CD86 (B7-2) molecules by CD28, resulting in expansion, differentiation, and survival. In contrast, the consequence of B7 interaction with CTLA4 is inactivation or anergy. CTLA4 is expressed on activated T cells and constitutively expressed on T regulatory cells (reviewed in [3]) (Figure 25.1). The most compelling evidence for the critical negative regulatory role of CTLA4 is the dramatic phenotype of CTLA4$^{-/-}$ mice. This has prompted several studies that demonstrate its role in regulating autoimmunity and peripheral tolerance. Most of the CTLA4 protein is retained intracellularly in lysosomes, endosomes, and the trans-Golgi network and is upregulated on cross-linking of the TCR and augmented intracellular calcium levels (reviewed in [3]). The constitutive expression of CTLA4 on Tregs has led to speculation on the importance of this molecule in the function of Tregs. Of note, mice defective in CTLA4 expression in Tregs succumb to lymphoproliferative disease

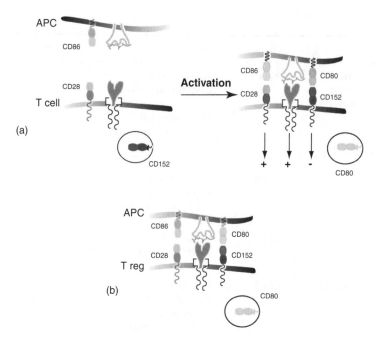

Figure 25.1 Expression of members of the C28 pathway. (a) Naïve T cells express low levels of CD28 and intracellular CTLA4. CD86 is expressed on APCs, including DC, B cells, and macrophages. Upon activation through the TCR, CD28 is upregulated and CTLA4 is translocated to the surface. Both CD86 and CD80 are expressed on APC after activation but the kinetics of CD80 expression is slower than CD86. The affinities of CD80 and CD86 are higher for CTLA4 than CD28 and it has been demonstrated that CD80 is responsible for the accumulation of CTLA4 at the surface. CD86 also can be expressed on murine T cells. (b) Tregs constitutively express CTLA4 and its expression may result in the downregulation of CD80 and CD86 on activated APCs.

by 7 weeks of age [4]. The study showed that B7 molecules were downregulated on dendritic cells (DC) in the presence of wild-type Tregs but not CTLA4$^{-/-}$ Tregs, indicating a cell-extrinsic role for CTLA4. The evidence thus far points to a complex mode of action of CTLA4 inhibition of T-cell activation, which may include competition for B7 binding, downregulation of B7 ligands through Tregs, and/or direct signaling through its cytoplasm tail. Other negative regulators such as PD1 and BTLA in the CD28 superfamily have prompted investigation into the role of these pathways, as the lack of compensatory signals in the CTLA4$^{-/-}$ mice indicates that these pathways may have distinct functions when compared to CTLA4.

Programmed cell death 1 (PD1, CD279)

Programmed cell death 1 (PD1, CD279) is a CD28 homolog that contains an immunoreceptor tyrosine-based inhibitory motif (ITIM) and an immunoreceptor tyrosine-based switch motif (ITSM) in its cytoplasmic tail. Unlike CD28 and CTLA4,

PD1 is not restricted in its expression and is upregulated on murine T cells, B cells, Tregs, myeloid cells, and NKT cells after their activation (reviewed in [5]) (Figure 25.2). PD-L1 (B7-H1, CD274) and PD-L2 (B7-DC, CD273) are the ligands for PD1. PD-L1 is constitutively expressed on T cells, B cells, and DC and upregulated by activation, while PD-L2 is tightly regulated and only upregulated on DC, monocytes, and B1 B cells [5]. PD-L1 and PD-L2 expression also has been detected in both human and mouse tissues and in nonlymphoid organs with high levels in placenta. PD1 mediates its negative regulatory effects via the ITIM and ITSM signaling motifs in its cytoplasmic tail. In addition, PD1 signaling blocks phosphatidylinositol-3-kinase (PI3K) kinase activity, unlike CTLA4, which targets AKT activity [6]. Thus far, negative signaling pathways such as CTLA4 and PD1 have shown separate mechanisms of action but probably are synergistic in their effects.

PD1$^{-/-}$ mice develop a lupus-like arthritis and glomerulonephritis or a fatal dilated cardiomyopathy, depending on the genetic background [5].

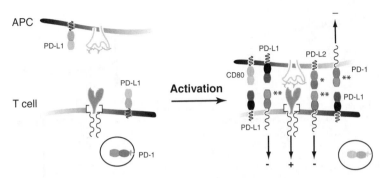

Figure 25.2 Expression of members of the PD1 pathway. Naïve T cells and APCs express low levels of PD-L1 and some studies have shown intracellular PD1. TCR together with CD28 signals upregulates PD1 and PD-L1 on T cells. Upon activation, PD-L1 is expressed on all APCs; however, PD-L2 (*) only is expressed on DC, myeloid, and B1 B cells. In addition, PD1 (**) is expressed on B cells and myeloid cells but not DC. PD-L1 interacts with CD80 with an affinity that is lower than PD-L1:PD1 interactions and CD80:CTLA4 interactions but higher than CD80:CD28 interactions. The interaction of CD80 and PD-L1 is likely to antagonize the CD28 pathway by removing the CD80 ligand.

Several studies using monoclonal antibodies against PD1-deficient mice have demonstrated acceleration in the course of disease in non-obese diabetic (NOD) mice and a murine model of experimental autoimmune encephalomyelitis (EAE) [5]. From these models of autoimmunity it is clear that PD-L1 expression on the host tissue is important for maintaining tolerance. These results demonstrate that PD-L1 on T cells, APCs, and host tissue inhibits naïve and effector T-cell responses and plays a critical role in T-cell tolerance.

There has been some controversy on the role of the ligands for PD1, with groups showing that both ligands were able to co-stimulate naïve T cells and this feature was independent of PD1 [7]. These results indicate an alternative yet unidentified CD28-like receptor for PD-L1 and PD-L2. Interestingly, Sharpe and colleagues have shown that CD80 interacts with PD-L1 to inhibit T-cell responses, indicating that antibodies to PD-L1 may block negative signal through PD1 as well as enhancing CD80:CD28 interactions [8]. Therefore, studies using blocking antibodies to PD-L1 and PD-L1$^{-/-}$ deficient mice may need to be reinterpreted to account for the interaction between PD-L1 and CD80. The inhibitory role of the PD1 pathway and its abil-

ity to influence both B and T cells indicates that this is an attractive pathway to target for augmenting the immune response. However, there is no data indicating if blocking PD-L1 rather than PD1 might be more advantageous.

B- and T lymphocyte attenuator (BTLA, CD272)

B- and T-lymphocyte attenuator (BTLA) is highly expressed on naïve B with a lower expression on T cells and myeloid cells. On activation, BTLA is upregulated on dendritic cells, Th1 cells, and anergic cells but not Th2 cells, and slightly downregulated on B cells (reviewed in [9]) (Figure 25.3). It has been shown that herpes virus-entry mediator (HVEM), a member of the TNF family, is a ligand for BTLA and not B7X as originally described. Interestingly, HVEM also interacts with LIGHT, another TNF family member, which downregulates its expression. The binding sites of BTLA and LIGHT on HVEM are distinct, which gives rise to the possibility that both receptors can bind at the same time; however, the *in vivo* consequences of these interactions have not been studied. The cytoplasmic tail of BTLA contains two ITIM sequences and both ITIM

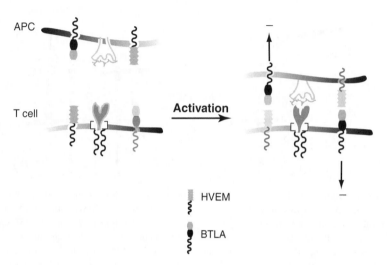

Figure 25.3 Expression of members of the BTLA pathway. BTLA is constitutively expressed on B cells and with lower levels on T cells and DC. Activation upregulates BTLA on T cells, myeloid, and DC but slightly downregulates its expression on B cells. HVEM is constitutively expressed on T cells, B cells, DC, and myeloid cells and downregulation occurs on activation. HVEM also interacts with LIGHT (not shown), another member of the TNF superfamily, resulting in a positive signal. Human HVEM interacts with CD160 (not shown) to give a negative signal. The affinity of HVEM for LIGHT is higher than the affinity for the BTLA and CD160.

motifs are necessary for the binding of SHP-1 and SHP-2 [9].

Anti-CD3 stimulation and antigen-specific responses from BTLA$^{-/-}$ T cells are increased compared to wild-type T cells [9]. It is noteworthy that HVEM$^{-/-}$ mice have a similar phenotype to BTLA-deficient mice, showing the importance of this negative regulatory pathway [10]. Cross-linking with antibodies against BTLA or CHO cells expressing HVEM has shown that this pathway is involved in downregulating T-cell responses. The HVEM:BTLA pathway has been shown to be important in several disease models, and HVEM and BTLA$^{-/-}$ mice have increased susceptibility to EAE induction [9]. These data are very similar to PD-L1$^{-/-}$ mice and necessitate investigation of whether these are independent or redundant pathways [11].

Negative regulatory pathways and enhancement of tumor immunity

To evade detection and recognition, tumor cells use various mechanisms, including downregulation of tumor and MHC antigens, secretion or expression of immunosuppressive factors, and upregulation of ligands of negative co-stimulation pathways. An understanding of avenues to perform checkpoint blockade of key immune system activation pathways together with how the immune system interacts with the tumor microenvironment will lead to better design of immunotherapies, which might involve a combination of methods to activate tumor-specific T cells. Blockade of negative regulators of the CD28 superfamily may be one valid strategy to design therapeutic vaccines due to the powerful inhibitory role they play on the activation of T cells.

CTLA4: from mouse to clinic

It was originally shown in mice that tumors expressing B7 were rejected by anti-CTLA4 blockade [12]. In a murine model of prostate cancer (TRAMP), partial or total regression was seen with subcutaneous tumors and reduced metastases, after treatment with anti-CTLA4 [13,14]. Since regression of tumors with anti-CTLA4 was not as successful with poorly immunogenic tumors such as B16, combination therapy was employed to facilitate a robust immune response. Vaccination with B16 tumor cells, breast carcinoma cells, or TRAMP tumor cells expressing GM-CSF together with anti-CTLA4 blockade has been successful in the eradication of tumor cells (reviewed in [15]). In addition, combination of anti-CTLA4 with tyrosinase-related protein-2 administered with CpG-ODN or chemotherapy or depletion of Tregs prolonged the survival of mice challenged with tumors [15]. In all the mouse models, a degree of autoimmunity has been induced and this has been associated with the regression of the tumors [16–18].

Results from mouse studies suggested that blockade of CTLA4 can lead to the rejection of transplanted tumor cells. These findings have led to several completed and ongoing clinical trials using combination strategies with anti-CTLA4 for several carcinomas, including melanoma, ovarian cancer, lung cancer, leukemia, and myelodysplastic syndromes (Table 25.2). Ipilimumab (MDX-010; Medarex/Bristol-Myers Squibb) and tremelimumab (CP-675205; Pfizer) are the two humanized antibodies against CTLA4 that have been evaluated in the clinic. The initial study with ipilimumab was a phase I study conducted by Dranoff and colleagues with nine patients with metastatic melanoma (MM) of whom five had previously received irradiated, autologous, GM-CSF-secreting tumor cells (GVAX) and four had received gp100 peptide-loaded DC or IL2 [19]. Although no tumor shrinkage occurred, there was necrosis of the tumor with increased neutrophil infiltrate. GVAX vaccination appeared to have an advantage over single antigen vaccination. Further studies have shown partial or complete responses in the presence of autoimmune adverse reactions [20–25]. A combination of ipilimumab and chemotherapy or radiotherapy has been reported in a small number of patients; although the results show some improvement over single moieties alone, the patient numbers have to be increased to validate these results [26]. Although many of the studies have been performed in patients with MM there are published data showing a beneficial

effect in prostate and renal cancer, and for treatment of relapsing malignancy after hematopoietic cell transplant [27–32]. Phase I/II clinical trials have also been observed with tremelimumab in MM [33–35]. A phase III clinical trial looking at the effectiveness of tremelimumab compared to chemotherapy in MM patients with no prior treatment was discontinued due to no survival benefit over standard treatment, indicating that anti-CTLA4 blockade requires combination therapy [36]. This might not be a reflection of an inherent difference between tremelimumab and ipilimumab treatments as their dosings are different and recent evidence has suggested that anti-CTLA4 treatment requires a longer duration of time to assess efficacy compared to standard treatments. This has led to an investigation of new assessments for endpoint parameters for biological agents used in cancer immunotherapy [37].

As mentioned, autoimmune adverse reactions have been associated with clinical response in MM patients in all clinical trials. These include severe rashes (50%), colitis grade III/IV (16%), and pituitary inflammation (5%). These adverse events induced by anti-CTLA4 therapy have been termed "immune-related adverse events" (irAE). Guidelines for the treatment of irAE have been published but as irAE have been linked with anti-tumor responses, a better understanding of the mechanism of action of anti-CTLA4 therapy is required to achieve the therapeutic dose that induces anti-tumor effects without irAE. Some insights have come from immunologic parameters measured during treatment with anti-CTLA4 therapy. Independent of the anti-CTLA4 antibody used, most studies show an increase in $CD8^+$ tumor-specific cells with tumor necrosis [38–40], and two studies have shown that the ratio between intra-tumor $CD8^+$ T cells and Tregs is important; however, another group has shown no correlation [40]. Increased NY-ESO-1 antibodies and NY-ESO-1-specific T cells also appear to correlate with tumor regression or stable disease [39,41]. In bladder cancer, treatment with anti-CTLA4 increased $CD4^+ICOS^{high}IFN-\gamma$ producing cells [42,43]. It is too early to define the mechanism responsible for the beneficial role of anti-CTLA4 antibody in

Table 25.2 Co-stimulatory moieties in clinical trials.

Published (Ref.) and ongoing (clinicaltrials.gov) studies	Treatment	Disease	Clinical response/phase	Immunologic response
	Anti-CTLA4			
[21]	Ipilimumab 0.1–3mg/kg + IL2	Metastatic melanoma	8/36 Complete or partial response	ND
[33]	Tremelimumab 1–15mg/kg	Melanoma, renal, colon	8/29 Complete or partial response, or stable disease	ND
[29]	Ipilimumab 3 mg/kg	Prostate cancer [3], colon cancer [4], non-Hodgkin's lymphoma [4]	2/4 non-Hodgkin's lymphoma patients: tumor regression	Prostate-specific T-cell responses not detected
[23]	Ipilimumab 9 mg/kg + peptide vaccination	Metastatic melanoma	23/129 Complete or partial response	ND
[30]	Ipilimumab 1–3 mg/kg	Renal cell cancer	1/21 (lower dose) 5/40 (higher dose) Partial response	ND
[41]	Ipilimumab 3 mg/kg	Metastatic melanoma	8/15 Complete or partial response, or stable disease	5/8 anti-NY-ESO-1 antibodies and anti-NY-ESO-1 T cells (two pre-existing). Correlated with response
[38]	Tremelimumab 10 mg/kg	Metastatic melanoma	3/12 Partial response	No significant change in percentage of MART1-specific T cells
[32]	Ipilimumab 3 mg/kg	Relapse of malignancy after stem cell transplantation	5/29 Complete or partial response	ND
[31]	Ipilimumab 0.5–3 mg/kg GM-CSF	Prostate cancer	3/24 Decrease in PSA (50%) 1/24 Partial response	5/24 anti-NY-ESO-1 antibodies (three prior to treatment), only one had a decrease in PSA
[45]	Tremelimumab 10–15 mg/kg or tremelimumab and DC pulsed with melanoma peptides	Metastatic melanoma	6/27 Complete or partial response	IL17 correlates with irAE

(Continued)

Table 25.2 Co-stimulatory moieties in clinical trials. (*Continued*)

Published (Ref.) and ongoing (clinicaltrials. gov) studies	Treatment	Disease	Clinical response/phase	Immunologic response
	Anti-PD1			
[50]	CT-011 0.2–6 mg/kg	Acute myeloid leukemia (AML), chronic lymphocytic leukemia, non-Hodgkin's lymphoma, Hodgkin's lymphoma, multiple myeloma	5/17 Complete response or stable disease	
[51]	MDX-1106 0.3–10 mg/kg	Advanced metastatic melanoma, colorectal cancer, castrate-resistant prostate cancer, non-small-cell lung cancer, renal cell carcinoma	3/39 Complete or partial response	
	Anti-CTLA4			
	Tremelimumab 3–15 mg/kg and Bicalutamide	Prostate cancer	I	
	Tremelimumab 3–15 mg/kg and BCG	Bladder cancer	I	
	Ipilimumab 10 mg/kg	After complete resection of high risk stage III melanoma	III Randomized, double blind placebo control	
	Ipilimumab 10 mg/kg and anti-CD137 0.1–3 mg/kg	Melanoma	I Non-randomized open label	
	Anti-PD1			
	MDX-1106-02, single dose	Hepatitis C	I	
	MDX-1106-02 + peptide vaccination	Melanoma	I	
	Anti-PD-L1			
	MDX-1105 3–15 mg/kg	Renal cell carcinoma, non-small-cell lung cancer, malignant melanoma, epithelial ovarian cancer	I Dose escalation	

(*Continued*)

Table 25.2 Co-stimulatory moieties in clinical trials. (*Continued*)

Published (Ref.) and ongoing (clinicaltrials. gov) studies	Treatment	Disease	Clinical response/phase	Immunologic response
	Anti CTLA and anti-PD1			
	Ipilimumab 3–10 mg/kg MDX-1106 0.3–3 mg/kg	Stage III or stage IV malignant melanoma	I Dose escalation	
	CTLA4Ig			
	Abatacept	Diabetes	II Randomized, double-blind, placebo-controlled	
	Abatacept	Psoriasis vulgaris	II Randomized, double-blind, placebo-controlled	
	Abatacept and cyclophosphamide	Lupus nephritis	II Randomized, double-blind, controlled,	
	Abatacept	Mild relapsing Wegener's granulomatosis	I/II Open-label pilot study	

ND, Not done.

anti-tumor therapy. However, it is clear that the treatment raises the threshold for the activation of low-affinity self-reactive T cells. Transgenic mice expressing human CTLA4 demonstrated that T effector enhancement and reduction in Treg suppression together were necessary for the anti-tumor effect observed with anti-CTLA4 [44]. Interestingly, Camacho's group have shown that IL17 producing CD4$^+$ T cells appear to be associated with irAE and not with clinical outcome. However, a detrimental role of Th17 cells in irAE during CTLA4 treatment has not been proven [45]. The success of CTLA4 has led to the exploration of other co-stimulatory pathways that may be as effective as CTLA4 without side effects.

PD1 pathway: next generation in anti-tumor therapy

In several tumor mouse models it has been shown that antibodies against PD-L1 or PD-L2 can increase anti-tumor immunity, and in addition tumor cell growth is suppressed in PD1$^{-/-}$ mice [15]. Combination strategies with murine anti-PD1 and B16 melanoma cells have proved successful in reducing tumor growth [15]. Using B16-OVA tumor cells, investigators demonstrated a decrease in conversion of tumor-infiltrating T cells to Tregs in the presence of anti-PD-L1 antibody, indicating a role for the PD-L1:PD1 pathway in the induction of adaptive Tregs [46]. In humans, PD-L1 and PD-L2 expression have been detected on many carcinomas, and some T cell tumors and tumor-associated DC express higher levels of PD-L1 [11,47,48]. In addition, PD-L1 expression on tumor cells correlates with poor prognosis in urothelial cancer, renal cell carcinoma, gastric carcinoma, breast cancer, ovarian cancer, esophageal cancer, and hepatocellular carcinoma (reviewed in [49]). Furthermore, using human tumor-specific T cells, a number of investigators have shown that blocking PD-L1:PD1 interactions simultaneously with antigen stimulation resulted in augmented T-cell responses [49]. These findings suggest that PD-L1:PD1-mediated inhibitory signals give tumors a selective advantage for growth by limiting CD8$^+$ T-cell clonal expansion and thereby attenuate tumor-specific responses. The emerging data of the role of PD-L1:PD1 signaling on various cell types, particularly its role in adaptive Treg induction, indicates that blocking this pathway together with stimulating the immune system will favor an improved anti-tumor response.

Humanized anti-PD1 and anti-PD-L1 antibodies are now in phase I clinical trials. MDX-1106/ONO-4538 (anti-PD1; Medarex, Inc. and Ono Pharmaceutical Ltd) is being used for advanced and recurrent malignancies and MDX-1105 (anti-PD-L1; Medarex, Inc) in solid tumors (Table 25.2). Cure Tech Ltd (CT-011; anti-PD1) has reported an escalating single dose clinical trial with CT-011, with seventeen patients with various hematologic malignancies, including acute myeloid leukemia (AML), chronic lymphocytic leukemia (CLL), and non-Hodgkin's lymphoma (NHL) [50]. The results showed that the antibody was well tolerated, with a third of the patients showing some improvement although this was not related to the dose of antibody received. Interestingly, the percentage of CD4$^+$ T cells but not CD8$^+$ T cells was increased 24 hours after antibody treatment but a trial with a larger number of patients and a placebo control group will have to be performed to see if this observation is accurate. Results from a dose-escalating clinical trial with anti-PD1 antibody (MDX-1106) in 39 patients with solid tumors showed that antibody was well tolerated and 3 patients showed complete or partial responses [51]. Interestingly, PD-L1 expression on the tumor seems to be indicative of response to treatment. A recent study combining PD1 and CTLA4 blockade in a murine model of melanoma illustrated the synergistic effects in tumor responses and has become the rationale for combining ipilimumab and MDX-1106 in a clinical trial for patients with advanced melanoma [52] (Table 25.2). In conclusion, the use of anti-CTLA4 in clinical trials has "opened the door" for co-stimulation blockade to be utilized in conjunctive with anti-tumor therapy. However, the trials are still in their early stages and more data is required to evaluate whether blocking negative pathways that may be involved in self-tolerance is devoid of side effects. The data on BTLA is limited in tumor immunity. However, this molecule might be a future target for immunotherapy as BTLA is highly expressed on tumor-specific cells and down-regulated by peptide vaccination together with CpG oligodeoxynucleotide [53].

Negative pathways and viral infections

Another area of active research is the role of the CD28 superfamily in viral infections. Some viruses use similar strategies as tumor cells to evade detection and elimination by the immune system. In HIV and hepatitis C virus (HCV), antiviral T cells can be detected but there is still replication of the virus, indicating deficiency in T-cell responses. This state of defective T-cell response with excessive antigen load has been defined as "T-cell exhaustion" [54]. The use of vaccines to attenuate anti-viral responses under these conditions will be beneficial in the clearance of persistent viruses.

PD1: new player in viral therapy

Ahmed and colleagues have shown in a mouse model of viral persistence, lymphocytic choriomeningitis virus (LCMV), that PD1 is upregulated on exhausted T cells [55,56]. Moreover, blockade of PD1 resulted in increased cytokine production and effector responses by anti-LCMV-specific T cells. Interestingly, blockade of CTLA4 had no effect, once again demonstrating the independent mechanisms of these two negative pathways. To date there are several publications showing the upregulation of PD1 in diseases such as HIV, HCV, and hepatitis B virus (HBV). In HIV, a number of investigators have shown that PD1 is expressed on CD8+ and CD4+ HIV-specific T cells and using antibodies against PD1 ligands increased the frequency of IFN-γ producing CD8+ T cells (reviewed in [57]). In addition, PD1 expression correlated with disease progression and viral load, and persistent viral load resulted in loss of polyfunctional HIV-specific CD8+ T cells and upregulation of PD1, and therefore an exhausted phenotype [57]. Data thus far indicates that antigen load drives the exhausted T cells and expression of PD1. In addition to PD1 expression on T cells, PD-L1 is also induced on APC during HIV infection [58–60]. Similar results to murine and human studies were obtained whereby PD1 was highly expressed on simian immunodeficiency virus (SIV)-specific CD8+ T cells and there was a higher expression in the lymph nodes and mucosal tissue [61–63]. Blocking PD1 *in vitro* increased the proliferation of SIV-specific CD8+ and CD4+ T cells [61]. More relevant to a therapeutic regime, vaccination with a replication-defective DNA/MVA vaccine expressing SIV resulted in SIV-specific CD8+ T cells with low PD1 expression and a memory phenotype [61]. Vaccination with SIV plasmid constructs together with IL12 also enhanced SIV-specific CD8 effector memory T-cell responses with low PD1 expression [64]. Two studies have tested anti-human PD1 antibodies in SIV-infected macaques [65,66] and showed an expansion of SIV-specific T cells in blood and mucosal tissue. In addition, Velu *et al.* showed an expansion in memory B cells and anti-SIV antibodies [66]. Interestingly, PD1 blockade did not expand specific T cells that were against escape mutants of SIV. This fact may be important when moving forward clinically with PD1 blockade in the treatment of HIV infection, and combination therapy with anti-retroviral agents may be necessary. In a prophylactic model using SIV-gag adenovirus vector vaccine, PD1 blockade increased the percentage of T cells against a Gag epitope [65]. Interestingly, CTLA4 blockade in SIV infection led to an increase in CD4+ T cells in one study and CD4+ and CD8+ SIV-specific T cells in another study but both showed no benefit in viral load [67,68]. This

was similar to the results seen in the murine LCMV model, indicating CTLA4 blockade in chronic viral diseases may not be as effective as PD1 blockade.

Similar to HIV infection, PD1 is expressed on HCV-specific T cells in the periphery, and blockade of PD1 leads to increased expansion and cytokine production by HCV-specific T cells (reviewed in [69]). Some groups have shown that levels of PD1 expression on HCV-specific T cells seem to be predictive of progression to chronic HCV infection, although other groups do not [70–72]. PD-L1 also has been shown to be upregulated on monocytes in chronic HCV infection, and hepatitis virus core protein upregulates both PD1 and PD-L1 on T cells of healthy donors, signifying the role of the virus in viral persistence and PD1 expression [73,74]. Although PD1 expression on HCV CD8+ T cells decreased on treatment with IFN-α or spontaneous remission, PD-L1 expression on DC was increased [75]. The authors suggest that synergizing PD1 blockade with IFN-α therapy may be important in regaining antiviral function. It is noteworthy that in a chimpanzee model of HCV infection, PD1 expression was low or negative on memory T cells of chimpanzees that had resolved their disease; however, on reinfection PD1 was re-expressed on functional memory T cells [76]. In this situation, PD1 blockade would have been detrimental to the clearance of the virus, highlighting the importance of investigating the role of PD1 on different subsets of T cells. Data thus far indicates that intrahepatic anti-HCV T cells were more resistant to PD1 blockade although the peripheral anti-HCV T cells were relieved of their exhaustion by anti-PD1 [77]. Blockade of PD1 and CTLA4 relieved the exhausted phenotype of intrahepatic anti-HCV CD8 T cells, indicating a role for both pathways in the "exhausted" phenotype of HCV-specific T cells [78]. Blockade of PD-L1:PD1 interactions would be a viable course of action in the treatment of persistent viral infections. However, blocking of other pathways together with PD1 might be more advantageous as blocking both lymphocyte-activating gene (LAG) and PD1 or T-cell Ig- and mucin-domain-containing molecule-3 (Tim-3) increased the function of exhausted LMCV-specific T cells [79,80]. Interestingly, BTLA was downregulated on exhausted

LMCV-specific T cells, indicating that this pathway may play no role in the "exhausted" T-cell phenotype. A phase I dose-escalating clinical trial with anti-PD1 (MDX-1106) as a monotherapy for patients with HCV infection is on its way (clinicaltrials.gov) and the results will give insight into the significance of blocking PD1 in persistent viral infections.

Blocking positive co-stimulation signals in autoimmunity

The incidence of autoimmune diseases is 2–3% of the general population and the frequency is on the rise [81]. Blockade of co-stimulatory signals has become an appropriate therapeutic choice by selectively inhibiting autoreactive T-cell responses, and offers the potential of inducing tolerance to specific autoimmune antigens. These therapeutic agents come in the shape of monoclonal antibodies, polyclonal antibodies, Fab fragments, and recombinant proteins. Drugs such as abatacept (CTLA4Ig) are now widely used as rheumatoid arthritis (RA) therapy for patients with an insufficient response to traditional therapy.

The key role for CD28 in mediating activation of naïve T cells has been heavily documented in the literature, as previously mentioned. Some of the early studies in animals indicated that blocking the CD28 pathway, through a fusion protein consisting of the extracellular domain of CTLA4 linked to the Fc portion of IgG (CTLA4Ig), in the presence of antigen rendered T cells anergic. Moreover, in the mouse model of RA (collagen-induced arthritis, CIA), CTLA4Ig treatment inhibited the production of anti-collagen IgG1 and IgG2, and the proliferation of T cells in the lymph nodes when administered prophylactically [82]. In other mouse models of autoimmune disease, CTLA4Ig has shown different mechanisms of action. For instance, in a lupus model of disease, CTLA4Ig suppressed the development of ds-DNA and prevented the shift from naïve T cell to memory/effector T cells [83]. In contrast, treatment of type I diabetes (the NOD model in mice) with CTLA4Ig resulted in an exacerbation of disease [84], possibly by reducing regulatory T cells.

In EAE the blockade of the CTLA4-CD28 pathway led to suppression of the initial phase of the disease but not of the relapse [85]. However, data on EAE is still controversial and while it is clear that blocking of the CD28:CD80 pathway leads to an improvement of disease, in some treatment contexts blockade of CD86 may lead to exacerbation of disease. These studies point to the essential role of CD28 in the maintenance of homeostasis of T-cell subsets in different models of autoimmunity.

CTLA4Ig: the good one

In 2006, abatacept became the first co-stimulatory moiety approved by the Food and Drug Administration for the treatment of severe RA. In 2007, the European Medicines Agency followed suit. It is a soluble recombinant protein, comprising the extracellular domain of CTLA4 linked to IgG1. One of the most important features of abatacept is that modifications in the hinge region of the Fc domain (CH3 CH2) impede the binding to CD16 and CD32, and to a lesser extent, CD64 [86]. Abatacept selectively inhibits the CD80/CD86:CD28 pathway of T cell co-stimulation. Immune responses are inhibited by CTLA4Ig by downregulating naive and memory T-cell responses, cytokine production, and humoral immunity. It had previously been used in psoriasis patients, and trials in Crohn's disease, ulcerative colitis, diabetes, and lupus nephritis are currently ongoing in the US (Table 25.2).

In RA, CTLA4Ig has proven to be effective for up to 5 years in follow-on clinical trials and has been shown to directly bind osteoclast precursor cells and inhibit monocyte differentiation into osteoclasts (reviewed in [87]). These findings may explain the anti-erosive effect of abatacept on bones. The CTLA4Ig therapy for RA has now became a safe and effective treatment for patients failing anti-TNF therapy. However, the long-term consequences of abatacept (opportunistic infections, increased number of malignancies) have not yet been evaluated. The use of abatacept in other autoimmune diseases has not been so promising. As previously mentioned, ongoing clinical trials include those for IBD, lupus nephritis, and diabetes. Despite a good start in an open-label phase I clinical trial in multiple sclerosis patients, a larger trial in relapsing-remitting MS in a randomized, double-blind, placebo-controlled phase II study had to be terminated because of differences in the baseline of the study [88,89]. Trials for systemic lupus erythematosus have been completed but the drug has not delivered the expected results, possibly because abacetept does not block co-stimulation in all T-cell subsets [90]. Interestingly, the first clinical study to evaluate the efficacy of abatacept was done in psoriatic patients with promising results; nevertheless, a larger and more comprehensive trial is now under way [91].

Anti-CD28: the bad one

While CTLA4Ig therapy has opened a myriad of co-stimulatory blockade therapy opportunities, other antibodies have not proven so successful and in fact have been life threatening. TGN1412 is a recombinant humanized superagonist anti-CD28 antibody and can stimulate T cells independently of ligation of the T-cell receptor. It appears to selectively act on regulatory T cells [92–95]. This results in a polyclonal T-cell expansion, activation, and IL2 production so that in diseases such as RA regulatory T cells can be expanded. In preclinical trial models, CD28 stimulation with TGN1412 activated Th2-type cells and regulatory T cells without any proinflammatory effects [96]. In 2006, this superagonistic antibody was tested in a phase I clinical trial. Six of the volunteers were given a single i.v. dose of anti-CD28 antibody and two were given placebo. Those volunteers receiving TGN1412 soon started to develop a systemic inflammatory response featuring an induction of proinflammatory cytokines, headache, nausea, myalgias, diarrhea, erythema, vasodilation, and hypotension. Unexpectedly, 24 hours after infusion there was a depletion of lymphocytes and monocytes [96]. The response to TNG1412 involved the increase of the TNF-α, IFN-γ, and IL6 cytokines, leading to multi-organ failure in the absence of infection or endotoxin contamination. Cytokine-storm-induced lymphopenia has been associated with other monoclonal antibodies such as OKT3, CAMPATH, and anti-CD20 [97–99]. However, it is unclear why the anti-CD28 monoclonal antibody activated pathogenic effector cells. The therapeutic targeting of the CD28 co-stimulatory molecule is challenging in principle due to the multiple and sometimes opposing biological roles of the receptor [100].

Conclusion

The blocking of negative and positive co-stimulatory pathways has great promise for use clinically for anti-tumor, antiviral therapy, and autoimmune diseases. However, there is still much research needed into the understanding of how co-stimulatory pathways are coordinated, and there is a need to find new markers for successful manipulation of co-stimulatory molecules. The discovery of new pathways within the CD28 superfamily and other co-stimulatory superfamilies and the interplay and redundancy of the pathways will be an area of active research. A detailed knowledge of co-stimulatory pathways will open new avenues for the use of co-stimulatory moieties in vaccine development.

References

1 Watts TH. Staying alive: T cell costimulation, CD28, and Bcl-xL. *J Immunol* 2010;**185**(7):3785–7.

2 Thompson CB, Allison JP. The emerging role of CTLA-4 as an immune attenuator. *Immunity* 1997; **7**(4):445–50.

3 Rudd CE, Taylor A, Schneider H. CD28 and CTLA-4 coreceptor expression and signal transduction. *Immunol Rev* 2009;**229**(1):12–26.

4 Wing K, Onishi Y, Prieto-Martin P, *et al.* CTLA-4 control over Foxp3+ regulatory T cell function. *Science* 2008;**322**(5899):271–5.

5 Francisco LM, Sage PT, Sharpe AH. The PD-1 pathway in tolerance and autoimmunity. *Immunol Rev* 2010;**236**:219–42.

6 Parry RV, Chemnitz JM, Frauwirth KA, *et al.* CTLA-4 and PD-1 receptors inhibit T-cell activation by distinct mechanisms. *Mol Cell Biol* 2005;**25**(21): 9543–53.

7 Dong H, Chen L. B7-H1 pathway and its role in the evasion of tumor immunity. *J Mol Med* 2003; **81**(5):281–7.

8 Butte MJ, Keir ME, Phamduy TB, Sharpe AH, Freeman GJ. Programmed death-1 ligand 1 interacts

specifically with the B7-1 costimulatory molecule to inhibit T cell responses. *Immunity* 2007;**27**(1): 111–22.

9 Murphy TL, Murphy KM. Slow down and survive: enigmatic immunoregulation by BTLA and HVEM. *Annu Rev Immunol* 2010;**28**:389–411.

10 Wang Y, Subudhi SK, Anders RA, *et al.* The role of herpesvirus entry mediator as a negative regulator of T cell-mediated responses. *J Clin Invest* 2005; **115**(3):711–17.

11 Latchman Y, Wood CR, Chernova T, *et al.* PD-L2 is a second ligand for PD-1 and inhibits T cell activation. *Nat Immunol* 2001;**2**(3):261–8.

12 Leach DR, Krummel MF, Allison JP. Enhancement of antitumor immunity by CTLA-4 blockade. *Science* 1996;**271**(5256):1734–6.

13 Kwon ED, Hurwitz AA, Foster BA, *et al.* Manipulation of T cell costimulatory and inhibitory signals for immunotherapy of prostate cancer. *Proc Natl Acad Sci U S A* 1997;**94**(15):8099–103.

14 Kwon ED, Foster BA, Hurwitz AA, *et al.* Elimination of residual metastatic prostate cancer after surgery and adjunctive cytotoxic T lymphocyte-associated antigen 4 (CTLA-4) blockade immunotherapy. *Proc Natl Acad Sci U S A* 1999;**96**(26):15074–9.

15 Weber J. Immune checkpoint proteins: a new therapeutic paradigm for cancer – preclinical background: CTLA-4 and PD-1 blockade. *Semin Oncol* 2010;**37**(5):430–39.

16 van Elsas A, Hurwitz AA, Allison JP. Combination immunotherapy of B16 melanoma using anti-cytotoxic T lymphocyte-associated antigen 4 (CTLA-4) and granulocyte/macrophage colony-stimulating factor (GM-CSF)-producing vaccines induces rejection of subcutaneous and metastatic tumors accompanied by autoimmune depigmentation. *J Exp Med* 1999;**190**(3):355–66.

17 Hurwitz AA, Foster BA, Kwon ED, *et al.* Combination immunotherapy of primary prostate cancer in a transgenic mouse model using CTLA-4 blockade. *Cancer Res* 2000;**60**(9):2444–8.

18 van Elsas A, Sutmuller RP, Hurwitz AA, *et al.* Elucidating the autoimmune and antitumor effector mechanisms of a treatment based on cytotoxic T lymphocyte antigen-4 blockade in combination with a B16 melanoma vaccine: comparison of prophylaxis and therapy. *J Exp Med* 2001;**194**(4): 481–9.

19 Hodi FS, Mihm MC, Soiffer RJ, *et al.* Biologic activity of cytotoxic T lymphocyte-associated antigen 4 antibody blockade in previously vaccinated metastatic melanoma and ovarian carcinoma patients. *Proc Natl Acad Sci U S A* 2003;**100**(8):4712–17.

20 Phan GQ, Yang JC, Sherry RM, *et al.* Cancer regression and autoimmunity induced by cytotoxic T lymphocyte-associated antigen 4 blockade in patients with metastatic melanoma. *Proc Natl Acad Sci U S A* 2003;**100**(14):8372–7.

21 Maker AV, Phan GQ, Attia P, *et al.* Tumor regression and autoimmunity in patients treated with cytotoxic T lymphocyte-associated antigen 4 blockade and interleukin 2: a phase I/II study. *Ann Surg Oncol* 2005;**12**(12):1005–16.

22 O'Day SJ, Hamid O, Urba WJ. Targeting cytotoxic T-lymphocyte antigen-4 (CTLA-4): a novel strategy for the treatment of melanoma and other malignancies. *Cancer* 2007;**110**(12):2614–27.

23 Downey SG, Klapper JA, Smith FO, *et al.* Prognostic factors related to clinical response in patients with metastatic melanoma treated by CTL-associated antigen-4 blockade. *Clin Cancer Res* 2007;**13**(22 Pt 1): 6681–8.

24 Weber JS, O'Day S, Urba W, *et al.* Phase I/II study of ipilimumab for patients with metastatic melanoma. *J Clin Oncol* 2008;**26**(36):5950–56.

25 Weber J, Thompson JA, Hamid O, *et al.* A randomized, double-blind, placebo-controlled, phase II study comparing the tolerability and efficacy of ipilimumab administered with or without prophylactic budesonide in patients with unresectable stage III or IV melanoma. *Clin Cancer Res* 2009;**15**(17): 5591–8.

26 Hersh EM, O'Day SJ, Powderly J, *et al.* A phase II multicenter study of ipilimumab with or without dacarbazine in chemotherapy-naive patients with advanced melanoma. *Invest New Drugs* 2011; **29**(3):489–98.

27 Theoret MR, Arlen PM, Pazdur M, *et al.* Phase I trial of an enhanced prostate-specific antigen-based vaccine and anti-CTLA-4 antibody in patients with metastatic androgen-independent prostate cancer. *Clin Genitourin Cancer* 2007;**5**(5):347–50.

28 Small EJ, Tchekmedyian NS, Rini BI, *et al.* A pilot trial of CTLA-4 blockade with human anti-CTLA-4 in patients with hormone-refractory prostate cancer. *Clin Cancer Res* 2007;**13**(6):1810–15.

29 O'Mahony D, Morris JC, Quinn C, *et al.* A pilot study of CTLA-4 blockade after cancer vaccine failure in patients with advanced malignancy. *Clin Cancer Res* 2007;**13**(3):958–64.

30 Yang JC, Hughes M, Kammula U, *et al.* Ipilimumab (anti-CTLA4 antibody) causes regression of

metastatic renal cell cancer associated with enteritis and hypophysitis. *J Immunother* 2007;**30**(8):825–30.

31 Fong L, Kwek SS, O'Brien S, *et al.* Potentiating endogenous antitumor immunity to prostate cancer through combination immunotherapy with CTLA4 blockade and GM-CSF. *Cancer Res* 2009;**69**(2): 609–15.

32 Bashey A, Medina B, Corringham S, *et al.* CTLA4 blockade with ipilimumab to treat relapse of malignancy after allogeneic hematopoietic cell transplantation. *Blood* 2009;**113**(7):1581–8.

33 Ribas A, Camacho LH, Lopez-Berestein G, *et al.* Antitumor activity in melanoma and anti-self responses in a phase I trial with the anti-cytotoxic T lymphocyte-associated antigen 4 monoclonal antibody CP-675,206. *J Clin Oncol* 2005;**23**(35):8968–77.

34 Ribas A, Hanson DC, Noe DA, *et al.* Tremelimumab (CP-675,206), a cytotoxic T lymphocyte associated antigen 4 blocking monoclonal antibody in clinical development for patients with cancer. *Oncologist* 2007;**12**(7):873–83.

35 Camacho LH, Antonia S, Sosman J, *et al.* Phase I/II trial of tremelimumab in patients with metastatic melanoma. *J Clin Oncol* 2009;**27**(7):1075–81.

36 Ribas A, Hauschild A, Kefford R, *et al.* Phase III, open-label, randomized, comparative study of tremelimumab (CP-675,206) and chemotherapy (temozolomide [TMZ] or dacarbazine [DTIC]) in patients with advanced melanoma. *J Clin Oncol* 2008; **26**(15S):LBA9011.

37 Hoos A, Eggermont AM, Janetzki S, *et al.* Improved endpoints for cancer immunotherapy trials. *J Natl Cancer Inst* 2010;**102**(18):1388–97.

38 Comin-Anduix B, Lee Y, Jalil J, *et al.* Detailed analysis of immunologic effects of the cytotoxic T lymphocyte-associated antigen 4-blocking monoclonal antibody tremelimumab in peripheral blood of patients with melanoma. *J Transl Med* 2008;**6**:22.

39 Hodi FS, Butler M, Oble DA, *et al.* Immunologic and clinical effects of antibody blockade of cytotoxic T lymphocyte-associated antigen 4 in previously vaccinated cancer patients. *Proc Natl Acad Sci U S A* 2008; **105**(8):3005–10.

40 Ribas A, Comin-Anduix B, Economou JS, *et al.* Intratumoral immune cell infiltrates, FoxP3, and indoleamine 2,3-dioxygenase in patients with melanoma undergoing CTLA4 blockade. *Clin Cancer Res* 2009;**15**(1):390–99.

41 Yuan J, Gnjatic S, Li H, *et al.* CTLA-4 blockade enhances polyfunctional NY-ESO-1 specific T cell responses in metastatic melanoma patients with clin-

ical benefit. *Proc Natl Acad Sci U S A* 2008;**105**(51): 20410–15.

42 Liakou CI, Kamat A, Tang DN, *et al.* CTLA-4 blockade increases IFNgamma-producing CD4$^+$ICOShi cells to shift the ratio of effector to regulatory T cells in cancer patients. *Proc Natl Acad Sci U S A* 2008; **105**(39):14987–92.

43 Chen H, Liakou CI, Kamat A, *et al.* Anti-CTLA-4 therapy results in higher CD4$^+$ICOShi T cell frequency and IFN-gamma levels in both nonmalignant and malignant prostate tissues. *Proc Natl Acad Sci U S A* 2009;**106**(8):2729–34.

44 Peggs KS, Quezada SA, Chambers CA, Korman AJ, Allison JP. Blockade of CTLA-4 on both effector and regulatory T cell compartments contributes to the antitumor activity of anti-CTLA-4 antibodies. *J Exp Med* 2009;**206**(8):1717–25.

45 von Euw E, Chodon T, Attar N, *et al.* CTLA4 blockade increases Th17 cells in patients with metastatic melanoma. *J Transl Med* 2009;**7**(1):35.

46 Wang L, Pino-Lagos K, de Vries VC, *et al.* Programmed death 1 ligand signaling regulates the generation of adaptive Foxp3$^+$CD4$^+$ regulatory T cells. *Proc Natl Acad Sci U S A* 2008;**105**(27): 9331–6.

47 Iwai Y, Ishida M, Tanaka Y, *et al.* Involvement of PD-L1 on tumor cells in the escape from host immune system and tumor immunotherapy by PD-L1 blockade. *Proc Natl Acad Sci U S A* 2002;**99**:12293–7.

48 Brown JA, Dorfman DM, Ma F, *et al.* Blockade of PD-1 ligands on dendritic cells enhances T cell activation and cytokine production. *J Immunol* 2003;**170**:1257–66.

49 Wolchok JD, Yang AS, Weber JS. Immune regulatory antibodies: are they the next advance? *Cancer J* 2010;**16**(4):311–17.

50 Berger R, Rotem-Yehudar R, Slama G, *et al.* Phase I safety and pharmacokinetic study of CT-011, a humanized antibody interacting with PD-1, in patients with advanced hematologic malignancies. *Clin Cancer Res* 2008;**14**(10):3044–51.

51 Brahmer JR, Drake CG, Wollner I, *et al.* Phase I study of single-agent anti-programmed death-1 (MDX-1106) in refractory solid tumors: safety, clinical activity, pharmacodynamics, and immunologic correlates. *J Clin Oncol* 2010;**28**(19):3167–75.

52 Curran MA, Montalvo W, Yagita H, Allison JP. PD-1 and CTLA-4 combination blockade expands infiltrating T cells and reduces regulatory T and myeloid cells within B16 melanoma tumors. *Proc Natl Acad Sci U S A* 2010;**107**(9):4275–80.

53 Derre L, Rivals JP, Jandus C, *et al.* BTLA mediates inhibition of human tumor-specific CD8$^+$ T cells that can be partially reversed by vaccination. *J Clin Invest* 2010;**120**(1):157–67.

54 Moskophidis D, Lechner F, Pircher H, Zinkernagel RM. Virus persistence in acutely infected immuno-competent mice by exhaustion of antiviral cytotoxic effector T cells. *Nature* 1993;**362**(6422):758–61.

55 Barber DL, Wherry EJ, Masopust D, *et al.* Restoring function in exhausted CD8 T cells during chronic viral infection. *Nature* 2006;**439**(7077):682–7.

56 Wherry EJ, Ha SJ, Kaech SM, *et al.* Molecular signature of CD8$^+$ T cell exhaustion during chronic viral infection. *Immunity* 2007;**27**(4):670–84.

57 Kaufmann DE, Walker BD. PD-1 and CTLA-4 inhibitory cosignaling pathways in HIV infection and the potential for therapeutic intervention. *J Immunol* 2009;**182**(10):5891–7.

58 Trabattoni D, Saresella M, Biasin M, *et al.* B7-H1 is up-regulated in HIV infection and is a novel surrogate marker of disease progression. *Blood* 2003;**101**(7):2514–20.

59 Rosignoli G, Cranage A, Burton C, *et al.* Expression of PD-L1, a marker of disease status, is not reduced by HAART in aviraemic patients. *AIDS* 2007;**21**(10):1379–81.

60 Meier A, Bagchi A, Sidhu HK, *et al.* Upregulation of PD-L1 on monocytes and dendritic cells by HIV-1 derived TLR ligands. *AIDS* 2008;**22**(5):655–8.

61 Velu V, Kannanganat S, Ibegbu C, *et al.* Elevated expression levels of inhibitory receptor programmed death 1 on simian immunodeficiency virus-specific CD8 T cells during chronic infection but not after vaccination. *J Virol* 2007;**81**(11):5819–28.

62 Petrovas C, Price DA, Mattapallil J, *et al.* SIV-specific CD8$^+$ T cells express high levels of PD1 and cytokines but have impaired proliferative capacity in acute and chronic SIVmac251 infection. *Blood* 2007;**110**(3):928–36.

63 Onlamoon N, Rogers K, Mayne AE, *et al.* Soluble PD-1 rescues the proliferative response of simian immunodeficiency virus-specific CD4 and CD8 T cells during chronic infection. *Immunology* 2008;**124**(2):277–93.

64 Halwani R, Boyer JD, Yassine-Diab B, *et al.* Therapeutic vaccination with simian immunodeficiency virus (SIV)-DNA + IL-12 or IL-15 induces distinct CD8 memory subsets in SIV-infected macaques. *J Immunol* 2008;**180**(12):7969–79.

65 Finnefrock AC, Tang A, Li F, *et al.* PD-1 blockade in rhesus macaques: impact on chronic infection and prophylactic vaccination. *J Immunol* 2009; **182**(2):980–87.

66 Velu V, Titanji K, Zhu B, *et al.* Enhancing SIV-specific immunity in vivo by PD-1 blockade. *Nature* 2009;**458**(7235):206–10.

67 Cecchinato V, Tryniszewska E, Ma ZM, *et al.* Immune activation driven by CTLA-4 blockade augments viral replication at mucosal sites in simian immunodeficiency virus infection. *J Immunol* 2008; **180**(8):5439–47.

68 Hryniewicz A, Boasso A, Edghill-Smith Y, *et al.* CTLA-4 blockade decreases TGF-beta, IDO, and viral RNA expression in tissues of SIVmac251-infected macaques. *Blood* 2006;**108**(12):3834–42.

69 Watanabe T, Bertoletti A, Tanoto TA. PD-1/PD-L1 pathway and T-cell exhaustion in chronic hepatitis virus infection. *J Viral Hepat* 2010;**17**(7):453–8.

70 Golden-Mason L, Klarquist J, Wahed AS, Rosen HR. Programmed death-1 expression is increased on immunocytes in chronic hepatitis C virus and predicts failure of response to antiviral therapy: race-dependent differences. *J Immunol* 2008;**180**(6): 3637–41.

71 Rutebemberwa A, Ray SC, Astemborski J, *et al.* High-programmed death-1 levels on hepatitis C virus-specific T cells during acute infection are associated with viral persistence and require preservation of cognate antigen during chronic infection. *J Immunol* 2008;**181**(12):8215–25.

72 Kasprowicz V, Schulze Zur Wiesch J, Kuntzen T, *et al.* High level of PD-1 expression on hepatitis C virus (HCV)-specific CD8$^+$ and CD4$^+$ T cells during acute HCV infection, irrespective of clinical outcome. *J Virol* 2008;**82**(6):3154–60.

73 Jeong HY, Lee YJ, Seo SK, *et al.* Blocking of monocyte-associated B7-H1 (CD274) enhances HCV-specific T cell immunity in chronic hepatitis C infection. *J Leukoc Biol* 2008;**83**(3):755–64.

74 Yao ZQ, King E, Prayther D, Yin D, Moorman J. T cell dysfunction by hepatitis C virus core protein involves PD-1/PDL-1 signaling. *Viral Immunol* 2007;**20**(2):276–87.

75 Urbani S, Amadei B, Tola D, *et al.* Restoration of HCV-specific T cell functions by PD-1/PD-L1 blockade in HCV infection: effect of viremia levels and antiviral treatment. *J Hepatol* 2008;**48**(4):548–58.

76 Bowen DG, Shoukry NH, Grakoui A, *et al.* Variable patterns of programmed death-1 expression on fully functional memory T cells after spontaneous resolution of hepatitis C virus infection. *J Virol* 2008;**82**(10):5109–14.

77 Nakamoto N, Kaplan DE, Coleclough J, *et al.* Functional restoration of HCV-specific CD8 T cells by PD-1 blockade is defined by PD-1 expression and compartmentalization. *Gastroenterology* 2008; **134**(7):1927–37, 1937 e1–2.

78 Nakamoto N, Cho H, Shaked A, *et al.* Synergistic reversal of intrahepatic HCV-specific CD8 T cell exhaustion by combined PD-1/CTLA-4 blockade. *PLoS Pathog* 2009;**5**(2):e1000313.

79 Blackburn SD, Shin H, Haining WN, *et al.* Coregulation of CD8$^+$ T cell exhaustion by multiple inhibitory receptors during chronic viral infection. *Nat Immunol* 2009;**10**(1):29–37.

80 Jin HT, Anderson AC, Tan WG, *et al.* Cooperation of Tim-3 and PD-1 in CD8 T-cell exhaustion during chronic viral infection. *Proc Natl Acad Sci U S A* 2010;**107**(33):14733–8.

81 Loftus EV, Jr. Clinical epidemiology of inflammatory bowel disease: incidence, prevalence, and environmental influences. *Gastroenterology* 2004;**126**(6):1504–17.

82 Webb LM, Feldmann M. Critical role of CD28/B7 costimulation in the development of human Th2 cytokine-producing cells. *Blood* 1995;**86**(9):3479–86.

83 Finck BK, Linsley PS, Wofsy D. Treatment of murine lupus with CTLA4Ig. *Science* 1994;**265**(5176):1225–7.

84 Salomon B, Lenschow DJ, Rhee L, *et al.* B7/CD28 costimulation is essential for the homeostasis of the CD4$^+$CD25$^+$ immunoregulatory T cells that control autoimmune diabetes. *Immunity* 2000;**12**(4):431–40.

85 Racke MK, Scott DE, Quigley L, *et al.* Distinct roles for B7-1 (CD-80) and B7-2 (CD-86) in the initiation of experimental allergic encephalomyelitis. *J Clin Invest* 1995;**96**(5):2195–203.

86 Davis PM, Nadler SG, Stetsko DK, Suchard SJ. Abatacept modulates human dendritic cell-stimulated T-cell proliferation and effector function independent of IDO induction. *Clin Immunol* 2008;**126**(1):38–47.

87 Solomon GE. T-cell agents in the treatment of rheumatoid arthritis. *Bull NYU Hosp Jt Dis* 2010;**68**(3):162–5.

88 Viglietta V, Bourcier K, Buckle GJ, *et al.* CTLA4Ig treatment in patients with multiple sclerosis: an open-label, phase 1 clinical trial. *Neurology* 2008;**71**(12):917–24.

89 Linsley PS, Nadler SG. The clinical utility of inhibiting CD28-mediated costimulation. *Immunol Rev* 2009;**229**(1):307–21.

90 Lipsky PE. The uncertain pathway to new therapeutics for SLE. *Nat Clin Pract Rheumatol* 2009;**5**(2):61.

91 Abrams JR, Lebwohl MG, Guzzo CA, *et al.* CTLA4Ig-mediated blockade of T-cell costimulation in patients with psoriasis vulgaris. *J Clin Invest* 1999;**103**(9):1243–52.

92 Beyersdorf N, Gaupp S, Balbach K, *et al.* Selective targeting of regulatory T cells with CD28 superagonists allows effective therapy of experimental autoimmune encephalomyelitis. *J Exp Med* 2005;**202**(3):445–55.

93 Beyersdorf N, Hanke T, Kerkau T, Hunig T. Superagonistic anti-CD28 antibodies: potent activators of regulatory T cells for the therapy of autoimmune diseases. *Ann Rheum Dis* 2005;**64**(Suppl 4):iv91–5.

94 Beyersdorf N, Balbach K, Hunig T, Kerkau T. Large-scale expansion of rat CD4$^+$ CD25$^+$ T(reg) cells in the absence of T-cell receptor stimulation. *Immunology* 2006;**119**(4):441–50.

95 Beyersdorf N, Hanke T, Kerkau T, Hunig T. CD28 superagonists put a break on autoimmunity by preferentially activating CD4$^+$CD25$^+$ regulatory T cells. *Autoimmun Rev* 2006;**5**(1):40–45.

96 Suntharalingam G, Perry MR, Ward S, *et al.* Cytokine storm in a phase 1 trial of the anti-CD28 monoclonal antibody TGN1412. *N Engl J Med* 2006;**355**(10):1018–28.

97 Gaston RS, Deierhoi MH, Patterson T, *et al.* OKT3 first-dose reaction: association with T cell subsets and cytokine release. *Kidney Int* 1991;**39**(1):141–8.

98 Wing MG, Moreau T, Greenwood J, *et al.* Mechanism of first-dose cytokine-release syndrome by CAMPATH 1-H: involvement of CD16 (FcgammaRIII) and CD11a/CD18 (LFA-1) on NK cells. *J Clin Invest* 1996;**98**(12):2819–26.

99 Winkler U, Jensen M, Manzke O, *et al.* Cytokine-release syndrome in patients with B-cell chronic lymphocytic leukemia and high lymphocyte counts after treatment with an anti-CD20 monoclonal antibody (rituximab, IDEC-C2B8). *Blood* 1999;**94**(7):2217–24.

100 Bluestone JA, St Clair EW, Turka LA. CTLA4Ig: bridging the basic immunology with clinical application. *Immunity* 2006;**24**(3):233–8.

CHAPTER 26

Toll Receptors in Relation to Adjuvant Effects

Dipshikha Chakravortty, Amit Lahiri, & Priyanka Das

Department of Microbiology and Cell Biology, Center for Infectious Disease Research and Biosafety Laboratories, Indian Institute of Science, Bangalore, India

One of the most remarkable features of the vertebrate immune system is its ability to discriminate between self and foreign antigens. The mechanism behind this discrimination became better understood after the discovery of the Toll-like receptors (TLRs). TLRs, a part of the innate immune mechanism (Chapter 2 gives a glimpse of innate immunity), are a family of evolutionarily conserved receptors capable of recognizing various pathogen-associated molecular patterns. Not only do these receptors serve as a first line of defense against invading organisms, but they also form the link between the innate and adaptive immune responses [1]. These dual functions played by TLRs undoubtedly make them a potential target that can be activated during vaccination. Hence, activating TLR signaling is one of the essential criteria that must be met during any effective vaccine design. Although the discovery of TLRs is a recent phenomenon, the use of this pathway is an age-old technique. Today we are quite convinced that the effectiveness of the BCG vaccine is due to the use of TLR signaling. TLRs can be activated by various bacterial ligands. If these ligands are used as an adjuvant with any vaccine, the resultant immune response will be highly effective.

This chapter first describes the detailed organization of the TLRs, their ligands, and the process by which TLR signaling leads to an enhanced immune response, then it examines how TLR agonists have

been used as adjuvants in various experimental and clinical vaccines, and the mechanism behind these adjuvant functions. The chapter concludes with a focus on open questions on how the better use of TLR adjuvants will lead to the generation of more efficient vaccines.

Toll-like receptors

In Drosophila a membrane protein involved in the antifungal response was termed Toll. Subsequently, a further eight similar Toll family proteins were identified that are involved in antifungal immunity in Drosophila. In the mid-1990s, a homolog of Drosophila Toll was identified in humans. The first implication of the human Toll in immune response came with the discovery of Toll-like receptor 4. To date, 10 TLRs in the human gene database have been identified, which are mainly transmembrane proteins with an extracellular domain having leucine-rich repeats (LRR) and a cytosolic domain called the Toll/IL1 receptor (TIR) domain [2]. The ligands for these receptors are highly conserved microbial molecules like lipopolysaccharides (recognized by TLR4), lipopeptides (recognized by TLR2 in combination with TLR1 or TLR6), flagellin (by TLR5), single- or double-stranded RNA (by TLR7 with TLR8 and by TLR3, respectively), and CpG motif containing DNA (recognized

Vaccinology: Principles and Practice, First Edition. Edited by W. John W. Morrow, Nadeem A. Sheikh, Clint S. Schmidt and D. Huw Davies.
© 2012 Blackwell Publishing Ltd. Published 2012 by Blackwell Publishing Ltd.

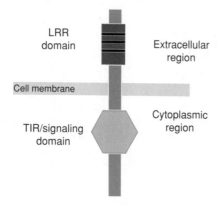

Figure 26.1 General structure of the TLRs.

by TLR9) [2]. Hence, the TLRs serve as pattern recognition receptors (PRR) capable of recognizing pathogen-associated molecular patterns (PAMPs). The general structure of the TLRs is shown in Figure 26.1 and the cognate ligands are listed in Table 26.1.

TLRs are mainly expressed in antigen-presenting cells (APC) such as macrophages and dendritic cells (DCs). However, in DCs the distribution of the TLRs depends on the origin of the dendritic cells. The expression pattern of the TLRs in the APCs is highly interesting. TLR1, −2, −4, −5, and −6 are ex-

Table 26.1 Known TLRs and their cognate ligands.

TLR	Adjuvants	Localization
TLR1 + TLR2	Pam3Cys MALP2	Cell membrane
TLR2 + TLR6	Pam2Cys	Cell membrane
TLR3	Poly I:C	Endosome
TLR4	MPL A E6020 LPS analogs Aminoalkyl glucosaminide phosphates	Cell membrane
TLR5	Flagellin	Cell membrane
TLR7/8	Resiquimod Imiquimod 3M-019 R-848	Endosome
TLR9	CpG DNA	Endoplasmic reticulum

pressed on the cell membrane. On the other hand TLR3, −7, and −9 are intracellular receptors expressed within the endosome.

TLR signaling

TLR activation by their ligands brings about the engagement of several downstream intermediates such as myeloid differentiation factor 88 (MyD88), Toll interleukin 1 receptor associated protein (TIRAP), Toll receptor associated activator of interferon (TRIF), Toll receptor associated molecule (TRAM), IL1 receptor associated kinases (IRAK), and tumor necrosis factor receptor associated factor 6 (TARF6) [3]. Then activated TRAF6 in turn activates nuclear factor-kB (NF-kB). This allows NF-kB to the nucleus and induces the expression of its target genes. The intracellular TLRs activate the IFN-γ promoter by activation of interferon response factor 3 (IRF3) by an MyD88 independent pathway. TLR4 can activate both NF-kB and IRF3. TLR3 in its turn activates IRF3 and IFN-β promoter whereas TLR7 and TLR9 activate interferon response factor 7 (IRF7) and IFN-α promoter [4]. The detailed signaling is illustrated in Figure 26.2.

TLRs in immunity

Before going into the case studies where TLR ligands have been used as adjuvants, a brief discussion of the TLR pathway in immunity is given below. The cumulative function is illustrated in Figure 26.3.

Phagocytosis
Phagocytosis of the foreign antigen is the first step for antigen presentation. The intersection of phagosome and major histocompatibility complex (MHC) class II containing cargo determines the course and character of antigen presentation. When an apoptotic body is phagocytosed TLR signaling does not take place. However, when the pathogens are phagocytosed, the subsequent TLR signaling leads to altered phagosome maturation [5], which ultimately leads to efficient and potent antigen

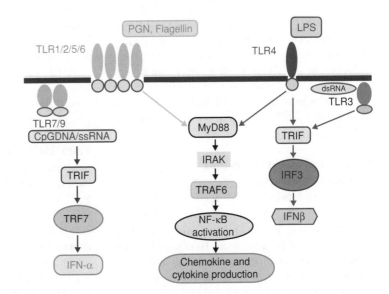

Figure 26.2 TLR signaling.

presentation [6]. It has been shown convincingly that the efficiency of antigen presentation from the phagocytosed cargo is dependent on the presence of the TLR ligands in the phagosome [7]. Thus, it can easily be speculated that when TLR ligands are used as adjuvant in any vaccine, the efficiency of the antigen presentation will be better as the microbial antigens get selected in a Toll-dependent manner for phagocytosis.

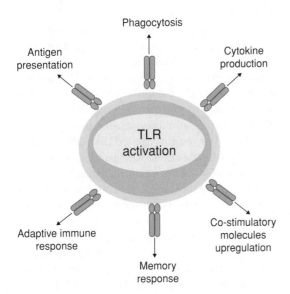

Figure 26.3 Benefits of using TLR agonists as adjuvant.

Cytokine production

As mentioned earlier, when a cognate ligand is recognized by any TLR, the downstream signaling leads to the transcriptional activation of various genes. For example, when NF-kB is activated, it translocates to the nucleus and induces the transcription of its target genes. Alternatively, IRF3 induction leads to production of IFN-β, and IRF7 induction leads to IFN-α production. The downstream genes of NF-kB are the various proinflammatory cytokines such as IL6, IL12, and TNF-α [8]. One study has found that TLR3, −7, and −9 ligand treatment leads to production of various cytokines and chemokines [9]. Thus, the engagement of microbial components as adjuvant should produce protective cytokine response after immunization. The question arises as to how this enhanced cytokine production can increase the effectiveness of the vaccine. This Th1-type response ultimately leads to adaptive immune response, which will be discussed below.

MHC and co-stimulatory molecule upregulation

There are various reports suggesting the critical role of TLR in linking innate and adaptive immunity [10]. This property can very well be utilized during vaccination by utilizing TLR ligands as adjuvant. The main mechanism by which TLR signaling activates adaptive immunity is by upregulating the expression of MHC and co-stimulatory molecules in the APCs. Co-stimulatory molecules like CD40, CD70, CD80, and CD86 are upregulated upon TLR activation [1]. Co-stimulatory molecule administration during vaccination is very effective (see Chapter 25).

Antigen presentation and memory response

For a potent vaccine, one of the essential criteria is that the antigen used for vaccination should be presented to the T cells and subsequent memory response should be generated. How can TLR ligands help in better antigen presentation and memory response? TLR ligands are involved in cross-presentation and cross-priming. Cross-presentation is the process by which exogenous antigen is presented by MHC I to CD8$^+$ T cells and the T-cell response generated is termed cross-priming [11]. TLR ligands have been proved to enhance the cross-presentation in several reports. In the B cell TLR9 ligand and in virus infected cells TLR3 ligand treatment increases the cross-presentation efficiency [12,13]. In an interesting study, the efficiency of all the TLR ligands for cross-presentation has been explored. It was suggested that a subset of TLR ligands, namely TLR3 and TLR9 ligands, induce cross-presentation in mature DCs [14].

Let us now consider the impact of TLR activation on the memory response in any experimental vaccine. Again, TLR3 and TLR9 ligand treatment have been shown to generate functional CD8$^+$ memory T cells. This process was further independent of the CD4$^+$ help, suggesting the critical role played by the Toll ligands [15]. Another interesting discovery in this field indicates that TLR ligands can increase the activated CD4$^+$ T-cell survival. It was observed that mouse CD4$^+$ cells express TLRs and thereby can increase the memory response [16].

TLR agonists as vaccine adjuvant

Keeping in mind the positive effects that TLR ligands can exert upon the response to a vaccine, as mentioned above, we now discuss how TLR ligands have been used successfully as adjuvants (Chapter 23 describes adjuvants and their function). The synthetic ligands for the TLRs that are used as adjuvants are listed in Table 26.1 and readers should familiarize themselves with these ligands before proceeding to the next section.

TLR1/2/4/6 agonists

The main function of these TLRs is to recognize bacterial cell-wall and cell-membrane components. For the Gram-positive bacteria the cell wall consists of a thick peptidoglycan (PGN) layer where different acylated forms of lipoproteins and lipoteichoic acids are embedded. TLR2 plays a very critical role in recognizing the peptidoglycan layer by pairing with distinct TLRs. Heterodimerization of TLR2 and TLR6 recognizes diacyl lipopeptides whereas TLR2 in combination with TLR1 recognizes bacterial triacyl lipopeptides [17]. To date the most characterized PAMP is lipopolysaccharide (LPS), a major component of the outer membrane of Gram-negative bacteria, composed of a lipid A moiety and a polysaccharide extension. TLR4 is involved in the recognition of LPS, and mice carrying a mutation in the TLR4 gene are hyporesponsive to LPS signaling [18]. Thus, if during vaccination TLR2 or TLR4 signaling needs to be induced, one should use either PGN or LPS as the adjuvant; this has been done by many groups. As LPS is a molecule that can cause septic shock, various analogs of LPS that can be less immunogenic are in use. A compound belonging to the family of synthetic lipid A mimetics (aminoalkyl glucosaminide phosphates [AGPs]) was evaluated in murine infectious disease to assess whether it can protect against pathogenic assault [19]. The result suggested that LPS mimetics can induce innate resistance against *Listeria monocytogenes* and influenza virus challenge. In the case of *Francisella tularensis* infection AGP-treated mice showed enhanced survival and were fully protected after rechallenge [20]. Another TLR4 synthetic ligand, E6020, also serves as a very potent adjuvant [21]. In a corollary finding, E6020 was shown to enhance vaccine efficacy in an experimental model of toxic-shock syndrome [22]. Bacterial lipoproteins such as outer surface lipoprotein A (OspA) have been used as adjuvant in Lyme disease vaccine. It was observed that the protection was antibody dependent [23]. In the case of *Mycobacterium bovis* cell wall cytoskeleton when used as adjuvant could induce effective immunity against tumors [24] in a TLR2-dependent way. The TLR2 agonist OspA has also proved to be an effective adjuvant in the case of *Borrellia burgdorferi* [25] and *Haemophilus influenzae* [26] type B vaccination.

TLR5 agonists

Flagellin, a component of the bacterial flagella, is one of the important PAMPs and is recognized by TLR5 [27]. In this regard, we will discuss two important findings wherein TLR5 signaling has been used to generate a better immune response after vaccine delivery. A recombinant protein conjugating flagellin and OVA (STF2.OVA) was compared for the adjuvant function with OVA emulsified in complete Freund's adjuvant. The results clearly indicated that fusing TLR5 agonist clearly increases antibody production and the results hint that flagellin is a better adjuvant than the conventional Freund's adjuvant [28]. The same group further made a recombinant protein comprising the flagellin fused to four tandem copies of the ectodomain of the conserved influenza matrix protein M2 (STF2.4xM2e). Similar to the previous finding, it was observed that engaging TLR5 signaling led to a better immune response when compared to vaccination when the influenza protein was delivered with alum as adjuvant [29]. *Salmonella enterica* serovar Typhimurium flagellin (FliC), a TLR5 agonist, has recently been used as an adjuvant in malaria vaccine. The results indicate that cytokine response and antibody production were enhanced with this adjuvant [30]. Additionally, TLR5 agonists are being tested by VaxInnate. The company's vaccines combine proteins of vaccine antigen (such as the influenza hemagglutinin) and bacterial flagellin. The method has been demonstrated by them to produce robust protective immune responses in animal models to several pathogens, including West Nile virus, Japanese encephalitis virus, and listeria, in addition to influenza.

TLR3/7/8/9 agonists

In addition to the cell-wall components, bacterial DNA and viral RNA can also function as PAMPs. Unmethylated CpG motifs in the bacterial DNA are recognized by TLR9 and viral RNA is recognized by TLR3 and TLR7 [31]. How can one use nucleic acids as adjuvants to induce these TLRs? The current use of stimulatory nucleic acids targeting TLRs is reviewed for applications ranging from vaccine adjuvants to anti-cancer, antiviral compounds. There has been an enormous number of trials for this purpose and the results are quite encouraging. Imiquimod and its related compound R848, which are synthetic TLR7 and/or TLR8 agonists, have been shown to be effective against *Leishmania* infection. The original FDA approval of imiquimod was on February 27, 1997. Imiquimod is approved to treat actinic keratosis, superficial basal cell carcinoma, and external genital warts. Adverse side effects have been reported, in some cases serious and systemic, resulting in the revision of warning labels. This drug is marketed by MEDA AB, Graceway Pharmaceuticals, and iNova Pharmaceuticals under the trade name Aldara and by Mochida as Beselna.

Further, the *Leishmania* antigen by itself was not protective against subsequent challenge infection unless it was administered with R848, clearly demonstrating the adjuvant activity of this agonist [32]. In the case of *Neisseria* outer membrane vaccine, various TLR agonists have been studied for their adjuvanting function, and TLR3, −7, and −9 ligands were found to produce an enhanced amount of bactericidal antibody [33]. The TLR3 ligand poly I:C also serves as an excellent adjuvant against cervical cancer [34]. Poly I:C (12)U, another analog, is less toxic but also less stable *in vivo* than poly I:C, and TLR3 is essential for its recognition. When this adjuvant was used it was able to induce an innate chemokine response and act as an adjuvant for virus-specific Th1 and humoral immune responses in nonhuman primates [35]. Ampligen is another synthetic analog of TLR3 ligand and has been proved to be safe in a human trial for cancer vaccines [36]. Interestingly, in the cases of HIV and influenza vaccines, TLR7/8 agonists improve the efficacy of the vaccines. In the case of HIV gag protein vaccination, TLR agonists enhance the CD8$^+$

T-cell response upon vaccination [37]. Further, it was also observed that poly I:C adjuvants used with attenuated recombinant H5N1 influenza virus vaccines could protect mice from lethal challenge [38].

The approach to immunotherapy has moved into the clinic based on the use of synthetic oligodeoxynucleotides (CpG ODN) as TLR9 agonists [39]. CpG ODN is used to treat infectious disease, cancer, and asthma. Let us consider the *Toxoplasma gondii* vaccine, where bradyzoite antigen is used as a vaccine candidate. When CpG ODN was used along with the vaccine there was enhanced protection against the disease and the survival of the mice increased [40]. In another study, CpG ODN and R-848 were used in combination with the hepatitis B surface antigen vaccine in mice. The vaccination resulted in increased cellular immune response as well as long-lasting immune memory [41]. In addition, for large tumors, CpG ODN served as an adjuvant in the DC vaccines, resulting in a transient control of tumor growth [42]. In a DNA vaccine against SIV, TLR9 ligand was used and it proved to be very effective [43]. When CpG was used as an adjuvant in the malaria vaccine, the memory B cell response was significantly increased [44]. Finally, in the case of respiratory syncytial virus immunization, TLR9 agonists were used and during rechallenge the disease severity was drastically reduced. Idera is conducting a phase I clinical trial of IMO-3100, a lead antagonist of TLR7 and TLR9 intended for application in autoimmune and inflammatory diseases. Its drug candidates include IMO-2125, a TLR9 agonist, which is in phase I clinical trial for hepatitis C virus infection.

Safety issues and open questions

Antibiotics are capable of controlling infectious disease but they bring the chance of multidrug-resistant organisms. Hence, the development of safe and efficient vaccines for cancer and various infectious diseases is still one of the major goals in global public health. The history of vaccination began with the use of attenuated and killed organisms to induce immunity. Slowly, the use of adjuvants gave rise to vaccines with enhanced mem-

ory response. TLR ligands when used as adjuvants increase the vaccine efficacy many-fold. Interestingly, in the case of chronic liver disease, treatment with TLR ligands has been shown to be very useful [45].

Future directions

However, much of the work described in this chapter has not been tested in proper model systems. It will be of interest to check whether these experimental discoveries can be reduced to practice in human vaccination for various diseases. One important point should be kept in mind in this regard. TLR ligands are potentially immunogenic and could prove to be toxic. Hence, critical choice of TLR ligands should be made. Studies to generate newer synthetic ligands for TLRs will be very useful. It will be of great interest to check whether using multiple TLRs can enhance the immune response in a better way than a single ligand. Thus, future work will determine the combinatorial use of TLR ligands that will prove to be much smarter adjuvants.

Acknowledgments

This work was supported by the grant Provision (2A) Tenth Plan (191/MCB) from the Director of Indian Institute of Science, Bangalore, India and Department of Biotechnology (DBT 197 and DBT 172), India.

References

1 Iwasaki A, Medzhitov R. Toll-like receptor control of the adaptive immune responses. *Nat Immunol* 2004;**5**(10):987–95.

2 Takeda K, Kaisho T, Akira S. Toll-like receptors. *Annu Rev Immunol* 2003;**21**: 335–76.

3 Akira S, Takeda K. Toll-like receptor signalling. *Nat Rev Immunol* 2004;**4**(7):499–511.

4 Seya T, Akazawa T, Tsujita T, Matsumoto M. Role of Toll-like receptors in adjuvant-augmented immune therapies. *Evid Based Complement Alternat Med* 2006;**3**(1):31–8; discussion 133–7.

5 Blander JM, Medzhitov R. Regulation of phagosome maturation by signals from toll-like receptors. *Science* 2004;**304**(5673):1014–18.

6 Blander JM. Coupling Toll-like receptor signaling with phagocytosis: potentiation of antigen presentation. *Trends Immunol* 2007;**28**(1):19–25.

7 Blander JM, Medzhitov R. Toll-dependent selection of microbial antigens for presentation by dendritic cells. *Nature* 2006;**440**(7085):808–12.

8 Lahiri A, Das P, Chakravortty D. Engagement of TLR signaling as adjuvant: towards smarter vaccine and beyond. *Vaccine* 2008;**26**(52):6777–83.

9 Matsushima H, Yamada N, Matsue H, Shimada S. TLR3-, TLR7-, and TLR9-mediated production of proinflammatory cytokines and chemokines from murine connective tissue type skin-derived mast cells but not from bone marrow-derived mast cells. *J Immunol* 2004;**173**(1):531–41.

10 van Duin D, Medzhitov R, Shaw AC. Triggering TLR signaling in vaccination. *Trends Immunol* 2006;**27**(1):49–55.

11 Groothuis TA, Neefjes J. The many roads to cross-presentation. *J Exp Med* 2005;**202**(10):1313–18.

12 Heit A, Huster KM, Schmitz F, *et al.* CpG-DNA aided cross-priming by cross-presenting B cells. *J Immunol* 2004;**172**(3):1501–7.

13 Schulz O, Diebold SS, Chen M, *et al.* Toll-like receptor 3 promotes cross-priming to virus-infected cells. *Nature* 2005;**433**(7028):887–92.

14 Datta SK, Redecke V, Prilliman KR, *et al.* A subset of Toll-like receptor ligands induces cross-presentation by bone marrow-derived dendritic cells. *J Immunol* 2003;**170**(8):4102–10.

15 Hervas-Stubbs S, Olivier A, Boisgerault F, Thieblemont N, Leclerc C. TLR3 ligand stimulates fully functional memory CD8$^+$ T cells in the absence of CD4$^+$ T-cell help. *Blood* 2007;**109**(12):5318–26.

16 Gelman AE, Zhang J, Choi Y, Turka LA. Toll-like receptor ligands directly promote activated CD4$^+$ T cell survival. *J Immunol* 2004;**172**(10):6065–73.

17 Takeda K, Takeuchi O, Akira S. Recognition of lipopeptides by Toll-like receptors. *J Endotoxin Res* 2002;**8**(6):459–63.

18 Poltorak A, He X, Smirnova I, *et al.* Defective LPS signaling in C3H/HeJ and C57BL/10ScCr mice: mutations in Tlr4 gene. *Science* 1998;**282**(5396):2085–8.

19 Cluff CW, Baldridge JR, Stover AG, *et al.* Synthetic toll-like receptor 4 agonists stimulate innate resistance to infectious challenge. *Infect Immun* 2005;**73**(5):3044–52.

20 Lembo A, Pelletier M, Iyer R, *et al.* Administration of a synthetic TLR4 agonist protects mice from pneumonic tularemia. *J Immunol* 2008;**180**(11):7574–81.

21 Ishizaka ST, Hawkins LD. E6020: a synthetic Toll-like receptor 4 agonist as a vaccine adjuvant. *Expert Rev Vaccines* 2007;**6**(5):773–84.

22 Morefield GL, Hawkins LD, Ishizaka ST, Kissner TL, Ulrich RG. Synthetic Toll-like receptor 4 agonist enhances vaccine efficacy in an experimental model of toxic shock syndrome. *Clin Vaccine Immunol* 2007;**14**(11):1499–504.

23 Alexopoulou L, Thomas V, Schnare M, *et al.* Hyporesponsiveness to vaccination with *Borrelia burgdorferi* OspA in humans and in TLR1- and TLR2-deficient mice. *Nat Med* 2002;**8**(8):878–84.

24 Murata M. Activation of Toll-like receptor 2 by a novel preparation of cell wall skeleton from *Mycobacterium bovis* BCG Tokyo (SMP-105) sufficiently enhances immune responses against tumors. *Cancer Sci* 2008;**99**(7):1435–40..

25 Yoder A, Wang X, Ma Y, *et al.* Tripalmitoyl-S-glyceryl-cysteine-dependent OspA vaccination of toll-like receptor 2-deficient mice results in effective protection from *Borrelia burgdorferi* challenge. *Infect Immun* 2003;**71**(7):3894–900.

26 Latz E, Franko J, Golenbock DT, Schreiber JR. *Haemophilus influenzae* type b-outer membrane protein complex glycoconjugate vaccine induces cytokine production by engaging human toll-like receptor 2 (TLR2) and requires the presence of TLR2 for optimal immunogenicity. *J Immunol* 2004;**172**(4):2431–8.

27 Hayashi F, Smith KD, Ozinsky A, *et al.* The innate immune response to bacterial flagellin is mediated by Toll-like receptor 5. *Nature* 2001;**410**(6832):1099–103.

28 Huleatt JW, Jacobs AR, Tang J, *et al.* Vaccination with recombinant fusion proteins incorporating Toll-like receptor ligands induces rapid cellular and humoral immunity. *Vaccine* 2007;**25**(4):763–75.

29 Huleatt JW, Nakaar V, Desai P, *et al.* Potent immunogenicity and efficacy of a universal influenza vaccine candidate comprising a recombinant fusion protein linking influenza M2e to the TLR5 ligand flagellin. *Vaccine* 2008;**26**(2):201–14.

30 Bargieri DY, Rosa DS, Braga CJ, *et al.* New malaria vaccine candidates based on the *Plasmodium vivax* merozoite surface protein-1 and the TLR-5 agonist *Salmonella* Typhimurium FliC flagellin. *Vaccine* 2008;**26**(48):6132–42.

31 Hemmi H, Takeuchi O, Kawai T, *et al.* A Toll-like receptor recognizes bacterial DNA. *Nature* 2000; **408**(6813):740–45.

32 Zhang WW, Matlashewski G. Immunization with a Toll-like receptor 7 and/or 8 agonist vaccine adjuvant increases protective immunity against *Leishmania major* in BALB/c mice. *Infect Immun* 2008;**76**(8):3777–83.

33 Fransen F, Boog CJ, van Putten JP, van der Ley P. Agonists of Toll-like receptors 3, 4, 7, and 9 are candidates for use as adjuvants in an outer membrane vaccine against *Neisseria meningitidis* serogroup B. *Infect Immun* 2007;**75**(12):5939–46.

34 Adams M, Navabi H, Jasani B, *et al.* Dendritic cell (DC) based therapy for cervical cancer: use of DC pulsed with tumour lysate and matured with a novel synthetic clinically non-toxic double stranded RNA analogue poly (I):poly (C(12)U) (Ampligen R). *Vaccine* 2003;**21**(7–8):787–90.

35 Stahl-Hennig C, Eisenblatter M, Jasny E, *et al.* Synthetic double-stranded RNAs are adjuvants for the induction of T helper 1 and humoral immune responses to human papillomavirus in rhesus macaques. *PLoS Pathog* 2009;**5**(4):e1000373.

36 Navabi H, Jasani B, Reece A, *et al.* A clinical grade poly I:C-analogue (Ampligen) promotes optimal DC maturation and Th1-type T cell responses of healthy donors and cancer patients in vitro. *Vaccine* 2009; **27**(1):107–15.

37 Wille-Reece U, Flynn BJ, Lore K, *et al.* HIV Gag protein conjugated to a Toll-like receptor 7/8 agonist improves the magnitude and quality of Th1 and CD8[+] T cell responses in nonhuman primates. *Proc Natl Acad Sci U S A* 2005;**102**(42):15190–94.

38 Asahi-Ozaki Y, Itamura S, Ichinohe T, *et al.* Intranasal administration of adjuvant-combined recombinant influenza virus HA vaccine protects mice from the lethal H5N1 virus infection. *Microbes Infect* 2006; **8**(12–13): 2706–14.

39 Krieg AM. Therapeutic potential of Toll-like receptor 9 activation. *Nat Rev Drug Discov* 2006;**5**(6): 471–84.

40 Zimmermann S, Dalpke A, Heeg K. CpG oligonucleotides as adjuvant in therapeutic vaccines against parasitic infections. *Int J Med Microbiol* 2008;**298**(1–2): 39–44.

41 Ma R, Du JL, Huang J, Wu CY. Additive effects of CpG ODN and R-848 as adjuvants on augmenting immune responses to HBsAg vaccination. *Biochem Biophys Res Commun* 2007;**361**(2):537–42.

42 Heckelsmiller K, Beck S, Rall K, *et al.* Combined dendritic cell- and CpG oligonucleotide-based immune therapy cures large murine tumors that resist chemotherapy. *Eur J Immunol* 2002;**32**(11): 3235–45.

43 Kwissa M, Amara RR, Robinson HL, *et al.* Adjuvanting a DNA vaccine with a TLR9 ligand plus Flt3 ligand results in enhanced cellular immunity against the simian immunodeficiency virus. *J Exp Med* 2007; **204**(11):2733–46.

44 Crompton PD, Mircetic M, Weiss G, *et al.* The TLR9 ligand CpG promotes the acquisition of *Plasmodium falciparum*-specific memory B cells in malaria-naive individuals. *J Immunol* 2009;**182**(5):3318–26.

45 Mencin A, Kluwe J, Schwabe RF. Toll-like receptors as targets in chronic liver diseases. *Gut* 2009; **58**(5):704–20.

PART 6

Regulatory Considerations

CHAPTER 27

Regulatory Issues (FDA and EMA)

Murrium Ahmad[1], Victoria Byers[2], & Peter Wilson[2]
[1]The John van Geest Cancer Research Centre, School of Science and Technology, Nottingham Trent University, Nottingham, UK
[2]NJM European Economic & Management Consultants Ltd, Gosforth, Newcastle Upon Tyne, UK

Vaccines: an overview

Immune interference has become a very important consideration with the ever-increasing complexity of vaccines (e.g., combined vaccines intended to confer protection against many of the common infectious diseases and the frequent need for the co-administration of multiple vaccines). The design and interpretation of studies intended to assess immune interference must be tailored to the antigens involved and should take into account any relevant experience about the possible effects of their combination and/or co-administration.

Special considerations are needed for the clinical development of vaccines when protective efficacy studies may not be feasible together with when there is no established immunologic correlate of protection. In some cases, it may not even be possible to generate sufficient amounts of data for new vaccines that are intended for use to prevent rare infections, which may carry considerable morbidity and mortality. Therefore in circumstances such as these, the data generated may require consideration on a case-by-case basis [1].

Vaccines designed for cancer, fight by stimulating the immune system and turning it against the cancer cells. Cancer vaccines are particularly challenging since the variety of scientific approaches used in their development is vast. The types of vaccines range from nonspecific immunostimulants to autologous tumor lysates vaccines [2].

The active immunotherapeutic strategies have the ability to elicit either nonspecific or specific anti-tumor reactions by stimulating the patient's immune system. The nonspecific immunostimulants aim to reverse immunosupression, which is induced by the patient's tumor. However, the specific cancer vaccines induce a tumor-specific immune response against the tumor or its antigenic components.

It has been shown that tumors can escape single-epitope vaccines if the tumor fails to express the target antigen. To overcome this, multi-epitope vaccines have been developed. In line with this approach, some vaccines have been developed using whole inactivated tumor cells that contain a spectrum of tumor-associated antigens in an ultravalent formulation [2].

It should be noted that cancer vaccines are being developed for both preventative and therapeutic use. Although the majority of cancer vaccine products are biotechnologically derived, some are not. Peptide vaccines may not be categorized as biologics as they are chemically synthesized and therefore can be regarded as small molecule drugs. This can have implications when it comes to regulatory issues.

The European Medicines Agency (EMA; formerly the European Agency for the Evaluation of Medicinal Products, EMEA) published a set of guidelines on clinical evaluation of vaccines [1]. This document covers the design of the clinical

Vaccinology: Principles and Practice, First Edition. Edited by W. John W. Morrow, Nadeem A. Sheikh, Clint S. Schmidt and D. Huw Davies.
© 2012 Blackwell Publishing Ltd. Published 2012 by Blackwell Publishing Ltd.

development program associated with a new vaccine that is intended for use in infectious diseases.

From the point of view of cancer and vaccines, GlaxoSmithKline (GSK) announced in October 2009 that the Food and Drug Administration (FDA) had finally approved the Cervarix® vaccine for the prevention of cervical pre-cancers and cervical cancer associated with human papillomavirus (HPV) types 16 and 18. The Cervarix® and Herceptin® case studies are discussed in more detail later.

DNA vaccines and monoclonal antibody vaccines

The two types of vaccines that this chapter will focus on are DNA vaccines and vaccines containing monoclonal antibodies.

DNA vaccines can be generated in a number of ways: they can use naked DNA, viral vectors, and/or bacterial immunizations [3,4]. The vectors encoding a specific tumor-associated antigen can enter a patient's cell, where it becomes the *in vivo* DNA template for the production of the specific protein antigen. Vaccination induces strong and long lasting immune responses against the expressed antigen, and the virus in the case of viral vector products, that involves both the humoral and cellular arms of the immune system [5,6].

The anti-idiotypic antibodies can potentially induce a human anti-anti-idiotypic response. These antibodies mimic the original antigen [7] and it is due to this mimicry that the anti-idiotype molecule can be used as a surrogate vaccine in place of natural tumor-associated antigens by stimulation of cellular and humoral immune responses. This strategy requires only small amounts of vaccine preparation and permits vaccination against nonprotein antigens that are difficult to clone [2].

As far as the regulatory issues are concerned, EU Directive 2004/27/EC [8] classifies cancer vaccines as "active substances for which the therapeutic indication is the treatment of cancer." The FDA regulation of cancer vaccines is not uniform and depends upon the nature of the individual vaccine.

It is known that a variety of approaches are used by companies to develop cancer vaccines and

this creates an enormous challenge for the regulatory agencies when discussing individual programs, and considering the required nonclinical studies. All regions (Europe, USA, and Japan) have now adopted a flexible case-by-case science-based approach to preclinical safety evaluation needed to support clinical development and marketing authorization. The recombinant DNA protein vaccines as well as the anti-idiotypic vaccines are specifically included in the International Conference on Harmonisation (ICH) 1997 guidelines, which have been approved by the EMA and the FDA, suggesting comparable expectations by both authorities.

Basically the regulatory environment for the preclinical development of cancer vaccines is not a very stringent one as no one guidance document or regulation exists that specifically deals with this product group.

However, the examples below describe how the Herceptin® drug was approved for licensing back in September 1998 for breast cancer and how the Cervarix® vaccine was also approved in 2009 for the prevention of cervical cancer. Moreover, this section of the chapter also discusses the more recently approved Provenge® vaccine, designed to treat patients with prostate cancer, as well as ipilimumab, which is used to treat patients with advanced melanoma.

Herceptin®

The breast cancer drug Herceptin® was originally licensed in September 1998 by the FDA, as a treatment for stage IV metastatic breast cancer, either in combination with paclitaxel or as a standalone treatment for women who had previously had chemotherapy. It was subsequently licensed in a number of countries including Argentina, Brazil, Canada, Israel, and Switzerland. It gained EU-wide approval in 2000. By 2006, successful clinical trial results in the US and internationally had demonstrated the drug's efficacy and safety as an adjuvant to treat early-stage Her2-positive breast cancer. (Herceptin® following standard chemotherapy significantly reduced the risk of cancer coming back by 46% compared to chemotherapy alone [9].) As a result, Genentech submitted a supplemental Biologics License Application (sBLA) to the FDA so that Herceptin® could be used to treat patients with early-stage breast cancer and requested a priority review. The FDA was required to make its assessment and response within six months. Genentech's sBLA was supported by data from two clinical trials sponsored by the US National Cancer Institute [10]. The sBLA was approved.

At the same time, Roche Pharmaceuticals (which markets Herceptin® in Europe) submitted a Marketing Authorization Application (MAA) to the EMA. Roche based its EMA application on clinical trial data from an international Herceptin® adjuvant, or HERA [11], study over a 3-year period. Collaborative partners for the HERA study include Roche and the Breast International Group (BIG) and its affiliated collaborative groups, plus non-affiliated collaborative groups, and independent sites. The drug won the recommendation from the EMA's CHMP in a record 27 days and a license was issued within 90 days.

Cervarix®

The Cervarix® vaccine, which has been manufactured by GSK [11], was licensed by the EMA in September 2007 and since September 2008 it has been used routinely to immunize against cervical cancer in the UK. Cervarix has since been approved in 67 other countries around the world and the FDA finally approved it in the USA in October 2009. The latter is in itself a very important development for this particular vaccine as it is used in the prevention of cervical cancer. The statistics show that the majority of cases (75%) are caused by HPV types 16 and 18 and the vaccine has been shown to be 93% efficacious in the prevention of cervical pre-cancers (cervical intraepithelial neoplasia 2+ or adenocarcinoma *in situ*).

The final approval by the FDA was based on data from clinical trials in more than 30 countries involving over 30 000 girls and young women. The vaccine is targeted at girls and women aged between 10 and 25 years.

Provenge®

In April 2010, the Sipuleucel-T (Provenge®) vaccine (made by Dendreon Corporation) was approved by the FDA for the treatment of asymptomatic or minimally symptomatic metastatic hormone-refractory prostate cancer. The primary efficacy endpoint of the trial was overall survival (OS). The treatment was shown to improve overall survival but had no effect on tumor progression [12]. The approval was based on the results obtained from a randomized double-blind placebo-controlled multicenter trial (Study 9902B, National Cancer Institute at the National Institutes of Health).

Sipuleucel-T is a form of cellular immunotherapy, which is made up of autologous peripheral blood mononuclear cells (PBMCs) activated with recombinant prostatic acid phosphotase linked to granulocyte-macrophage colony stimulating factor (PAP-GM-CSF). Eligible patients either had bony metastatic disease or soft tissue metastatic disease and evidence of disease progression. The patients were randomly assigned to receive either the Sipuleucel-T treatment or control (un-activated PBMCs). Patients receiving Sipuleucel-T exhibited an OS of 25.8 months as compared to 21.7 months for patients on the control treatment [13].

Provenge® is designed to stimulate the patient's immune system to target the prostate cancer cells and it was anticipated that in the first year of FDA approval, Dendreon would manufacture treatment to support 2000 patients [14]. However, in September 2011, Dendreon dropped GlaxoSmithKline as a Provenge® manufacturer due to implementation difficulties. Moreover, the uptake of the treatment has been slow due to a combination effect of (i) the complexity of drug administration being a major issue, and (ii) reimbursement issues.

Yervoy™ (ipilimumab)

In August 2010, Bristol-Myers Squibb (BMS) announced that its Biologics License Application (BLA) for ipilimumab had been accepted for filing by the FDA and it had also been granted a priority review designation. This type of designation is usually granted to agents that either offer major advances in the treatment of disease or provide treatment where no adequate therapy exists. The projected FDA action date was scheduled for December 25, 2010 [15]. However, they finally approved ipilimumab (Yervoy™, made by BMS) on March 25, 2011 for the treatment of unresectable or metastatic melanoma.

Ipilimumab (MDX-010) is a fully human monoclonal antibody directed toward CTLA4, which acts as a "brake" on T cells. Therefore, this antibody overcomes the CTLA4-mediated T-cell suppression to enhance the immune response against tumors [16].

Early preclinical and clinical studies of patients with advanced melanoma have shown that ipilimumab promotes anti-tumor activity both as a monotherapy and in combination with other therapy such as chemotherapy, vaccines, or cytokines [16]. The phase III trial for ipilimumab was co-funded by BMS and it showed patients who received ipilimumab together with the glycoprotein peptide vaccine had a median survival of 10 months as compared to 6.4 months for patients receiving peptide alone. Patients receiving the monoclonal antibody alone (monotherapy) had a survival of 10.1 months too.

Swine flu vaccine

In 2009, swine flu caused by the H1N1 influenza virus became a real threat worldwide and in a drive to vaccinate people against swine flu before winter, many European governments fast-tracked their testing of a new flu vaccine, which aroused concerns by experts on the safety and proper use of the vaccine doses.

In September 2009, the EMA recommended two vaccines for licensing by the European Commission [17]. The Agency's committee fast-tracked the assessment of the vaccines Focetria® (Norvartis) and Pandemrix® (GlaxoSmithKline). A third recommendation for the vaccine Celvapan® by Baxter followed in October 2009.

The Focetria® vaccine was developed and launched by Norvartis within 3 months of the

swine flu pandemic being declared by the World Health Organization (WHO). This vaccine was formulated with the MF59® adjuvant, which boosts the body's immune response and increases the protective antibody levels with less H1N1 antigen (7.5 µg viral antigen) being needed as compared to the non-adjuvant vaccines (15 µg viral antigen) [18].

The Pandemrix® vaccine was developed and launched by GSK. This vaccine delivers 3.75 µg of the viral antigen together with the GSK proprietary adjuvant AS03 and was designed to be given in two doses at three-week intervals [19].

The Celvapan® vaccine differs from the other two in that this is a non-adjuvated vaccine and it is recommended that this be administered in two doses at three-week intervals [20].

All the influenza vaccines mentioned above were developed using the "mock-up" approach, which means they were made ahead of a pandemic by using available viral strains to which the general population was considered immunologically "naïve." The vaccines were all developed for use in children older than 6 months and adults, including pregnant women.

Use of transgenic animals in vaccine development

With regard to animals, the selection of animal species for the pharmacologic and/or toxicologic evaluation of cancer vaccines depends on the underlying mechanisms of action and specificities of each product. The complexity of vaccine development may necessitate the use of more than one animal model for the entire preclinical program. Generally the selection of animal models may differ depending on the use of the vaccine.

The factors that are taken on board when choosing an animal model include the efficacy and toxicity testing of cancer vaccines requiring an intact immune system and a product that is pharmacologically active within the selected species.

For cancer vaccines an animal species that shows a relevant immune response to the vaccine is needed.

EU licensing system

The EMA, established by the European Commission on January 1, 1995, re-established 2004, is a decentralized scientific agency (as opposed to a regulatory authority) of the European Union, with headquarters in London. Its main responsibility is the protection and promotion of public and animal health, through the evaluation and supervision of medicines for human and veterinary use. It acts as a secretariat, bringing together the scientific resources of over 40 national authorities in 30 EU and EEA-EFTA countries and a network of over 4500 European experts.

The EMA is responsible for the scientific evaluation of applications for European marketing authorization for medicinal products under the centralized procedure, which requires a company to submit a single MAA to the EMA. The EMA Committee for Medicinal Products for Human Use (CHMP) undertakes the scientific evaluation of vaccines. If a positive opinion is advised by CHMP, the European Commission grants the final approval of the centralized (or "Community") marketing authorization, which is valid in all EU Member States and the EEA-EFTA states (Iceland, Liechtenstein, and Norway). The EMA coordinates marketing authorizations for the EU nations, but the Member States are responsible for enforcement. In addition, each of the Member States has at least one drug regulatory agency and in some cases as many as two. Figure 27.1 summarizes the main steps involved in seeking approval at the EU level.

Alternative marketing authorization procedures are available to a company, which may be selected depending on the product involved and the company's marketing strategy. The centralized procedure is mandatory for biotechnology products and biosimilar products, as well as for orphan drugs and a growing list of innovative drugs for certain diseases. The decentralized or mutual recognition procedure generally is sought when a company wishes to limit the markets in which it offers the product. A company may also apply for a national marketing authorization, which covers the market in the selected country only. The majority of existing medicines and vaccines throughout the Member States remain authorized nationally, but the majority of genuinely novel medicines are authorized through the EMA.

The EMA also provides scientific advice and guidance relating to the quality, safety, or efficacy of medicinal products, and protocol assistance to companies during the research and development phase of medicinal products. The safety of medicines is monitored constantly by the Agency through a pharmacovigilance network and the regulatory framework has the flexibility to function in emergency situations, when needed, such as a pandemic of a human disease. The Agency increasingly cooperates closely with international partners, contributing to global harmonization, and is involved in initiatives with key regulatory agencies across the globe including the WHO, the ICH, and the US FDA.

Centralized procedure

All medicinal products, including vaccines, that have been made using biotechnology (including recombinant DNA technology) and new medicinal products intended to treat cancer, AIDS, neurodegenerative diseases, and diabetes must use the centralized procedure. The marketing authorization (MA) is valid for up to five years. However, it is optional for others [21].

During the pre-submission phase, the proposer can obtain scientific advice from the EMA. These meetings are seen as critical in the product development and regulatory approval process. A company that wishes to follow the centralized procedure must submit its MAA dossier to the EMA. The scientific evaluation is required to be completed within a 210-day period (not including time for queries). Two rapporteurs are appointed in the CHMP for each medicinal product, who monitor the product throughout its life cycle and assess the MAA, together with an assessment team called a Scientific Advisory Group (SAG) comprising six to eight experts in a particular therapeutic field. There are currently seven SAGs. Other experts may be appointed, where necessary.

The CHMP also consults with a number of permanent working parties, comprising members selected from the EMA's European Experts lists.

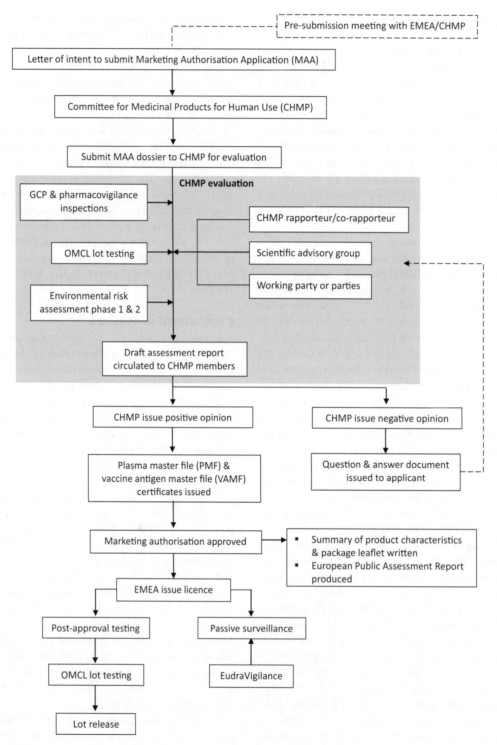

Figure 27.1 Summary of the processes involved in licensing a product with the EMA.

Currently there are 12 permanent working parties and one temporary working party, including the Vaccine Working Party (VWP) (other key working groups include biologics, safety, and gene therapy). The VWP and other working groups can be involved in the scientific evaluation of the MAA, address product specific regulatory issues, develop guidance documents, and communicate with external parties.

In the preclinical development phase, a company must comply with the Good Laboratory Practice Directive. During clinical development, the Clinical Trials Directive [22] and ICH Good Clinical Practices (GCPs) apply. The Agency carries out inspections to verify specific aspects of clinical or laboratory testing or manufacture and control of a product to ensure compliance. GCP and pharmacovigilance inspections may be undertaken during the assessment of the MAA or in accordance with EU legislation. EMA also carries out particular analysis of data and clinical trial conditions for those companies that carry out clinical trials in non-EU countries, where it is perceived that the application of GCP is not as well established as in Europe, the US, and other developed countries. The EU direct clinical trial database records those trials carried out in Member States.

The EMA also issues plasma master file (PMF) and vaccine antigen master file (VAMF) certificates of a medicinal product through assessment of the application dossier. The documents describe the manufacturing facility including general data, the premises, equipment, personnel, sanitation, manufacturing control, quality control, packaging material testing, finished product testing, records, samples, and stability.

The CHMP may recommend that certain products, such as a live vaccine, may need testing before they are released for sale, in the interest of public health. The applicant would be required to submit samples from each batch before release onto the market for testing by an EU official medicines control laboratory (OMCL). A batch of a medicinal product cannot be placed on the market until the OMCL has examined the batch (within a 60-day period) by issuing a European Community certificate of batch compliance. The initial review of vaccine lots is done during the licensing process when the methods of manufacture and testing, and the consistency of production of several (usually consecutive) lots are evaluated. Legal provisions are in place that allows EU regulations for marketing authorization to be modified temporarily to enable very rapid review and release of much-needed products. The accelerated assessment procedure can reduce the process from 210 days to 150 days. A market authorization holder who wishes to renew a product license must submit a dossier for CHMP assessment, which can take up to 120 days.

An environmental risk assessment (ERA) is required as part of the MAA, registering new active pharmaceutical ingredients (APIs) or new uses of APIs, to determine the environmental impact of a proposed vaccine's storage, use, and disposal. The first phase (Phase I) estimates the exposure of the environment to the drug substance. Based on an action limit, the assessment may be terminated. In the second phase (Phase II), data on the impact and effects in the environment is obtained and assessed. Separate ERA guidance is issued for live vaccines containing genetically modified organisms (GMOs), which are susceptible to being released into the environment.

Once a marketing authorization has been approved by the Commission, the Summary of Product Characteristics and the package leaflet are written and a European Public Assessment Report (EPAR) is produced. Each product approved is given a European marketing authorization number. However, if the product is rejected, information is provided on why this conclusion was reached.

Decentralized procedure

Companies may apply via the decentralized procedure for simultaneous authorization of most conventional medicinal products in more than one EU country, and which have not yet been authorized in any EU country. It requires several marketing authorizations and several trade names. The Coordination Group for Mutual Recognition and Decentralized Procedures – Human, CMD(h), set up by the revised pharmaceutical Directive [8], has responsibility for the decentralized procedure and mutual recognition procedure and is composed of the Heads of Medicines Agencies (HMA). It can discuss any procedural or scientific questions in the procedure and settles any disagreements arising from the procedures. The company selects a Reference Member State (RMS) and market. The RMS evaluates the dossier submitted by the company and prepares the assessment report on behalf of the other Member State(s) (Concerned Member State [CMS]) for both the decentralized and mutual recognition procedures. The RMS has 210 days to complete the evaluation. The RMS has a pivotal role in both procedures, undertaking scientific evaluation, providing regulatory advice to the company, and facilitating discussions between the RMS, CMS, and the applicant. The submission subsequently enters the mutual recognition phase, where other CMSs nominated by the applicant have up to 90 days to raise concerns, before establishing a final decision on the application. Disputed decisions go to the CHMP, for binding arbitration. On approval, the RMS prepares the final assessment report and the public assessment report, which will be published on the HMA website.

Mutual recognition procedure

The mutual recognition procedure, which is under the decentralized procedure, is used to obtain a marketing authorization in several Member States for a medicinal product that has already received a license in at least one other Member State. As such, each country may, or may not, choose to recognize each other's authorizations. The RMS's assessment report forms the basis for requesting the other CMSs' mutual recognition of the marketing authorization (including the Summary of Product Characteristics [SPC], package leaflet, and labeling text). At the end of the mutual recognition procedure involving identical applications submitted to CMSs, a national marketing authorization will be issued in the other CMSs, unless they have objections on the grounds of a potentially serious risk to public health. The procedure is completed within 90 days.

The decentralized or mutual recognition procedure allows a company to select markets, a famil-

iar procedure, and more access and flexibility. The disadvantages of this approach include long review periods, lack of harmonization or Member State consensus, risks and problems with mutual recognition, industry avoidance of arbitration processes, and a lack of a single market. At present, legislation seeks to strengthen the decentralized procedure to make it harder for Member States to object to the mutual recognition of products. In addition, it aims to make it more difficult for companies to withdraw their products from a Member State that makes requests the company is unwilling to comply with.

If a company wishes to alter an aspect of a vaccine under the centralized, decentralized, and mutual recognition procedures, it follows a standard administrative process under the Variations Regulation (1084/2003/EC). Minor variations such as a change of address are classified as Type IA or IB. Changes in dosage or safety warnings are considered Type II, major variations. A company with a vaccine authorized nationally can face an array of administrative procedures in that country.

Post-licensing

In 1991 the EMA set up EudraVigilance, an electronic database, for the reporting of adverse reactions during the development and following the marketing authorization of medicinal products, in the European Economic Area (EEA). The reports related to these adverse events following immunization (AEFI) are referred to as Individual Case Safety Reports (ICSRs). In addition, clinical trials should report suspected, unexpected serious adverse reactions (SUSARs) electronically.

UK licensing system

Applicants who follow the UK national procedure will be granted a marketing authorization by the Medicines and Healthcare products Regulatory Agency (MHRA). Since this marketing authorization is not based on the recognition of another marketing authorization for the same product awarded by an assessment authority of another EU/EEA Member State, the product can only be placed on the UK market. The national procedure can also serve as the first phase of a mutual recognition procedure if the UK is going to act as the RMS in that procedure. The national procedure is not available for categories of medicinal products where the EMA centralized procedure is compulsory. Similarly, the national procedure is not available if the same applicant has already obtained marketing authorization in another Member State, or has previously submitted an application dossier that is under consideration for marketing authorization in another Member State. In the latter case, applicants must follow the mutual recognition procedure. An MHRA marketing authorization is valid for five years.

US licensing system

The FDA is a government agency of the United States Department of Health and Human Services. It is the single approval and regulatory body responsible for regulating and supervising the safety of biologics products, including vaccines, to be marketed in the US. The regulations cover efficacy, safety, product quality, conduct of clinical trials, good manufacturing practices and controls, facilities, holding of vaccines, labeling and packaging, advertising, marketing, and licensing. The regulations are found at Title 21 of the Code of Federation Regulations (21 CFR) and Title 45 Part 46, as part of Section 351 of the Public Health Service Act, and cover the requirements of the Food, Drug, and Cosmetic Act (FD&C). The Agency publishes guidance to support manufacturers and those involved in developing new biologics products. The Center for Biologics Evaluation and Research (CBER), Office of Vaccines Research and Review (OVRR) is responsible for the licensing of vaccines.

Investigational New Drug (IND) process

The clinical development of a new product normally begins when the company formally submits an Investigational New Drug (IND) application to the CBER. The IND comprises all known information about the compound, including how it is manufactured, a description of the clinical research plan for the product, and the specific protocol for phase I human clinical trials. The IND is an on-

going file, which contains data on the proposed drug as it passes through the development process. The CBER has 30 days to review the IND to determine whether study participants will be exposed to unacceptable risk. The main steps following the submission of an application are highlighted in Figure 27.2.

Early-phase clinical trials evaluate safety, optimize the dose and schedule, and identify evidence of biologic drug activity. Later phase efficacy studies evaluate the clinical benefit. Purity and preclinical safety are the first regulatory requirements for vaccine development, which must be demonstrated before beginning clinical trials. An IND is not required at the preclinical stage but pre-IND discussions are encouraged with the FDA to expedite the IND submission process. The FDA recommends that randomized and well-controlled trials be designed to evaluate the safety, immunogenicity, and efficacy of vaccines [23]. The design of phase III trials should, if possible, be discussed with CBER to ensure they meet intended goals and in relation to marketing requirements.

Biologics License Application (BLA)

Once the phase I–III clinical trials have been successfully completed, the manufacturer submits the BLA dossier to the FDA for marketing authorization. A company that already has a licensed vaccine, which now has changes to the manufacturing process, facilities, labeling, or its efficacy, must submit a supplemental BLA (sBLA). The FDA may grant fast-track, accelerated approval, or priority review of therapeutically important drugs that meet certain conditions so that they are made available earlier than standard treatments, especially for serious illnesses such as cancer. In addition, specific provisions make some treatments available to patients with special needs even before the approval process is complete. This may reduce the approval time from the standard of ten months down to six months but does not affect the clinical trial period. The BLA comprises information on the applicant, product, manufacturing information, preclinical studies, clinical studies, and labeling.

A pre-BLA meeting is held between the applicant and CBER reviewers regarding the general

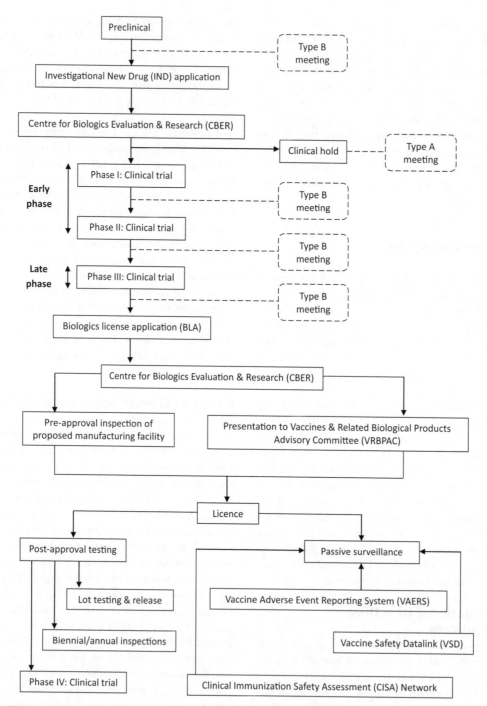

Figure 27.2 Summary of the processes involved in licensing a product with the FDA.

information that will be submitted in the application. This meeting may take place without an IND when the entire development of the drug has been outside the US and there will be no studies conducted under IND in the application. As part of the dossier, the CBER team (of microbiologists, medical officers, chemists, biostatisticians, etc.) will review the clinical trial results and manufacturing information, as well as efficacy and safety data. The information is used to carry out a risk/benefit assessment and results in the recommendation or rejection of the vaccine license.

Well-defined manufacturing methods (Good Manufacturing Practice [GMP] compliant) and controls are critical to the evaluation of the safety and purity of the vaccine and must be documented in the BLA. CBER experts make pre-approval inspections of the manufacturing plant where the vaccine will be made to review the production process and the critical clinical studies sites during which the progress of the production of the vaccine is examined in detail. This includes a review of all production equipment, utility systems, personnel, and batch records.

Prior to the licensing of a new vaccine, the sponsor will often be invited to present their data to the FDA's Vaccines and Related Biological Products Advisory Committee (VRBPAC), which is a non-FDA expert committee (comprising scientists, physicians, biostatisticians, and a consumer representative). The VRBPAC provides advice to the Agency regarding the production, testing, safety, and efficacy of the vaccine for the proposed indication.

In order to respond to scientific and technological advances in vaccines, the BLA includes all the appropriate testing methods for in-process and release testing for each specific vaccine. When the CBER is satisfied that the vaccine has provided satisfactory documentation with regard to its safety, efficacy, manufacturing process, facilities, testing, and clinical data, the license is approved. The BLA also requires adequate product labeling. If the application is unsatisfactory, additional review cycles are undertaken lasting between four and six months until adequate documentation is provided. The overall licensing process from drug development to license approval can be between eight and twelve years.

Post-approval surveillance

Upon license approval, the FDA continues to monitor the vaccine's production and performance to ensure its continuing safety and efficacy. Vaccine manufacturers must comply with strict manufacturing standards. Periodic facility inspections for compliance with current GMP guidance are carried out as long as the manufacturer holds a license for the product. Extensive in-process quality control and product testing (such as for potency and purity) are required at multiple stages of the manufacturing process. Each lot of vaccine manufactured must be reviewed and tested by the manufacturer, and results and samples of every lot must be provided to the FDA. No lot can be used until testing is completed and it is released by the manufacturer and FDA. Manufacturers may be asked to perform post-marketing studies to further assess less common or rare adverse events or to assess the duration of protection induced by the approved vaccine. Many vaccines also undergo phase IV studies.

If requested by the FDA, manufacturers are required to submit to the results of their own tests for potency, safety, and purity for each vaccine lot. They may also be required to submit samples of each vaccine lot to the CBER for testing. However, if the sponsor describes an alternative procedure that provides continued assurance of safety, purity, and potency, CBER may determine that routine submission of lot release protocols (showing results of applicable tests) and samples is not necessary.

The FDA and the US Centers for Disease Control and Prevention (CDC) closely monitor the safety of all licensed vaccines through the nationwide Vaccine Adverse Event Reporting System (VAERS). VAERS receives reports from health care professionals, manufacturers, and the general public, which supports the detection of rare adverse events and rapid detection of possible signals. The Vaccine Safety Datalink (VSD) project is a collaborative effort between CDC and eight managed care organizations that participate in a linked database, which monitors vaccine safety and addresses the gaps in scientific knowledge about rare and serious side effects following immunization. VSD stores the complete medical records for the 8.8 million members and monitors for possible side effects. In 2005, the VSD project team launched an active surveillance system called Rapid Cycle Analysis (RCA). Its goal is to monitor adverse events following vaccination (possible side effects) in near real time, so the public can be informed quickly of possible risks. RCA is used to monitor newly licensed vaccines and new vaccine recommendations.

Reforms within the EMA and FDA

Both the EMA and FDA have been taking action both independently and in some cases jointly that increases their focus on safety and enforcement issues with clinical research. The both announced that greater importance must be placed on regulatory control and procedures, especially with regard to GCP when conducting clinical trials outside of the EU and US.

In addition, the EMA and FDA also launched the EMA-FDA GCP Initiative. This will be a joint effort between the CDER and the EMA to ensure that clinical trials submitted in Europe and the US are conducted uniformly, appropriately, and ethically. It began on September 1, 2009 as an 18-month pilot phase. The Initiative covers three main key objectives:
• conducting information exchange between the USA and the EU on GCP information;
• conducting collaborative GCP inspections;
• sharing information in interpretation of GCP.

The Initiative is a step toward the continuing globalization of regulation of human medicines and the GCP will be the international standard used in conducting clinical trials.

Conclusion

This chapter has highlighted both the similarities and differences between the EMA and FDA when it comes to authorizing and licensing a new product and the different steps involved in the process. We have also discussed by example the licensing of

a number of vaccine products, namely Herceptin®, Cervarix®, Provenge®, and Yervoy™).

Now that the FDA and EMA have started to approve cancer vaccines, it can be said that the scientific, regulatory, and commercial hurdles that were an obstacle for so many products are now becoming a thing of the past.

Acknowledgment

Murrium Ahmad wishes to acknowledge the support of the John and Lucille van Geest Foundation.

References

1 EMA (2005). Guideline on clinical evaluation of new vaccines (EMEA/CHMP/VWP/164653/2005). Available at: www.ema.europa.eu/pdfs/human/vwp/16465305enfin.pdf. Accessed Feb 2012.

2 Mocellin S, Mandruzzato S, Bronte V, *et al.* Vaccines for solid tumours. *Lancet Oncol* 2004;**5**: 681–9.

3 Conry RM, Khazaeli MB, Saleh MN, *et al.* Phase I trial of a recombinant vaccinia virus encoding carcinoembryonic antigen in metastatic adenocarcinomas: comparison of intradermal versus subcutaneous administration. *Clin Cancer Res* 1991;**5**:2330–37.

4 Marshall JL, Hoyer RJ, Toomey MA, *et al.* Phase I study in advanced cancer patients of a diversified prime-and-boost vaccination protocol using recombinant vaccinia virus and recombinant nonreplicating avipox virus to elicit anti-carcinoembryonic antigen immune reponses. *Clin Oncol* 2000;**18**:3964–73.

5 Hipp JD, Hipp JA, Lyday BW, *et al.* Cancer vaccines: an update. *In vivo* 2000;**14**:571–81.

6 Kim JJ, Yang JS, Nottingham LK, *et al.* Induction of immune responses and safety profiles in rhesus macaques immunised with a DNA vaccine expressing human prostate specific antigen. *Oncogene* 2001; **20**:4497–506.

7 Perelson AS. Immune network theory. *Immunol Rev* 1989;**110**:5–36.

8 Directive 2004/27/EC of the European Parliament and of the Council amending Directive 2001/83/EC on the Community code relating to medicinal products for human use. *Official Journal of the European*

Union 2004 Apr 30;L 136/34–57. Available at http://eur-lex.europa.eu/LexUriServ/LexUriServ.do?uri=OJ:L:2004:136:0034:0057:EN:PDF. Accessed Feb 2012.

9 Piccart-Gebhart M, Procter M, Leyland-Jones B, *et al.* Trastuzumab after adjuvant chemotherapy in HER2-positive breast cancer. *N Engl J Medicine* 2005; **353**: 1659–72.

10 Breast Cancer International Research Group. Taxotere®-based regimes with Herceptin® in women with early-stage HER2-positive breast cancer demonstrate the highest reduction in the risk of death to date and provide a treatment option without anthracyclines. NCCTG N9831 (US), NSABP B-31 (US), BCIRG 006 (international). Available at www.bcirg.org/NR/rdonlyres/eeisn6nnhvy6yuaxl5ctdii7uynkgxlmiiljimo7tsttocqlg5dr5vxcbbcinwuceyp7ge4e3omw5mpcgwiatqcsc2d/TAXOTERE+BCIRG+006+ENG.pdf. Accessed Feb 2012.

11 GSK. FDA approves Cervarix, GlaxoSmithKline's cervical cancer vaccine, Oct 16, 2009. Available at www.gsk.com/media/pressreleases/2009/2009_pressrelease_10112.htm. Accessed Feb 2012.

12 Glare J. Drug in development: Sipuleucel-T in advanced prostate cancer. *N Engl J Med* 2010; **363**:411–22, 479–81.

13 National Cancer Institute. FDA approval of Sipuleucel-T, Apr 30, 2010. Available at www.cancer.gov/cancertopics/druginfo/fda-sipuleucel-T. Accessed Feb 2012.

14 Dendreon. PROVENGE® (sipuleucel-T) is FDA approved. Available at www.dendreon.com/products/provenge/default.asp. Accessed Feb 2012.

15 Mulcahy N. FDA fast tracks ipilimumab for metastatic melanoma. Aug 19, 2010. Available at www.medscape.com/viewarticle/727137. Accessed Feb 2012.

16 Weber J. Anti-CTLA-4 antibody ipilimumab: case studies of clinical response and immune-related adverse events. *Oncologist* 2010;**12**(7):864–72.

17 Cook S. European Agency approves swine flu vaccine for licensing. *BMJ* 2009; **339**:b3992.

18 Novartis. A(H1N1) pandemic influenza vaccine Focetria® receives positive opinion from CHMP, Sep 25, 2009. Available at http://insciences.org/article.php?article_id=6929. Accessed Feb 2012.

19 GSK. Pandemic (H1N1) 2009 influenza update: GSK's H1N1 "Pandemrix" vaccine receives positive opinion from European Regulators, Sep 25, 2009. Available at www.gsk.com/media/pressreleases/2009/2009_pressrelease_10089.htm. Accessed Feb 2012.

20 Baxter. Baxter receives European Commission approval for Celvapan H1N1 pandemic influenza vaccine. Oct 7, 2009. Available at www.baxter.com/press_room/press_releases/2009/10_07_09-celvapan.html. Accessed Feb 2012.

21 Regulation (EC) No. 726/2004 of the European Parliament and of the Council of 31 March 2004 laying down Community procedures for the authorisation and supervision of medicinal products for human and veterinary use and establishing a European Medicines Agency. *Official Journal of the European Union* 2004 Apr 30;L 136/1–33. Available at http://eur-lex.europa.eu/LexUriServ/LexUriServ.do?uri=OJ:L:2004:136:0001:0033:EN:PDF. Accessed Feb 2012.

22 Directive 2001/20/EC of the European Parliament and of the Council of 4 April 2001 on the approximation of the laws, regulations and administrative provisions of the Member States relating to the implementation of good clinical practice in the conduct of clinical trials on medicinal products for human use. *Official Journal of the European Union* 2001 May 1;L 121/34–44. Available at www.eortc.be/services/doc/clinical-eu-directive-04-april-01.pdf. Accessed Feb 2012.

23 FDA. Draft Guidance for Industry: Integrated Summary of Effectiveness, Aug 2008, 21 CFR 324 126. Available at www.fda.gov/downloads/Drugs/GuidanceComplianceRegulatoryInformation/Guidances/UCM079803.pdf. Accessed Feb 2012.

PART 7

Evaluating Vaccine Efficacy

CHAPTER 28

Immune Monitoring Design within the Developmental Pipeline for an Immunotherapeutic or Preventive Vaccine

Sylvia Janetzki[1], Pedro Romero[2], Mario Roederer[3], Diane L. Bolton[3], & Camilla Jandus[2]

[1]Zellnet Consulting, Inc., Fort Lee, NJ, USA
[2]Division of Clinical Onco-Immunology, Ludwig Institute for Cancer Research, Lausanne, Switzerland
[3]Vaccine Research Center, National Institute of Allergy and Infectious Diseases (NIAID), National Institutes of Health (NIH), Bethesda, MD, USA

Introduction

Immunotherapy is defined as the treatment of disease by inducing, enhancing, or suppressing an immune response, whereas preventive vaccination is intended to prevent the development of diseases in healthy subjects. Most successful prophylactic vaccines rely on the induction of high titers of neutralizing antibodies. It is generally thought that therapeutic vaccination requires induction of robust T-cell mediated immunity. The diverse array of potential or already in use immunotherapeutic and preventive agents all share the commonality of stimulating the immune system. Hence, measuring those vaccination-induced immune responses gives the earliest indication of vaccine take and its immune modulating effects. Obviously, vaccination modes have changed since its introduction by Jenner in the 1770s with the inoculation of whole organisms (cowpox) to elicit protection against smallpox [1], via Coley's vaccine, which elicits an infection-triggered nonspecific immune response used for the treatment of cancer [2], to today's vaccines, complex in design, which are expected to elicit potent and specific T- or B-cell responses [3–5].

The development of vaccines aimed to generate strong T-cell immune responses implies not only the search for new treatment modalities, but also concomitant optimization of robust methods for successful immunomonitoring of the induced responses. Both novel strategies of immunization as well as new readout methodologies are currently under investigation: the former might allow finding more potent ways to achieve long-lasting specific immune activation; the latter should lead to a standardized multiparametric way of assessing vaccine-induced responses. This is necessary to both increase our knowledge of the contribution of distinct components of the immune system to specific immunity and to find positive correlates between immune and clinical outcomes.

Various immunotherapeutic vaccines have shown some success in the treatment of cancer

Vaccinology: Principles and Practice, First Edition. Edited by W. John W. Morrow, Nadeem A. Sheikh, Clint S. Schmidt and D. Huw Davies.
© 2012 Blackwell Publishing Ltd. Published 2012 by Blackwell Publishing Ltd.

and infectious and autoimmune diseases. Just recently, long-awaited first positive reports about immunotherapeutic cancer vaccines have revitalized the field [6–8], while the AIDS vaccine field has experienced both a serious setback [9] and exciting advances [10] in the pursuit of a preventive vaccine.

But, by and large, there is still much to learn about the action and clinical effectiveness of immunotherapeutic vaccines. It is likely that the best strategy to prevent or combat disease via the immune system is to combine specific and nonspecific methods with a variety of antigens and approaches. The need for a detailed understanding of how vaccines work should therefore include the evaluation of responses from the innate as well as the adaptive immune system. The more we know and the earlier, the more effectively we can adapt and develop our strategies, and establish successful prevention or immunotherapy of cancer, HIV, and other infectious and autoimmune diseases. This process has recently been described as immunoguiding [11].

Here we present a comprehensive review of immune monitoring techniques that can provide information on innate as well as specific immune responses, including humoral, helper, and cytotoxic responses, and give recommendations on how to best incorporate these techniques into the developmental pipeline of immunotherapeutic vaccines (Table 28.1).

Challenges for immune monitoring

Despite tremendous technological advances made during the past decade, a variety of challenges exist for effective and comprehensive immune monitoring. One of the key questions pertains to the "what, where, and when" issue: which cells from what compartment should be monitored when and for how long? Further complicating is the lack of clearly defined correlates of protection and the notion that the qualitative features of immune responses could be more important than their quantitative features [12]. Evidence exists that even high numbers of circulating effector cells do not correlate with clinical benefit [13,14]. When the immune monitoring approach for a vaccine candidate is being determined, it needs to be taken

Table 28.1 Overview of immune monitoring techniques applied to assess different arms of the immune system, arranged by their trend toward higher difficulty in performance and validation.

Innate	B-cell	T-cell	
ELISA	ELISA	BrdU proliferation assays	
ADCC	ADCC	ELISA	
Assessment of:	ELISpot	^{51}Cr release assays	
• phagocytosis	Antibody neutralization	ELISpot	
• complement cascade activation	ICS	CFSE proliferation assays	
• neutrophilic function	Multiplex bead arrays	Other cytotoxicity assays:	Validation complexity and difficulty
• NK cell function (e.g., ELISpot)		• CD107 degranulation	
• macrophages, dendritic cells		• caspase activation	
		• co-culture labeling assays	
		HLA-multimer staining	
		ICS	
		Multiplex bead arrays	
		Multiparametric functional flow analysis	

into account where immune responses are induced, where cells are expected to migrate to and act, and, most importantly, which immunologic features are expected to be induced and which are unwanted. A recent report demonstrates the importance of accurate delivery and trafficking of dendritic cells (DCs) for a successful induction of immune responses [15]. Further, potent immune responses have been measured in compartments other than blood [16,17], and correlation with clinical outcome has been reported when testing delayed-type hypersensitivity (DTH) skin biopsies for tumor-specific T cells following vaccination [18].

To obtain thorough information about induced immune responses that can guide the development and further use of vaccines, multiple assays need to be utilized, especially in early testing phases, at multiple time points [19]. Certainly, this bears many logistic challenges. Assays have to be established in the appropriate laboratory. Necessary equipment, materials, and reagents often represent a large monetary burden. Good laboratory practices need to be introduced [20,21]. Staff have to be trained and periodically assessed for the quality of assay performance [22]. All of these steps may slow down the routine operations of a laboratory, and final decisions might be determined by assay expertise and existing preferences. Large immune monitoring core facilities and outsourcing options could present an acceptable solution for some of these challenges.

Further, despite the fact that many assays are well established, an abundance of protocols exist, reflecting local protocol preferences and adjustments to experimental systems worked in. The dispersion of assay protocols and the varying training and experience status of scientists performing the assays have led at least partially to high interlaboratory variability, as recently demonstrated in large international proficiency panels [23–26]. These challenges are currently tackled by standardization across laboratories within specific trial networks [27], or via assay harmonization across different laboratories and fields [25,26,28,29].

The lack of a gold standard (test) for many assays assessing single immune cells, like ELISpot, intracellular cytokine staining (ICS), and HLA-peptide multimer staining, to name the most commonly used assays, is setting further hurdles. Even though well-characterized peripheral blood mononuclear cell (PBMC) reference samples are commercially available today, the true number of antigen-specific cells or subtypes of cells remains to be determined. Perhaps the currently most straightforward and effective way to create an alternate gold standard is through participation in large proficiency panels, in which the same donor samples are tested for their reactivity against the same antigen(s) by a consortium of laboratories using different assay protocols [30]. Laboratory-specific results will accumulate around a hypothetical value that can, depending on size and setup of such panels, be assumed with good probability to present a good estimate of the actual frequency of antigen-specific cells within the sample tested. Hence, participation in well-designed proficiency panels can provide information about a laboratory's ability to provide accurate immune monitoring results with assays lacking a direct gold standard.

Finally, no agreement exists on the information that needs to be provided when reporting immune monitoring results to allow a thorough and objective interpretation of presented data by reviewers and readers alike. Orienting on the Minimal Information for Biological and Biomedical Investigations (MIBBI) objectives [31], the project on Minimal Information About T cell Assays (MIATA) was announced in 2009 [32]. The goal of this project is to establish a field-wide consensus document on a reporting framework for data from T-cell assays in the immunomonitoring context. Through a public consultation phase and workshop, during which feedback and suggestions were obtained from many peers in different areas of immunology, the initial guidelines were updated and are currently undergoing a second round of vetting to reach wide acceptability and maturity [33]. The implementation of the MIATA reporting framework will add transparency about how and under what quality measures immune monitoring data were obtained, and with that serve the scientific community in data analysis and exchange to enhance immunotherapeutic programs. Further, it provides the foundation for an expanded framework for annotations required for openly accessible databases, which enables unprejudiced analysis of data generated in immune monitoring studies.

Immune monitoring design along the vaccine pipeline

Example of an imaginary cancer vaccine: LSPs + CpGs + αCTLA4 administered in nanoparticles

The most important variables in therapeutic vaccine development seem to be antigenic composition, delivery system, and adjuvant choice. Moreover, the delivery includes variables such as the injection site, frequency, and modality of administration.

Although remarkable advances have been achieved in the past few years, current therapeutic vaccination protocols might induce detectable specific T-cell responses, but none of the strategies tested so far has emerged as universally applicable and sufficiently potent as standard treatment modality in established infections or cancer.

A novel interesting approach in immunotherapy might be the use of long synthetic peptides (LSPs), usually 20–30 amino acid long antigenic peptides, in combination with powerful adjuvants (e.g., activators of Toll-like receptors). LSPs represent a compromise between short synthetic peptide vaccination and the use of recombinant proteins, and offer several advantages. First, in contrast to exact major histocompatibility complex (MHC)-binding peptides, LSPs are generally unable to directly bind to MHC class I molecules so that their presentation to naïve T cells depends on uptake and processing by professional antigen-presenting cells (APCs). This precludes suboptimal presentation (e.g., without co-stimulation) by non-professional APCs, which may induce specific tolerance rather than immunity. Second, LSPs generally carry both MHC-I and MHC-II epitopes, thus enabling efficient CD4 T-cell-mediated help in initiating robust CD8 T-cell responses. Third, LSPs are generally amenable to rigorous purification. Fourth, parallel generation of T-cell responses against different MHC-I and MHC-II epitopes is crucial for the prevention of

potential immune escape mechanisms, in the context of both viral infections and cancer. In this regard, injection of pools of LSPs would go across any human leukocyte antigen (HLA) barrier and induce a large panel of T-cell responses in unselected individuals. Inclusion in the vaccination cocktail of LSPs derived from different antigens (e.g., several viral or tumor antigens, depending on the underlying disease) might be a valuable way to directly target the largest spectrum of possible immune players, while avoiding immune escape. Sustained responses and specific memory T cell generation are expected to result from this type of immunization. Fifth, similarly to short peptide immunization, clinical-grade production of LSPs is feasible and not prohibitively expensive, as generation and pharmacologic conditioning of recombinant proteins might be.

One of the shortcomings of immunotherapy in its earliest phases has been the lack of induction of robust responses and long-lasting memory. Addition of adjuvants to the vaccine composition seems to lead to both higher T-cell frequencies and longer persistence of expanded T cells. One of the most potent adjuvants tested so far is DNA containing demethylated CpGs (ODN-CpG). In fact, in immunotherapy trials in cancer patients, addition of synthetic ODN-CpGs, known to trigger Toll-like receptor 9 (TLR9) and activate plasmacytoid dendritic cells (pDCs), B lymphocytes, and macrophages, gave increased frequencies of tumor-specific T cells and promoted effector T-cell differentiation, if injected in conjunction with antigens (e.g., short peptides or recombinant proteins) [14,34].

However, despite activation of specific immune cells, lack of vaccine efficiency might eventually be observed, mainly due to the presence of established complex tolerogenic conditions at infectious/tumor sites. Moreover, responding T cells not only acquire effector functions but, simultaneously, express co-inhibitory receptors that enable control of potential immune pathology. Therefore, addition of molecules blocking co-inhibitory receptors within the ingredients of the vaccine formulations might dramatically augment the induced response. In this regard, a multimodal therapeutic strategy including administration of LSPs, ODN-CpGs, and, for example, humanized αCTLA4 antibodies could prove to be a powerful treatment. CTLA4 is a major checkpoint in adaptive immune responses, as illustrated by the severe lymphoproliferative disease in the absence of this gene. Unfortunately, clinical experience with intravenous administration of blocking antibodies to CTLA4 has shown it causes systemic toxicity in more than one third of patients, whose main manifestations are colitis and severe skin rashes as well as hypophysitis [35]. These side effects are to be expected and emphasize the need to selectively place the blocking agent at the lymph nodes for the priming phase, and at the tumor tissues for the effector phase. In this imaginary example of an ideal vaccine, nanoparticles would be used to directly target the tissue of interest. Compared to other delivery systems, nanoparticles would have several advantages. First, it has recently been shown in murine models that ultra-small (25 nm) particles injected intradermally efficiently get trapped in the lymph node vasculature and selectively reach lymph nodes via the slow-rate lymphatic flow [36]. Once in the lymph nodes, nanoparticles are retained there relatively long after injection, preferentially co-localize at sites of high-density lymph node resident DCs and macrophages, and if engineered to deliver antigens and activate complement, they efficiently induce both cellular and humoral immunity. Second, for the specific targeting of tumor tissues, one might imagine decorating nanoparticles with addresins. Certain peptides identified by phage display would function as "ZIP codes" addressing nanoparticles to tissues selectively expressing receptors for such peptides [37]. Third, the slow release rate of nanoparticles in the tissue may constitute an additional advantage by prolonging the bioavailability of αCTLA4 antibodies within target tissues, if compared to other targeting systems. Fourth, the depot effect in vaccines has emerged as a critical parameter. The best delivery vehicle thus far is the use of emulsions with mineral oil. A drawback is, however, the induration of the depot site, which may last for long periods of time and even lead to formation of uncomfortable, even painful, granulomas [13,14]. Nanoparticles would provide a solution to the depot effect, by releasing antigen and adjuvants in a controlled manner to the subcutaneous tissue.

Sample logistics

With the preceding paragraphs in mind, questions arise about the origin and amount of test specimen needed, and how often specimen samples should be obtained. Obviously, blood offers the easiest access, and repeated sample collection is feasible. It has been recommended to obtain the maximum justifiable amount that allows for repeated testing with at least two different assays [19]. Even though DTH skin biopsies, tumor, or draining lymph node samples present an attractive choice for obtaining information about cell migration and immune responses at the actual desired place of action, feasibility, logistics, and limited availability confine their use to a few, specifically designed studies. Today the preferred specimen choice for immune monitoring is PBMC. Numerous factors around the isolation and storage of PBMC determine their usefulness for immune assays.

Blood collection tubes

The choices for anti-coagulated blood collection to isolate PBMC are tubes supplemented with heparin (most commonly sodium heparin), ethylenediamine tetraacetic acid (EDTA), or acid citrate dextrose (ACD). After collection, Ficoll gradient centrifugation allows the separation of PBMC from erythrocytes, platelets, and granulocytes. Another choice is the use of CPT Vacutainers, which allow blood collection and PBMC isolation in the same tube by combining sodium citrate or heparin with a Ficoll density fluid and a polyester gel barrier. Numerous reports exist about the negative influence of EDTA on PBMC function and phenotype [38–41]. Thus, heparin- and ACD-supplemented blood collection tubes are the preferred choice for PBMC isolation [42,43].

PBMC isolation

The single most important factor for yielding functionally proper PBMC is the time elapsed between blood collection and PBMC isolation. It has been compellingly demonstrated that PBMC need to be isolated within 8 hours of blood draw [44–46]. The PBMC isolation method of choice is the Ficoll gradient centrifugation [47]. The use of Accuspin or Leucosep tubes, which contain a porous membrane frit that allows the fast addition of blood to tubes prefilled with Ficoll, can save time and possibly increase the PBMC yield. It has been noted that blood should not be diluted with PBS when using these tubes, in order to allow the erythrocytes that accumulate at the bottom of the tube to push the PBMC ring above the membrane frit. The overall efficiency of PBMC isolation using the traditional Ficoll method, Accuspin/Leucosep tubes, or CPT tubes appears to be similar [44,48].

Cryopreservation and thawing of cells

Cryopreservation of PBMC allows simultaneous testing of cells from different time points, as well as safe transport of cells between collection and testing sites. It has been demonstrated that freshly isolated and cryopreserved cells can perform comparably in cellular immune assays [49–51]. To date, various factors related to freezing of cells are known to influence PBMC functionality, like the choice of freezing medium or the temperature of washing medium after thawing cells [52]. While sporadic reports about freezing media for PBMC rely on observations with unique batches of sera, a study is currently being conducted by the Association for Immunotherapy of Cancer (CIMT) in collaboration with the Cancer Immunotherapy Consortium (CIC) systematically investigating the influence of different freezing media [53].

Cells should be frozen in the presence of a cryoprotectant such as dimethyl sulfoxide (DMSO), at a rate of approximately 1 °C/min, optimally provided by automated controlled rate freezers. An acceptable cheaper alternative is the use of Mr. Frosty™, a plastic container that relies on a similar cooling rate of isopropanol in a –80 °C freezer [54].

When thawing PBMC, it can be of advantage to use a DNase to eliminate DNA released from dying cells. Released DNA serves as a sticky matrix for cells, leading to cell clumps that cannot be dissolved, and cell recovery decreases. Benzonase has

been demonstrated to work reliably when thawing PBMC [51]. Further, it is recommended to add medium slowly to thawing cells, and to use warm medium for washing, in order to prevent an osmotic shock [52,55].

With knowledge of the variety of factors that can influence the functionality of PBMC in further testing, a quality assurance protocol for PBMC should be implemented in immune monitoring labs [56].

Multicenter trials and shipping of cells

An increasing number of clinical trials are performed by involving multiple centers for donor recruitment. While centralized testing for immune responses is an accepted and common procedure, logistic difficulties surround the collection, cryopreservation, and shipment of cells. The fact that collected blood needs to be processed within 8 hours prohibits its overnight shipment. Various options exist:

1 All participating centers are trained for PBMC isolation and freezing. Optimally, preassembled kits containing all materials necessary are provided, and centers are trained following the same Standardized Operating Procedure (SOP). An encouraging example has been set by Immatics, a biopharmaceutical company, which established a large network of laboratories for sample processing across Europe [57].

2 Core facilities in close proximity to participating centers, trained and specialized in sample processing, are identified and contractually involved. Transport of blood samples is guaranteed by using specialized messenger services.

3 Commercial services, yet limited, might be able to take on sample processing per the laboratory's specification.

Once cells have been frozen, they can be shipped to the central laboratory for monitoring purposes. Domestic shipment up to 48 hours on dry ice is possible [51]. Cycling of PBMC from liquid nitrogen to dry ice back to liquid nitrogen is acceptable once, but should not be repeated [56]. Most reliable shipment of frozen PBMC is obtained with the use of liquid nitrogen shippers. Cells are stored in the vapor phase of liquid nitrogen, and temperature is typically consistent for more than one week. Overall, the avoidance of temperature fluctuations is crucial to ensure good recovery rates and proper function of PBMC.

Current established assays

Screening assays

Proliferation assay using ^{3H}thymidine

The classical way to assess T-cell proliferation capacities is the use of a radioactive ^{3H}thymidine assay, which is based on the incorporation of ^{3H}thymidine into the DNA of replicating cells. Bulk proliferation of T cells stimulated polyclonally or with the antigen(s) of interest can be measured: the more cell division, the more ^{3H}thymidine will be incorporated into the cells' DNA. After incubation, cells are harvested on a membrane and the amount of radioactivity is counted in a scintillation counter. This proliferation assay has the advantage of being an easy procedure that can be validated without too many hurdles for the clinical setting: it does not require expensive equipment and is simple in terms of collection and processing of the data. Major limitations of this method are the need to use a radioactive agent, the impossibility of enumerating proliferation at a single-cell level or of combining other markers in the analysis, and the lack of visualization of the number of cell divisions.

Cytotoxicity assays

The most common assessment of the cytotoxic potential of T cells consists of measuring cytotoxic T lymphocyte (CTL)-induced killing of antigen-pulsed target cells or tumor cells in a ^{51}Cr release assay. Appropriately selected target cells lend themselves to perform quantitative assays of efficiency of antigen recognition by specific CTL lines or clones (Figure 28.1). Moreover, many tumor cell lines are amenable to ^{51}Cr labeling for assessment of recognition by tumor antigen specific CTL. Recently, nonradioactive, flow cytometric-based methods have been proposed to replace the standard ^{51}Cr release assay. Among others, FATAL (fluorometric assessment of T-lymphocyte antigen-

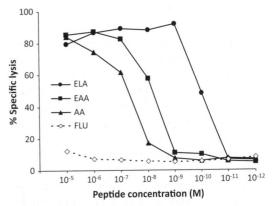

Figure 28.1 Efficiency of antigenic peptide recognition by cloned human CTL. Target cells are from the T2 line (a B × T lymphocyte hybrid lacking TAP expression). These cells offer the double advantage of labeling well with ^{51}Cr and being highly receptive to exogenous peptide binding to HLA-A2 on the cell surface. Effector cells are CD8 T cells from a CTL clone specific for the melanocyte/melanoma tumor antigen Melan-A. The effector to target cell ratio is set at 10:1. Titrated amounts of peptides Melan-A$_{26-35}$ A27L (filled circles), Melan-A$_{26-35}$ (filled squares), Melan-A$_{27-35}$ (filled triangles), and influenza matrix$_{58-66}$ (empty diamonds) are added and the plates incubated for 4 h at 37 °C before harvesting the supernatants and counting on a beta-counter. It is noteworthy that the peptide titration curves are sigmoid, and a direct comparison of the efficiency of antigen recognition is possible by calculating the ratio between the concentration of each peptide needed to obtain 50% of maximal lysis, provided that the slopes of curves are parallel, as illustrated in this example.

specific lysis) [58], VITAL (versatile fluorometric technique for assessing CTL- and NKT-mediated cytotoxicity) [59], and an alternative approach based on the measurement of caspase activity as an indicator of early apoptotic events have been applied as methods for the *in vitro* evaluation of T-cell cytotoxicity. However, all these approaches only offer an indirect assessment of T cell killing capacity, since they exclusively rely on the analysis of target cell death, and not on the direct measurement of CTL functions. In this regard, novel assays have been developed: detection of the lysosomal-associated membrane glycoproteins CD107a and CD107b on the cell surface of degranulating CD8 T cells seems to directly correlate with their functional activity [60,61]. However, it has to be noted that not all degranulated cells are cytotoxic [62], and, inversely, some cytotoxic cells kill in a granule-independent way. Further, if CD107a/b measurement is combined with pMHCI-multimer staining, direct enumeration of cytotoxic antigen-specific cells is feasible and isolation of viable functional cells is possible using a multiparameter cell sorter. In an even more complex setting, the recently proposed live count assay (LCA) provides the possibility for the concomitant visualization of both degranulation and phenotypic markers on single antigen-specific T cells with the detection of fluorescently labeled dying target cells by multiparametric flow-cytometry [63]. Optimization of this assay for very low cell numbers allows it to be used directly with *ex vivo* sampled material, for example from vaccinated patients. Finally, measurement of direct *in vivo* CTL activity is also possible by infusion of CFSE-labeled target cells [64], and it might be the best way, at least in animal models, to directly monitor cytotoxicity, in particular in terms of kinetics and mechanisms.

Antibody-dependent cell-mediated cytotoxicity assays

The classical antibody-dependent cell-mediated cytotoxicity (ADCC) is mediated by natural killer (NK) cells activated by antibodies bound to antigen. The FcγRIII (CD16) receptors of NK cells bind to the Fc portion of the antibodies, and upon cross-linking a cytotoxic effector cascade is initiated that mirrors CTL-mediated apoptosis and cell death. Hence, the classical assay to monitor ADCC is the ^{51}chromium release assay, as described earlier. A common problem, however, is high background signaling due to cellular "leakiness." This can be prevented by implementing the ^{35}sulfur release assay, during which target cells are incubated with radiolabeled methionine or cysteine, which are incorporated into newly translated peptides [65]. In addition, a flow cytometry-based method was described using target cells labeled with enhanced green fluorescent protein (EGFP) [66].

The advantage of ADCC assays is that they allow monitoring of antibody-directed and antigen-specific attacks by NK cells, which lack antigen specificity. The importance of developing and introducing newer ADCC assays to measure appropriate responses correlated to HIV prevention has recently been emphasized [67].

Antibody neutralization assay

Neutralizing antibodies play a key role in protection from viral infection. Thus, the development of vaccines that can effectively generate neutralizing antibodies against viruses that cause such devastating diseases as HIV or influenza would be of major importance. The gold standard assay to measure neutralizing antibodies is the antibody neutralization assay, which measures the reduction in viral infectivity. The impressive variety of antibody neutralization assays mainly represents variations, even though often of considerable extent, of the plaque reduction neutralization test (PRNT). In HIV-related studies, the MT-2 cell-killing assay is used to assess different T-cell-line-adapted HIV strains [68]. In order to test for neutralization of primary HIV isolates, PBMC-based neutralization assays monitoring the p24 Gag core synthesis or other viral proteins are employed [69]. The extracellular expression of these proteins is quantified by ELISA, which provides the final readout. These assays have been reported to be labor intensive and time consuming, with questionable reproducibility [70,71]. To overcome these disadvantages, a flow-based *in vitro* PBMC neutralization assay was developed that enumerates the infected target cells after the addition of a protease inhibitor [72]. This fast, direct quantification of first-round infected PBMC exhibits high precision and reproducibility. Constant assay modifications and refinements have led to a newly developed micro-neutralization assay that in combination with a standard binding assay allowed the recent identification of two broadly neutralizing antibodies for HIV [10].

ELISA

The enzyme-linked immunosorbent assay (ELISA) presents a classical assay for the quantification of particular molecules in fluids, like serum or cell culture supernatant. It is widely used in diagnostics and research, including the initial testing for HIV antibodies. Two general principles of the ELISA technique exist: the indirect and the direct methodology. The indirect ELISA is used for the quantification of specific antibodies. For that, serum is added to an antigen-coated plastic microtiter plate, and bound antigen-specific immunoglobulins are made visible with an anti-immunoglobulin antibody typically coupled with an enzyme, followed by the addition of a substrate. Chromogenic substrates change the color of the assay buffer, which can be translated into the amount of immunoglobulin bound. In the case of the hypothetical cancer vaccine described above, LSPs would be used to cover ELISA microtiter plates and the post-vaccination serum (or plasma) samples would be expected to contain peptide-specific IgG antibodies, at levels far superior to those measured in the pre-vaccination samples. Newer ELISA formats employ fluorogenic substrates that provide higher sensitivity.

With the direct or "sandwich" ELISA, the microtiter plate is coated with an antibody against a specific molecule, such as a cytokine, then serum or culture supernatant is added, and bound molecules are made visible with another enzyme-linked antibody, followed by the addition of substrate. The release of cytokines into the culture medium by T cells specifically activated by their cognate antigen (i.e., the LSPs in our example) lends itself to monitoring of vaccine activity at the T-cell level. The most commonly measured cytokines by ELISA are IFN-γ, TNF-α, and IL2. IFN-γ is the most robust as the majority of antigen-specific T cells produce this cytokine, which is stable in culture medium at 37 °C.

In addition to its specificity, versatility, and ease of automation, the main advantage of an ELISA is the ability to detect very small amounts of antibodies or other molecules. Today, the introduction of specific amplification steps enables the detection of proteins in the femtogram range. Further, the intracellular ELISA technique, which requires the lysis of cells added to the microplate, can be used for the detection of signal transduction and apoptosis-related molecules. Moreover, cell-based

ELISAs have been developed, allowing the simultaneous detection of two proteins after the fixation of cells in the microplate well, followed by fluorescent detection. This method can be applied for the analysis of protein phosphorylation. The ELISA technique is probably one the most commonly used immunologic assays, and can and should be applied for immune monitoring if the total amount of specific antibodies or other molecules in fluids or cell culture supernatants is of specific interest and value. It does not, however, provide information about the phenotype or function of cells on a single-cell level.

ELISpot

The principle of ELISpot (enzyme-linked immunosorbent spot) assays originates from the ELISA technique. Even though first developed for the quantification of immunoglobulin-secreting B cells, it was fast adopted for the enumeration of cytokine-secreting T cells [73]. Today, ELISpot is being used for the enumeration of immune cells secreting a large variety of cytokines [74]. Undoubtedly the most commonly utilized assay is the IFN-γ ELISpot. Cells and antigens are incubated in high-protein-binding membrane-based microtiter plates coated with antibodies against the cytokine(s) of interest. Secreted and bound cytokine is made visible via an antibody-avidin-biotin-enzyme-substrate cascade. The localized enzyme causes precipitation of the substrate, which forms spots. Each spot represents an indirect imprint of a cell that secreted cytokine in response to antigen exposure. The size and staining intensity of spots can give further information about the amount of cytokine and the avidity of cells [75]. The recent combination of ELISpot and ELISA assays has been used for the quantification of antibody secretion on the individual plasma cell level [76].

One advantage of this technique is its outstanding sensitivity, which allows detection of antigen-specific cells at very low frequencies. With excellent tools available for its standardization, the assay is fairly easy to perform and to adapt to different experimental conditions [45]. Multiple samples can be analyzed in a short time, allowing for high-throughput sample processing. The recent identification of crucial protocol steps and their harmonization efforts across laboratories without imposing strict standardization on individual laboratories has decreased inter-laboratory variability substantially [25]. Recently, these systematic efforts proved the suitability of serum-free media for use in the IFN-γ ELISpot [77], providing a practical solution to overcome the leading reason for suboptimal performance in ELISpot.

Additionally, recent developments have made it possible to detect two cytokines simultaneously in one assay [78], and the introduction of fluorescent detection systems allows easy enumeration of cells secreting two or even three cytokines [79,80].

Noteworthy is the renaissance of the B-cell ELISpot, driven by the ease and sensitivity of the assay itself and the availability of newly standardized reagents and improved protocols. A B-cell ELISpot assay allows the identification and enumeration of both the total number of antibody-secreting cells as well as the number of cells that secrete antibody in response to specific antigens.

In addition to the countless studies that use a cytokine ELISpot assay for vaccination-related immune monitoring, an increasing number of reports exist for the successful application of B-cell ELISpot assays in the context of vaccination [81,82]. In the case of our cancer vaccine, care should be taken in ensuring appropriate processing and presentation of the LSPs to the specific T cells. The ability to challenge the test PBMC sample with pools of peptides (even large pools) simplifies the initial screening and reduces the need of PBMCs for performing the assay.

While the strength of ELISpot lies in its superb early screening abilities, this assay can also be used in later stage testing of vaccines, keeping in mind that it is limited to the robust detection of only a single, or possibly two, predefined cytokines per test. With a growing number of clinical reports identifying polyfunctionality as a positive correlate for disease protection, methods that allow concomitant detection of multiple cytokines need to be considered. In addition, no or limited information, for example concerning phenotype or differentiation state, about the cytokine-secreting cell can be collected using ELISpot.

Multimer assay

Fluorescent peptide MHC class I (pMHCI) multimers represent a powerful flow-cytometry-based technique to directly investigate a series of T-cell parameters at the antigen-specific level. pMHCI multimers allow the direct *ex vivo* identification, enumeration, phenotyping, and isolation of antigen-specific T cells, without any prior *in vitro* expansion or treatment [83]. Clear advantages of this assay are the ability to detect specific T cells at a frequency down to 1 specific cell in 10 000 (0.01%), the possibility to characterize antigen-specific viable T cells with a parallel combination of markers for phenotypic analysis (Figure 28.2) or functional competence (e.g., cytokine secretion, Figure 28.3), and the feasibility to successively isolate specific T-cell populations of interest for more in-depth investigations at the clonal level. Combination with CFSE labeling and short-term stimulation also enables assessment of the proliferative capacity of antigen-specific T cells (Figure 28.4). Major shortcomings, however, include limited application to only those samples with a matching haplotype, restriction of the analysis to the given epitope carried by the multimer used, requirement for large amounts of biological samples to monitor different specific responses, and the need to load each specific peptide onto the corresponding MHC molecule. Finally, in terms of detection of antigen-specific CD4 T-cell responses, development of pMHCII multimers has also been pursued in recent years; however, technical difficulties in their generation as well as the physiological lower frequency of antigen-specific CD4 T cells in the peripheral circulation compared to antigen-specific CD8 T cells limit *ex vivo* use of these reagents in the majority of the diseases studied [84,85]. Previous step(s) of *in vitro* stimulation with the cognate peptide is (are) needed to promote the proliferation/expansion of the antigen-specific CD4 T cells so as to bring them into relative frequencies that fall within the flow cytometry detection range using tetramers (generally 1 in 10 000). However, if the *in vitro* stimulation is performed in a limiting dilution setting, readout using pMHCII multimers allows estimating the precursor frequency of antigen-specific CD4 T cells. In the case of our cancer

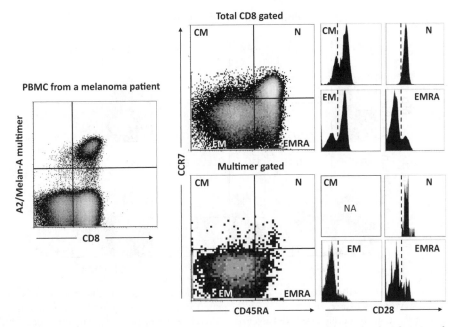

Figure 28.2 Example of direct enumeration and phenotyping of HLA-A2 restricted Melan-A$_{26-35}$ A27L specific CD8 T cells in a melanoma patient using "tetramers" (these are arrays of MHC-I/peptide complexes, the ligands of specific TCRs that are attached to a streptavidin-fluochrome conjugate via biotin. Since streptavidin has four biotin binding sites of very high affinity [10^{-14} M], each array carries four MHC-I/peptide complexes, hence the name of tetramers. However, it is clear that these arrays tend to aggregate into higher order multimers and that T cells can selectively pick up the latter. Hence, a more appropriate name would be multimers). PBMCs were analyzed in six-color flow cytometry using HLA-A2/Melan-A$_{26-35}$ A27L peptide multimers [111] and fluorescent antibody conjugates against the cell surface markers CD8, CCR7, CD45RA, and CD28. This example shows a high frequency of Melan-A$_{26-35}$ A27L antigen-specific CD8 T cells in peripheral blood (left dot plot) which are mostly, but not totally, of the effector memory type (CD45RA$^-$CCR7$^-$, deemed EM, middle lower dot plot). The majority of these EM cells in turn are CD28$^-$ (lower right histograms), indicating advanced differentiation into effector T cells [112].

vaccine, the deconvolution of the results obtained with pools of LSPs needs to be done in order to identify the target epitopes and their corresponding presenting MHC molecules. Only then can tetramers of defined MHC-peptide complexes be prepared for monitoring T cells of defined epitope specificity.

"Few (3–4) color" ICS assays

ICS is a highly informative means of assessing T-cell responses elicited by a candidate vaccine. Like ELISpot and tetramer analysis, it provides quantitative information about the magnitude of the antigen-specific response. And while T cells are the most common cell type interrogated by this method, application of ICS to B cells or other APCs has revealed that their cytokine production can greatly influence the developmental fate (Th1 or Th2) of uncommitted T-helper cells [10,86].

Similar to ELISpot, ICS typically involves *ex vivo* stimulation of a cell suspension with protein or peptides derived from the immunogen. Cytokine secretion is blocked, allowing detection by intracellular staining with cytokine-specific antibodies conjugated to fluorochromes following cell fixation and permeabilization. Simple flow cytometric instruments measure four colors, which is sufficient to distinguish expression of a single cytokine (e.g. IFN-γ, IL2, or TNF-α) in different T-cell subsets defined by antibodies specific for CD3, CD4, and CD8,

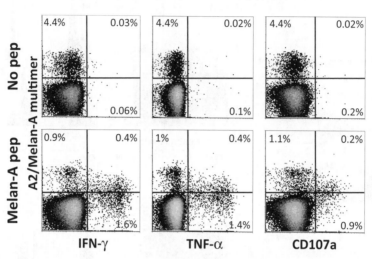

Figure 28.3 This example shows the use of multiparameter flow cytometry to assess effector functions directly at the antigen-specific CD8 T cell level. PBMCs from the same melanoma patient shown in Figure 28.2 were first labeled with HLA-A2/peptide multimers and immediately challenged with the Melan-A$_{26-35}$ $_{A27L}$ antigenic peptide for 6 hours at 37 °C. Brefeldin A was added after the first hour of incubation to block secretion of cytokines. Cells were then fixed, permeabilized, and incubated with anti-IFN-γ (left dot plots) or anti-TNF-α (middle dot plots) (for details of this labeling procedure see [113]). Anti-CD107a conjugate was added just before fixing and permeabilization to label the LAMP-1 protein that is put on the surface of the effector cells during degranulation (right dot plots). Therefore this marker is directly correlated with lytic activity of the effector CD8 T cells. The upper dot plots show the results with control cells incubated in exactly the same manner but in the absence of the antigenic peptide. The lower dot plots show that substantial proportions of HLA-A2/Melan-A$_{26-35}$ $_{A27L}$ multimer$^+$ CD8 T cells produce IFN-γ and TNF-α, and degranulate in response to short-term antigenic challenge. This is typical of EM CD28-effector CD8 T cells. It should be noted that multimer reactivity is variably downregulated because T-cell activation triggers internalization of TCRs.

or directly by antigen-specific T cells if combined with tetramers as mentioned above (Figure 28.3). This is a major advantage over ELISpot, which requires dividing often limited samples into separate CD4 and CD8 assays to obtain similar information. And, unlike tetramer analysis, there is no limitation of analysis to samples with certain MHC alleles. However, since both *ex vivo* ICS and ELISpot assays depend on the ability of T cells to produce cytokines, these assays may underestimate the magnitude of a response compared to results obtained by tetramer analysis [10,87]. In certain cases, individuals may use MHC molecules other than the known restricting one for peptide presentation. The result would be a clear dissociation between a negative tetramer assay and positive ICS and ELISpot assays.

Other assays

Other functional markers of lymphocyte activation that are relatively simple in that they involve expression of a single indicator include CD154 (CD40L; for CD4 T cells), CD137 (for CD8 T cells), CD138 (for B cells), and Ki67 (for any cell type). CD154 is essential for CD4 T cell help to APCs, including monocytes, dendritic cells, and B cells. While it is rapidly induced on CD4 T cells following antigen exposure, CD154 expression can decrease dramatically within 4–6 hours due to internalization [10,88], complicating detection by surface staining. To circumvent this, fluorescent antibody is added to culture media at the beginning of *in vitro* stimulation assays to detect transient surface CD154, while addition of the chemical monensin prevents degradation of internalized

Gated on A2/NY-ESO-1 multimer+

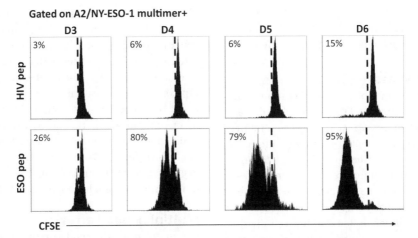

Figure 28.4 Illustration of flow cytometry-based assay of antigen-specific CD8 T cell proliferation. Cells were labeled with CFSE and immediately placed in culture with a control peptide (HIV-derived, upper row of histograms) or with the cognate NY-ESO-$1_{157-165}$ peptide [114]. Aliquots of cultures were harvested at the indicated days (Dx) and labeled with HLA-A2/NY-ESO-$1_{157-165}$ multimers. The lower left histogram shows that 26% of the multimer$^+$ cells have undergone at least one cell division. This is antigen dependent as no CFSE dilution is detectable in cells cultured with the unrelated HIV peptide (upper row).

antibody within endosomes [88]. A major advantage of CD154 staining is that it is expressed by nearly all CD4 T cells responding to cognate antigen, including those producing a wide range of cytokines, and thus serves as a global marker of CD4 T cell functionality.

There is also a single marker for measuring functional antibody-secreting B lymphocytes. While ELISpot works well to enumerate B cells secreting antibody specific for antigen, further characterization of the reactive cells is not feasible. Quantitating antigen-specific B cells by surface staining with fluorescent antigen overcomes this limitation, but can underestimate their frequency due to poor detection of B cells that have matured to plasmocytes and downregulated the B-cell receptor. However, a novel plasma cell marker, CD138 or syndecan-1, specifically identifies these cells as it is uniquely expressed at the precursor and plasma cell stages of B cell differentiation [89]. Surface staining for CD138 in conjunction with memory markers can thus reveal the phenotypic composition of a B-cell response. Of particular note, CD138, CD107a/b, and CD154 staining are all performed on live unfixed cells, which has the distinct advantage of permitting subsequent analyses such as cell sorting for nucleic

acid measurements, *in vitro* expansion in culture, and adoptive transfer.

And finally, the proliferation marker Ki67 is a valuable tool for detecting lymphocytes capable of expanding, an important indicator of protection for some diseases. Expression of this nuclear antigen, whose function is unknown, is restricted to active phases of the cell cycle (non-G_0) and thus present only in cells that recently underwent cell division [90]. It is revealed by intracellular staining with a Ki67-specific antibody. The primary advantage of Ki67 staining over other proliferative indices is that it can be measured directly on *ex vivo* specimens without any experimental manipulation (e.g., labeling or stimulation).

Complex assays

Once a vaccine demonstrates elicitation of an adaptive immune response using one or more of the above screening assays, more complex immunoassays may be employed to probe additional functional and phenotypic properties of the antigen-specific cells. In addition, alternatives to some of the classical assays described above have been developed to avoid use of hazardous radioisotopes. This section details these contemporary assays as well as more involved polyfunctional analyses.

Proliferation assay (CFSE)

Due to the importance of T-cell proliferation in controlling some pathogens [10], it may be of use to assess the proliferative capacity of vaccine-induced responses. The most common of these alternative approaches involves labeling cells with the fluorescent dye carboxyfluorescein succinimidyl ester (CFSE). This membrane-permeable dye is deacetylated in the cytoplasm, where it then covalently binds to intracellular proteins. Upon cell division, dye concentration is diluted by half as protein is equally distributed to the two daughter cells. Quantitation of the ensuing reduction in fluorescence by flow cytometry can distinguish up to seven daughter generations, making this a very powerful tool for calculating not only the proportion of cells that proliferate in response to antigen, but also the extent to which they are capable of expanding. As shown for vaccinia vaccinees, CFSE-based detection of antigen-specific cells can be more sensitive than ^{3}H-thymidine and ^{51}Cr-release assays [91]. Furthermore, dye labeling can be used in conjunction with other flow cytometric analyses, including tetramers (Figure 28.4), ICS, and memory phenotyping.

Polyfunctional assays

Multicolor ICS assays

Important qualitative information can also be gleaned from complex ICS analysis that incorporates additional phenotypic and functional markers relative to standard 3–4 color ICS. In particular, a growing body of evidence suggests that pathogen-specific T cells that concurrently express multiple Th1 cytokines are correlated with disease control or protection [10,92,93]. To measure these polyfunctional cells, panels of at least six antibodies are generally necessary to assess three cytokines (e.g., IL2, IFN-γ, and TNF-α) on CD4^{+} and CD8^{+} T cell (CD3^{+}) subsets. Staining is then measured by flow cytometry to simultaneously quantify all parameters for each individual cell to enumerate all possi-

ble combinations of cytokine production. This assay also enables measurement of the amount of each cytokine produced by each cell using fluorescence intensity, which correlates with protection in some disease models [93]. Finally, the memory phenotype of the antigen-specific population may be relevant for some diseases [94], so it may be useful to incorporate markers such as CD45RA, CD62L, and CCR7 into the multiparametric functional flow analysis (Figure 28.3). With commercially available instruments able to measure up to 18 different parameters, such complex analysis is feasible.

Multiplex bead arrays

For many diseases, good correlates of protection remain unknown. To expand the range of functions assayed and potentially define such correlates [95], multiplex bead arrays are a complementary approach to multicolor ICS. Typically, bead populations coated with cytokine-specific antibodies or antigen are used to detect secreted cytokine or antigen-specific humoral responses, respectively. A unique fluorescent spectral signature for each bead population tracks specificity, while a secondary fluorescent-revealing reagent quantifies the amount of analyte bound to each bead. Together, this allows simultaneous determination of the amount of multiple soluble factors present in a specimen [96]. Commercially available cytokine bead array kits combine 6 to 32 bead populations readily distinguished by a variety of cytometers (Figure 28.5). Alternatively, up to 500 different bead populations can be differentiated by the Luminex® system using a specialized data collection platform that identifies bead populations labeled with different proportions of fluorophores. These approaches are particularly suitable for assessing the content of mucosal secretions from vaccinees or supernatant from antigen-specific lymphocytes stimulated *ex vivo*.

New technologies

In an attempt to overcome the current hurdles in the use of multimers, a novel methodology has recently been described that allows simultaneous

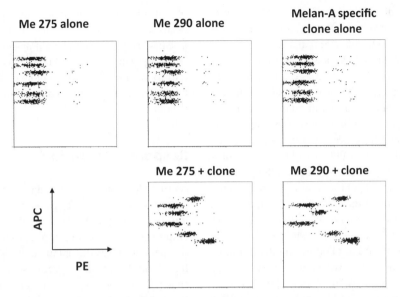

Figure 28.5 Example of six-cytokine bead array-based detection of cytokines in culture supernatant. The upper row of dot plots shows the negative cytokine profiles in supernatants (50 µl) collected from control cultures of two tumor cell lines, both expressing the tumor antigen (Melan-A presented by HLA-A2), and of the CTL specific for the Melan-A antigen alone. The lower dot plots show the profile of six cytokines present in the supernatants from CTL mixed in culture with each one of the two tumor cell lines. The incubation took place for 16 h at 37 °C. Together, these results indicate that tumor antigen recognition by cloned CD8 T cells triggers the release of variable amounts of all six cytokines tested.

detection of many T-cell specificities in a single biological sample. Using a mix of pMHC multimers labeled with different fluorochromes, combinatorial analysis can reveal T cells with different specificity and restriction in parallel within the same biological sample, as well as concomitantly visualizing the phenotype and the function of the specific cells [97,98]. In the context of clinical monitoring, this method allows a direct and broad analysis of antigen-specific T cells, without the need for large amounts of biologic material. In the near future, additional applications of this technology will likely include identification of responses to novel epitopes from potential antigen candidates and assessment of epitope spreading upon patient immunization.

Systems biology approaches have been recently advocated to gather as much information as possible to obtain a rich and sophisticated description of the perturbations taking place in the immune system upon vaccination. A promising new technology combines flow cytometry and mass spectrometry, allowing the simultaneous analysis of many parameters [99]. Genomics and proteomics at high throughput need to be matched by good bioinformatics platforms and the use of appropriate algorithms [100,101]. This new way of immunomonitoring is expected to provide biomarkers of vaccination. Obvious current drawbacks are cost and the hurdles associated with expanding its applicability, particularly in the clinical setting. Nonetheless, if gene or protein signatures predicting clinical outcome upon therapeutic vaccination are eventually identified, they will for sure find their way into the clinical arena.

Qualification and validation of immune monitoring assays

All immunologic methods used for endpoint analysis in clinical trials need to be appropriately validated according to ICH guidelines [102]. During the validation process, sources of potential assay variability are identified and quantified, and the likelihood of their occurrence is determined. The goal is to describe the performance characteristics of an assay in quantifiable terms, namely accuracy, precision, limit of detection and quantification, repeatability, linearity, robustness, and ruggedness [102]. However, the currently available guidance documents address the validation of immune assays only in a limited way, and specific challenges arise due to the absence of gold standards for many commonly used assays. Hence, accuracy cannot be reliably determined in such cases. Further, since the actual analyte in most assays relies on the interaction of antigens and antibodies, the definition of precision for those assays will be more relaxed than for biochemical methods, for instance [103]. Therefore the appropriate validation approach has to be established by each laboratory, with consideration of the nature of the immune assay(s) and the intended use [104].

Since immune assay protocols are not standardized across the entire immunotherapy field, demonstration of the method's validity is currently the responsibility of the researcher involved. Sufficient practical experience and knowledge of the assay are essential in order to make sound and logical decisions.

Assay validation is preceded by assay optimization and qualification experiments. These steps consist of experiments that determine how a range of matrix elements (everything but the analyte), as well as assay conditions, affect assay parameters and performance. The optimization data together with the scientific judgment set the acceptance criteria for the final assay validation. The qualification procedure is similar to an assay validation, but does not require predefined assay acceptance criteria.

Some reports about validation of cellular immune monitoring assays are available [105–107]. The need for laboratories to establish a suitable environment, specifically good laboratory practice (GLP), is well known and described [21,108,109]. The earlier the appropriate quality measurements are taken, the easier the transition for a laboratory from preclinical studies to progressive phases of clinical trials. While assay validation is not necessary for preclinical settings, it should be started in early trial phases and is an absolute necessity in late-stage clinical trials (Figure 28.6). It is important to keep in mind that a biologic license application might not be approved due to missing bioassay validation.

Response definition

As of today, there is little agreement on the definition of a positive immune response based on immunomonitoring data. Numerous statistical and empiric tests are being applied, complicating the comparison of results obtained by different groups. Based on results from various large-scale proficiency panels as well as simulation studies, it is now recommended to apply a nonparametric statistical test for defining positive responsiveness in ELISpot [110], which is able to control the overall false positive rate when testing multiple antigens. Importantly, a Web-based user interface is now openly available to allow easy access to and use of the proposed method (www.scharp.org/zoe/runDFR).

For ICS assays, positivity can be far more complex. Often, there are multiple outcome measures. For example, a typical ICS assay might quantify the production of IL2, IFN-γ, and/or TNF within CD4 or CD8 cells. The simplest positivity measure would be to enumerate cells that make any cytokine in either CD4 or CD8 cells – reducing the system to a single value. However, this puts the assay at the mercy of the highest background: often, TNF has far more background than the other cytokines. Another approach is to separately determine positivity for each cytokine within each lineage; in this case, that would comprise six outcomes. This has the advantage of allowing for far greater sensitivity for certain measures (e.g., IFN-γ) by lowering the threshold for positivity where there is less background. The disadvantage is the definition of sample positivity – since multiple measures are involved, the probability of false positivity increases significantly. Finally, this does not account even for the full range of outcome measures; for example, one might quantify separately every combination

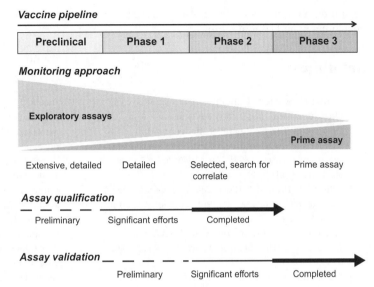

Figure 28.6 Requirement for immune monitoring along vaccine pipeline. While there needs to be as much information extracted during early phases (exploratory assays), the focus on late-stage trials is on primary assay(s), which optimally provide correlative biomarker information. Qualification and validation need to start early on, and have to be completed before entering phase III trials.

of the three cytokines (7 possibilities) within the two lineages – for a total of 14 possible outcomes. Similar to the ELISpot assay positivity, one can use a nonparametric test, or a combination of this together with a minimum threshold. Any such positivity definition should, at a minimum, be qualified and possibly validated.

In general, for any assay, whether it is a single-measure such as ELISpot or CFSE proliferation, or multiple measures such as complex ICS, positivity must be defined by a standardized approach using statistically based assessments. In general, this approach will include three major steps:

1 A pre-qualification assessment, where typically about 30 (non-immune, negative) test samples are assayed to determine potential thresholds for positivity. A smaller number of immune-reactive test samples are also run in multiple replicates, to define potential values for maximum variability.

2 A qualification assessment, where anywhere from 50 to 200 negative samples are assayed to confirm the positivity thresholds, possibly fine-tuning them. The number of samples required will depend on the desired false positive value; 100 or more are needed to set a threshold that is likely to give a reasonably accurate 5% false positive threshold. In addition, a few positive samples (typically derived from leukapheresis) are run as multiple aliquots per

day, by multiple operators, across multiple days, to fully assess variability.

3 If needed, a validation, which will be sized about the same as the qualification, and will test the *a priori* defined cutoff thresholds for positivity and maximum variance.

Validating immune assays is a difficult, laborious, and time-consuming process; only one report of a validated ICS assay has been published [105].

Summary

Many techniques exist to assess the immunologic signature of preventive or immunotherapeutic vaccines. With the combination of different techniques, disadvantages of single assays can be overcome, and advantages combined. In the light of the vaccine development pipeline, the most effective and beneficial immunomonitoring approach is to assess the breadth and magnitude of responses across various arms of the immune system early on. By defining markers of vaccine take, immunologic action, and finally correlation of protection, specific prime bioassays are chosen for advanced-stage clinical trials. Those assays need to be optimized, qualified, and finally validated under GLP guidance, including the specimen preparation. Well-designed immunomonitoring is an integral part of vaccine development and clinical testing.

References

1 Cartwright K. From Jenner to modern smallpox vaccines. *Occup Med (Lond)* 2005;**55**(7):563.

2 Coley WB. The treatment of malignant tumors by repeated inoculations of erysipelas. With a report of ten original cases. 1893. *Clin Orthop Relat Res* 1991 Jan;(262):3–11.

3 Allison JP, Dranoff G (Eds). *Cancer Immunotherapy (Advances in Immunology*, vol. 90). Elsevier Academic Press, San Diego, CA, 2006.

4 Fauci AS, Johnston MI, Dieffenbach CW, *et al*. HIV vaccine research: the way forward. *Science* 2008; **321**(5888):530–32.

5 Feldmann M, Steinman L. Design of effective immunotherapy for human autoimmunity. *Nature* 2005;**435**(7042):612–19.

6 Kantoff PW, Higano CS, Shore ND, *et al*. Sipuleucel-T immunotherapy for castration-resistant prostate cancer. *N Engl J Med* 2010;**363**(5):411–22.

7 Schuster SJ, Neelapu SS, Gause BL, et al. (Eds). Idiotype vaccine therapy (BiovaxID) in follicular lymphoma in first complete remission: phase III clinical trial results. *J Clin Oncol* 2009;**27**(18s): abstr 2.

8 Hodi FS, O'Day SJ, McDermott DF, *et al*. Improved survival with ipilimumab in patients with metastatic melanoma. *N Engl J Med* 2010;**363**(8):711–23.

9 Cohen J. AIDS research. Did Merck's failed HIV vaccine cause harm? *Science* 2007;**318**(5853): 1048–9.

10 Walker LM, Phogat SK, Chan-Hui PY, *et al*. Broad and potent neutralizing antibodies from an African donor reveal a new HIV-1 vaccine target. *Science* 2009;**326**(5950):285–9.

11 van der Burg SH. Therapeutic vaccines in cancer: moving from immunomonitoring to immunoguiding. *Expert Rev Vaccines* 2008;**7**(1):1–5.

12 Appay V, Douek DC, Price DA. CD8$^+$ T cell efficacy in vaccination and disease. *Nat Med* 2008; **14**(6):623–8.

13 Rosenberg SA, Sherry RM, Morton KE, *et al*. Tumor progression can occur despite the induction of very high levels of self/tumor antigen-specific CD8$^+$ T cells in patients with melanoma. *J Immunol* 2005;**175**(9):6169–76.

14 Speiser DE, Lienard D, Rufer N, *et al*. Rapid and strong human CD8$^+$ T cell responses to vaccination with peptide, IFA, and CpG oligodeoxynucleotide 7909. *J Clin Invest* 2005;**115**(3):739–46.

15 Verdijk P, Aarntzen EH, Punt CJ, de Vries IJ, Figdor CG. Maximizing dendritic cell migration in cancer immunotherapy. *Expert Opin Biol Ther* 2008;**8**(7): 865–74.

16 Jacobs JF, Aarntzen EH, Sibelt LA, *et al*. Vaccine-specific local T cell reactivity in immunotherapy-associated vitiligo in melanoma patients. *Cancer Immunol Immunother* 2009;**58**(1):145–51.

17 Slingluff CL, Jr, Yamshchikov GV, Hogan KT, *et al*. Evaluation of the sentinel immunized node for immune monitoring of cancer vaccines. *Ann Surg Oncol* 2008;**15**(12):3538–49.

18 de Vries IJ, Bernsen MR, Lesterhuis WJ, *et al*. Immunomonitoring tumor-specific T cells in delayed-type hypersensitivity skin biopsies after dendritic cell vaccination correlates with clinical outcome. *J Clin Oncol* 2005;**23**(24):5779–87.

19 Hoos A, Parmiani G, Hege K, *et al*. A clinical development paradigm for cancer vaccines and related biologics. *J Immunother* 2007;**30**(1):1–15.

20 Ezzelle J, Rodriguez-Chavez IR, Darden JM, *et al*. Guidelines on good clinical laboratory practice: bridging operations between research and clinical research laboratories. *J Pharm Biomed Anal* 2008; **46**(1):18–29.

21 Sarzotti-Kelsoe M, Cox J, Cleland N, *et al*. Evaluation and recommendations on good clinical laboratory practice guidelines for phase I–III clinical trials. *PLoS Med* 2009;**6**(5):e1000067.

22 Landay AL, Fleisher TA, Kuus-Reichel K, et al. *Performance of Single Cell Immune Response Assays; Approved Guideline*. Clinical and Laboratory Standards Institute, Wayne, PA, 2004, pp. 1–71.

23 Cox JH, Ferrari G, Kalams SA, *et al*. Results of an ELISPOT proficiency panel conducted in 11 laboratories participating in international human immunodeficiency virus type 1 vaccine trials. *AIDS Res Hum Retroviruses* 2005;**21**(1):68–81.

24 Britten CM, Gouttefangeas C, Welters MJ, *et al*. The CIMT-monitoring panel: a two-step approach to harmonize the enumeration of antigen-specific CD8$^+$ T lymphocytes by structural and functional assays. *Cancer Immunol Immunother* 2008;**57**(3): 289–302.

25 Janetzki S, Panageas KS, Ben-Porat L, *et al*. Results and harmonization guidelines from two large-scale international Elispot proficiency panels conducted by the Cancer Vaccine Consortium (CVC/SVI). *Cancer Immunol Immunother* 2008;**57**(3):303–15.

26 Britten CM, Janetzki S, Ben-Porat L, *et al.* Harmonization guidelines for HLA-peptide multimer assays derived from results of a large scale international proficiency panel of the Cancer Vaccine Consortium. *Cancer Immunol Immunother* 2009;**58**(10):1701–13.

27 Boaz MJ, Hayes P, Tarragona T, *et al.* Concordant proficiency in measurement of T-cell immunity in human immunodeficiency virus vaccine clinical trials by peripheral blood mononuclear cell and enzyme-linked immunospot assays in laboratories from three continents. *Clin Vaccine Immunol* 2009;**16**(2):147–55.

28 Britten CM, Janetzki S, van der Burg SH, Gouttefangeas C, Hoos A. Toward the harmonization of immune monitoring in clinical trials: quo vadis? *Cancer Immunol Immunother* 2008;**57**(3):285–8.

29 Hanekom WA, Dockrell HM, Ottenhoff TH, *et al.* Immunological outcomes of new tuberculosis vaccine trials: WHO panel recommendations. *PLoS Med* 2008;**5**(7):e145.

30 Tholen DW, Berte LM, Cooper WG, et al. *Using Proficiency Testing to Improve the Clinical Laboratory; Approved Guideline—Second edition.* Clinical and Laboratory Standards Institute, Wayne, PA, 2007, pp. 1–41.

31 Taylor CF, Field D, Sansone S-A, *et al.* Promoting coherent minimum reporting guidelines for biological and biomedical investigations: the MIBBI project. *Nat Biotechnol* 2008;**26**(8):889–96.

32 Janetzki S, Britten CM, Kalos M, et al. "MIATA" – minimal information about T cell assays. *Immunity* 2009;**31**(4):527–8.

33 Britten CM, Janetzki S, van der Burg SH, *et al.* Minimal information about T cell assays (MIATA): the process of reaching the community of T cell immunologists in cancer and beyond. *Cancer Immunol Immunother* 2011;**60**(1):15–22.

34 Valmori D, Souleimanian NE, Tosello V, *et al.* Vaccination with NY-ESO-1 protein and CpG in Montanide induces integrated antibody/Th1 responses and CD8 T cells through cross-priming. *Proc Natl Acad Sci U S A* 2007;**104**(21):8947–52.

35 Weber J. Ipilimumab: controversies in its development, utility and autoimmune adverse events. *Cancer Immunol Immunother* 2009;**58**(5):823–30.

36 Reddy ST, van der Vlies AJ, Simeoni E, *et al.* Exploiting lymphatic transport and complement activation in nanoparticle vaccines. *Nat Biotechnol* 2007;**25**(10):1159–64.

37 Trepel M, Pasqualini R, Arap W. Chapter 4. Screening phage-display Peptide libraries for vascular targeted peptides. *Methods Enzymol* 2008;**445**:83–106.

38 Kumar P, Satchidanandam V. Ethyleneglycol-bis-(beta-aminoethylether)tetraacetate as a blood anticoagulant: preservation of antigen-presenting cell function and antigen-specific proliferative response of peripheral blood mononuclear cells from stored blood. *Clin Diagn Lab Immunol* 2000;**7**(4):578–83.

39 Nicholson JK, Green TA. Selection of anticoagulants for lymphocyte immunophenotyping. Effect of specimen age on results. *J Immunol Methods* 1993;**165**(1):31–5.

40 Shalekoff S, Page-Shipp L, Tiemessen CT. Effects of anticoagulants and temperature on expression of activation markers CD11b and HLA-DR on human leukocytes. *Clin Diagn Lab Immunol* 1998;**5**(5):695–702.

41 Weinberg A, Betensky RA, Zhang L, Ray G. Effect of shipment, storage, anticoagulant, and cell separation on lymphocyte proliferation assays for human immunodeficiency virus-infected patients. *Clin Diagn Lab Immunol* 1998;**5**(6):804–7.

42 Cox JH, D'Souza M, Ratto-Kim S, *et al.* Cellular immune assays for evaluation of vaccine efficacy in developing countries. In NR Rose, RG Hamilton, B Detrick (Eds) *Manual of Clinical Laboratory Immunology.* ASM Press, Washington, DC, 2005, p. 301.

43 D'Souza P Cox JH, Ferrari G, *et al.* Endpoint assays in HIV-1 vaccine trials: functioning in a Good Laboratory Practices environment. In U Prabhakar, M Kelley (Eds) *Validation of Cell-Based Assays in the GLP Setting: A Practical Guide.* John Wiley & Sons, Chichester, 2008, pp. 239–75.

44 Bull M, Lee D, Stucky J, *et al.* Defining blood processing parameters for optimal detection of cryopreserved antigen-specific responses for HIV vaccine trials. *J Immunol Methods* 2007;**322**(1–2):57–69.

45 Janetzki S, Cox JH, Oden N, Ferrari G. Standardization and validation issues of the ELISPOT assay. *Methods Mol Biol* 2005;**302**:51–86.

46 Kierstead LS, Dubey S, Meyer B, *et al.* Enhanced rates and magnitude of immune responses detected against an HIV vaccine: effect of using an optimized process for isolating PBMC. *AIDS Res Hum Retroviruses* 2007;**23**(1):86–92.

47 Böyum A. Isolation of mononuclear cells and granulocytes from human blood. Isolation of monuclear cells by one centrifugation, and of granulocytes by combining centrifugation and sedimentation at 1 g. *Scand J Clin Lab Invest Suppl* 1968;**97**:77–89.

48 Ruitenberg JJ, Mulder CB, Maino VC, Landay AL, Ghanekar SA. VACUTAINER CPT and Ficoll density gradient separation perform equivalently in maintaining the quality and function of PBMC from HIV seropositive blood samples. *BMC Immunol* 2006;**7**:11.

49 Kreher CR, Dittrich MT, Guerkov R, Boehm BO, Tary-Lehmann M. CD4$^+$ and CD8$^+$ cells in cryopreserved human PBMC maintain full functionality in cytokine ELISPOT assays. *J Immunol Methods* 2003;**278**(1–2):79–93.

50 Russell ND, Hudgens MG, Ha R, Havenar-Daughton C, McElrath MJ. Moving to HIV-1 vaccine efficacy trials: defining T cell responses as potential correlates of immunity. *J Infect Dis* 2003;**187**:226–42.

51 Smith JG, Liu X, Kaufhold RM, Clair J, Caulfield MJ. Development and validation of a gamma interferon ELISPOT assay for quantitation of cellular immune responses to varicella-zoster virus. *Clin Diagn Lab Immunol* 2001;**8**(5):871–9.

52 Disis ML, dela Rosa C, Goodell V, *et al.* Maximizing the retention of antigen specific lymphocyte function after cryopreservation. *J Immunol Methods* 2006;**308**(1–2):13–18.

53 Filbert H, Attig S, Bidmon N, *et al.* Serum-free freezing-media support high cell quality and excellent ELISPOT assay performance across a wide variety of different assay protocols. Poster presentation, CIMT Annual Meeting 2011, Mainz, Germany, abst 117. Available at: http://meeting.cimt.eu/cimt-meeting/files/dl/CIMT_Abstractbook_2011.pdf. Accessed Feb 2012.

54 Weinberg A. Cryopreservation of peripheral blood mononuclear cells. In N Rose, RG Hamilton, B Detrick (Eds) *Manual of Clinical Laboratory Immunology.* ASM Press, Washington, DC, 2002.

55 Weinberg A, Song LY, Wilkening C, *et al.* Optimization and limitations of use of cryopreserved peripheral blood mononuclear cells for functional and phenotypic T-cell characterization. *Clin Vaccine Immunol* 2009;**16**(8):1176–86.

56 Smith JG, Joseph HR, Green T, *et al.* Establishing acceptance criteria for cell-mediated-immunity assays using frozen peripheral blood mononuclear cells stored under optimal and suboptimal conditions. *Clin Vaccine Immunol* 2007;**14**(5):527–37.

57 Immatics. Immatics Company Fact Sheet, Sep 19, 2009. Available at www.immatics.net/index.php?action=download&id=421. Accessed Feb 2012.

58 Sheehy ME, McDermott AB, Furlan SN, Klenerman P, Nixon DF. A novel technique for the fluorometric assessment of T lymphocyte antigen specific lysis. *J Immunol Methods* 2001;**249**(1–2):99–110.

59 Hermans IF, Silk JD, Yang J, *et al.* The VITAL assay: a versatile fluorometric technique for assessing CTL- and NKT-mediated cytotoxicity against multiple targets in vitro and in vivo. *J Immunol Methods* 2004;**285**(1):25–40.

60 Betts MR, Ambrozak DR, Douek DC, *et al.* Analysis of total human immunodeficiency virus (HIV)-specific CD4$^+$ and CD8$^+$ T-cell responses: relationship to viral load in untreated HIV infection. *J Virol* 2001;**75**(24):11983–91.

61 Rubio V, Stuge TB, Singh N, *et al.* Ex vivo identification, isolation and analysis of tumor-cytolytic T cells. *Nat Med* 2003;**9**(11):1377–82.

62 Wolint P, Betts MR, Koup RA, Oxenius A. Immediate cytotoxicity but not degranulation distinguishes effector and memory subsets of CD8$^+$ T cells. *J Exp Med* 2004;**199**(7):925–36.

63 Devêvre E, Romero P, Mahnke YD. LiveCount Assay: concomitant measurement of cytolytic activity and phenotypic characterisation of CD8(+) T-cells by flow cytometry. *J Immunol Methods* 2006;**311**(1–2):31–46.

64 Oehen S, Brduscha-Riem K. Differentiation of naive CTL to effector and memory CTL: correlation of effector function with phenotype and cell division. *J Immunol* 1998;**161**(10):5338–46.

65 Andoins C, de Fornel D, Fontet P, Dutartre P. Use of [35S]methionine-labelled rat lymphoblasts in microcytotoxic and limiting dilution assays. *J Immunol Methods* 1996;**192**(1–2):117–23.

66 Kantakamalakul W, Jaroenpool J, Pattanapanyasat K. A novel enhanced green fluorescent protein (EGFP)-K562 flow cytometric method for measuring natural killer (NK) cell cytotoxic activity. *J Immunol Methods* 2003;**272**(1–2):189–97.

67 Chung A, Rollman E, Johansson S, Kent SJ, Stratov I. The utility of ADCC responses in HIV infection. *Curr HIV Res* 2008;**6**(6):515–19.

68 Bures R, Gaitan A, Zhu T, *et al.* Immunization with recombinant canarypox vectors expressing membrane-anchored glycoprotein 120 followed by glycoprotein 160 boosting fails to generate antibodies that neutralize R5 primary isolates of human immunodeficiency virus type 1. *AIDS Res Hum Retroviruses* 2000;**16**(18):2019–35.

69 Pilgrim AK, Pantaleo G, Cohen OJ, *et al.* Neutralizing antibody responses to human immunodeficiency virus type 1 in primary infection and

long-term-nonprogressive infection. *J Infect Dis* 1997; **176**(4):924–32.

70 Burns DP, Desrosiers RC. A caution on the use of SIV/HIV gag antigen detection systems in neutralization assays. *AIDS Res Hum Retroviruses* 1992; **8**(6):1189–92.

71 Mascola JR, Burke DS. Antigen detection in neutralization assays: high levels of interfering anti-p24 antibodies in some plasma. *AIDS Res Hum Retroviruses* 1993;**9**(12):1173–4.

72 Mascola JR, Louder MK, Winter C, *et al.* Human immunodeficiency virus type 1 neutralization measured by flow cytometric quantitation of single-round infection of primary human T cells. *J Virol* 2002;**76**(10):4810–21.

73 Czerkinsky C, Andersson G, Ekre HP, *et al.* Reverse ELISPOT assay for clonal analysis of cytokine production. I. Enumeration of gamma-interferon-secreting cells. *J Immunol Methods* 1988; **110**(1):29–36.

74 Cox JH, Ferrari G, Janetzki S. Measurement of cytokine release at the single cell level using the ELISPOT assay. *Methods* 2006;**38**(4):274–82.

75 Hesse MD, Karulin AY, Boehm BO, Lehmann PV, Tary-Lehmann M. A T cell clone's avidity is a function of its activation state. *J Immunol* 2001; **167**(3):1353–61.

76 Bromage E, Stephens R, Hassoun L. The third dimension of ELISPOTs: quantifying antibody secretion from individual plasma cells. *J Immunol Methods* 2009;**346**(1–2):75–9.

77 Janetzki S, Price L, Britten CM, *et al.* Performance of serum-supplemented and serum-free media in IFNgamma Elispot assays for human T cells. *Cancer Immunol Immunother* 2010;**59**(4):609–18.

78 Boulet S, Ndongala ML, Peretz Y, *et al.* A dual color ELISPOT method for the simultaneous detection of IL-2 and IFN-gamma HIV-specific immune responses. *J Immunol Methods* 2007;**320**(1–2):18–29.

79 Gazagne A, Claret E, Wijdenes J, *et al.* A Fluorospot assay to detect single T lymphocytes simultaneously producing multiple cytokines. *J Immunol Methods* 2003;**283**(1–2):91–8.

80 Rebhahn JA, Bishop C, Divekar AA, *et al.* Automated analysis of two- and three-color fluorescent Elispot (Fluorospot) assays for cytokine secretion. *Comput Methods Programs Biomed* 2008;**92**(1):54–65.

81 Byers AM, Tapia TM, Sassano ER, Wittman V. In vitro antibody response to tetanus in the MIMIC system is a representative measure of vaccine immunogenicity. *Biologicals* 2009;**37**(3):148–51.

82 Doria-Rose NA, Klein RM, Manion MM, *et al.* Frequency and phenotype of human immunodeficiency virus envelope-specific B cells from patients with broadly cross-neutralizing antibodies. *J Virol* 2009;**83**(1):188–99.

83 Altman JD, Moss PA, Goulder PJ, *et al.* Phenotypic analysis of antigen-specific T lymphocytes. *Science* 1996;**274**(5284):94–6.

84 Vollers SS, Stern LJ. Class II major histocompatibility complex tetramer staining: progress, problems, and prospects. *Immunology* 2008;**123**(3):305–13.

85 Ayyoub M, Dojcinovic D, Pignon P, *et al.* Monitoring of NY-ESO-1 specific CD4$^+$ T cells using molecularly defined MHC class II/His-tag-peptide tetramers. *Proc Natl Acad Sci U S A* 2010;**107**(16):7437–42.

86 Gagro A, Servis D, Cepika AM, *et al.* Type I cytokine profiles of human naive and memory B lymphocytes: a potential for memory cells to impact polarization. *Immunology* 2006;**118**(1):66–77.

87 Sun Y, Iglesias E, Samri A, *et al.* A systematic comparison of methods to measure HIV-1 specific CD8 T cells. *J Immunol Methods* 2003;**272**(1–2):23–34.

88 Chattopadhyay PK, Yu J, Roederer M. A live-cell assay to detect antigen-specific CD4$^+$ T cells with diverse cytokine profiles. *Nat Med* 2005;**11**(10): 1113–17.

89 Wijdenes J, Vooijs WC, Clement C, *et al.* A plasmocyte selective monoclonal antibody (B-B4) recognizes syndecan-1. *Br J Haematol* 1996;**94**(2):318–23.

90 Gerdes J, Lemke H, Baisch H, *et al.* Cell cycle analysis of a cell proliferation-associated human nuclear antigen defined by the monoclonal antibody Ki-67. *J Immunol* 1984;**133**(4): 1710–15.

91 Abate G, Eslick J, Newman FK, *et al.* Flow-cytometric detection of vaccinia-induced memory effector CD4(+), CD8(+), and gamma delta TCR(+) T cells capable of antigen-specific expansion and effector functions. *J Infect Dis* 2005;**192**(8):1362–71.

92 Betts MR, Nason MC, West SM, *et al.* HIV nonprogressors preferentially maintain highly functional HIV-specific CD8$^+$ T cells. *Blood* 2006;**107**(12): 4781–9.

93 Darrah PA, Patel DT, De Luca PM, *et al.* Multifunctional TH1 cells define a correlate of vaccine-mediated protection against Leishmania major. Nat Med 2007;**13**(7):843–50.

94 Hansen SG, Vieville C, Whizin N, *et al.* Effector memory T cell responses are associated with protection of rhesus monkeys from mucosal simian immunodeficiency virus challenge. *Nat Med* 2009;**15**(3):293–9.

95 Chattopadhyay PK, Hogerkorp CM, Roederer M. A chromatic explosion: the development and future of multiparameter flow cytometry. *Immunology* 2008;**125**(4):441–9.

96 Chen R, Lowe L, Wilson JD, *et al.* Simultaneous quantification of six human cytokines in a single sample using microparticle-based flow cytometric technology. *Clin Chem* 1999;**45**(9):1693–4.

97 Hadrup SR, Bakker AH, Shu CJ, *et al.* Parallel detection of antigen-specific T-cell responses by multidimensional encoding of MHC multimers. *Nat Methods* 2009;**6**(7):520–26.

98 Newell EW, Klein LO, Yu W, Davis MM. Simultaneous detection of many T-cell specificities using combinatorial tetramer staining. *Nat Methods* 2009;**6**(7):497–9.

99 Maecker HT, Nolan GP, Fathman CG. New technologies for autoimmune disease monitoring. *Curr Opin Endocrinol Diabetes Obes* 2010;**17**(4):322–8.

100 Gaucher D, Therrien R, Kettaf N, *et al.* Yellow fever vaccine induces integrated multilineage and polyfunctional immune responses. *J Exp Med* 2008;**205**(13):3119–31.

101 Shen-Orr SS, Goldberger O, Garten Y, *et al.* Towards a cytokine-cell interaction knowledgebase of the adaptive immune system. *Pac Symp Biocomput* 2009:439–50.

102 (ICH) ICoH. Guidance for Industry: Q2B Validation of Analytical Procedures: Methodology, Sep 21, 2009. Available at www.fda.gov/downloads/ RegulatoryInformation/Guidances/UCM128049.pdf. Accessed Feb 2012.

103 Findlay JW, Smith WC, Lee JW, *et al.* Validation of immunoassays for bioanalysis: a pharmaceutical industry perspective. *J Pharm Biomed Anal* 2000;**21**(6):1249–73.

104 Lee JW, Devanarayan V, Barrett YC, *et al.* Fit-for-purpose method development and validation for successful biomarker measurement. *Pharm Res* 2006;**23**(2):312–28.

105 Horton H, Thomas EP, Stucky JA, *et al.* Optimization and validation of an 8-color intracellular cytokine staining (ICS) assay to quantify

antigen-specific T cells induced by vaccination. *J Immunol Methods* 2007;**323**(1):39–54.

106 Mander A, Chowdhury F, Low L, Ottensmeier CH. Fit for purpose? A case study: validation of immunological endpoint assays for the detection of cellular and humoral responses to anti-tumour DNA fusion vaccines. *Cancer Immunol Immunother* 2009;**58**(5):789–800.

107 Xu Y, Theobald V, Sung C, *et al.* Validation of a HLA-A2 tetramer flow cytometric method, IFNgamma real time RT-PCR, and IFNgamma ELISPOT for detection of immunologic response to gp100 and MelanA/MART-1 in melanoma patients. *J Transl Med* 2008;**6**:61.

108 Prabhakar U, Kelley M (Eds). *Validation of Cell-Based Assays in the GLP Setting: A Practical Guide.* John Wiley & Sons, Chichester, 2008.

109 Kalos M. An integrative paradigm to impart quality to correlative science. *J Transl Med* 2010;**8**:26.

110 Moodie Z, Price L, Gouttefangeas C, *et al.* Response definition criteria for ELISPOT assays revisited. *Cancer Immunol Immunother* 2010;**59**(10):1489–501.

111 Romero P, Dunbar PR, Valmori D, *et al.* Ex vivo staining of metastatic lymph nodes by class I major histocompatibility complex tetramers reveals high numbers of antigen-experienced tumor-specific cytolytic T lymphocytes. *J Exp Med* 1998;**188**(9):1641–50.

112 Romero P, Zippelius A, Kurth I, *et al.* Four functionally distinct populations of human effector-memory CD8$^+$ T lymphocytes. *J Immunol* 2007;**178**(7):4112–19.

113 Pittet MJ, Zippelius A, Speiser DE, *et al.* Ex vivo IFN-gamma secretion by circulating CD8 T lymphocytes: implications of a novel approach for T cell monitoring in infectious and malignant diseases. *J Immunol* 2001;**166**(12):7634–40.

114 Derre L, Bruyninx M, Baumgaertner P, *et al.* Distinct sets of alphabeta TCRs confer similar recognition of tumor antigen NY-ESO-1157-165 by interacting with its central Met/Trp residues. *Proc Natl Acad Sci U S A* 2008;**105**(39):15010-15.

CHAPTER 29

Clinical Development Strategy: Nuts and Bolts

Candida Fratazzi & Claudio Carini

Boston Biotech Clinical Research, Cambridge, MA, USA

Introduction

Infectious diseases remain major causes of illness, disability, and death worldwide. Increases in international travel, importation of foods, inappropriate use of antibiotics as treatments for both humans and animals, and environmental changes multiply the potential for global epidemics. International cooperation on disease surveillance, research, and training is essential to prevent or control these epidemics. Actions taken to vaccinate subjects in one country may affect disease epidemics in neighboring countries or across the world. Vaccines protect more than the vaccinated individuals.

Knowledge of vaccine safety is essential to assess accurately the risks and benefits in formulating vaccine use recommendations. In collaboration with several health maintenance organizations, the Centers for Disease Control and Prevention (CDC) has linked anonymous vaccination and medical records in a large database that is used to: (i) monitor vaccine safety, (ii) conduct active surveillance of vaccine-preventable diseases, (iii) carry out vaccine safety and immunogenicity trials, (iv) evaluate vaccine economics, and (v) assess vaccine coverage. CDC also co-sponsors the Vaccine Adverse Event Reporting System (VAERS; see Chapter 33), which is a post-marketing safety surveillance program, with the US Food and Drug Administration (FDA).

Rotavirus

Background

Rotavirus (RV) infection is the leading cause of severe acute gastroenteritis (GE) in infants and young children worldwide. In the United States, RV infection causes 2.7 million GE episodes, over 400 000 outpatient visits, up to 70 000 hospitalizations, and 60 deaths in children under 5 years of age [1,2]. RV infection is primarily transmitted via close person-to-person contact by the fecal-oral route [3]; respiratory droplets may be another mode of transmission [4]. RV disease occurs from winter to spring in temperate climates, and year-round in tropical and subtropical areas [5–8]. The varieties of different patterns of disease that occur in different parts of the world do not affect the severe nature of the disease. G and P serotypes of RV strains are mainly responsible for infection worldwide. G serotype distribution differs geographically (Figure 29.1a,b) [9].

Initial RV infection in children causes serum and mucosal antibody (Ab) response that protects against subsequent infections. The Ab response against all proteins, structural and nonstructural, is considered to be the key protection mechanism against infection. Immunoglobulin (Ig) M followed by IgA and IgG is the typical pattern of the Ab response observed in RV infection. Serum-specific IgA Abs are monitored and are considered the standard measure of immunity in vaccine clinical

---

Vaccinology: Principles and Practice, First Edition. Edited by W. John W. Morrow, Nadeem A. Sheikh, Clint S. Schmidt and D. Huw Davies.
© 2012 Blackwell Publishing Ltd. Published 2012 by Blackwell Publishing Ltd.

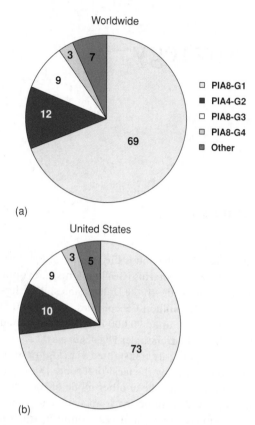

(a)

(b)

Figure 29.1 The G serotypes (G1, G2, G3, and G4) are (a) >88% (1989–2004) and (b) >97% (1973–2003) of RV strains worldwide and in the US, respectively. The P serotype (PIA) is >80% of RV strains.

trials. In children 0–24 months old, RV immunity protects against RV reinfection even if caused by a different G type [10]. It has been demonstrated that an RV asymptomatic infection induces the same level of protection as a symptomatic infection, thereby allowing the assumption that RV vaccination may provide adequate protection against RV infections [11–13].

After an incubation period of 2–4 days, RV disease manifests with abrupt onset of fever, abdominal distress, diarrhea, and vomiting. Diarrhea stools are often frequent, loose, and watery. The symptoms typically tend to last between 3 and 9 days, leading to severe dehydration with a fatal outcome in untreated infants with severe GE. Most RV infections occur in the first and second year of life,

while severe GE occurs mainly in 3–35-month-old children [1,14,15]. Viral shedding can be measured by enzyme-linked immunosorbent assay (ELISA) and reverse transcriptase-polymerase chain reaction (RT-PCR), and typically persists up to 57 days after disease onset in immunocompetent infants [16,17].

Biomarkers

Markers of RV infection are specific IgA and IgM Abs present in duodenal juice. However, both salivary and fecal anti-RV Abs can be taken as indicators of intestinal immune responses in young children [18,19]. Studies in mice have shown that a single inoculation of live virus in Ab-negative animals elicited a long-lasting protective immunity. That protection correlates with the presence of IgA intestinal Abs, while high levels of serum-neutralizing Abs of the IgG type were not related to protection [20].

Furthermore, the detection of such Abs in stool samples from both symptomatic and asymptomatic children can be taken as a marker of recently acquired infections. IgM and IgA copro-Abs remain for long periods of time after the onset of clinical disease has occurred and in the absence of viral shedding. Consistent with these findings, that fluctuations in levels of RV-IgA copro-Abs are sensitive indicators of RV reinfection, a greater-than-threefold increase of copro-IgA was detected in stool samples from young children [19].

A study of serum, fecal, and breast milk RV-Abs determined in 68 mother-infant pairs demonstrated that IgA copro-conversion was the most sensitive method for detection of symptomatic and asymptomatic RV infection in children [18]. Furthermore, it was demonstrated that, after a primary RV infection with serotype G2P [21] followed by a reinfection with a different serotype, G4P [22], 12 months later, a large increase in copro-IgA Abs occurred in the stool samples at the onset of each infection. However, copro-IgA Abs did not persist for >2 weeks after primary infection, whereas copro-IgA antibody increase persisted for >10 weeks after reinfection, resulting in a long-lasting copro-IgA response (IgA plateau).

The importance of intestinal IgA and cellular immunity, such as CD8 lymphocytes, in protecting against RV disease was confirmed by other groups [21], and correlated with titers of serum or stool anti-RV antibodies following natural infection [23,24].

Clinical development

RotaShield® by Wyeth

Clinical development of RV vaccines began in the 1980s. In August 1998, RotaShield®, a tetravalent (G1–4) rhesus-human reassortant vaccine, became the first FDA-approved RV vaccine [25]. This vaccine was studied in 9 countries and 10 816 subjects, including 5733 infants, who received the vaccine in placebo-controlled studies. Between September 1998 and July 1999, fifteen cases of intussusception (IS), an uncommon type of bowel obstruction, were reported in vaccine recipients. Case-control study, case series analysis, and observational cohort study found [26] that the rate was higher than expected when compared to the estimated attributable risk of 1/10 000 vaccines [27]. Wyeth voluntarily withdrew the vaccine from the market, and the Advisory Committee on Immunization Practices (ACIP) voted to discontinue use of RotaShield for infants in October 1999 [28].

RotaTeq® by Merck

RotaTeq is composed of five human-bovine reassortant strains of RV that are propagated in Vero cells. The vaccine was derived from the Wistar Calf 3 RV strain evaluated in clinical studies in the 1980s. Immunogenicity in animals was not evaluated due to the lack of an appropriate model. No genotoxicity, carcinogenicity, reproductive toxicity, or local tolerance studies were performed.

In 2006, RotaTeq® was licensed in the US, and has shown no safety concerns [29]. RotaTeq's Biologic License Application [30] and European Public Assessment Report [31] contained three phase III studies conducted in the US and 10 other countries. Overall 72 324 infants were treated with this oral vaccine for administration in a three-dose series, with the first dose given to healthy infants at 6–12 weeks of age followed by two subsequent doses separated by 4–10 week intervals. The GE evaluations in these studies included: (i) prevention of any grade of severity of RV-GE; (ii) prevention of severe RV-GE; and (iii) reduction in hospitalizations due to RV-GE. Primary vaccine effectiveness (VE) against RV-GE caused by naturally occurring serotypes G1, G2, G3, or G4 through the first RV season after vaccination was 74.0%, 98.0%, and 95.0% for any grade of severity, severe RV GE, and reduction of hospitalization, respectively. RotaTeq induced a three-fold or higher rise in serum anti-RV-IgA formation in 92.2–100% of infants after a three-dose regimen when compared to placebo recipients. The detected anti-RV Abs neutralized serotypes G1, G2, G3, and G4, and a selection of serotypes that contain P1. Fecal shedding was evaluated in infants. The percentage of infants who shed vaccine-virus in the stool following vaccination visit 1 was 13%. No virus was shed following the second and third doses.

Safety data from the three pivotal phase III trials demonstrated that administration of RotaTeq, when compared to placebo, conferred no increased risk for IS at 42 and 60 days post-vaccination. There was no evidence of clustering of IS cases within a seven-day window post-vaccination. Also, there did not appear to be an increased incidence of fever in infants who received RotaTeq compared to placebo. All infants in the phase III trials were permitted to receive licensed poliovirus 1, 2, 3, hepatitis B, *Haemophilus influenzae* type b, pneumococcal serotype 4, 6B, 9V, 14, 18C, 19F, and 23F, diphtheria, and tetanus vaccines. Antibody responses to these vaccines were measured after the three doses at approximately 7–8 months old; the noninferiority statistical criteria for declaring similarity between the RotaTeq and placebo group were met.

Rotarix® by GlaxoSmithKline

Rotarix is a live, attenuated strain of a human RV that is propagated in Vero cells. The vaccine is formulated with calcium carbonate as antacid, and has a shelf life of 3 years at 2–8 °C. No genotoxicity, carcinogenicity, reproductive toxicity, or local tolerance studies of Rotarix were performed.

Rotarix has been approved in 99 countries since 2004. Rotarix is indicated for the prevention of

RV-GE caused by G1 and non-G1 types. Rotarix is to be administered as a two-dose series, at $10^{6.5}$ cell culture infective dose (CCID)^{50} per dose, to healthy infants 6–24 weeks of age, with doses separated by a minimum interval of four weeks. Rotarix's Biologics License Application [32] and European Public Assessment Report [33] included eleven clinical trials, six phase II studies, and five phase III studies, and post-marketing surveillance data. Two phase III studies were considered pivotal efficacy studies. The vaccine was approved in April 2008 for marketing in the US. The first trial was conducted in 11 Latin American countries and Finland and included over 63 000 infants, who received either Rotarix or placebo; assessment of efficacy and safety was the primary objective. The second study, in 3990 infants, was conducted in 6 European countries with a primary objective being the assessment of VE against any RV-GE during the first follow-up period from two weeks after the second dose until the end of the RV epidemic season. The efficacy outcome was tested in 20 000 infants, and determination of whether two doses of Rotarix could prevent severe RV-GE caused by circulating wild-type RV strains during the period starting from two weeks post-second dose until 1 year of age was based on the rationale that the disease burden of severe RV is maximal between 5 and 11 months of age. Clinical trials showed that approximately 26% of infants shed live virus at day 7 post-first dose. In addition, live RV was detected in fewer samples from Rotarix vaccinated infants than samples from wild-type RV-GE episodes. Rotarix was effective in preventing naturally occurring RV-GE of any grade of severity during the first year of life when administered to children 6–13 weeks of age at one- or two-month intervals. Overall, vaccine efficacy was high (>80%) from first dose to 1 year of age and remained high (up 70%) during the second year of follow-up. VE was reported to be 87.1% against any RV-GE, including against G1 and G9 wild strains (>90%). VEs against severe RV-GE were 95.8% and 84.7% in trials conducted in different countries, and the anti-RV IgA sero-conversion rate, at 1–2 months post-second dose, was 86.5% and 76.8%, respectively. These results suggest that geographical or ethnic factors may affect the anti-RV IgA immune response and clinical efficacy. Two doses of Rotarix appeared immunogenic in infants.

The safety outcome measure was tested in 60 000 infants with respect to IS within 31 days after each dose based on the rationale that IS was expected to occur when vaccine virus replication and host responses are maximal. An increased risk of defined IS following Rotarix was not observed within 31 days after any dose. Pooled safety data from 36 755 infants included in eight clinical studies indicated that Rotarix demonstrated similar frequency of adverse events compared to placebo-treated infants. Rotarix appeared also to be safe when administered to preterm infants. GSK initiated an active IS surveillance in 2007 in Germany and the United Kingdom, and committed to continue it for at least two years. Co-administration of routine vaccines was allowed, with the choice of vaccines determined according to national recommendations in each country: DTPw, DTPa, HBV, Hib, IPV, MMR, and BCG. Oral polio vaccine was administered two weeks apart from RV vaccine. Two doses of hepatitis A vaccine (Havrix 720 junior, GSK), was offered to a subset of subjects between 15 and 22 months. Unrestricted feeding pre- and post-vaccination was also allowed. Another important factor was the value physician and payers put on Rotarix's two-dose regiment compared to RotaTeq's requirement for three doses. In addition to convenience and compliance advantages, Rotarix dosing could be completed, and therefore provide full protection, at a young age [9].

Post-approval clinical trials

As these RV vaccines became licensed and used in the US, Europe, and Latin America, global interest focused on the effect of these vaccines in Africa and Asia. The key question for the global community was to determine whether these vaccines worked equally well among the poorest infants in the developing world [34]. There are two issues: the first is cross-protection against the G9 serotype, which is becoming increasingly important in Asia and was not identified when the two vaccines were designed, and the G8 serotype, which is mainly prevalent across Africa. The second concern is how host factors, including malnutrition, interfering bacterial and viral agents, and breast-feeding and maternal antibodies, might neutralize the live oral vaccines. To answer these questions, both GSK and Merck started phase III trials in these areas with the support of global health agencies [35,36].

Human papillomavirus

Background

A variety of cancers have been shown to be associated with oncogenic human papillomavirus (HPV), including cervical, vulvar, anal, penile, and oropharyngeal cancers. Cervical cancer is the most common HPV-related malignancy and after breast cancer, the most commonly occurring cancer in women worldwide [37]. Infection with an oncogenic HPV type is a necessary prerequisite for the development of cervical cancer and HPV DNA can be found in virtually all cervical carcinomas [38–40].

Fourteen HPV types are considered oncogenic. The five most common oncogenic types (HPV-16, HPV-18, HPV-31, HPV-33, and HPV-45) (Figure 29.2) account for the vast majority (approximately 88%) of all cervical cancer in North America [41], with HPV-16 and -18 responsible for 76% of these

cases. HPV-18 and -45 have a relatively greater contribution to adenocarcinoma (ADC) and, combined with HPV-16, account for approximately 90% of ADC cases worldwide [40]. The underlying discoveries required to develop HPV vaccines were made in the early 1990s [42–45]. By the mid-1990s, Merck and GSK had cross-licensed the patents and began development of Gardasil and Cervarix, respectively.

Longitudinal studies suggest that acquisition of oncogenic HPV occurs rapidly following sexual debut. Approximately 50% of women who are initially HPV negative will acquire an infection within 3–4 years after onset of sexual activity [46,47]. Acquisition of HPV is highest among women younger than 25, but continues throughout life in sexually active women and remains substantial in older age groups [48–52]. Although HPV infections are very common, most are transient in nature and 70–90% will clear [53–55]. Infections that persist are at the highest risk of developing into precancerous lesions and cancer [56–59] (Figure 29.3).

Guidelines published by the World Health Organization (WHO) [60,61] concluded that virologic endpoints, including persistent infection, have predictive value. Both sequential and simultaneous infections with multiple oncogenic HPV types are common in sexually active young women, and those with cytological abnormalities [62–64].

Biomarkers

Biomarkers that correlate with progression to neoplasia in HPV infection have been identified. These biomarkers can be used to diagnosis, assist in the diagnosis of HPV-induced cancer [65,66], and increase the positive predictive value of current screening modalities [66]. In addition, they can provide insights into the biology of HPV-induced cancer that may lead to development of nonsurgical therapies [66]. Preferred biomarkers for HPV-induced cancer include cornulin, DJ-l, PA28α and PA28β, trp-tRNA synthetase, HSPβ6, creatine kinase B, aflatoxin reductase, GST p, transthyretin, transferrin, a2-type 1 collagen, and combinations of them [67,68].

Cervical cancer cells and HPV head and neck cancer cells express three testis-specific genes not

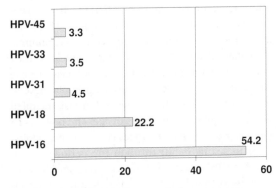

Figure 29.2 North American cervical cancer cases (percentage attributed to oncogenic HPV types). The five most common oncogenic types (HPV-16, HPV-18, HPV-31, HPV-33, and HPV-45) account for the vast majority (~88%) of all cervical cancer in North America [41].

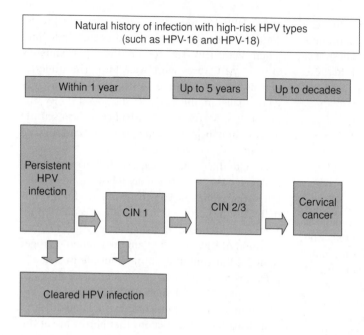

Figure 29.3 Natural history of persisting HPV-16 and HPV-18 infections are at the highest risk of developing into precancerous lesions and cancer. CIN, cervical intraepithelial neoplasm; HPV, human papilloma virus.

normally observed in somatic cells: testicular cell adhesion molecule 1 (TCAM1), synaptosomal complex protein 2 (SYCP2), and stromal antigen 3 (STAG3) [69]. Increased expression of these three genes compared to a normal standard is indicative of disease [68,70–72]. Among those three markers, TCAM1 and SYCP2 are considered early detection markers. Diagnosis of cervical cancer has been based on methods determining the expression level of TCAM1, SYCP2, and STAG3 genes in either cervical smear sample or fluid sample collected by vaginal rinsing. The idea of using methods with a combinatory approach of including biomarkers such as hTERT, IGFBP-3, transferrin receptor, beta-catenin, Myc-HPV E6 interaction, HPV E7, and telomere length has been proven potentially successful for diagnosis [72] and for evaluating the treatment efficacy of cervical cancer [67,70].

Clinical development

Gardasil® by Merck

Gardasil is a quadrivalent vaccine composed of the major capsid protein (L1) of four HPV types (6, 11, 16, and 18), each of which is produced separately in recombinant *Saccharomyces cerevisiae*, adsorbed on an adjuvant (amorphous aluminum hydroxyphosphate sulfate) [73]. The product was found to be extremely stable, with a half-life of over 10 years when the vaccine is kept at room temperature [74,75].

The clinical development program for Gardasil®, which was FDA-approved in October 2009, included six phase I and II clinical studies conducted between 1997 and 2004 to characterize safety and immune responses among different doses. Two larger phase II studies were also conducted between 2000 and 2004, and included clinical endpoints. Two phase III studies evaluating the clinical efficacy and safety were included in the Biologics License Application [76], and the European Public Assessment Report [77]. The studies of Gardasil included girls and women, 9–26 years of age, and boys, 9–15 years of age. These age ranges cover the period just prior to sexual debut through the period of peak risk for HPV infection. Subjects were enrolled regardless of baseline HPV status because vaccination programs will be population-based. Inclusion of subjects with prior or ongoing HPV infection also allowed for evaluation of the effect of such infection on the efficacy, immunogenicity, and safety of Gardasil. The clinical program was conducted in

5 continents and 33 countries. Efficacy was assessed in 20 887 randomized women in the 16–26 year age range. Efficacy was durable through at least 2.5 years with respect to diseases caused by HPV-6, -11, and -18, and at least 3.5 years with respect to disease caused by HPV-16. Long-term study with a 15-year follow-up was part of the post-approval commitment and is still ongoing. Immunogenicity was tested in 12 344 subjects from 1 month after completion of the three-dose vaccination regimen and up to 3.5 years thereafter.

Safety was evaluated in 16 014 subjects with regard to: (i) injection site reaction and systemic tolerability, (ii) impact on long-term health status, and (iii) interaction with pregnancy and lactation. There was no signal with respect to allergic reaction and the proportions of subjects reporting new medical conditions were comparable between Gardasil and placebo subjects. No impact on pregnancy outcomes and nursing mother or child was observed. The concomitant administration of hepatitis B vaccine also showed no interference with mounting of the immune response.

Cervarix® by GlaxoSmithKline

Cervarix is a bivalent vaccine composed of HPV types 16 and 18, each of which is produced separately using a recombinant Baculovirus expression system and the insect cell line Hi-5 Rix4446. The antigens are formulated with AS04 adjuvant comprising aluminum hydroxide and 3-O-desacyl-4-monophosphoryl lipid A (MPL).

Cervarix was FDA-approved in March 2007. Studies included women naïve (without current infection and without prior exposure) or non-naïve (with current infection and/or prior exposure) to HPV at the time of vaccination. The clinical development program included approximately 30 000 healthy women, with over 16 000 women having received at least one dose of Cervarix with a long-term follow-up to 6.4 years included in the Biologics License Application [78] and European Public Assessment Report [79]. Studies were conducted in over 30 countries from different geographical regions, and included 4332 subjects from the US. Data were collected from six controlled phase II/III studies and four uncontrolled or consistency phase

II/III studies. The efficacy of the vaccine was evaluated in women 15–25 years old; however, Cervarix is targeted for girls 10–14 years of age. Efficacy studies could not be conducted in girls 10–14 years of age as endpoints evaluation required gynecological evaluation, which was not feasible in this age group. Therefore, immune-bridging was performed in girls below 15 years of age. As the study population was pre-screened prior to vaccination, these data provide insights into the vaccine benefits against HPV infection and diseases progression in a population presumed naïve to oncogene HPV prior to vaccination, which is closely representative of the young adolescents targeted for primary prevention of cervical cancer. In women presumed to be HPV naïve, the high level of efficacy correlated with 6-month and 12-month persistent infection with HPV-16 and -18 following Cervarix administration. The observed vaccine efficacy against CIN1+ and CIN2+ associated with HPV-16 and -18 was 100% (Figure 29.3) and showed maintenance of high vaccine efficacy up to 6.4 years postvaccination. Cervarix is currently licensed in over 95 countries worldwide.

The safety profile of Cervarix and the adjuvant system was further confirmed by data from over 57 000 women, with over 33 000 of them receiving at least one dose of Cervarix, and a meta-analysis of more than 68 000 subjects with over 36 000 subjects receiving Cervarix or other AS04-containing vaccines. Approximately 7 million doses of Cervarix have been distributed (May 2009) [78] and the number of subjects exposed is estimated to be over 2 million. With the majority of subjects in the clinical database consisting of women 15–25 years of age, safety was evaluated with regard to: (i) pregnancy and pregnancy outcomes, and (ii) incidence of autoimmune disorders. Similar overall rates of pregnancy outcomes, spontaneous pregnancy loss, and events of potentially autoimmune etiology were observed in vaccine and control groups. An extensive risk management program to further monitor the safety of Cervarix, including clinical trials among HIV-positive women, long-term immunogenicity, and co-administration trials, is still ongoing. Indeed, the immune response detected in the women 15–25 years of age was compared with the immune response detected in the 10–14-year-old group, which also provided additional safety and immunogenicity data in this younger age group. Finally, an extension study, up to 18 months post-vaccination, supported extension of indication from 10 years through 25 years of age.

Summary

A high standard of safety is expected of vaccines since they are recommended for, and administered to, millions of healthy people, including infants. Vaccine developments have been shown to have a significant impact on global disease burden and are an important strategy to control disease morbidity and mortality. Clinical trial confirmatory data must prove that the vaccine is efficacious in the broad study groups, who were representative of the population. Therefore, vaccines undergo an extensive clinical development program in a diverse population, with a broad age range, nutritional status, and routine vaccinations. Furthermore, vaccines must induce an immune response regardless of gender, ethnicity, national origin, body mass index, smoking status, sexual partners, and many other parameters according to the target population.

Each vaccine development offers specific challenges; in the case of RV vaccines Merck and GSK started the development of RotaTeq and Rotarix, following the experience with RotaShield. For both companies, the first order of business was to show that their vaccines did not trigger IS, a task that was hugely complicated. Attempting to prove the absence of a very small risk forced the companies to conduct some of the most massive and expensive clinical trials ever undertaken. These two tests are the largest vaccine trials conducted by drug companies and the largest by any sponsor since the March of the Dimes trials in the 1950s, which led to the eradication of polio in the western world. Their phase III clinical trials were watched closely by an independent safety panel that would have halted the trials if an increased risk of IS was detected.

In the case of HPV vaccines, although implementation of cervical screening programs has drastically reduced the lifetime risk of cervical cancer in the US, the absolute burden of cancerous and precancerous lesions still remains considerable. Cervical screening practices can frequently miss the precursor lesions of adenocarcinoma, the most aggressive form of cervical cancer, resulting in an increase in its incidence to approximately 20% of all cervical cancers in the US. Recent studies have shown that HPV can be detected in 98.7% of all cervical carcinomas. HPV infections are responsible for sexually transmitted infections in 25% of the population of many European countries, 70% of the US population, and 95% of the population in Africa.

In conclusion, in its complexity, any vaccine development program should prove that geographical and ethnic factors do not affect the immune response.

Acknowledgment

We thank Janice M. Reichert, PhD, Senior Research Fellow, Tufts CSDD; Editor-in-Chief mAbs; VP and Board of Directors, The Antibody Society, for her contribution to the development and review of this chapter.

References

1 Charles MD, Holman RC, Curns AT, et al. Hospitalizations associated with rotavirus gastroenteritis in the United States, 1993–2002. Pediatr Infect Dis J 2006;**25**(6):489–93.

2 Kilgore PE, Holman RC, Clarke MJ, Glass RI. Trends of diarrheal disease-associated mortality in US children, 1968 through 1991. JAMA 1995;**274**(14):1143–8.

3 Butz AM. Prevalence of rotavirus on high risk fomites in day care facilities. Pediatrics 1993;**92**:202–5.

4 Santosham M, Yolken RH, Wyatt RG, et al. Epidemiology of rotavirus diarrhea in a prospectively monitored American Indian population. J Infect Dis 1985; **152**:778–83.

5 Visikari T, Rautanen T, Von Bonsdorff CH. Rotavirus gastroenteritis in Finland: burden of disease and epidemiological features. Acta Paediatr Suppl 1999; **88**(426):24–30.

6 Frühwirth M, Heininger U, Ehlken B, et al. International variation in disease burden of rotavirus

gastroenteritis in children with community- and nososcomial acquired infection. *Pediatr Infect J.* 2001; **20**(8):784–91.

7 Ruggeri FM, Declich S. Rotavirus infection among children with diarrhoea in Italy. *Acta Peadiatr Suppl* 1999;**88**(426):66–71.

8 Yaluapari JP, Alvarez C, Kurt P, *et al.* Epidemiological surveillance of rotavirus diarrhea in Mexico. 3rd World Congress of the World Society for Pediatric Infectious Diseases, Santiago, Chile, Nov 19–23, 2002, abst.

9 Santos N, Hoshino Y. Global distribution of rotavirus serotypes/genotypes and its implication for the development and implementation of an effective rotavirus vaccine. *Rev Med Virol* 2005;**15**(1):29–56.

10 Velázquez FR, Matson DO, Calva JJ, *et al.* Rotavirus infections in infants as protection against subsequent infections. *N Engl J Med* 1996;**335**(14):1022–8.

11 Bernstein DI, Sander DS, Smith VE, Schiff GM, Ward RL. Protection from rotavirus reinfection:two year prospective study. *J Infect Dis* 1991;**164**:277–83.

12 Ward RL, Bernstein DI. Protection against rotavirus diseases after natural rotavirus infection. *US Rotavirus Vaccine Efficacy Group.* J Infect Dis 1994;**69**:900–904.

13 Ward RL. Mechanism of protection against rotavirus in humans and mice. *J Infect Dis* 1996;**174**:51–8.

14 Ehlken B, Laubereau B, Karmaus W, *et al.* Prospective population-based study on rotavirus diseases in Germany. *Acta Paediatr* 2002;**91**(7):769–75.

15 Parashar UD, Alexander JP, Glass RI. Prevention of rotavirus gastroenteritis among infants and children: recommendations of the Advisory Committee on Immunization Practices (ACIP). *MMWR Morb Mortal Wkly Rep* 2006;**55**(RR12):1–13.

16 Vesikari T, Sarkkinen HK, Mäki M. Quantitative aspects of rotavirus excretion in childhood diarrhea. *Acta Peadiatr Scand* 1981;**70**(5):33–6.

17 Richardson K, Grimwood K, Gorrell R, *et al.* Extended excretion of rotavirus after severe diarrhea in young children. *Lancet* 1998;**351**:1844–8.

18 Bishop RF, Bugg HC, Masendycz PJ, *et al.* Serum, fecal, and breast milk rotavirus antibodies as indices of infection in mother-infant pairs. *J Infect Dis* 1996;**174**(Suppl 1):S22–9.

19 Coulson BS, Grimwood K, Hudson IL, Barnes GL, Bishop RF. Role of coproantibody in clinical protection of children during reinfection with rotavirus. *J Clin Microbiol* 1992;**30**:1678–84.

20 Estes MK. Advances in molecular biology: impact on rotavirus vaccine development. *J Infect Dis* 1996;**174**(Suppl 1):S37–46.

21 Burns WB, Siadat-Pajouh M, Krishnaney AA, Greenberg HB. Protective effect of rotavirus VP6-specific IgA monoclonal antibodies that lack neutralizing activity. *Science* 1996;**272**(5258):104–7.

22 Cukor G, Blacklow NR. Human viral gastroenteritis. *Microbiol Rev* 1984;**48**(2):157–79.

23 Coulson BS. Typing of human rotavirus VP4 by an enzyme immunoassay using monoclonal antibodies. *J Clin Microbiol* 1993;**31**(1):1–8.

24 Gómez J, Estes MK, Matson DO, *et al.* Serotyping of human rotavirus in Argentina by ELISA with monoclonal antibodies. *Arch Virol* 1990;**112**(3–4): 249–59.

25 Advisory Committee on Immunization Practices. Rotavirus vaccine for the prevention of rotavirus gastroenteritis among children. *MMWR Morb Mortal Wkly Rep* 1999;**48**:1–20.

26 Murphy T, Gargiullo PM, Massoudi MS, *et al.* Intussusception among infants given an oral rotavirus vaccine. *N Engl J Med* 2001;**344**:1564–8.

27 Peter G, Myers MG. Intussusception, rotavirus, and oral vaccines: summary of a workshop. *Pediatrics* 2002;**110**:67–9.

28 CDC. Withdrawal of rotavirus vaccine recommendation. *MMWR Morb Mortal Wkly Rep* 1999;**48**(43): 1007–8.

29 Vesikari T, Matson DO, Dennehy P, *et al.* Safety and efficacy of a pentavalent human-bovine (WC3) reassortant rotavirus vaccine. *N Engl J Med* 2006;**534**(1): 23–33.

30 Tiernan R. FDA Briefing Document, RotaTeq™ (rotavirus vaccine, live, oral, pentavalent), Merck & Co, Inc., STN125122, Dec 14, 2005.

31 European Medicines Agency. RotaTeq European Public Assessment Report (EMEA/H/C/669). Available at www.ema.europa.eu/ema/index.jsp?curl=pages/ medicines/human/medicines/000669/human_med_ 001045.jsp. Accessed Feb 2012.

32 Kitsutani P. Clinical Review for STN 125265/0 Rotarix: Rotavirus Vaccine, Live, Oral, GlasoSmithKline Biologicals, FDA, STN125265/0, Mar 10, 2008. Available at www.fda.gov/downloads/biologicsblood vaccines/vaccines/approvedproducts/ucm133580.pdf. Accessed Feb 2012.

33 European Medicines Agency. Rotarix European Public Assessment Report (EMEA/526825/2009; EMEA/ H/C/639). Available at www.ema.europa.eu/ema/ index.jsp?curl=pages/medicines/human/medicines/ 000639/human_med_001043.jsp. Accessed Feb 2012.

34 Dennehy PK. Rotavirus vaccines:an overview. *Clin Microbiol Rev* 2008;**21**(1):198–208.

35 Glass RI, Parashar UD. The promise of new rotavirus vaccines. *New Engl J Med* 2006;**354**:75–7.

36 Roberts L. Vaccines. Rotavirus vaccines' second chance. *Science* 2004;**305**(5692):1890–93.

37 Ferlay J, Bray F, Pisani P, Parkin DM. *GLOBOCAN 2002: Cancer Incidence, Mortality and Prevalence Worldwide*. IARC CancerBase No. 5, version 2.0, Lyon: IARC Press, 2004.

38 Bosch FX, Manos MM, Muñoz N, *et al.* Prevalence of human papillomavirus in cervical cancer: a worldwide perspective. International biological study on cervical cancer (IBSCC) Study Group. *J Natl Cancer Inst* 1995;**87**(11):796–802.

39 Walboomers JM, Jacobs MV, Manos MM, *et al.* Human papillomavirus is a necessary cause of invasive cervical cancer worldwide. *J Pathol* 1999;**189**:12–19.

40 Bosch FX, Burchell AN, Schiffman M, *et al.* Epidemiology and natural history of human papillomavirus infections and type-specific implications in cervical neoplasia. *Vaccine* 2008;**26**(Suppl 10):K1–16.

41 Smith JS, Lindsay L, Hoots B, *et al.* Human papillomavirus type distribution in invasive cervical cancer and high-grade cervical lesions: a meta-analysis update. *Int J Cancer* 2007;**121**(3):621–32.

42 McNeil C. Who invented the VLP cervical cancer vaccines? *J Natl Cancer Inst* 2006;**98**(7):433–6.

43 Giannini SL, Hanon E, Moris P, *et al.* Enhanced humoral and memory B cellular immunity using HPV16/18 L1 VLP vaccine formulated with the MPL/aluminum salt combination (AS04) compared to aluminum salt only. *Vaccine* 2006;**24**:5937–49.

44 Lowe RS, Brown DR, Bryan JT, *et al.* Human papillomavirus type 11 (HPV-11) neutralizing antibodies in the serum and genital mucosal secretions of African green monkeys immunized with HPV-11 virus-like particles expressed in yeast. *J Infect Dis* 1997;**6**:11–16.

45 Palker TJ, Monteiro JM, Martin MM, *et al.* Antibody, cytokine and cytotoxic T lymphocyte responses in chimpanzees immunized with human papillomavirus virus-like particles. *Vaccine* 2001;**19**:3733–43.

46 Winer RL, Kiviat NB, Hughes JP, *et al.* Development and duration of human papillomavirus lesions, after initial infection. *J Infect Dis* 2003;**191**:731–8 .

47 Moscicki AB, Ma Y, Holland C, Vermund SH. Cervical ectopy in adolescent girls with and without human immunodeficiency virus infection. *J Infect Dis* 2001;**183**(6):865–70.

48 Muñoz N, Méndez F, Posso H, *et al.* Incidence, duration and determinants of cervical human papillomavirus infection in a cohort of Colombian women

with normal cytological results. *J Infect Dis* 2004;**190**(2):2077–87.

49 Bory JP, Cucherousset J, Lorenzato M, *et al.* Recurrent HPV infection detected with the hybrid capture II assay selects women with normal smears at risk for developing high grade cervical lesions: a longitudinal study of 3,091 women. *Int J Cancer* 2002;**102**:519–25.

50 Dalstein V, Riethmuller D, Prétet JL, *et al.* Persistence and load of high-risk HPV are predictors for development of high-grade cervical lesions: a longitudinal French cohort study. *Int J Cancer* 2003;**106**:396–403.

51 Franco EL, Villa LL, Sobrinho JP, *et al.* Epidemiology of acquisition and clearance of cervical human papillomavirus infection in women from a high-risk area for cervical cancer. *J Infect Dis* 1999;**180**:1415–23.

52 Grainge MJ, Seth R, Guo L, *et al.* Cervical human papillomavirus screening among older women. *Emerg Infect Dis* 2005;**11**(11):1680–85.

53 Brown DR, Shew ML, Qadadri B, *et al.* A longitudinal study of genital human papillomavirus infection in a cohort of closely followed adolescent women. *J Infect Dis* 2005;**191**(2):182–92.

54 Richardson K, Kelsall G, Tellier P, *et al.* The natural history of type-specific human papillomavirus infections in female university students. *Cancer Epidemiol Biomarkers Prev* 2003;**12**:485–90.

55 Moscicki AB, Shiboski S, Broering J, *et al.* The natural history of human papillomavirus infection as measured by repeated DNA testing in adolescent and young women. *J Pediatr* 1998;**132**:277–84.

56 Ho GY, Burk RD, Klein S, *et al.* Persistent genital human papillomavirus infection as a risk factor for persistent cervical dysplasia. *J Natl Cancer Inst* 1995;**87**:1365–71.

57 Hildesheim A, Schiffman MH, Gravitt PE, *et al.* Persistence of type-specific human papillomavirus infection among cytological normal women. *J Infect Dis* 1994;**169**:235–40.

58 Schiffman M, Herrero R, Desalle R, *et al.* The carcinogenicity of human papillomavirus types reflects viral evolution. *Virology* 2005;**337**(1):76–84.

59 Schlecht NF, Platt RW, Duarte-Franco E, *et al.* Human papillomavirus infection and time to progression and regression of cervical intraepithelial neoplasia. *J Natl Cancer Inst* 2003;**95**:1336–43.

60 Pagliusi SR, Teresa Aguado M. Efficacy and other milestones for human papillomavirus vaccine introduction. *Vaccine* 2004;**23**:569–78.

61 WHO. *Guidelines to Assure the Quality, Safety and Efficacy of Recombinant HPV Virus-Particle Vaccine.* Geneva, Switzerland, 2006.

62 Ho GY, Palan PR, Basu J, *et al.* Viral characteristics of human papillomavirus infection and antioxidant levels as risk factors for cervical dysplasia. *Int J Cancer* 1998;**78**:594–9.

63 Herrero R, Hildesheim A, Bratti C, *et al.* Population-based study of human papillomavirus infection in cervical neoplasia in rural Costa Rica. *J Natl Cancer Inst* 2000;**92**:464–74.

64 Rousseau MC, Villa LL, Costa MC, *et al.* Occurance of cervical infection with multiple HPV types is associated with age and cytologic abnormalities. *Sex Transm Dis* 2003;**30**:581–7.

65 Boulet GA, Horvath CA, Depuydt CE, Bogers JJ. Biomarkers in cervical screening: quantitative reverse PCR analysis of P16NK4a expression. *Eur J Cancer Prev* 2010;**19**(1):35–7.

66 Wentzensen N, Schiffman M, Dunn ST, *et al.* Grading the severity of cervical neoplasia based on combined histopathology, cytopathology, and HPV genotype distribution among 1,700 women referred to colposcopy in Oklahoma. *Int J Cancer* 2009;**124**(4): 964–67.

67 Boulet GA, Benoy IH, Depuydt CE, *et al.* Human papilloma virus 16 load and E2/E6 ratio in HPV16-positive women: biomarkers for cervical intraepithelial neoplasia greater than or equal to 2 in a liquid based cytology setting? *Cancer Epidemiol Biomark Prev* 2009;**18**(11):2992–6.

68 Chung YL, Lee MY, Horng CF, *et al.* Use of combined molecular biomarkers for prediction of clinical outcome in locally advanced tonsillar cancer treated with chemoradiotherapy alone. *Head Neck* 2009;**31**(1):9–20.

69 Pyeon D, Newton MA, Lambert PF, *et al.* Fundamental differences in cell cycle deregulation in human papillomavirus-positive and human papillomavirus-negative head/neck and cervical cancers. *Cancer Res* 2007;**67**(10):4605–19.

70 Kiviat NB, Hawes SE, Feng Q. Screening for cervical cancer in the era of the HPV vaccine – the urgent need for both new screening guidelines and new biomarkers. *J Natl Cancer Inst* 2008;**100**(5):290–96.

71 Ruiz W, McClements WL, Jansen KU, Esser MT. Kinetics and isotype profile of antibody responses in rhesus macaques induced following vaccination with HPV 6, 11, 16 and 18 L1-virus-like particles formulated with or without Merck aluminum adjuvant. *J Immune Based Ther Vaccines* 2005;**3**(1):1–11.

72 De Wilde J, Wilting SM, Meijer CJ, *et al.* Gene expression profiling to identify markers associated with deregulated hTERT in HPV transformed keratinocytes and cervical cancer. *Int J Cancer* 2008;**112**(4):8–11.

73 Bryan JT. Developing an HPV vaccine to prevent cervical cancer and genital warts. *Vaccine* 2007; **25**:3001–6.

74 Shank-Retzlaff ML, Zhao Q, Anderson C, *et al.* Evaluation of the thermal stability of Gardasil. *Hum Vaccin* 2006;**2**:147–54.

75 Shi L, Sings HL, Bryan JT, *et al.* GARDASIL: prophylactic human papillomavirus vaccine development – from bench top to bed-side. *Clin Pharmacol Ther* 2007; **81**:259–64.

76 FDA Briefing Document. Human Papillomavirus (Types 6, 11, 16, 18) recombinant vaccines, STN125126, 2006.

77 Gardasil European Public Assessment Report (EMEA/ H/C/703). Available at www.ema.europa.eu/ema/ index.jsp?curl=pages/medicines/human/medicines/ 000703/human_med_000805.jsp. Accessed Feb 2012.

78 FDA Briefing Document. Human Papillomavirus Bivalent (Types 16 and 18) Vaccine, Recombinant/ CERVARIX®, STN125259, 2010.

79 Cervarix European Public Assessment Report (EMEA/ H/C/721). Available at www.ema.europa.eu/ema/ index.jsp?curl=pages/medicines/human/medicines/ 000721/human_med_000694.jsp. Accessed Feb 2012.

CHAPTER 30

Current Approaches to Identify and Evaluate Cancer Biomarkers for Patient Stratification

Robert Rees[1,3], Stephanie Laversin[1], Cliff Murray[2], & Graham Ball[1,3]

[1]The John van Geest Cancer Research Centre, School of Science and Technology, Nottingham Trent University, Nottingham, UK
[2]Source BioScience, Nottingham, UK
[3]CompandX Ltd, Nottingham, UK

General overview

As a consequence of the unacceptably high attrition rates seen in taking new cancer therapies through to phase III and ultimately licensing, the US Food and Drug Administration (FDA) has identified a need for better "product evaluation tools" in the drug development process. Such tools will hopefully lead to safer and more effective drugs and, in turn, improved patient outcome [1]. Similar sentiments are expressed in the EU's latest research program (European Union Seventh Framework Programme, 2007–2013). Pressure, therefore, from the FDA and the EU is helping to drive an emerging market for biomarkers and other tools for stratifying patients according to likely response to new treatments. Of course this search is also driven by economic pressure on the pharma/biotech sector to make earlier go/no-go decisions on new therapeutics.

This need to provide more effective therapies for the treatment of cancer translates in practice into a requirement for more "targeted" therapies, based on an understanding of the molecular profile of the individual cancer as well as knowledge of that patient's ability to respond to a specific treatment. In this regard, a holistic approach to being able to predict the outcome of treatment, whether this is based on conventional therapy, such as surgery, radiotherapy, or chemotherapy, or on gene or immunotherapy, is required. Cancer, and breast cancer in particular, is recognized as a highly heterogeneous disease. Sorlie *et al.* [2] proposed five different forms based on genomic profiling. Since then, based on further genomic profiling, it has been hypothesized that up to 80 forms may exist [3], each of these having a different response to therapy.

Historically there has been a need to stratify patients into prognostic groups and into therapeutic response groups. Given the primary treatment for many cancers is surgery, the opportunity arises for molecular and genomic profiling of tumors. However, breast cancer is only one example, among many, where there is an underlying requirement to stratify patients for therapy into subgroups. Detailed analysis of the tumor tissues and blood samples of patients using genomic, proteomic, or transcriptomic technologies offers the potential for development of new prognostic, diagnostic, and

Vaccinology: Principles and Practice, First Edition. Edited by W. John W. Morrow, Nadeem A. Sheikh, Clint S. Schmidt and D. Huw Davies.
© 2012 Blackwell Publishing Ltd. Published 2012 by Blackwell Publishing Ltd.

predictive tools based on biomarker genes and proteins.

The data generated by these approaches is, however, extremely complex and of high dimensionality. Care must be taken that the assumptions of the statistical approaches employed remain valid under these conditions. Thus, generation of predictive tools will require the development and application of new statistical methods that deal with this complexity, reduce the rate of false detection, and result in a parsimonious set of biomarkers. Furthermore, addressing such issues necessitates validation of individual technological platforms and the resulting biomarkers using multiple blinded datasets.

Once identified, the results of these developments will allow identification and modeling of disease-related pathways important not only for patient stratification, but also for the design of new intervention therapies. Molecular definition of disease, which in some cases is capable of defining the optimal treatment for a patient, is rapidly replacing traditional pathology-based assessment; this is especially true for cancer and many common chronic diseases. The application of current therapies for personalized medicine is driven by biomarkers that identify patients who are likely to benefit from a given treatment and it is important that we identify how we can effectively integrate robust biomarkers in drug development and clinical practice. The qualitative and quantitative expression of biomarkers relevant to disease status and predicted outcome of therapy will contribute to their acceptance in patient management.

Breast cancer: developmental risk

Globally, breast cancer has the fifth highest mortality of all cancers, according to the World Health Organization (WHO). Breast cancer is the most commonly diagnosed cancer in women under the age of 35, with the highest incidence in postmenopausal women. Improvements have been made in survival, largely due to patient management and wider treatment options. In 2005, the five-year survival rate was 80%, compared with only 50% in the 1970s (see http://info.cancerresearchuk.org).

Genetically, 5–10% of all breast cancer cases have inherited one or several gene mutations associated with a predisposition to the disease. The genes BReast CAncer susceptibility 1 and 2 (BRCA1 and BRCA2) [4], p53, and the Cowden disease gene PTEN/MMAC1 are tumor suppressor genes and their ineffective mutated forms have been linked to a high risk of developing breast cancer [5]. BRCA1 and BRCA2 are the best-known inherited "high-risk" breast cancer genes [6,7], responsible for about 80% of the familial breast cancers and 5–6% of all breast cancers [8].

The majority of breast cancers develop sporadically (no familial history), often due to somatic mutations or incorrectly regulated genes in the breast cells [9–11]. Overexpression of oncogenic epidermal growth factor receptors (EGFR, HER2, ERBB3, ERBB4) and intracellular signaling molecules (c-Src, h-Ras) and inactivation of tumor suppressor genes such as cell cycle regulators (RB1, p53) are frequently found in sporadic cases of breast cancer. In conclusion, the predisposition to breast cancer for a woman is determined by the inheritance of different penetrance gene variants, which may weaken the cell's defense mechanisms against carcinogens and the accumulation of unrepaired somatic mutations. It is important therefore to understand the molecular events in order to subclassify patients and recommend appropriate treatment.

Molecular heterogeneity of breast cancer

Breast tumors exhibit a characteristic cellular and molecular heterogeneity [2] and it is globally accepted that the molecular differences among cancers are responsible for the different clinical courses in patients with histologically similar tumors [12]. An increasingly more accurate molecular classification of breast tumors into subtypes has been developed since the beginning of the century through the extensive use of DNA microarrays [2,13,14]. To date, the definitive five clinically relevant molecular subgroups are: luminal subtype A (ER$^+$, PR$^+$, HER2$^-$; 45% of breast cancer cases, better prognosis), luminal subtype B (ER$^+$, PR$^+$, HER2$^-$;

Table 30.1 Biomarkers used in breast cancer prognosis, pathological typing, and treatment.

Pathological type	Marker usage										
	ER	PGR	Her2	Her3	Her4	CK5/6	CK14	P53	Ki67	Grade	Stage
Luminal A	Pos	Pos	–	Pos	Pos	–	–	–	–	–	–
Luminal N	Pos	Pos	–	Neg	Neg	–	–	–	–	–	–
Luminal B	Pos	Neg	–	Pos	Pos	–	–	–	–	–	–
HER2	Neg	–	Pos	–	–	–	–	–	–	–	–
Basal	Neg	Neg	Neg	–	–	Pos	Pos	Neg	–	–	–
Basal altered	Neg	Neg	Neg	–	–	Pos	Pos	Pos	–	–	–
Prognostic outcome	y/n	y/n	y/n	–	–	–	–	y/n	y/n	y/n	y/n
Treatment	y/n	y/n	y/n	–	–	–	–	–	y/n	y/n	y/n

Ki67 >10%, poor prognosis), HER2$^+$ (ER$^-$, PR$^-$, HER2$^+$; aggressive tumors), basal subtype (ER$^-$, PR$^-$, HER2$^-$; 15% of breast cancer cases, aggressive tumors), and normal breast-like. In 2005, using tissue microarray (TMA) technology and hierarchical clustering methodology with 1076 cases of invasive breast cancer, Abd El-Rehim and colleagues uncovered five groups with distinct patterns of protein expression from a large panel of well-characterized commercially available biomarkers, which illustrated the biological heterogeneity of breast cancer [15]. Further analysis using multiple layer perceptron (MLP) artificial neural network (ANN) identified two large groups based on their expression of luminal epithelial cell phenotypic characteristics, hormone receptors positivity, absence of basal epithelial phenotype characteristics, and lack of HER2 protein overexpression. Two other groups were defined by high HER2 positivity and negative or weak hormone receptors expression. The fifth group was identified by strong basal epithelial characteristics, p53 positivity, absence of hormone receptors, and weak to low luminal epithelial cytokeratin expression. According to the authors, this classification, not yet accepted in clinical practice, provides information for revision of current traditional classification systems for breast cancer [15]. In 2008, Meijnen and colleagues successfully categorized ductal carcinoma in situ (DCIS) into two main groups and five subgroups using six published molecular markers defining breast cancer subtypes and an immunohistochemistry approach [16].

Table 30.1 summarizes the known biomarkers used for pathological typing as proposed from available data.

Prediction of outcome based on clinicopathological features

Nottingham Prognostics Index (NPI)

Historically a number of approaches have been used in the development of prognostic indices. One example is the Nottingham Prognostics Index (NPI), which assigns a score to breast cancer patients who have an operable primary invasive breast carcinoma less than 5 cm in size and are less than 70 years old [17]. The index calculates a score based on the following formula:

$$NPI = Grade\ (Elston - Ellis\ criteria)$$
$$+ Lymph\ node\ stage\ (based\ on\ number$$
$$of\ lymph\ nodes\ infiltrated)$$
$$+ 0.2 \times tumor\ size$$

Grades are determined by the Elston-Ellis method [18], which assesses tubule formation, mitochondrial index, and nuclear pleomorphism, and are classified into three types: grade 1 (low grade, slow growing cells), grade 2 (intermediate grade), and grade 3 (high grade, fast growing cells). High-grade tumor cells are more aggressively proliferating than low-grade tumor cells, and patients with grade 3 tumor cells are given a worse prognosis.

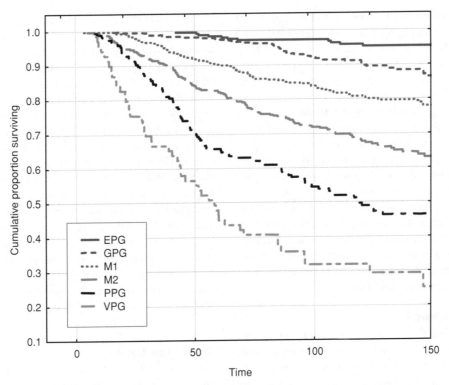

Figure 30.1 Kaplan Meier curves of six Nottingham Prognostic Index groups. Data by kind permission of Graham Ball, Ian Ellis, and Roger Blamey: the Nottingham Prognostic Index.

The score then bands patients into six prognostic groups: excellent (EPG), good (GPG), moderate 1 (M1), moderate 2 (M2), poor (PPG), and very poor (VPG) (Figure 30.1). This approach is commonly used to determine the prognostic outcome for patients but also in the treatment decision-making process. The approach has been widely validated for a range of patient cohorts globally [19].

The NPI does have some limitations. It is somewhat subjective, particularly when considering grade determination, and it does not consider treatment. A second-generation NPI, which will combine clinicopathological with molecular features of the tumor, is currently in development.

Adjuvant! Online

Similar clinicopathological features, such as age of the patient, tumor grade, and hormone receptor status, are incorporated into another computer program freely available online for assessing the prognosis of individual breast cancer cases (www.adjuvantonline.com). The purpose of Adjuvant! Online is to assist health professionals and patients with early cancer discuss the risks and benefits of getting additional therapy after surgery. This program considers risk from the perspective of negative outcome (cancer-related mortality or relapse) without systemic adjuvant therapy, estimates of the reduction of these risks afforded by therapy, and risks of side effects of the therapy.

Prediction of outcome based on molecular features and profiling

Despite many years of research, there is little evidence of a single marker providing a robust prognosticator for breast cancer. Serum or urine from breast cancer patients can be used in an ELISA assay to detect the presence of the protein mammaglobin, which would indicate that breast tumor cells have spread through peripheral blood and lymph nodes to other parts of the body [20]. The expression of EpCAM or HER2 antigens may also be indicators of micrometastases in peripheral blood and bone marrow of breast cancer patients [21,22]. Urokinase-type plasminogen activator (PAl-1 and PAl-2) and cathepsins B and L are biomarkers for breast cancer recurrence [23,24].

In the postgenomic era, where the expression patterns of large number of genes may be reproducibly evaluated in a single assay, a number of groups have now used microarray profiling techniques to determine prognostic risk in breast cancer patients. This in turn has led to the development of prognostic tests based on sophisticated statistical manipulation of the data to reduce the gene set required to maintain significance.

MammaPrint®

MammaPrint® is a gene microarray-based test from Agendia BV used to categorize breast cancer patients (lymph-node negative, ER-positive or -negative tumors) who have only received surgery as treatment, into a low- or a high-risk group based on distant metastases of the disease within or after a 5-year period [25,26]. This clearly has implications for prognosis. The test uses computational approaches to identify a genomic profile of 70 genes that predict the likelihood an individual will develop metastatic disease. The MammaPrint test measures the level of expression of each of these genes in a sample of a woman's surgically removed breast tumor and then uses a specific algorithm to produce a score that determines whether the patient is deemed low risk or high risk for spread of the cancer to another site. This test, approved by FDA in 2007, is the first cleared product that profiles genetic activity.

Questions concerning the ultimate utility of this test arise from the fact that (i) it requires frozen tissue to be shipped to a central laboratory, when without forward planning, usually only fixed material is available, and (ii) it stratifies patients into high- and low-risk groups only, presenting problems for those whose risk lies somewhere in the middle.

More recently Lancashire *et al.* [27] have further analyzed the datasets upon which the MammaPrint assay is based, using ANN to identify a panel of nine genes with prognostic performances of 96% correct classification of the data. In this study, more advanced computational approaches were applied to the data, resulting in a more parsimonious model. Furthermore, the panel identified had improved performance on the van't Veer validation set [25]. This model showed a performance of 84% on this dataset, which was blind to the initial model. The key marker identified in this study was carbonic anhydrase IX. This was subsequently validated on an independent cohort using immunohistochemistry on an alternative cohort from Nottingham, UK. The approaches adopted in this study apply an approach that extensively cross-validated models developed on blind data, using performance on this basis to identify predictive biomarker genes.

Oncotype DX®

Oncotype DX® was developed by Genomic Health, Inc. to provide a quantitative test for the likelihood of a cancer recurring in a specific subset of breast cancer patients, namely those whose tumors are ER-positive and who have no evidence of lymph node involvement. While many of these patients have a very good prognosis, a significant proportion will ultimately develop secondary tumors and therefore might well have benefited from chemotherapy. The Oncotype DX test, which, unlike the MammaPrint test, is suitable for archival (conventionally fixed) tissue samples, assesses the expression of 21 genes using real-time PCR, and provides a "Recurrence Score." The Recurrence Score is a number between 0 and 100 that corresponds to a specific likelihood of breast cancer recurrence within 10 years of the initial diagnosis [28,29].

Interestingly, subsequent analysis of accumulated data gathered from the use of this test indicted that it also provides *predictive* information concerning the likely response to chemotherapy in this group of patients. Therefore the Oncotype DX test can now be said to be of both prognostic and predictive value.

Prediction of response to therapy

As pointed out above, current usage distinguishes between "prognostic" and "predictive" tests, a predictive test being one that provides information about likely response to a treatment. Current interest in biomarkers reflects the growing demand for predictive tests, which will enjoy an extended lifespan, accompanying new drugs from the early phases of development, through patient stratification for phase III clinical trials, to licensing and routine clinical testing prior to prescribing.

Prior to the 1980s the predominant method of second-line treatment was radiotherapy. However, in the late 1980s the use of adjuvant therapies such as chemotherapy became more prevalent. Such treatments had no identifiable biomarkers indicative of response, and due to side effects, use was often restricted to patients with the worst prognosis.

Vascular endothelial growth factor-receptor (VEGFR-1) has been associated both with prognostic outcome and with response to chemotherapy [30]. This study specifically indicated that high VEGF levels related to shortened progression-free interval, a shortened overall survival, and a poor decreased response rate in first-line chemotherapy. It is likely that this effect is largely due to the role of VEGF in angiogenesis [31]. Paradiso et al. [32] indicated that beta tubulin III was a strong indicator of progression post-treatment with taxol-based chemotherapies. Hormonal (endocrine) therapies such as tamoxifen or aromatase inhibitors [33] and the monoclonal antibody trastuzumab [34] are well-accepted therapies. With the identification of estrogen receptor status of tumors and development of subsequent tests for estrogen receptor status, endocrine therapies such as anti-estrogens were developed. These stratified patients who were estrogen receptor positive and allowed treatment showing a strong response for a subgroup of patients [35]. Tamoxifen, an anti-estrogen, blocks the estrogen receptor by binding to it instead of estrogen, thus inhibiting the effect of estrogen on the cancer cell [36]. According to many trials, tamoxifen greatly diminishes the risk of a recurrent cancer and furthermore it improves the survival

for women by 10 years [37]. Other hormonal therapies include progestogens (artificial progesterone) and aromatase inhibitors (given to postmenopausal women only), both blocking the production of estrogen.

The reintroduction of maspin expression [38] and wild-type p53 expression [39] are potential treatments for breast cancer. EpCAM, cyclin E, the platelet-derived growth factor (PDGF), and Flk-1 (a growth factor receptor) are potential targets for immunotherapies [21,40–42]. Cancer cell growth can be inhibited in around 90% of breast cancer patients tested positive for the vitamin D receptor (nuclear steroid hormone receptor) when tumor cells are treated with the vitamin D analog 1a,25-(OH)2D3 [43]. Wu and colleagues stated that receptor-selective retinoids, which have a role in growth inhibition and induction of apoptosis, could be used in novel therapies for breast cancer patients whose tumor tested positive for these but negative for ER [44]. Also, ligands for the peroxisome proliferator-activated receptor (PPAR), such as the natural prostaglandin 15-deoxy-delta-12,14-prostaglandin J2 (PGJ2) and the synthetic anti-diabetic thiazolidenediones troglitazone (TGZ), could be of interest for use in novel therapies targeting breast cancer cell growth [45]. Another receptor that could be a good candidate for therapy is the growth factor receptor Flk-1. It has been shown that when Flk-1 mRNA molecules are cleaved by ribozymes the growth rate of microvasculature endothelial cells decreases, making Flk-1 a potential target in novel strategies against angiogenesis [41]. In 2004, Castelli and colleagues stated that heat shock proteins are potential biomarkers for breast cancer treatment due to their ability to chaperone tumor antigens and to break the immune tolerance to these, thus inducing specific regression of the tumor [46].

In 2000, an antigen specific to a subgroup of breast cancers was developed [47]. This antigen was c-erbB-2 (HER2/neu). An immunotherapy was developed to this antigen called trastuzumab (Herceptin™). Approximately 25% of patients diagnosed with breast cancer present a high level of HER2 receptors on their tumors (Herceptest scores of 3). HER2-positive tumors are commonly of higher grade, more likely to be ER negative, and present a more aggressive phenotype, therefore patients have a poorer prognosis. HER2-positive patients can be treated with trastuzumab or lapatinib. Trastuzumab (Herceptin™), manufactured by Genentech, is a humanized monoclonal antibody directed against the growth factor receptor HER2. Lapatinib (Tykerb™), manufactured by GlaxoSmithKline, is a small-molecule inhibitor of the growth factor receptors HER2 and EGFR. Trastuzumab and lapatinib, both molecular therapies, were the only two targeted breast cancer therapeutics approved in 2007 and, to date, no immunotherapy for breast cancer has been approved. An alternative approach to targeting HER2/neu utilized a specific vaccine approach, designed to promote T-lymphocyte response to MHC-associated HER2/neu class I restricted peptides expressed on HER2/neu-positive breast cancer cells. A UK clinical trial is currently being tested in phase I and is based on a novel DNA-based vaccine called polyHER2neu for immunotherapy of metastasized breast cancer, with the aim to activate the immune system to recognize one or more T-cell epitopes on antigen-bearing breast cancer cells (see www.cancerhelp.org.uk/trials).

Breast cancer patients diagnosed with triple negative tumors (ER negative, PR negative, HER2 not overexpressed) have a really poor prognosis since these will not respond to hormonal therapies (tamoxifen, aromatase inhibitors) or targeted therapies (trastuzumab, lapatinib) and can only be treated with chemotherapies. Many studies are currently focusing on the molecular characteristics of the tumor cells of this group of patients in order to develop alternative targeted therapies [48].

Toward personalized medicine for breast cancer patients

While many biomarkers have been shown to have utility in breast cancer, there are few multi-biomarker models. Truly personalized medicine requires the integration of patient profiling techniques (such as mass spectrometry, gene microarrays, and/or patient DNA sequencing) with computational modeling and data mining techniques. This approach will lead to the development of multi-marker models that can cope with the heterogeneity associated with cancer.

Early diagnosis is key to survival and is more significant than any treatment [49]. The tumors detected early (either by self-diagnosis or by screening programs) tend to be smaller in size and more importantly have no lymph node involvement. Up to 70% of breast cancer patients will have recurrent disease following treatment [50], and reports from Cancer Research UK suggest that out of all female breast cancer patients diagnosed in the UK in 2006, around 20% will not survive beyond five years. These statistics highlight the limitations of accepted prognostic tools in predicting recurrence of the disease. Consequently, in a significant number of breast cancer cases, women are overtreated as they are given aggressive therapies in which associated side effects actually outweigh benefits [51]. Also, the major drawbacks of a number of current therapies such as chemotherapy and hormonal therapy are undeniably the inefficacy and toxicity of treatments.

Omic technologies

High-throughput "omic" technologies such as genomics and proteomics have been extensively used in the identification of breast-cancer-specific biomarkers, exemplified by recent gene expression profiling studies [52,53]. Additional techniques to study the proteome include mass spectrometry analysis, which is used to compare the levels of protein expression between samples from healthy and cancer patients with the objective to discover breast-cancer-associated biomarkers for diagnosis, prognosis, and prediction of treatment outcome. The samples used include serum, urine, and tissue lysates. Ideally, lysates are produced from laser microdissected tissue, allowing morphologically distinct cell populations from tissue sections to be retrieved [54], thus allowing a more targeted and accurate analysis of the samples by proteomic or genomic means. Matrix-assisted laser desorption/ionization mass spectrometry (MALDI) and surface-enhanced laser desorption/ionization mass spectrometry (SELDI) technologies have been extensively used for biomarker discovery in the past few years [55,56]. These are combined with downstream bioinformatics in order to identify proteins through the analysis of relevant links and database interrogation [27]. The application of microarray and proteomic platforms is set to revolutionize the way we stratify patients into diagnostic and prognostic groups, but more importantly into subgroupings that bear the hallmark molecular signatures of response to therapy.

Patient modeling based on genomic and proteomic data

The identification of multiple markers that exist in a panel and predict patient outcome requires a truly interdisciplinary approach. However, there exists the potential for development of predictive medicine, which utilizes different treatment strategies for specific patients. Furthermore, through the modeling of information derived from postgenomic technologies and through systems biology approaches, disease biomarkers and patient-specific disease pathways may be derived. Thus a greater understanding of disease is gained and new therapies may be derived that block or stimulate elements associated with the disease-causing process.

Modeling and analysis of patient profiles has been illustrated in a number of studies employing ANNs. Matharoo-Ball *et al.* [57] used an approach based on ANN to analyze data generated from tryptic-digested serum samples of staged melanoma patients. In this study, they were able to stratify patients based on markers that were validated using alternative assays. The workflow typically used for high-throughput analysis to achieve sequence data is shown in Figure 30.2. Samples are subjected to ZipTip chromatography clean-up to remove abundant high molecular mass proteins prior to tryptic digestion and concentration. The mass spectra of samples, consisting of at least two groups, for example patients and controls, are analyzed by bioinformatics to achieve a rank order of discriminatory "ions of importance." The top-ranked ions can then be sequenced using ESI mass spectrometry to achieve identity and further validated by independent biological tests.

The same approach was use by Lancashire *et al.* [27] for analysis of gene microarray data from the van't Veer study indicating risk of metastases. This study was extended further by Lemetre *et al.* [58], where the authors took the top 100 genes identified by Lancashire *et al.* and incorporated them into an ANN-based pathway analysis (a systems biology methodology). Differential pathways for the metastatic and nonmetastatic groups were identified. Lancashire *et al.* also re-analyzed the West dataset [59] to identify genes associated with lymph node positivity risk and with estrogen receptor positivity. Interestingly, this approach identified the ER gene as a key predictor (out of several thousand genes) for ER status defined by immunohistochemistry. This indicates the validity of the approach for identifying predictive genes of relevance. These ANN-based approaches have also been used in the analysis of immunotherapy clinical trials as a part of the ENACT EU FP6 program. In this instance, they have been shown to predict response to therapy in a number of trials based on mass spectrometry based patient blood profiles prior to vaccination. This is an extension of an earlier study by Michael *et al.* [60], which used cytokine profiles to predict response and demonstrates the utility of this bioinformatic approach.

There is a clear opportunity for "omic" technologies to substantially increase our ability to generate results that will allow the stratification of patients in a meaningful way, which leads to a better understanding of treatment benefits as well as further awareness of the biological processes and molecular pathways involved in cancer progression and response to therapy. There are principally two approaches that can be adopted as we work toward personalized medicine: (i) to utilize complex genomic, transcriptomic, and proteomic data directly for patient classification, and (ii) to abstract the identified pivotal molecular features to develop alternative and more easily used biological assays. Whichever technology is applied, the consensus view is that panels of markers are more likely

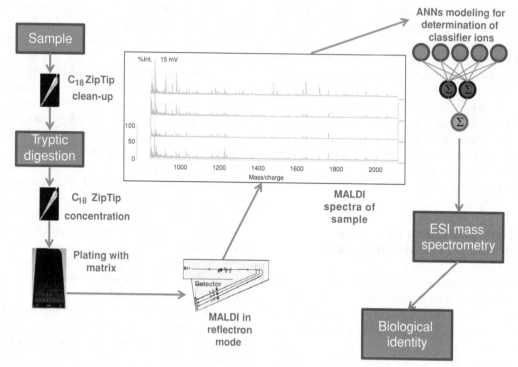

Figure 30.2 Process flow diagram for the identification of biomarkers from samples by mass spectrometry.

to be of patient benefit than individual, single marker tests.

Perspective on biomarkers in personalized medicine

With the increasing demand for diagnostic tests for cancer it is especially interesting to consider the value and clinical utility of PSA screening for prostate cancer and whether or not general population screening, using the current PSA test, is of real benefit in the diagnostic arena. In particular, available data suggests that the widespread screening of men in the USA detects an increasing number of patients with low-risk prostate cancer who receive aggressive treatment that carries with it a high risk of side effects. It can be argued that this policy is not beneficial for patients, since there does not appear to be evidence that PSA screening reduces the mortality rate. Although screening will increase the detection rate of early-stage prostate cancer, this

provides a dilemma and uncertainty about the optimum treatment in this cohort. PSA is a valuable biomarker for monitoring patient response to therapy and as an indicator of disease recurrence following therapy. There are, however, no reliable assays that indicate spread of disease outside the confines of the prostate, where at present pathological scoring (Gleeson grade) is used to determine disease status and treatment options. In particular, Gleeson 7 patients offer the greatest challenge to clinicians, since a score of $3 + 4$ (indicative of confined disease) and $4 + 3$ (used to indicate disease progression beyond the prostate capsule) is determined by subjective pathological assessment. The identification of prognostic markers for these patients would offer considerable clinical benefit.

New therapeutic modalities will also require patient stratification and the need for biomarkers that predict response to treatment and associate with response parameters. The cell-based dendritic cell (DC) therapy sipuleucel-T (Provenge®, Dendreon), consisting of autologous, patient-derived DCs programmed to activate T-cell immunity against the prostate cancer-associated antigen PAP, became the first FDA-approved cancer vaccine for human use in 2010, based on the outcome of clinical trials. CD54, also known as intracellular adhesion molecule 1 (ICAM-1), shows a cumulative upregulation on activated DCs administered to patients sequentially and represents a perspective marker of potency, since ICAM-1 is an adhesion molecule important for antigen-presenting (DC) cell/T-cell binding. CD54 expression levels, used as a continuous variable in assessing patient survival, showed a strong correlation with clinical response [61] and can be considered as a biomarker, indicative of therapeutic efficacy.

Assessing the clinical and biological response to new therapies will require robust and validated biomarkers and an additional example is the use of anti-CTLA4 therapy to target T regulatory (Treg) cells. An increased clinical efficacy was observed in melanoma patients, determined by progression-free and overall survival, which correlated with the restoration of T-cell proliferation capacity and the induction of effector-memory $CD4^+$ and $CD8^+$ cells; interestingly, T-cell proliferation following treatment proved to be totally resistant to the influence of Treg cell-mediated suppression [62]. Linking biomarkers with immunologic competence and clinical outcome will be important in realizing the potential of targeted therapy.

There are several lessons to be learned from the above studies if we are to develop robust strategies for early detection and prognosis and work toward personalized medicine. Given recent advances in genomic, proteomic, and bioinformatic technologies, there is the very real possibility that in the future the widespread introduction of biomarkers and assays that are able to stratify patients to derive optimal therapeutic benefit will be realized.

Acknowledgments

The authors at the John van Geest Cancer Research Centre wish to acknowledge the support of the John and Lucille van Geest Foundation.

References

1 FDA. Critical Path Opportunities Report, March 2006. Available at www.fda.gov/downloads/Science Research/SpecialTopics/CriticalPathInitiative/Critical PathOpportunitiesReports/UCM077254.pdf. Accessed Feb 2012.

2 Sorlie T, Perou CM, Tibshirani R, et al. Gene expression patterns of breast carcinomas distinguish tumor subclasses with clinical implications. Proc Natl Acad Sci U S A 2001;**98**(19):10869–74.

3 Caldas C, Aparicio SA. The molecular outlook. Nature 2002;**415**(6871):484–5.

4 Ponder BA. Inherited predisposition to breast cancer. Biochem Soc Symp 1998;**63**:223–30.

5 Ellisen LW, Haber DA. Hereditary breast cancer. Annu Rev Med 1998;**49**:425–36.

6 Miki Y, Swensen J, Shattuck-Eidens D, et al. A strong candidate for the breast and ovarian cancer susceptibility gene BRCA1. Science 1994;**266**(5182):66–71.

7 Wooster R, Bignell G, Lancaster J, et al. Identification of the breast cancer susceptibility gene BRCA2. Nature 1995;**378**(6559):789–92.

8 Greene MH. Genetics of breast cancer. Mayo Clin Proc 1997;**72**(1):54–65.

9 Lerebours F, Lidereau R. Molecular alterations in sporadic breast cancer. Crit Rev Oncol Hematol 2002;**44**(2):121–41.

10 Ross JS, Linette GP, Stec J, et al. Breast cancer biomarkers and molecular medicine. Expert Rev Mol Diagn 2003;**3**(5):573–85.

11 Widschwendter M, Jones PA. DNA methylation and breast carcinogenesis. Oncogene 2002;**21**(35):5462–82.

12 Pusztai L, Cristofanilli M, Paik S. New generation of molecular prognostic and predictive tests for breast cancer. Semin Oncol 2007;**34**(2 Suppl 3):S10–16.

13 Perou CM, Sorlie T, Eisen MB, et al. Molecular portraits of human breast tumours. Nature 2000;**406**(6797):747–52.

14 Sorlie T, Tibshirani R, Parker J, et al. Repeated observation of breast tumor subtypes in independent gene expression data sets. Proc Natl Acad Sci U S A 2003;**100**(14):8418–23.

15 Abd El-Rehim DM, Ball G, Pinder SE, et al. High-throughput protein expression analysis using tissue microarray technology of a large well-characterised series identifies biologically distinct classes of breast cancer confirming recent cDNA expression analyses. Int J Cancer 2005;**116**(3):340–50.

16 Meijnen P, Peterse JL, Antonini N, Rutgers EJ, van de Vijver MJ. Immunohistochemical categorisation of ductal carcinoma in situ of the breast. *Br J Cancer* 2008;**98**(1):137–42.

17 Haybittle JL, Blamey RW, Elston CW, *et al.* A prognostic index in primary breast cancer. *Br J Cancer* 1982;**45**(3):361–6.

18 Elston CW, Ellis IO. Pathological prognostic factors in breast cancer. I. The value of histological grade in breast cancer: experience from a large study with long-term follow-up. *Histopathology* 2002;**41**(3A):154–61.

19 Galea MH, Blamey RW, Elston CE, Ellis IO. The Nottingham Prognostic Index in primary breast cancer. *Breast Cancer Res Treat* 1992;**22**(3):207–19.

20 O'Brien N, Maguire TM, O'Donovan N, *et al.* Mammaglobin a: a promising marker for breast cancer. *Clin Chem* 2002;**48**(8):1362–4.

21 Gastl G, Spizzo G, Obrist P, Dunser M, Mikuz G. EpCAM overexpression in breast cancer as a predictor of survival. *Lancet* 2000;**356**(9246):1981–2.

22 Andersen TI, Paus E, Nesland JM, McKenzie SJ, Borresen AL. Detection of c-erbB-2 related protein in sera from breast cancer patients. Relationship to ERBB2 gene amplification and c-erbB-2 protein overexpression in tumour. *Acta Oncol* 1995;**34**(4):499–504.

23 Borstnar S, Vrhovec I, Svetic B, Cufer T. Prognostic value of the urokinase-type plasminogen activator, and its inhibitors and receptor in breast cancer patients. *Clin Breast Cancer* 2002;**3**(2):138–46.

24 Foekens JA, Kos J, Peters HA, *et al.* Prognostic significance of cathepsins B and L in primary human breast cancer. *J Clin Oncol* 1998;**16**(3):1013–21.

25 van de Vijver MJ, He YD, van't Veer LJ, *et al.* A gene-expression signature as a predictor of survival in breast cancer. *N Engl J Med* 2002;**347**(25):1999–2009.

26 van't Veer LJ, Dai H, van de Vijver MJ, *et al.* Gene expression profiling predicts clinical outcome of breast cancer. *Nature* 2002;**415**(6871):530–36.

27 Lancashire LJ, Lemetre C, Ball GR. An introduction to artificial neural networks in bioinformatics – application to complex microarray and mass spectrometry datasets in cancer studies. *Brief Bioinform* 2009;**10**(3):315–29.

28 Cronin M, Pho M, Dutta D, *et al.* Measurement of gene expression in archival paraffin-embedded tissues: development and performance of a 92-gene reverse transcriptase-polymerase chain reaction assay. *Am J Pathol* 2004;**164**(1):35–42.

29 Paik S, Shak S, Tang G, *et al.* A multigene assay to predict recurrence of tamoxifen-treated, node-negative breast cancer. *N Engl J Med* 2004;**351**(27):2817–26.

30 Foekens JA, Peters HA, Grebenchtchikov N, *et al.* High tumor levels of vascular endothelial growth factor predict poor response to systemic therapy in advanced breast cancer. *Cancer Res* 2001;**61**(14):5407–14.

31 Ohta Y, Shridhar V, Bright RK, *et al.* VEGF and VEGF type C play an important role in angiogenesis and lymphangiogenesis in human malignant mesothelioma tumours. *Br J Cancer* 1999;**81**(1):54–61.

32 Paradiso A, Mangia A, Chiriatti A, *et al.* Biomarkers predictive for clinical efficacy of taxol-based chemotherapy in advanced breast cancer. *Ann Oncol* 2005;**16**(Suppl 4):iv14–19.

33 Cristofanilli M, Hortobagyi GN. Molecular targets in breast cancer: current status and future directions. *Endocr Relat Cancer* 2002;**9**(4):249–66.

34 McKeage K, Perry CM. Trastuzumab: a review of its use in the treatment of metastatic breast cancer overexpressing HER2. *Drugs* 2002;**62**(1):209–43.

35 Holmes FA, Fritsche HA, Loewy JW, *et al.* Measurement of estrogen and progesterone receptors in human breast tumors: enzyme immunoassay versus binding assay. *J Clin Oncol* 1990;**8**(6):1025–35.

36 Ward HW. Anti-oestrogen therapy for breast cancer: a trial of tamoxifen at two dose levels. *Br Med J* 1973;**1**(5844):13–14.

37 Wishart GC, Gaston M, Poultsidis AA, Purushotham AD. Hormone receptor status in primary breast cancer – time for a consensus? *Eur J Cancer* 2002;**38**(9):1201–3.

38 Maass N, Nagasaki K, Ziebart M, Mundhenke C, Jonat W. Expression and regulation of tumor suppressor gene maspin in breast cancer. *Clin Breast Cancer* 2002;**3**(4):281–7.

39 Liu TJ, el-Naggar AK, McDonnell TJ, *et al.* Apoptosis induction mediated by wild-type p53 adenoviral gene transfer in squamous cell carcinoma of the head and neck. *Cancer Res* 1995;**5**(14):3117–22.

40 Ariad S, Seymour L, Bezwoda WR. Platelet-derived growth factor (PDGF) in plasma of breast cancer patients: correlation with stage and rate of progression. *Breast Cancer Res Treat* 1991;**20**(1):11–17.

41 Hasan J, Jayson GC. VEGF antagonists. *Expert Opin Biol Ther* 2001;**1**(4):703–18.

42 Hunt KK, Keyomarsi K. Cyclin E as a prognostic and predictive marker in breast cancer. *Semin Cancer Biol* 2005;**15**(4):319–26.

43 Friedrich M, Rafi L, Tilgen W, Schmidt W, Reichrath J. Expression of 1,25-dihydroxy vitamin D3 receptor in breast carcinoma. *J Histochem Cytochem* 1998; **46**(11):1335–7.

44 Wu K, Zhang Y, Xu XC, *et al.* The retinoid X receptor-selective retinoid, LGD1069, prevents the development of estrogen receptor-negative mammary tumors in transgenic mice. *Cancer Res* 2002;**62**(22): 6376–80.

45 Pignatelli M, Cortes-Canteli M, Lai C, Santos A, Perez-Castillo A. The peroxisome proliferator-activated receptor gamma is an inhibitor of ErbBs activity in human breast cancer cells. *J Cell Sci* 2001;**114**(Pt 22):4117–26.

46 Castelli C, Rivoltini L, Rini F, *et al.* Heat shock proteins: biological functions and clinical application as personalized vaccines for human cancer. *Cancer Immunol Immunother* 2004;**53**(3):227–33.

47 Slamon DJ, Leyland-Jones B, Shak S, *et al.* Use of chemotherapy plus a monoclonal antibody against HER2 for metastatic breast cancer that overexpresses HER2. *N Engl J Med* 2001;**344**(11):783–92.

48 Irvin WJ, Jr, Carey LA. What is triple-negative breast cancer? *Eur J Cancer* 2008;**44**(18):2799–805.

49 Hu Y, Zhang S, Yu J, Liu J, Zheng S. SELDI-TOF-MS: the proteomics and bioinformatics approaches in the diagnosis of breast cancer. *Breast* 2005;**14**(4): 250–55.

50 Chatterjee SK, Zetter BR. Cancer biomarkers: knowing the present and predicting the future. *Future Oncol* 2005;**1**(1):37–50.

51 Chia SK, Wykoff CC, Watson PH, *et al.* Prognostic significance of a novel hypoxia-regulated marker, carbonic anhydrase IX, in invasive breast carcinoma. *J Clin Oncol* 2001;**19**(16):3660–68.

52 Chang JC, Wooten EC, Tsimelzon A, *et al.* Gene expression profiling for the prediction of therapeutic response to docetaxel in patients with breast cancer. *Lancet* 2003;**362**(9381):362–9.

53 Esteban J, Baker J, Cronin M, *et al.* Tumor gene expression and prognosis in breast cancer: multi-gene RT-PCR assay of paraffin-embedded tissue [abstract]. *Proc Am Soc Clin Oncol* 2003;**22**:A3416.

54 Emmert-Buck MR, Bonner RF, Smith PD, *et al.* Laser capture microdissection. *Science* 1996;**274**(5289): 998–1001.

55 Laronga C, Drake RR. Proteomic approach to breast cancer. *Cancer Control* 2007;**14**(4):360–68.

56 Garrisi VM, Abbate I, Quaranta M, *et al.* SELDI-TOF serum proteomics and breast cancer: which perspective? *Expert Rev Proteomics* 2008;**5**(6):779–85.

57 Matharoo-Ball B, Ratcliff L, Lancashire L, *et al.* Diagnostic biomarkers differentiating metastatic melanoma patients from healthy controls identified by an integrated MALDI-TOF mass spectrometry/ bioinformatic approach. *Proteomics Clin Appl* 2007; **1**(6):605–20.

58 Lemetre C, Lancashire L, Rees RC, Ball GR. Artificial neural network based algorithm for biomolecular interactions modeling. *IWANN* 2009;**1**:877–85.

59 West M, Blanchette C, Dressman H, *et al.* Predicting the clinical status of human breast cancer by using gene expression profiles. *Proc Natl Acad Sci U S A* 2001;**98**(20):11462–7.

60 Michael A, Ball G, Quatan N, *et al.* Delayed disease progression after allogeneic cell vaccination in hormone-resistant prostate cancer and correlation with immunologic variables. *Clin Cancer Res* 2005; **11**(12):4469–78.

61 Higano CS, Schellhammer PF, Small EJ *et al.* Integrated data from 2 randomized, double-blind, placebo-controlled, phase 3 trials of active cellular immunotherapy with sipuleucel-T in advanced prostate cancer. *Cancer* 2009;**115**(16):3670–79.

62 Menard C, Ghiringhelli F, Roux S, *et al.* CTLA-4 blockade confers lymphocyte resistance to regulatory T-cells in advanced melanoma: surrogate mark efficacy of tremelimumab? *Clinical Cancer Res* 2008;**14**:5242–9.

PART 8
Implementing Immunizations/Therapies

CHAPTER 31

Mass Immunization Strategies

David L. Heymann[1], R. Bruce Aylward[2], & Rudolf H. Tangermann[2]
[1]Infectious Disease Epidemiology, London School of Hygiene and Tropical Medicine, London, UK
[2]World Health Organization, Geneva, Switzerland

Mass immunization: history and concept

Variolation, the purposeful infection of a person with material from vesicles of smallpox patients to prevent serious smallpox infection, was first used in China and India around AD 1000 [1]. In 1796, Edward Jenner first inoculated humans with material from lesions of cowpox from milkmaids, rather than from smallpox patients, which meant that direct vaccination from a person with smallpox was no longer required. The practice of vaccination was further refined in the United Kingdom in the early 19th century when material from cowpox lesions, dried on threads, was used to vaccinate. This "vaccine" could be transported throughout the country and to other parts of the world [2] in order to vaccinate persons at risk.

Between 1807 and 1816, smallpox vaccination laws were passed in Bavaria, Denmark, and Sweden, and vaccination against smallpox soon became compulsory in Europe. Later in the 19th century, Great Britain adopted Vaccination Acts, which made free smallpox vaccination universal and mandatory for all. By enforcement through vaccination officers, those who refused vaccination for any reason were fined. Mandatory smallpox vaccination was soon introduced in many other countries, either through school entry laws or legislation pertaining to young children and families [3].

As demand for vaccination grew, general vaccination days were conducted in Europe and elsewhere in the world, where vaccination directly from cowpox lesions on cows replaced person-to-person vaccination or vaccination through impregnated threads. These vaccination days were effectively early mass immunization campaigns, which, over a short time period, rapidly and efficiently protected large numbers of non-immune persons against disease. Already by 1820, mass immunization in Sweden had led to an over hundredfold [4] decrease in the number of smallpox cases.

It soon became clear that vaccination not only protected individuals against the disease, but that mass immunization, through an overall decrease in the number of infected persons and in smallpox transmission rates, even provided some degree of protection to those who remained unvaccinated. The observed effect – "herd immunity" – became an important benefit of mass immunization campaigns. Mass campaigns protect the targeted population either directly through vaccination of susceptible persons, or indirectly through reducing the risk of infection for those who remain unvaccinated, as the intensity of transmission of the infectious agent decreases in the target population.

Since Jenner's time, mass immunization campaigns have become a commonly used tool for disease control programs in both developing and industrialized countries. This chapter presents a brief review of the evolution and current use of mass immunization strategies, including the sometimes "uneasy," but important and necessary, alliance between mass immunization and routine

Vaccinology: Principles and Practice, First Edition. Edited by W. John W. Morrow, Nadeem A. Sheikh, Clint S. Schmidt and D. Huw Davies.
© 2012 Blackwell Publishing Ltd. Published 2012 by Blackwell Publishing Ltd.

immunization programs. The presented broad framework should be helpful for policy makers in assessing the role that mass immunization can play in vaccine-preventable disease control.

Smallpox eradication

All member states of the World Health Organization (WHO) in 1967 resolved to intensify smallpox eradication efforts globally [5]. Countries where smallpox transmission had not yet been interrupted agreed to adopt the search and containment strategy in addition to routine immunization. Despite the risks from complications associated with primary smallpox vaccination (from local vaccinal eruption to generalized vaccinia infection and post-vaccinal encephalitis, leading to permanent disability), there were clear benefits of eradication. Thirty-one countries were still endemic for smallpox at the time of the 1967 World Health Assembly resolution. Without accelerated efforts, an estimated two to three million deaths from smallpox would have occurred that year, with many more suffering severe facial and corneal scarring, and blindness. It was clear that smallpox eradication would lead to considerable prevention of death and disability, and be associated with significant savings from reduced costs for treatment and for vaccine, once vaccination against smallpox could be stopped [6,7].

The achievement and certification of the eradication of smallpox by 1980 was accomplished to a large extent by routine smallpox vaccination (prior to the 1970s), supplemented in some countries by mass vaccination campaigns. During the 1970s, however, the strategy was changed to one of active surveillance – which consisted of searching for persons with smallpox and isolation of cases, followed by vaccination of their immediate contacts and of a ring of households around each case. Active surveillance was quite effective in identifying all smallpox infections because each infection was clinically expressed, and ring containment was sufficient to create sufficient herd immunity to interrupt transmission.

The last smallpox case resulting from a naturally occurring virus transmission chain occurred in Somalia, in 1977, after 10 years of intensified eradication activities. Global smallpox eradication was certified three years later, in 1980, by an independent global commission. The smallpox eradication effort became the first public health program to achieve worldwide equity in the benefits of a vaccine.

By the late 20th century it had become clear that vaccination and herd immunity, whether in a ring of households surrounding a person infected with smallpox or in the general population in the case of other pathogens, could be enough to interrupt person-to-person transmission. It was also increasingly understood that if the infectious agent, such as the smallpox virus, had no other reservoir except humans, the decrease and eventual interruption of transmission would mean the eradication of both the pathogen and the disease it caused.

Routine and mass immunization as complementary strategies

Mass vaccination strategies were a critical component of the smallpox eradication program mainly because routine immunization services in most developing countries were not yet strong enough to achieve the immunization coverage levels needed for herd immunity to interrupt smallpox virus transmission. Consequently, the success of smallpox eradication also provided a critical stimulus for the establishment of strong national routine immunization services through the WHO Expanded Programme on Immunization (EPI).

The Expanded Programme on Immunization (EPI)

Interest in immunization was greatly boosted by progress toward smallpox eradication during the 1970s. WHO expert advisory groups increasingly discussed the need to ensure equitable access for children in all countries to other vaccines, such as diphtheria-pertussis-tetanus (DPT) combination vaccine, or the newly developed measles and rubella vaccines. The use of mass immunization was an obvious choice. However, there was emerging consensus that the effort required to implement and sustain mass immunization strategies would be intense, with high cost, and that routine provision of immunization services, as part of other maternal and child health services, would be more sustainable [8–10]. As a result, the EPI was established in 1974, to assist developing countries in establishing and strengthening routine immunization services.

The overall strategy of the EPI was to assist developing countries in increasing the proportion of children under the age of 12 months who were protected against selected diseases for which vaccines existed. In 1977, the World Health Assembly resolved to provide six vaccines to children in all countries: BCG and trivalent oral polio vaccine, and vaccines against diphtheria, pertussis, tetanus, and measles. The EPI established common strategies for planning, implementation, and evaluation of national immunization programs, and implemented standardized EPI training programs in developing countries.

The EPI immunization goal was further reinforced by the Alma-Ata Declaration in 1978 [11], which identified immunization as a key component of primary health care. As progress toward improving overall coverage was slow in the first half of the 1980s, the UN Secretary-General in 1985 called for all countries to reach at least 80% infant coverage (Universal Child Immunization, UCI) by the end of the decade. With renewed efforts in developing countries and by immunization partner agencies, the UCI goal was declared as achieved in 1990, 16 years after the EPI was established. To reach the UCI goal, some countries added supplementary mass immunization campaigns to their routine service delivery. These campaigns received substantial support from bi- and multilateral donors, and from nongovernmental and international organizations.

Up until the late 1980s, the EPI concentrated on establishing the necessary infrastructure to deliver vaccines to children in tropical, developing country settings (e.g., appropriate vaccine cold chain, transportation, training of staff) and on monitoring coverage. To maintain support and increase attention to "missed" populations, specific disease control goals were added, beginning mainly in 1988 with targets for polio eradication, accelerated control of measles, and maternal and neonatal tetanus (MNT) elimination.

Since 2000, the Global Alliance for Vaccine and Immunization (GAVI) has supported the 75 poorest countries in the world with low immunization coverage to introduce new and underutilized vaccines, and to overcome obstacles to improving and strengthening immunization services [12]. GAVI's incremental funding for immunization services strengthening is made contingent on improvements in immunization coverage. GAVI also co-finances the introduction and procurement of new vaccines into routine immunization systems.

Since the late 1990s, several successful initiatives have been launched to assist district health managers in improving immunization services, often building on lessons learned through accelerated disease control initiatives. In 2003, for example, WHO and UNICEF jointly launched the "Reach Every District" (RED) strategy, which has been implemented by 53 countries. The RED approach uses lessons learned through polio eradication to encourage supportive supervision, strengthen district immunization management, conduct regular outreach services, enhance community links with service delivery, improve data management, and improve data-based planning.

While efforts to strengthen routine immunization through EPI strategies and GAVI continue, the need for mass immunization campaigns, also referred to as "supplemental immunization activities" (SIAs), remains, for outbreak prevention and accelerated disease control, and to achieve disease elimination and eradication goals.

Preventing and responding to emerging outbreaks

One of the most widely accepted reasons to implement a mass immunization campaign is to respond to, or limit the morbidity and mortality associated with, a manifest emerging or re-emerging communicable disease outbreak by rapidly increasing population immunity. The use of mass immunization strategies is increasingly justified when surveillance data show that the incidence of an epidemic-prone disease is beginning to rise, particularly if the disease is not targeted by routine immunization or if there are large known or suspected immunity gaps. Mass immunization campaigns may also be needed to prevent outbreaks of EPI target diseases, such as measles, in settings where routine immunization was disrupted, such as in camps for internally displaced people (IDPs) during humanitarian emergencies.

Meningitis

Meningococcal meningitis is a disease found all over the world; however, large epidemics occur regularly in a number of semi-arid countries in sub-Saharan Africa designated as the "African meningitis belt" [13]. Transmission in most countries of the meningitis belt increases each year during the dry period, with large epidemics recorded every 8–12 years during the past 50 years, particularly in more populated regions with frequent population movements. African meningitis epidemics can be very large, with attack rates ranging from 100 to 800 per 100 000 population and reaching as high as 1 per 100. During the 6-year period 2003–2009, epidemics in the meningitis belt alone resulted in close to 270 000 cases and 25 000 deaths. The 2008–2009 meningitis epidemic in the African meningitis belt was the largest since 1996, with more than 80 000 reported cases and >5000 deaths [14].

Meningitis epidemics in sub-Saharan Africa are generally caused by serogroup A meningococci bacteria, although W135 serogroups have been recently shown to also play a role. Conventional meningococcal vaccines are based on capsular polysaccharide antigens. While awaiting the introduction of a conjugate meningococcal vaccine (see below), mass immunization campaigns with the appropriate polysaccharide vaccine continue to be used as a standard and effective tool to control meningitis epidemics. Early detection of epidemics and rapid identification of circulating pathogens are crucial to determine when the threshold of transmission that generally leads to epidemics has been reached, and to mount an effective response. Mass meningitis campaigns target a large age range, which sometimes includes the whole population. Provided the campaign can be rapidly organized and conducted, it is possible to effectively protect susceptible individuals, and to interrupt epidemic transmission within weeks.

Although infants and young children are at greatest risk of meningitis infection and disease, polysaccharide meningitis vaccines are not routinely used in that age group because of their limited efficacy in very young children [15]. Intensive efforts are ongoing to introduce and scale up the use of a newly developed conjugate meningitis

A vaccine [16] that is affordable for countries of the African meningitis belt. It is hoped that this new vaccine, with good efficacy in both young children and older individuals [17], will establish herd immunity and broad community protection. This could potentially lead to the eventual elimination of serogroup A meningococcal meningitis epidemics as a public health problem [18] in the African meningitis belt.

The introduction strategy for the new conjugate meningitis A vaccine consists of providing an initial single dose during mass campaigns to all persons aged 1–29 years to rapidly reduce bacterial carriage and transmission, thereby reducing disease-related morbidity and mortality. Following these initial mass campaigns, to protect birth cohorts throughout infancy, it is planned that countries with a well-performing EPI will introduce the vaccine into their routine immunization program. Regular follow-up campaigns, targeting children aged 1–4 years old, may still be required in countries with low-performing immunization programs.

Yellow fever

Yellow fever is caused by a virus that is endemic in tropical regions of Africa and South America, where 44 countries (33 in Africa and 11 in South America) are considered to be at risk. In francophone Africa, intensive preventive mass vaccination campaigns nearly eliminated yellow fever during the 1950s but subsequently vaccine coverage waned, with epidemics occurring in the 1980s. Currently, 500 million people are considered at risk for the disease in Africa.

A severe epidemic of human-to-human transmission is most likely to occur when conditions allow the density of the mosquito vector populations to substantially increase, as often happens during the rainy season. Epidemiologic surveillance is a key strategy for limiting yellow fever epidemics by rapidly identifying human infections when they occur. Mosquito control is an effective supplemental prevention strategy.

The most effective means of preventing yellow fever epidemics is through vaccination at 9 months of age using the vaccine as part of routine immunization programs [19]. However, routine yellow fever vaccine coverage is generally poor in Africa

(<50%), lagging behind measles vaccine coverage even though both vaccines should be given at the same visit.

If routine immunization at 9 months of age does not reach the level needed to achieve herd immunity in the general population, epidemic transmission is a risk and mass vaccination is required to fill the gap in immunity. The target population for mass vaccination, once yellow fever has been identified in human populations, is the entire population living or working in the area where the infection has been identified. In the event of limited financial resources or limited vaccine supply, the primary target population is usually children aged from 9 months to 14 years, after which adults at risk are also vaccinated. Vaccinations are generally provided through house-to-house campaigns, during which there is also active questioning (i.e., an "active case search") to detect additional human infections.

Influenza

Influenza viruses cause annual epidemics and sometimes global pandemics. Each year, seasonal influenza occurs during the winter months in both the northern and southern hemispheres. It is estimated that up to 500 000 persons, mainly over the age of 60, die annually from seasonal influenza. Because of frequent mutations ("antigenic drift") in circulating influenza virus strains, the composition of the vaccine needs to be modified annually, followed by the rapid annual re-vaccination of the populations at risk, in time before the start of the influenza epidemic season.

In some industrialized countries vaccination against seasonal influenza is only recommended for the elderly, while in others it is also offered to health workers and/or military personnel. In a few areas (see below) the vaccine is being offered to the general population over 6 months of age. Because of the seasonal nature of the disease, and the need to produce a new vaccine formulation each year, influenza vaccine is provided by mass immunization at fixed health facilities, most frequently at doctor's offices; however, clinics, the workplace, or other gathering points in the community (pharmacies, stores) may also be used [20].

"Universal" vaccination of all persons older than 6 months of age against seasonal influenza has been recommended as a strategy to increase overall coverage and also to indirectly protect older persons by decreasing infection and transmission among children. This approach requires further expanding mass immunization in the community and into schools and has so far not been widely adopted. However, universal influenza vaccination was introduced in 2000 in the provinces of Ontario in Canada. An evaluation of that program in 2008 [21] showed that the introduction of universal vaccination had been followed by greater increases in vaccination coverage in Ontario, and greater decreases in influenza-related mortality and health-facility usage in that province, compared to other Canadian provinces; the universal vaccination approach introduced in Ontario province was also found to be cost effective [22].

Following the introduction of a new or novel influenza A subtype into human populations, usually from an avian source ("antigenic shift"), a global influenza pandemic may result, since most or all of the population is susceptible and there is little or no cross-immunity from existing influenza vaccines. The most recent global pandemic occurred in 2009–2010, with the emergence of the new H1N1 strain. In such cases, the pandemic virus strain is used to develop a new vaccine, of which two doses may be required to produce an acceptable antibody response to a subtype that has not circulated previously. Following global and national pandemic preparedness and response plans, the entire population is targeted using mass immunization, beginning with defined high-priority groups such as those providing essential services (including health care workers), and groups identified at highest risk of severe illness and death.

Emergency settings: displaced populations

War, civil disturbance, and natural disasters can lead to a sudden and massive internal or international displacement of populations. During the initial phase of the emergency, primary health care and immunization services are often not available. The risk of infectious disease outbreaks, particularly due to vaccine-preventable diseases, increases once refugees or internally displaced groups start to congregate in camp settings; the risk may be further exacerbated by very close living conditions, compromised water supplies, and poor sanitation.

To respond to the high risk of outbreaks in such settings, it is standard practice for agencies responsible for the health of refugees and for groups of internally displaced persons (IDPs) to conduct mass immunization campaigns with the main EPI vaccines, which will, depending on local circumstances, include vaccines against measles, meningococcal meningitis, and yellow fever [23].

The most critical vaccine to use in refugee and IPD camp settings during the early phase of an emergency is measles vaccine – particularly where previous routine measles vaccine coverage is low. To assure protection of the most vulnerable age groups against measles, the target age group is often extended to include children from 6 months up to 14 years of age; for very young children, a second dose of measles vaccine is given at 12 months of age due to the lower efficacy of the vaccine before that age.

Mass vaccination for meningitis and yellow fever is conducted if risk factors for epidemics are present. Studies on the usefulness of new cholera and typhoid vaccines in mass campaigns in displaced populations are ongoing, with initial results suggesting that they may be useful as supplements to the provision of safe drinking water and proper sanitation in such settings.

Responding to threats of deliberately caused outbreaks

Under certain circumstances, public health authorities may decide to initiate preventive action to avert the risk of a deliberately caused epidemic, or respond to the threat of "bioterrorism." In the resulting scenario, mass immunization campaigns may be conducted as a deterrent, or to prevent a planned or impending intentionally caused infectious disease outbreak. Responding to a perceived threat from deliberately caused outbreaks of diseases such as smallpox and anthrax, some countries have begun to stockpile vaccines against these perceived threats to prepare for mass immunization of the entire population should such a threat become real [24].

Different countries have formulated different strategies for mass immunization responses to bioterrorism threats. Most countries, however, prioritize first vaccinating and protecting staff involved in primary response activities, such as health workers, followed by mass immunization of the general population if the intentionally used infectious agent is shown to be capable of person-to-person spread.

Compared to other indications, mass immunization activities in response to the threat of a deliberately caused outbreak will be a deterrent and preventive in nature. Consequently, they must be as safe as possible, often requiring more complex strategies than other campaigns. Smallpox vaccination of persons infected with HIV, for example, has been associated with generalized vaccinia and death [25]. Until a safer smallpox vaccine becomes available, preventive mass immunization strategies that use smallpox vaccine will therefore need to be designed to avoid vaccination of HIV-infected persons, while providing these individuals with protection by other means, such as passive immunization with vaccinia immune globulin.

Accelerated disease control

Immunization campaigns to supplement routine vaccination programs and increase coverage – now often referred to as supplementary immunization activities (SIAs) – were used during the early phase of the EPI to rapidly increase coverage and reach the 1990 "universal child immunization" (UCI) goal. However, the approach at that time was associated with both positive and negative effects [26].

More recently, SIAs have been used less to boost overall coverage than as important tools for disease eradication and elimination initiatives, including global polio eradication, measles mortality reduction (e.g., in Africa [27]), measles elimination (in WHO Regions with an elimination goal [28]), and MNT elimination.

Polio and measles SIAs have often been used to provide additional interventions, most commonly vitamin A supplementation [29], but also, for example, insecticide-treated bed nets for malaria prevention [30] or deworming medication. Over the past decade, a growing number of African and South Asian countries have adopted "Child Health Days" (CHDs) [31] to offer a wider package of child health interventions, including immunizations through a mass campaign approach. Typically, vitamin A supplementation and one or more other child health services, usually childhood immunizations and deworming medication, are offered to children <5 years of age. A recent study of CHDs in six sub-Saharan countries [32] found that CHDs can quickly increase coverage of key child survival interventions, but that the conduct of CHDs contributes little toward establishing effective primary health care systems. Therefore, mass immunization campaigns (SIAs) and accompanying CHDs should not be used to replace weak immunization and primary health care delivery systems.

Mass immunization against measles

Measles is one of the most contagious of human diseases. An estimated 2.6 million deaths from measles occurred in 1980, before the widespread use of measles vaccine [33]. In view of the potential of measles vaccination to help reduce mortality of young children, measles immunization coverage was selected as an indicator of progress toward reaching the Millennium Development Goal 4 (reduction of child mortality).

Measles vaccination has been included in routine immunization programs in developing countries for over 40 years, targeting children between 9 and 12 months of age. At this age, measles vaccine efficacy is about 85–90% (i.e., 10–15% of children remain unprotected), most likely due to the presence of maternal antibodies that in effect "protect" against the vaccine virus, and due to the relative immaturity of the immune system.

While high coverage with one dose of measles vaccine will substantially reduce measles morbidity and mortality in a population, a second vaccine dose is needed to achieve higher levels of measles reduction and especially to achieve measles elimination [34]. This second dose is intended to give a "second opportunity" to seroconvert for children who did not respond to or who missed the first dose.

WHO recommends [35] that reaching all children with two doses of measles vaccine, either through routine immunization services or through periodic mass immunization campaigns, should be the standard for all national immunization programs.

In countries with low-performing immunization services, an initial "catch-up" measles mass campaign targeting a large age group (all children 9 months to <15 years of age) is recommended, followed by regular follow-up campaigns (in children aged 9 months to <5 years of age). This has proven to be an effective strategy to protect children and achieve substantial reductions in measles mortality and morbidity by rapidly increasing population immunity, especially if done during the pre-epidemic season.

Because the risk of measles outbreaks is determined by the rate of accumulation of susceptible individuals in the population, the WHO Region of the Americas developed a strategy recommending that programs conduct their follow-up mass campaigns before the number of susceptible children of pre-school age reaches the size of a birth cohort, effectively every 3–5 years, depending on routine immunization coverage. This approach has contributed significantly to lower overall child mortality. During 2000–2008, global mortality attributed to measles declined by 78%, from an estimated 733 000 deaths in 2000 to 164 000 in 2008 [36].

As of 2008, a "two-dose measles vaccine opportunity" strategy is used by 192 of 193 WHO Member States: 60 countries use a routine first dose plus regular mass campaigns, while 132 countries use a routine two-dose schedule. Of this latter group, 49 also conduct regular nationwide campaigns and 39 have conducted a one-time catch-up campaign; 44 rely only on the delivery of two routine doses. Though mass immunization campaigns against measles can rapidly increase herd immunity, they must not be used as a substitute for strengthening weak routine immunization programs.

Maternal and neonatal tetanus elimination

Routine EPI immunization schedules in developing countries include maternal immunization with tetanus toxoid (TT) to prevent MNT, in conjunction with the promotion of clean birth and delivery practices. To compensate for low routine TT coverage of women of childbearing age, and to accelerate progress toward MNT elimination, a high-risk approach has been adopted that includes supplementary mass immunization campaigns with

TT and promotion of clean delivery practices, targeting women of childbearing age in high-risk areas identified through neonatal tetanus surveillance.

Since WHO called for global MNT elimination in 1989 [37], progress has been substantial, with the number of estimated deaths from neonatal tetanus worldwide reduced from >800 000 in the 1980s to 180 000 in 2002. Between 1999 and June 2008, 45 countries implemented supplemental TT immunization campaigns, immunizing more than 81 million women with two or more doses of TT vaccine. However, the goal of MNT elimination has not yet been achieved. By 2008, MNT had not yet been eliminated from 46 countries [38].

Introduction of new vaccines

More than 20 new vaccines have become available during the past 60 years. Often when a new vaccine is introduced into routine immunization programs, mass immunization is an important tool for the initial rapid reduction, or "mopping up," of the number of persons susceptible to the vaccine target disease. The objective of mass immunization in such situations is to equalize the levels of population immunity to avoid the sudden changes in target disease transmission patterns that might occur when only a subgroup of susceptible people is covered when routine immunization begins. After the initial mass immunization campaign, the new vaccine can then be incorporated into the routine program to protect all susceptible newborns.

One example in which mass immunization campaigns were used to introduce a new vaccine was for the inactivated poliovirus or Salk vaccine (IPV) after its first licensure in the US in the 1950s. Initially, mass campaigns were used to target all population groups considered at risk of polio, before integrating the vaccine into routine immunization programs.

Another example is the rubella vaccine, which has long been used in routine programs in industrialized countries, but until recently had not been introduced widely in developing countries. The reasons for this include concerns that the use of rubella vaccine in routine infant immunization programs could shift the age of rubella infection to older girls, which in turn could increase the risk of disease in susceptible pregnant women, and thereby

lead to a higher incidence of congenital rubella syndrome (CSR). For this reason, one-time mass campaigns are recommended to accompany the introduction of routine rubella vaccination [39]. These campaigns typically target girls under 15 years of age, but in some countries include all women of childbearing age.

In the western hemisphere, many countries were already conducting mass campaigns targeting children up to 15 years as part of their measles elimination strategies. The use of combination products containing rubella and measles and/or mumps vaccines (MR, MMR) in measles routine and supplementary immunization campaigns greatly facilitated the introduction of routine rubella vaccination and the conduct of initial rubella vaccine mass campaigns.

As outlined above, one-time mass campaigns are also used to facilitate the introduction of routine yellow fever vaccination by rapidly reducing susceptibility to yellow fever infection in multiple birth cohorts, usually by targeting all children <15 years [40]. The objective is to "fill immunity gaps" in older age groups and prevent yellow fever outbreaks that would otherwise continue to occur until birth cohorts immunized as infants reach adulthood. A similar approach, using even larger initial mass campaigns targeting all individuals under 30 years of age, will soon be used to introduce the new conjugate meningitis A vaccine into routine immunization programs in sub-Saharan African countries.

Mass immunization for disease eradication: example polio eradication

Effective vaccines against poliomyelitis became available in the mid-1950s (IPV) and early 1960s (OPV). Early polio control efforts with IPV in the US used mass campaigns, which were conducted in public gathering places like schools, worksites, and churches. This led to dramatic decreases in the incidence of poliomyelitis [41]. Following licensure in industrialized countries in the early 1960s, monovalent OPVs were also used extensively in mass campaigns, called "SOS" (Sabin Oral Sundays) in the USA [42]. Subsequently, trivalent oral poliovirus vaccine (tOPV) became the main vaccine used in routine infant immunization programs in both industrialized and developing countries.

As early as the 1960s, Cuba demonstrated that regular, high-coverage nationwide campaigns with OPV could rapidly interrupt indigenous poliovirus transmission. During the 1980s, mass immunization campaigns with tOPV ("National Immunization Days," or NIDs), in addition to routine polio immunization, interrupted wild poliovirus transmission in a number of other tropical and semi-tropical developing countries of Latin America. Following the success of smallpox eradication and in view of rapid progress toward interrupting wild poliovirus transmission in the WHO Region of the Americas, the World Health Assembly resolved in 1988 to eradicate poliomyelitis globally [43].

Since then, nationwide or subnational mass supplementary immunization days (NIDs or sub-NIDs), providing oral poliovirus vaccine to children under the age of 5 years, irrespective of prior polio vaccination history, became one of the four core strategies for polio eradication. An increasing number of countries were able to interrupt the transmission of indigenous wild poliovirus, using vaccine delivery at fixed sites, with intense house-to-house "mop-up" vaccination in the last remaining foci of virus transmission.

Initial progress in polio eradication was remarkable. The last case of polio in the Americas was reported in 1991, followed by certification of the Region as polio-free by an international certification commission in 1994 [44]. The Western Pacific and European Regions of the WHO were certified as polio-free in 2000 and 2001, respectively [45,46].

Since 2006, however, four countries remain where wild poliovirus transmission has never been interrupted: India, Pakistan, Afghanistan, and Nigeria. In addition, wild virus derived from these countries, especially Nigeria and India, has repeatedly reinfected previously polio-free countries, mainly in West and Central Africa.

To complete global eradication, a range of operational and technical innovations have been introduced since the late 1990s to improve both the impact and coverage of polio campaigns, with implications and lessons for all SIAs. To improve OPV coverage, for example, several large countries with persistent transmission (e.g., Egypt, India, Pakistan) switched to mainly house-to-house vaccine delivery; independent monitoring of campaign performance was introduced globally; "finger-marking" of vaccinated children with indelible ink was used to improve coverage estimates; and areas found to be covered poorly were systematically targeted for immediate re-vaccination.

To improve the impact of each vaccination contact, monovalent type 1 and type 3 oral polio vaccines (mOPV1, mOPV3) were reintroduced in 2005 for countries with persistent wild poliovirus transmission that required very high levels of population immunity, and for countries with new outbreaks due to reinfection with a single serotype. Building on the regulatory experience and safety of mOPVs, a new bivalent OPV formulation (types 1 and 3) was licensed in mid-2009 to accelerate eradication in areas of concomitant transmission of both type 1 and type 3 wild poliovirus.

Just over 1600 polio cases were reported in 2009 [47], with the most intense transmission in northern Nigeria and northern India. In India, nearly all polio cases in 2009 were limited to high-risk districts in western Uttar Pradesh and central Bihar. In Afghanistan and Pakistan, difficulties in accessing children in conflict-affected areas and operational limitations in parts of Pakistan allowed continuing wild polio virus circulation in a relatively small number of high-risk districts.

By mid-2010, however, the number of cases reported from both India and Nigeria had fallen to the lowest levels since eradication efforts began, and the majority of African countries that had been reinfected in 2009 again appeared to be polio-free. Building on the lessons learned over the past 20 years, in June 2010 a new Strategic Plan for polio eradication was launched to address the local barriers to interrupting transmission in each of the remaining infected areas and scale up the use of the new bivalent oral poliovirus vaccine (bOPV) in SIAs, which will be key to further progress. By end-2011, the impact of the new strategic approaches and area-specific tactics had been demonstrated, by the absence of wild poliovirus in India, arguably one of the most technically challenging places from where to eradicate polio. And although positive developments were also seen in the remaining three endemic countries Nigeria, Pakistan and Afghanistan, all three suffered a significant and unexpected surge in new cases in 2011. Reviewing the latest epidemiological evidence and the opportunity which presented itself to achieving a polio-free world, the Executive Board of the World Health Assembly in January 2012 declared the completion of eradication a programmatic emergency for global public health. Subsequently, national emergency action plans were launched in all three remaining endemic countries, the implementation of which will be overseen by the highest levels of the governments, and focusing on urgently addressing the remaining obstacles to achieving a polio-free world.

Mass immunization campaigns: programmatic issues

The impact of mass immunization campaigns depends on their quality (i.e., their ability to reach and vaccinate a very high proportion of the target population), which in turn depends on the quality of planning and preparation, on ensuring well-supervised and monitored campaign implementation, and on conducting appropriate post-campaign evaluation, to assess coverage and identify operational problems to better target "mopping-up" vaccination.

The most critical questions that need to be answered when planning and implementing a mass immunization campaign are the age range and size of the target population group (e.g., children aged <5 years for polio campaigns versus persons of all ages for meningitis campaigns), the geographical size of the targeted area (nationwide versus subnational campaigns), the type of vaccine to be used, the vaccine delivery strategy (e.g., immunization at fixed posts versus house-to-house vaccine delivery), and who will be the main groups to conduct the actual campaign field work (trained health workers versus community volunteers).

Some planning, operational, and logistic issues that critically determine the quality of a mass immunization campaign are outlined below.

Campaign planning committee

In many countries, national-level campaign planning committees, often the existing Interagency Coordinating Committees (ICCs) for immunization, chaired by the Ministry of Health, have played a critical role in planning, preparing, and financing mass campaigns. Such committees, with the participation of different sectors of government as well as other national and international agencies with an interest in immunization, should have overall responsibility for preparing campaign plans and budgets, and for coordinating subcommittees in charge of operational planning, vaccine procurement, and communications/social mobilization. There should be sufficient lead time from the first planning meeting to campaign implementation. In countries where no campaign has been done for several years, planning should start up to 6 months ahead of the campaign date, though in emergency situations this can be as short as a few weeks.

Engaging and obtaining local government support

Ownership and engagement of health and political leaders at all levels, but particularly at the district level, is the most critical factor to assure campaign quality. Mass campaigns, often targeting 20% or more of the total population, cannot be run by the health department alone. District campaign management teams with multisectoral representation (e.g., education, labor, police) and including other civic organizations and nongovernmental groups have proven invaluable to ensure a successful activity.

Detailed "microplanning" process

Microplanning, ideally conducted together with campaign workers from the grassroots level, is critical to translate overall planning into practical and locally implementable action plans. Microplanning starts with confirming, and where necessary adjusting, the target population, taking particular care to include high-risk groups and areas (see below). Microplans typically break the targeted area into basic operational units, often the area covered by one field supervisor and his/her teams during the campaign, and document and list all logistical requirements, required vaccination teams, supervisors, local volunteers, and social mobilization activities. The development of simple, usually hand-drawn, maps is a critical element of a good microplanning process.

Identification of "high-risk" groups and areas

Both for routine and supplementary immunization activities, certain population groups are known to be at higher risk of being missed. These groups, often underserved by government health services, can include ethnic or religious minorities, nomads and other mobile populations, refugees, internally displaced persons and other marginalized groups, or groups with low socioeconomic status, who are often found in the more remote and/or harder to access areas (i.e., border and mountainous areas, but also peri-urban slum areas). The quality of campaigns and their impact on disease transmission depends considerably on the extent to which these groups can be identified and vaccinated. Priority campaign implementation elements through which to assure the inclusion of high-risk groups are microplans, maps, communication and social mobilization strategies, and even the selection of culturally appropriate vaccination team members.

Communication and social mobilization

Timely communication and social mobilization activities among the general public are important to assure awareness of the immunization campaign and its objectives, and to mobilize communities to participate and support activities. Communication and mobilization activities increase in importance when campaigns target wider age groups, especially if adults are to be vaccinated. Communication and social mobilization activities also need to be adjusted and targeted to reach and vaccinate high-risk groups (see above), particularly those who may have concerns about the vaccine, or even refuse to accept it.

Strengthening routine immunizations

Mass immunization should be used temporarily or intermittently to increase herd immunity for specific public health program needs, and in such a way as to strengthen routine immunization services. It should not be used to replace weak immunization programs.

Implementation: team selection, training, supervision, and monitoring

The success of a mass campaign depends on the quality of fieldwork, which is largely determined by the selection of appropriate vaccinators and supervisors, and by their training and motivation, particularly in areas with weak health services. In many areas it is important to assure the recruitment of vaccination team members who are from the local community, who speak the local language and belong to the same ethnic or religious group. In culturally conservative areas of Islamic countries, for example, only female vaccinators will be able to enter homes during house-to-house work and completely identify and vaccinate all target children.

Field supervisors need to be mobile and actively follow their teams to assure all target children are vaccinated. Monitors independent of campaign implementation can provide critical information by monitoring both campaign processes and outcomes; they should provide immediate feedback on problems to campaign managers to facilitate and ensure corrective action.

Technical support from partner agencies

Both at the national and provincial level, but particularly in districts and areas with weak health infrastructure and limited numbers of trained health staff, strong support from partner agencies, specifically from WHO and UNICEF, has been critical to successfully implement campaigns.

Mass immunization: future outlook

Since the first use of mass immunization during the Jenner era, major progress has been made in establishing and strengthening routine childhood immunization as a key component of primary health care services at the community level. However, mass immunization campaigns, conducted over short time periods, remain a critical tool for optimizing the control of vaccine-preventable diseases in both developing and industrialized countries (Table 31.1).

Mass campaigns are particularly important for the prevention of and early response to vaccine-preventable disease outbreaks, to rapidly protect vulnerable groups in emergency settings, to optimize the impact of a newly introduced vaccine, to achieve the very high levels of population

Table 31.1 Uses of mass immunization in public health.

Public health need	Specific disease
Preventing and responding to outbreaks	Meningitis, yellow fever, influenza, vaccine preventable disease in displaced populations, deliberately caused infectious disease outbreak
Accelerated disease control	Measles mortality reduction, maternal and neonatal tetanus elimination, new vaccine introduction
Eradication	Polio

immunity required to achieve disease elimination and eradication goals, and, sometimes, to supplement routine infant immunization. Routine and mass immunization remain equally valuable and complementary tools to attain national and international vaccine-preventable disease objectives – the key to their joint success is to optimize the opportunities afforded by mass campaigns to also strengthen routine immunization services rather than for them to serve as a substitute.

References

1 Hopkins DR. *Princes and Peasants: Smallpox in History*. University of Chicago Press, Chicago, IL, 1983.

2 Fenner F, Henderson DA, Arita I, Jezek Z, Ladnyi ID. Early efforts at control: variation, vaccination, and isolation and quarantine. In *Smallpox and its Eradication*. World Health Organization, Geneva, 1988, ch. 6, p. 263.

3 McLeod RM. Law, medicine and public opinion: the resistance to compulsory health legislation 1870–1907. *Public Law* 1967;**6**:107–28, 189–211.

4 Edwards EJ. *A Concise History of Smallpox and Vaccination in Europe*. Lewis, London, 1902.

5 World Health Organization. World Health Assembly resolution 19.16, 1966.

6 Fenner F, Henderson DA, Arita I, Jezek Z, Ladnyi ID. Lessons and benefits. In *Smallpox and its Eradication*. World Health Organization, Geneva, 1988, ch. 31, pp. 1363–5.

7 Barrett S, Hoel M. Optimal disease eradication (HERO working paper 23/2003). Frisch Centre, University of Oslo, 2003.

8 Sencer JD, Axnick NW. Cost benefit analysis. In *Proceedings of the International Symposium on Vaccination against Communicable Disease*, March, 1973. Symposium Series on Immunobiological Standardization, Karger, Basel, 1973, vol. 22, pp. 37–46.

9 Gonzalez CL. *Mass Campaigns and General Health Services*, Public Health Papers, no. 29. World Health Organization, Geneva, 1965.

10 Mills A. Mass campaigns versus general health services: what we have learnt in 40 years about vertical versus horizontal approaches. *Bull World Health Org* 2005;**83**(4):315–16.

11 World Health Organization. Declaration of Alma-Ata. International Conference on Primary Health Care, Alma-Ata, USSR, Sep 6–12, 1978.

12 Muraskin W. The Global Alliance for Vaccines and Immunization: is it a new model for effective public-private cooperation in international public health? *Am J Public Health* 2004;**94**(11):1922–25.

13 Greenwood BM. The epidemiology of acute bacterial meningitis in tropical Africa. In JD Williams, J Brunie (Eds) *Bacterial Meningitis*. Academic Press, London, 1987, pp. 61–91.

14 World Health Organization. Meningitis in Chad, Niger and Nigeria: 2009 epidemic season. *WHO Wkly Epidemiol Rec* 2009;**85**:57–63.

15 Reingold AL, Broome CV, HightowerA, *et al*. Age specific differences in duration of clinical protection after vaccination with meningococcal polysaccharide A vaccine. *Lancet* 1985;**2**:112–18.

16 LaForce FM, Konde K, Viviani S, Préziosi MP. The Meningitis Vaccine Project. *Vaccine* 2007;**25**(Suppl 1):A97–100.

17 Kshirsagar N, Mur N, Thatte U, *et al*. Safety, immunogenicity, and antibody persistence of a new meningococcal group A conjugate vaccine in healthy Indian adults. *Vaccine* 2007;**25**(Suppl 1):A101–7.

18 World Health Organization and UNICEF. Eliminating serogroup A meningococcal meningitis epidemics as

a public health problem in Africa. An investment case for the GAVI Alliance, Apr 3, 2008. Available at www.who.int/entity/immunization/sage/Meningitis_Investment_Case_Exec_summary.pdf. Accessed Feb 2012.

19 World Health Organization. Yellow Fever. WHO/EPI/GEN/98.11, WHO/CDS/EDC/2000.2, 2000.

20 Stohr K. Influenza. In DL Heymann (Ed.) *Control of Communicable Diseases Manual*, 18th edn. American Public Health Association, Washington, DC, 2004.

21 Kwong JC, Stukel TA, Lim J, *et al.* The effect of universal influenza immunization on mortality and health care use. *PLoS Med* 2008;**5**(10):e211.

22 Sander B, Kwong JC, Bauch CT, *et al.* Economic appraisal of Ontario's Universal Influenza Immunization Program: a cost-utility analysis. *PLoS Med* 2010;**7**(4):e256.

23 Connolly MA, Gayer M, Ryan MJ, *et al.* Communicable diseases in complex emergencies – impacts and challenges. *Lancet* 2004;**364**:1974–83.

24 World Health Organization. *Public Health Response to Biological and Chemical Weapons*, 2nd edn. WHO, Geneva, 2004.

25 Redheid RR, Wright DK, James WJ, *et al.* Disseminated vaccinia in a military recruit with human immunodeficiency virus (HIV) disease. *N Engl J Med* 1987;**316**:673–6.

26 Dietz V, Cutts F. The use of mass campaigns in the expanded programme on immunization: a review of reported advantages and disadvantages. *Int J Health Services* 1997;**27**(4):766–90.

27 Bielik R, Madema S, Taole A, *et al.* First 5 years of measles elimination in southern Africa: 1996–2000. *Lancet* 2002;**359**(9137):1564–8.

28 Expanded Programme on Immunization. Progress in reducing global measles deaths, 1999–2004. *Wkly Epidemiol Rec* 2006;**81**:90–94.

29 Ching P, Birmingham M, Goodman T. Childhood mortality impact and costs of implementing vitamin A supplementation in immunization campaigns. *Am J Public Health* 2000;**90**:1526–9.

30 Centers for Disease Control and Prevention. Distribution of insecticide-treated bednets during an integrated nationwide immunization campaign – Togo, West Africa, December 2004. *MMWR Morb Mortal Wkly Rep* 2005;**54**:994–6.

31 UNICEF. Results from the Child Health Days Assessments. Preliminary Findings: Ethiopia, Tanzania and Uganda. Presentation at the Global Immunization Meeting, Feb 13–15, 2007, New York.

32 Doherty T, Chopra M, Tomlinson M, *et al.* Moving from vertical to integrated child health programmes: experiences from a multi-country assessment of the Child Health Days approach in Africa. *Trop Med Int Health* 2010;**15**(3):206–305.

33 Wolfson L, Strebel P, Gacic-Dobo M, *et al.* Has the 2005 measles mortality reduction goal been achieved? A natural history modelling study. *Lancet* 2007;**369**: 191–200.

34 World Health Organization. Strategies for reducing global measles mortality. *Wkly Epidemiol Rec* 2000;**75**:409–16.

35 World Health Organization. Measles vaccines: WHO position paper. *Wkly Epidemiol Rec* 2009;**84**:349–60.

36 CDC. Global Measles Mortality 2000–2008, *MMWR Morb Mortal Wkly Rep* 2009;**58**(47):1321–6.

37 World Health Organization. Tetanus vaccine. WHO position paper. *Wkly Epidemiol Rec* 2006;**81**:198–208.

38 UNICEF. Elimination of Maternal and Neonatal Tetanus. Available at www.unicef.org/health/index_43509.html. Accessed Feb 2012.

39 World Health Organization. Control of rubella and congenital rubella syndrome in developing countries. WHO/V&B/00.03, 2003.

40 World Health Organization. Yellow Fever. WHO/EPI/GEN/98.11, WHO/CDS/EDC/2000.2, 2000.

41 Sutter RW, Kew OM, Cochi SL. Poliovirus vaccine – live. In SA Plotkin, WA Orenstein (Eds), *Vaccines*, 4th edn. WB Saunders, Philadelphia, PA, 2003, pp. 651–705.

42 Sabin AB. Oral poliovirus vaccine: history of its development and use and current challenge to eliminate poliomyelitis from the world. *J Infect Dis* 1985; **151**:420–36.

43 41st World Health Assembly. Resolution WHA41.28. Call for the worldwide eradication of poliomyelitis, 1988.

44 CDC. Certification of polio eradication – the Americas, 1994. *MMWR Morb Mortal Wkly Rep* 1994; **43**:720–22.

45 CDC. Certification of polio eradication – Western Pacific Region, 2000. *MMWR Morb Mortal Wkly Rep* 2001;**50**:1–3.

46 WHO. Certification of poliomyelitis eradication, European Region, June 2002. *Wkly Epidemiol Rec* 2002;**77**: 221–3.

47 WHO. Progress in interrupting wild poliovirus transmission worldwide, 2009. *Wkly Epidemiol Rec* 2010; **85**:177–84

The Role of Mathematical Models in Vaccine Development and Public Health Decision Making

Marie-Claude Boily[1], Marc Brisson[2], Benoit Mâsse[3], & Roy M. Anderson[1]

[1]Division of Epidemiology, Public Health and Primary Care, School of Public Health, London, UK
[2]Unité de Recherche en Santé des Populations, Centre de Recherche Fonds de la Recherche en Santé du Québec du Centre Hospitalier affilié Universitaire de Québec, Canada
[3]Public Health Sciences Division, Biostatistics, Fred Hutchinson Cancer Research Center, Seattle, Washington, USA

Introduction

Since Daniel Bernouilli applied mathematical methods nearly 300 years ago to evaluate the effectiveness of variolation techniques against smallpox, mathematical models have been applied widely to understand the spread of infections and potential impact of control interventions such as vaccination [1–4]. A theoretical framework provides a template to explore how different factors – both biologic and epidemiologic factors, and public health interventions – impact on the prevalence and incidence of morbidity and mortality caused by an infectious agent [1,4–7]. Early work by Hamer [8], Ross [9], Kermack and McKendrick [10], and others, summarized in [1], employed simple mathematical models to improve understanding of various factors and processes, including what factors determine transmission success, what are the key determinants of the prevalence of infection, and how infections are transmitted between individuals, to derive key concepts such as the basic reproductive number and the herd immunity threshold, with important implications for control by vaccination. With the advent of powerful computers, more complex simulation models have been used to explore the im-

portance of various forms of heterogeneity, including variation in infectiousness and susceptibility to infection, and host movement as well as mixing patterns [1,11–13]. Over the past two decades various events have stimulated the use of mathematical templates to explore how best to control the spread of infection, both nationally and internationally. These include the AIDS pandemic, the 2001 foot and mouth (FMD) epidemic in cattle and sheep in the UK, the 2003 SARS epidemic, and most recently the 2009 H1N1 influenza A pandemic [14–17]. Models are increasingly being used both to address a wide range of issues in public health and disease control and, combined with economic analyses, to identify optimal control strategies [18,19]. Perhaps the most developed area of application is that of vaccination. Models can provide many insights of relevance to the optimal design of mass vaccination programs. For example, they can yield insights on who and how many to vaccinate to induce a defined reduction in the incidence or prevalence of infection. They can also be used to assess the risks and benefits of immunization. All vaccines carry some small risk of inducing morbidity in those vaccinated. An inescapable truth is that vaccination is always beneficial to the majority when the target

Vaccinology: Principles and Practice, First Edition. Edited by W. John W. Morrow, Nadeem A. Sheikh, Clint S. Schmidt and D. Huw Davies.
© 2012 Blackwell Publishing Ltd. Published 2012 by Blackwell Publishing Ltd.

disease is common, but when it is rare the incidence of vaccine-induced morbidity may exceed that of disease-induced morbidity. Models can also be used to inform vaccine trial design and analysis to help identify promising vaccine candidates [20,21]. Simulating trials before implementation is a very valuable and cost effective tool to try to maximize the likelihood of identifying the true efficacy of a candidate under field trial (phase III) conditions [20,21]. In this chapter, we summarize key principles governing the impact of vaccines on infectious disease transmission and discuss how an understanding of these principles can be used to optimize the design of mass or targeted vaccination programs. The chapter also discusses how economic factors can be incorporated into mathematical models of infectious agent transmission and intervention impact. We also describe new developments in the use of mathematical models at different stages of vaccine development and efficacy assessment.

Key concepts of infectious disease spread and control

Spread of infection

Models of the transmission dynamics of microparasites often divide the population into a number of compartments such as Susceptible (S), Exposed (E), Infected (I), and Recovered/Immune (R) to describe the natural history of infection (Figure 32.1a) [1,4,5,22,23]. The natural history of the virus or bacterium within an infected person strongly influences the dynamics of infection in populations. For example, infections that confer long-lasting immunity tend to display oscillations due to exhaustion and renewal by new births in the number of susceptibles over time. In contrast, infections that do not confer long-lasting immunity tend to settle to a constant prevalence (Figure 32.1b,c) [1,5]. The central parameter of transmission dynamics models is the force of infection, $\lambda(t)$ (i.e., the incidence rate of new infections per susceptible per unit time) because it describes the transmission process between infected and susceptible individuals. In simple models representing a homogeneous population all individuals have the

same characteristics and make contacts with other individuals randomly (i.e., with equal probability – a concept referred to as the mass action principle [1]). Under these assumptions, $\lambda(t)$ depends on the prevalence of infection in the population at time t, $\frac{Y(t)}{N(t)}$, the average effective contact rate per unit time (c), and the transmission probability of infection per contact, β (Equation 32.1a) [1,4, 5,22]. The type of contacts considered are those that can lead to transmission, and they vary by infectious agent (e.g., droplets for the influenza virus; sexual contact for HIV; vector bites for malaria). The number of newly infected individuals depends on the force of infection and the number of susceptible in the population, $S(t)$ (Equation 32.1b).

$$\lambda(t) = \beta \cdot c \cdot \frac{Y(t)}{N(t)} \qquad (32.1a)$$

$$NewInfections(t) = \lambda(t) \cdot S(t) \qquad (32.1b)$$

When a pathogen is newly introduced into a fully susceptible population, it can either die out soon after its introduction or establish and spread to create an epidemic. In the longer term, depending on the natural history of infection and the supply of new susceptibles, the infectious agent may persist and settle to an endemic prevalence or die out. The outcome strongly depends on the maximum reproductive potential of the infection – that is, its basic reproductive number (R_0) – and whether there are enough new susceptibles to sustain transmission in the longer term (the reproductive number $R(t)$) [1,5–7,20,21]. R_0 is defined as the average number of secondary infections generated by one primary infected individual in a totally susceptible population (i.e., when the fraction of susceptibles $x(t) = 100\%$) [1,5–7]. In an open and stable homogeneous population, R_0 depends on the transmission parameter, β, the contact rate, c, and the average duration of the infectious period D (Equation 32.2) [1,21].

$$R_0 = \beta \cdot c \cdot D \qquad (32.2)$$

It should be noted that R_0 varies in value for different infections, in different populations, and over time due to variation in contact rates (Table 32.1) [1]. For example, a short duration infection such as

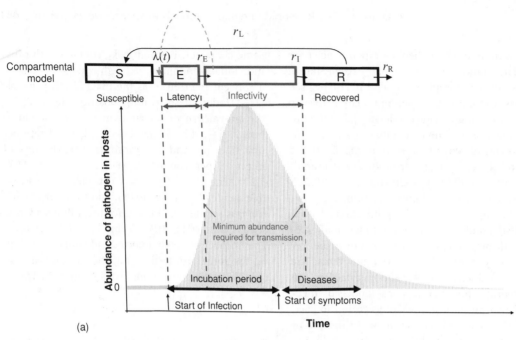

(a)

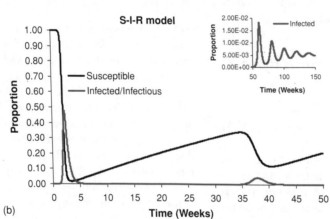

(b)

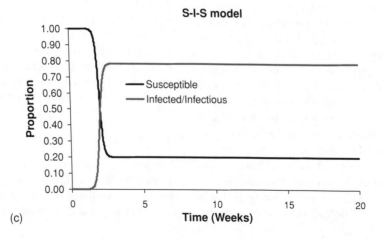

(c)

Figure 32.1 (a) Flowchart of the stages of infection of an S-E-I-R-S compartmental model that captures the effect of the abundance of the pathogen replicating inside individuals. The transmission process starts when susceptible individuals (S) are exposed and get infected with the pathogen, which multiplies in individuals but not sufficiently to be transmitted (E). Exposed individuals become infectious to others, if the pathogen is shed in sufficient quantity (I), after which they can recover from infection if the pathogen is adequately controlled by the immune system or successful treatment, or die if the infection is not controlled [23]. Depending on the pathogen, individuals can become immune (R) for life, or for some limited duration and become susceptible again (S). In the flow chart, each compartment represents the number of individuals in each infection stage at time t (i.e., state variable). More compartments can be added to the model to include more complexity. For example, additional compartments can be added to better reflect that individuals develop symptoms some time after infection depending on the duration of the incubation period (time period between infection and disease), which does not always correspond to the infectious period. Typically, three compartments are used to reflect the three main infectivity stages of, for example, HIV infectivity/infection: acute/primary, low/asymptomatic, and medium/symptomatic. The compartmental model can be translated in mathematical terms using differential equations to represent the change of individuals in the different states at time t [5]. The flow of individuals between stages of infection occurs at an average state-specific per capita rate per time unit: r_E = rate of becoming infectious, r_I = rate of developing protective immunity, r_L = rate of loss of immunity, r_R = rate of deaths. The inverse of these rates $(1/r_c)$ gives the average duration in each state. The force of infection, $\lambda(t)$, which is the rate at which susceptibles become infected, depends on the number/prevalence of infectious individuals in the population (as represented by the curved dotted line). Adapted from [23]. Different combinations of these compartments and the progression rates between them influence disease spread over time. Graphs show the fraction of susceptible and infectious individuals over time in stable open population. (b) Infections that confer long lasting immunity (S-I-R) will tend to display long-term oscillations due to the depletion and replenishment of susceptibles over time (e.g., measles, syphilis). (c) Infections that do not confer long lasting immunity (S-I-S) tend to settle to a constant prevalence (e.g., gonorrhea).

Table 32.1 Estimates of the basic reproductive rate and the eradication fraction for different diseases, countries, and time period.

Infection	Location	Period	R_0	Eradication fraction (herd immunity), p_h
Measles	England and Wales	1950–1968	16–18 [1]	90–95% [1]
	Kansas, USA	1918–1921	5–6 [1]	83–94% [24]
	Ontario, Canada	1912–1913	11–12 [1]	
	Willesden, England	1912–1913	11–12 [1]	
	Ghana	1960–1968	14–15 [1]	
	Eastern Nigeria	1960–1968	16–17 [1]	
	Senegal	1964	18	94% [31]
Chicken pox	England and Wales	1944–1968	10–12 [1]	85–90% [1]
	Baltimore, USA	1943	10–11 [1]	
Malaria			5–100 [24]	80–99% [1,24]
	Multi-strains		6–7 [5]	
Rubella	England and Wales	1960–1970	6–7 [1]	82–87% [1,24]
	West Germany	1970–1977	6–7 [1]	
	USA	1967	6	83% [31]
	Gambia	1976	15–16 [1]	
Smallpox			5–7 [24]	70–80% [1]
			3.5–6 [5]	80–85% [24]
	West Africa	1960s	2.3	57% [31]
Poliomyelitis	USA	1955	5–6 [1]	80–87% [1,24]

gonorrhea ($D < 6$ months) requires a higher contact rate, c, to establish compared to an infection like HIV with a longer period of infectivity, sometimes lasting many years. The R_0 of some childhood viral and bacterial infections is often larger in developing than developed countries because of greater crowding and higher birth rates, which favors infection like measles and rubella, or poorer hygiene, which favors transmission of infections like cholera, poliomyelitis, or hepatitis A through the fecal-oral route [1,4,5,24]. R_0 and $R(t)$ are important concepts which define threshold conditions for establishment and persistence. If $R_0 > 1$, infected individuals on average transmit their infection to more than one individual and an epidemic usually occurs. However, even when R_0 exceeds unity in value in small populations or communities stochastic effects may result in extinction because the probability of the index case not leading to transmission (e.g., if it dies) is larger. If $R_0 < 1$, only a few secondary transmissions occur and the infection eventually dies out. When the infection spreads in the population, the fraction of susceptibles decreases and some contacts are eventually "wasted" on individuals already infected and/or immune. Consequently, the average number of new transmissions per infected individual declines over time [1]. The quantity $R(t)$ reflects this dependence on the fraction of susceptibles (Equation 32.3a).

$$R(t) = R_0 \times x(t) \tag{32.3a}$$

At equilibrium:

$$R(t) = R_0 \times x(t) = 1 \tag{32.3b}$$

The critical fraction of susceptibles for the spread of infection is given by:

$$x_{min} > 1/R_0 \tag{32.3c}$$

When an epidemic persists in the longer term due to adequate replenishment of susceptibles through new births, immigration, recovery, or loss of immunity, it is said to have reached an endemic equilibrium. In this situation, each infected individual on average transmit its infection to one individual ($R(t) = 1$, Equation 32.3b). By rearranging Equation 32.3b, we obtain Equation 32.3c, which

Table 32.2 Estimates of the age at first infection for measles and rubella in different countries.

Infection	Location	Period	A (years)
Measles	England and Wales	1950–1968	~4–6
	Kansas, USA	1918–1921	~4.0–6.0
	Ghana	1960–1968	2.0–3.0
	Eastern Nigeria	1960–1968	2.0–3.0
Rubella	England and Wales	1960–1970	~9–10
	West Germany	1970–1977	11–12
	Gambia	1976	2–3
	India	1848–1968	12
	England and Wales	1948–1965	11–12

Reproduced from Anderson and May [1] with permission from OUP.

gives the minimum fraction of susceptibles necessary for an infection to establish and persist.

In practice, R_0 can be estimated directly if each parameter is known or indirectly if the relationship between R_0 and the average age at first infection (A) is known [1,5]. In simple models of childhood infection in an open and stable homogeneous population with a force of infection and mortality rate constant with age (i.e., exponential age distribution), R_0 is approximated by Equation 32.4 [1,4,5, 24]. The age at first infection of childhood infections is often estimated from age-stratified serological surveys (the most reliable information) or from case reports [1,5] (Table 32.2). Figure 32.2a shows that R_0 increases rapidly as the age of infection declines; a low average age at infection reflects a high force of infection.

$$R_0 = 1 + L/A \tag{32.4}$$

where L is the average life expectancy [1].

Elimination and eradication

Vaccination against an infectious disease protects individuals and populations in two ways. First, it directly protects adequately immunized individuals against infection. Second, it also confers indirect protection to nonvaccinated susceptibles by the creation of herd immunity. In other words, if sufficient individuals are effectively immunized by vaccination, the transmission rate of the infectious agent declines and hence the remaining susceptibles have a reduced chance of infection [1,4,5, 24–26]. In order to eradicate an infection it is necessary to reduce and maintain $R(t)$ below 1 (Equation 32.5a). To achieve this, not all susceptible individuals need to be vaccinated but only a critical fraction or herd immunity threshold, p_h, which depends on R_0 [1,5,7,24,26]. For a "perfect" vaccine, which perfectly protects 100% of those vaccinated for life, the fraction of susceptible newborns that needs to be vaccinated is given by Equation 32.5b. Figure 32.2b shows that the eradication fraction increases rapidly as R_0 rises in value. Infectious agents with high R_0 values such as measles and rubella are more difficult to control and eradicate than those such as influenza A, which typically has R_0 values in the range of 1.2–1.8 (Figure 32.2b).

$$\text{Eradication if } R(t) = R_0 \times x(t) < 1 \qquad (32.5a)$$

$$\text{Eradication fraction:} p_h = 1 - 1/R_0 \qquad (32.5b)$$

A population is said to have herd immunity once the eradication fraction has been achieved [24]. However, herd immunity effects can also occur even if coverage is below the eradication fraction due to the indirect protection (i.e., reduction in the risk of infection) conferred to unvaccinated and vaccinated individuals because the prevalence of infection is reduced among immunized individuals, which reduces exposure to infection of the whole population [1,4,5,24–26]. The herd/indirect effect is larger for larger vaccination coverage and lower R_0, and modest when vaccination coverage, or similarly vaccine efficacy, is poor because the force of infection acting on those who remain unvaccinated will remain essentially unchanged (Figure 32.2c).

However, in practice it is important to distinguish between elimination and eradication [31]. Elimination requires maintaining the vaccination coverage above the eradication fraction to eliminate endemic transmission and ensure that outbreaks will only be localized following the importation of new cases [25,34]. It can therefore be achieved only regionally. Eradication is more ambitious. It requires

the elimination of infection worldwide in order to eventually cease all control measures [1,5,24, 27–31].

Over the past 50 years different diseases (e.g., yellow fever, yaws, malaria, dracunculiasis [guinea worm], poliomyelitis) have been targeted for global eradication [27,28]. However, only smallpox has been certified eradicated [27–31]. This is in part because smallpox had a lower R_0, and lower eradication fraction, than many infections (Table 32.1, Figure 32.2b). For example, estimates of the measles eradication fraction range between 83% and 95% (compared to 70–85% for smallpox), depending on model assumptions, with estimates above 90% believed to be more realistic due to the younger average age at infection for measles (~2–3 years) than smallpox (around teenage to early 20s years) (Table 32.1, Figure 32.2) [1,4,5,24,27–30]. Other reasons for the effective smallpox eradication campaign include the ease with which cases of disease could be identified and reported. In contrast, despite considerable progresses and long-term efforts, measles has been eliminated in many parts of the world but has not yet been eradicated. Reviews of key global eradication requirements are ongoing to decide if it is really feasible [33,34]. Global eradication is obviously challenging since it depends on biologic and epidemiologic factors, as well as logistic/operational, political (the desire to allocate the required funds for repeated mass vaccination), and economic issues (Table 32.3) [27–31, 33,35–37]. Indeed, to maintain vaccination coverage above the eradication threshold and be able to reach often difficult to access high-transmission areas, the initial burden of disease (morbidity and mortality) needs to be large, and sufficient societal and political will is required to sustain the intense efforts required over several years, especially when the disease becomes rare following an effective vaccination campaign [27–31]. For example, even though smallpox was eliminated early in industrialized countries, soon after the first global eradication efforts began in 1959, vaccination had to continue until 1970 to prevent outbreaks due to reintroduction of the virus from countries in less developed regions with poor health care infrastructure [29–31]. Smallpox eradication was

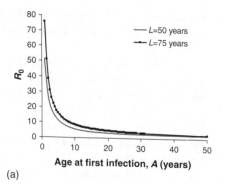

(a)

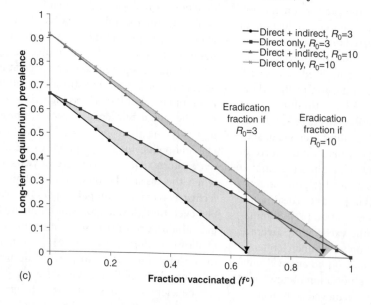

(b)

(c)

facilitated by a low herd immunity threshold that was relatively easy to achieve initially by mass vaccination, in less dense populations, and because infectious cases, and their contacts, were easy to diagnose, isolate, or vaccinate due to obvious disease manifestations (ring vaccination) (Table 32.3) [1,5,27–31]. There was also no known non-human reservoir of the variola virus, which limited reintroduction in controlled areas. In contrast, despite significant progresses since 1988, the feasibility of eradicating wild poliomyelitis virus in order to stop all control measures has been questioned despite the existence of the cheap, easily administered, and effective live-attenuated oral poliomyelitis vaccine (OPV) [31,35–39]. Polio is a highly infectious viral disease that attacks the nervous system and can cause paralysis and even death, especially among children. However, case finding and containment can be difficult because polio is often asymptomatic and because the virus can be transmitted by different routes (e.g., contaminated drink, food, or contact with contaminated fecal matter, saliva) that are influenced by hygiene levels [39–43]. The estimated average age at infection ranges from 2 years in developing countries to 10 years in the industrialized world [4,24,39]. Determining the eradication fraction and monitoring vaccination coverage is difficult because the efficacy of OPV is not perfect and varies by location, serotype (three strains

of the virus cause paralysis), and vaccine formulation [24,39–44]. In the US, polio is reported to have been successfully eliminated, with 65% of children being fully vaccinated. In reality vaccine coverage may have exceeded the eradication fraction due to the long history of vaccination, the long-term vaccine protection, and the potential transmission of the vaccine virus types [5,24,39]. Vaccinated individuals can shed and secrete the live virus in the feces and oropharynx sufficiently to transmit the "vaccine virus," indirectly increasing the fraction of the population effectively immunized/vaccinated, especially if hygiene is poor [5, 24,39–41]. Unfortunately, the excreted "vaccine virus" occasionally reverts to a pathogenic type, causing paralytic disease among vaccinated individuals [24,36,39,42,45,47–49]. Despite, the low risk (~1 per 400 000–750 000 immunized infants) [48] it becomes increasingly important as a "reservoir" of infection, especially if OPV use was reduced or replaced by the Salk inactivated vaccine (SIV), which is believed to protect against disease rather than infection [35–38,41,46–48]. In the absence of sufficient immunity, the poliovirus can circulate silently, eventually re-emerge, and cause outbreaks of vaccine-associated paralytic polio, months or even years after the vaccine has been administered due to continuous circulation of undetected "vaccine" live viruses [46,47].

Figure 32.2 (a) The basic reproductive rate, R_0, as a function of the average age at first infection for childhood infection based on Equation 32.4, which assumed an open and stable homogeneous population with a force of infection and mortality rate constant with age. Equation 32.4 also assumes that the distribution of the population declines exponentially with age, as is the case for developing countries [1]. For developed countries with a more uniform age distribution, $R_0 = L/A$ [1]. (b) Relationship between the eradication fraction, p_h, and the basic reproductive rate, R_0. The figure also presents estimates of the eradication fraction for selected diseases and populations based on Equation 32.5b and R_0 values reported in Table 32.1. (c) Herd immunity effects (shaded areas) on the long-term endemic prevalence of a sexually transmitted infection (STI) as a function of the fraction vaccinated (f_c) for a low and high R_0. The vaccine is assumed to protect 100% of the individuals vaccinated perfectly and for life in a homogeneous

population. These are based on the following formulas. Endemic prevalence (p^*) ignoring the herd effects of vaccination (direct effects only): $p^* = (1 - f_v)(1 - 1/R_0)$. This is equivalent to assuming that the force of infection remains constant over time following vaccination. Thus, only those receiving the intervention are directly protected. Endemic prevalence taking into account the direct and indirect effects of vaccine: $p^* = (1 - 1/R_0) - f_v$. This reflects that non-vaccinated individuals also benefit from vaccination because the force of infection is reduced for all members of the population after vaccination. For each R_0, the shaded areas between the curves show the indirect impact of vaccination (indirect effects = f_c/R_0) [5]. In the absence of indirect effect, 100% of the population needs to be vaccinated to reduce the prevalence to 0%. When the indirect effects are taken into account the eradication fraction can be much less than 100%, especially if R_0 is slow.

Table 32.3 Important factors to consider before targeting an infectious disease for global eradication [24,27–31,33,34,38,41,46]

	Disease	
Factors	Smallpox	Polio
1 Biological and technical		
Theoretically feasible	✓	✓
Absence of non-human reservoir of the causative organism (to prevent constant reintroduction of the virus in the population)	✓	✓[1]
Low R_0 (i.e. low infectiousness and transmissibility of infection) = low eradication fraction, p_h	✓	×
No chronic carrier state	✓	×[2]
Infectious cases easy to identify: simple tools to diagnosis infectious cases or evident symptoms easy to recognize are present when cases are infectious (to identify and isolate infectious cases and vaccinate contacts)	✓	×
Effective and safe prevention tool (e.g., vaccine, treatment, etc.)	✓	✓[3]
2 Economic and logistic		
Availability of simple and affordable prevention tools (inexpensive, long-lasting, and easily deployed intervention (e.g., vaccine)	✓	✓
Must be more cost-effective than effective control	✓	✓[4]
Operational and technical feasibility of implementing eradication strategies: What fraction of the population must be immunized, at what age? Is it easy to deliver the vaccine?	✓	×
Global capacity for political, financial, managerial, and technical support needed for a worldwide initiative	✓	✓
Surveillance system to effectively adequately monitor outbreak post-eradication	✓	×
Long-term commitment	✓	×
3 Political		
Prevent important burden of disease, severity, disability, and death	✓	✓
Sufficient societal and political will to start and sustain this massive undertaking over several years	✓	×

✓ Criteria met; × criteria not met or challenging.
[1] However, some individual can shed the polio vaccine virus even for years and therefore they can act as a human reservoir [31].
[2] Many cases are asymptomatic for many years.
[3] The OPV vaccine is not always safe since the "vaccine virus" sometimes reverts to a neurovirulent form, which can cause diseases [31].
[4] Some studies suggest that the economics of polio eradication would be favorable but all the studies have limitations and the economics is less favorable than for smallpox [31].

Post-vaccination dynamics

The introduction of mass vaccination can change the epidemiological landscape of both infection and disease over time and across age groups. In general, the prevalence of an infection that does not confer natural immunity, like many sexually transmitted infections (STIs), will tend to decline gradually over time until it reaches a new post-vaccination endemic prevalence level below pre-vaccination level, provided there is no compensatory risk behavior [1,26].

In contrast, the introduction of routine infant vaccination against directly transmitted viruses and bacteria often produces three main dynamic effects (Figure 32.3a,b). First, shortly after the start of mass vaccination at high levels of coverage, the number

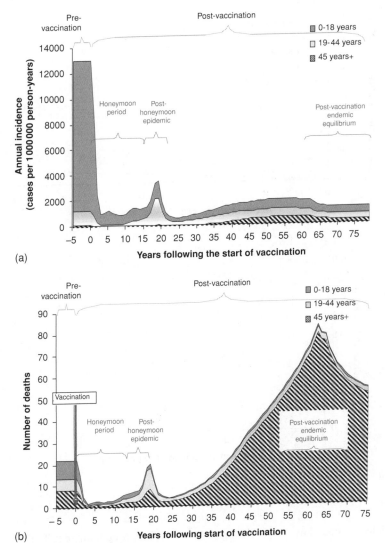

Figure 32.3 Pre- and post-vaccination dynamics of varicella infection. (a) Predicted age-specific incidence of natural varicella cases. (b) Number of deaths annually in a population of 50 million after the introduction (at time zero) of infant vaccination, assuming 80% coverage with a perfect vaccine (100% protection for life). The various epidemiological phases are: (i) pre-vaccination; (ii) honeymoon period; (iii) post-honeymoon epidemic; and (iv) equilibrium. Vaccination pushes the age at infection to older age, and reduces the number of varicella cases in all age groups. However, vaccination reduces varicella deaths among 0–44-year-olds but increases deaths among older people (45+ years). (c) Increase in average age at first infection following infant vaccination with a perfect vaccine (VE = 100%, lifelong protection) assuming a homogeneous population and a constant force of infection with age (Equation 32.7). (d) Increase of the eradication fraction (p_h) when the age of vaccination (V) is delayed by a few months for childhood infection with different average age at infection (A), using formula $p_h = (L - A)/(L - V)$ and $L = 50$ years (see Equation v in Table 32.4), and a perfect vaccine.

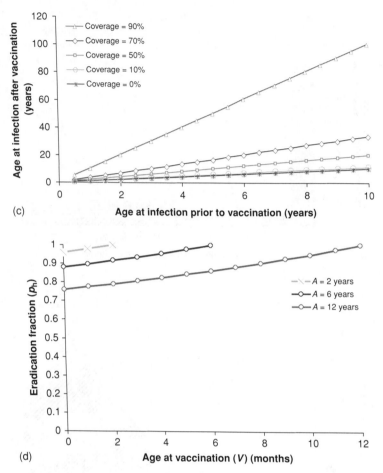

Figure 32.3 (*Continued*)

of susceptibles falls to such low levels that continued transmission is no longer possible. This results in a period of very low incidence, which is commonly called the "honeymoon period." Second, over time, the low incidence of infection allows the slow renewal of susceptible unvaccinated individuals through births, loss of immunity, or inadequate response to vaccine. This gives rise to an epidemic once the critical threshold of susceptibles required to sustain transmission is again exceeded. This is called the "post-honeymoon epidemic" [32,49]. Third, the infection eventually settles to a new and much lower equilibrium incidence than before vaccination. This is often called the "post-

vaccination endemic equilibrium." Patterns of this type have been observed following mass vaccination against measles and mumps viruses [1,5,25, 32,49]. When the number of infected individuals falls to very low levels, an infection can become "stochastically extinct" due to chance fluctuations, even with suboptimal coverage. Heterogeneity in host density can result in local extinction but with the continued risk of reintroduction from denser populations or those with low vaccine uptake [1].

In addition, routine infant vaccination often results in an increase in the average age of infection approximately as defined by Equation 32.6, for a homogeneous population with a constant force of infection across age classes and a vaccine efficacy VE, where f_c is the fraction vaccinated (Figure 32.3c) [1,5,24].

$$A' = A/(1 - VE \times f_c) \qquad (32.6)$$

The average age at infection increases only marginally when coverage is low. Very high coverage with a very effective vaccine will result in barely any infection over a lifetime. However, at intermediate coverage, vaccination can push the age at infection from early childhood to adolescence or adulthood because infections become concentrated in the older unvaccinated cohorts as the population ages. Vaccination reduces the circulation of infection and the overall force of infection (at sufficiently high levels of coverage) such that susceptible individuals tend to be older when they are exposed and become infected. The shift in the age at infection can have beneficial or detrimental effects if disease severity varies by age (Figure 32.3b).

Rubella is a classical example of an infection that is benign among infants but can be serious for women of childbearing age as it can result in a disease condition known as congenital rubella syndrome (CRS) in the newborn [1,4,24,50]. Before vaccination, it was estimated that approximately 85% and nearly 100% of the population experienced infection before 16 years of age in developed and developing countries, respectively [1,4,5, 24]. As a result fewer women of childbearing age remained susceptible to infection, and fewer CRS cases were reported in developing as opposed to developed countries [1,4,5].

Complex age-stratified models have been employed to assess the population-level risks and benefits of two different rubella vaccination strategies: a selective or a universal strategy [1,5,24,51,52]. The universal policy aims to eliminate transmission among children by achieving very high vaccination coverage of boys and girls in order to protect pregnant women through herd immunity effects and ultimately eliminate CRS. However, the risk associated with this strategy is to increase the average age at infection and the number of CRS cases if coverage is too low and too many pregnant women remain susceptible [4]. The selective strategy only vaccinates 10–14-year-old girls in order to directly reduce their risk of infection. This strategy does not increase the average age at infection and CRS rates because the disease remains endemic and a large fraction of girls still acquire infection at a young age and become naturally immune. However, all susceptible women need to be vaccinated to eliminate CRS because there is no significant herd immunity effect created by this selective strategy, as illustrated in Figure 32.2c. Early modeling studies suggested that CRS would increase if universal coverage was below 60% and that more CRS cases would be prevented under the universal policy when coverage exceeded 75% [1,24,51,52]. Interestingly, in the US universal rubella vaccination was introduced following the licensing of the vaccine in 1969, achieved high coverage, and successfully reduced the number of reported CRS cases from 57 686 in 1969 to fewer than 10 annual cases since 2003. CRS was declared no longer endemic in 2004 [53]. In the UK, the selective strategy was initially implemented. As it had a poor impact on CRS incidence, it was successfully replaced in 1988 by a universal vaccination strategy [54,55]. Unfortunately, in Greece, universal vaccination resulted in a period during which susceptibility to rubella among women of childbearing age increased because essentially insufficient vaccination coverage was achieved [56]. Detailed studies of how rubella mass vaccination influences herd immunity have been carried out in Finland via longitudinal age-stratified serological surveys [57,58]. Similar large-scale serological surveys for measles, mumps, and rubella virus antibodies have been conducted in Switzerland post the introduction of MMR mass vaccination [59]. Methods for the estimation of R_0 from age-stratified serology are described in [1] and [60].

More realistic assumptions

The basic theory outlined above is based on simplifying assumptions such as homogeneous mixing populations, a constant force of infection by age, vaccination at birth (or at onset of sexual activity for STI), perfect vaccine (100% efficacy), and no immunity conferred by maternally derived antibodies. All these complications influence both the estimation of R_0 and the critical eradication fraction (see equations in Table 32.4). For example,

Table 32.4 Summary of formula for R_0 or the eradication fraction (p_h) for the vaccination of childhood infections[a] for different model specifications and assumptions [1,4,5,24,32].

Equation number	Threshold formula	Main assumptions			
		Population characteristics	Force of infection	Vaccination	Vaccine efficacies
Establishment					
i	$R_0 = \beta \cdot c \cdot D$ β, transmission probability per contact; c, contact rate; D, duration of infectivity	Homogeneous contact rate, open, stable population (i.e., death balances births)	Constant with age	NA	NA
ii	$R_0 = 1 + (L - M)/(A - M)^a$ M, average age at loss of maternal antibody; A, average age at first infection; L, average life expectancy	Homogeneous contact rate; exponential age distribution of the population	Constant with age; maternal immunity	NA	NA
iii	$R_0 \propto \left(m + \dfrac{variance}{m}\right)$ m, average contact rate or infectivity; $variance$, = variance in contact rates or infectivity by risk groups, geography, etc.	Heterogeneous population with proportionate mixing[b]	Depends on heterogeneity in contact rates	NA	NA
Eradication					
iv	$p_h = \left(1 - \dfrac{1}{R_0}\right)$	Homogeneous	Constant with age	At birth[c]	Perfect (VE = 100%), lifelong protection
v	$p_h = (L - A)/(L - V)^b$ A, average age at first infection; V, average age at vaccination	Homogeneous contact rate	Constant with age	At age V^c	Perfect (VE = 100%), lifelong protection
vi	$p_h = \dfrac{1}{VE}\left(1 - \dfrac{1}{R_0}\right)$ VE, vaccine efficacy	Homogeneous contact rate	Constant with age	At birth[c]	Imperfect (VE < 100%), lifelong protection
vii	$p_h = \dfrac{1}{VE \cdot \mu/(\mu + \omega)}\left(1 - \dfrac{1}{R_0}\right)$ ω, per capita rate of loss of vaccine immunity ($1/\omega$ = average duration of protection); μ, per capita mortality rate ($L = 1/\mu$)	Homogeneous contact rate	Constant with age	At birth[c]	Imperfect (VE < 100%), limited duration of vaccine protection

[a]For sexually transmitted infection one must consider that individuals only become susceptible once sexually active.
[b]Proportionate mixing implies that individuals mix proportionately to their contact rate and therefore the expression for R_0 includes a variance term that reflects the heterogeneity in contact rate, which contributes to increase R_0.
[c]Ignores maternal antibodies.

ignoring the protective maternally derived immunity of newborns during the first few months (e.g., an average duration of protection of roughly 6 months for many viruses) slightly underestimates the value of R_0, and the eradication fraction, because of the slight overestimation of the age at infection since newborns only enter the susceptible pool once they have lost their maternally derived antibodies (Equation ii in Table 32.4) [1,5,24,32,34].

So far we have assumed that the population mixes homogeneously and makes contacts with other individuals randomly. In reality, infection risk may vary across individuals due to differences in susceptibility, contact rates, or infectiousness, resulting in clusters or groups of highly infected and/or infectious individuals by age, spatially dispersed, or risk groups compared to the overall population. This is particularly relevant for STIs because, in most populations, the majority have a few sexual partners and the few who form many partnerships contribute disproportionately to the transmission of infection, which concomitantly increases the value of R_0 (see Equation iii in Table 32.4 for proportionate mixing) [1,5,6,22,26]. Additional heterogeneity may also occur when individuals make contact preferentially by age, social group, geographic locations, or risk behavior category [12,61–64]. For example, men often prefer female sexual partners who are on average 5–10 years younger than themselves [62,63]. The common cold or influenza spreads more easily during the winter season when children gather at schools [64–68]. Note, however, that the prevalence is usually lower in heterogeneously mixed populations than in homogeneously mixing populations (for the same R_0 or average transmission rate) because infections are concentrated in a smaller fraction of the overall population [1].

Because heterogeneity increases the value of R_0, it also increases the fraction that must be immunized for eradication, which concomitantly makes the infection more difficult to control. In presence of heterogeneity, uniform vaccination across all strata of the population is no longer the most effective strategy. The overall vaccination coverage necessary to eradicate the infection can be reduced below that of uniform coverage ($p_h^{\text{targeted}} \leq p_h^{\text{uniform}}$) by targeting vaccination and increasing coverage among high-risk groups or transmission clusters, provided they can be identified [1,5,7,26]. Age is often a useful guide to risk for infections such as influenza A, since most transmission occurs in schools, as illustrated by the recent H1N1 pandemic [64,66].

We have also assumed that vaccines confer perfect (VE = 100%) and lifelong protection against infection, which is often not the case. Many vaccines confer adequate protection to only a fraction of vaccinated individuals or for a limited duration. Vaccines of low efficacy or short duration can render eradication difficult or impossible ($p_h > 100\%$), especially for high R_0 values, even if everybody is vaccinated (Figure 32.4). For example, eradication is not possible (i.e., $p_h > 100\%$) unless a vaccine that confers lifelong protection has an efficacy of over 80% if R_0 is 5 (Figure 32.4a). For comparison, if the efficacy is 33% eradication is only possible if R_0 is less than 1.5 in value. For an infection with an $R_0 = 1.5$ and human life expectancy of 60 years, eradication is not possible unless the protection lasts more than 30 years, even with a vaccine efficacy of 100% (Figure 32.4b). Interestingly, under these conditions, a 100% efficacious vaccine with an average duration of protection of 60 years is not better than a lifelong vaccine with 50% efficacy, since the predicted eradication fraction is 67% for both cases. This highlights the disproportionate importance of the duration of vaccine protection [20,32,67,68]. Importantly, imperfect vaccines that are not sufficiently effective to eradicate infection are still useful to control infection and reduce the burden of disease caused by infection (Figure 32.2). In addition, multiple doses or boosters can also be given (e.g., at birth and later in life) to improve the effectiveness of imperfect vaccine (Table 32.5) [5].

Vaccines act in many different ways. Some confer sterilizing immunity, and protect vaccinated individuals perfectly or imperfectly against infection, while others provide protection against disease but not infection. For example, the poliovirus vaccine OPV protects against infection whereas the Salk polio vaccine is believed to protect mostly again

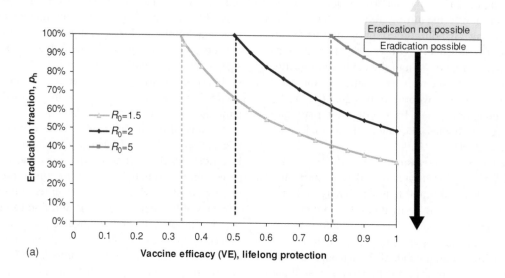

(a) Vaccine efficacy (VE), lifelong protection

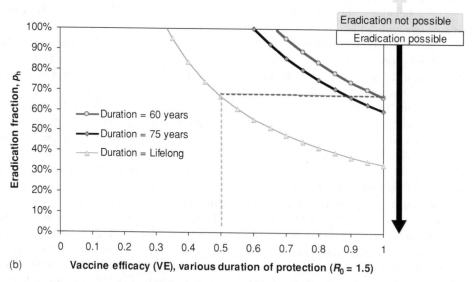

(b) Vaccine efficacy (VE), various duration of protection ($R_0 = 1.5$)

Figure 32.4 Eradication fraction (p_h) as a function of the vaccine efficacy (VE) for (a) different R_0 and lifelong vaccine protection and (b) different duration of vaccine protection and low R_0 based on Equation vii in Table 32.4 and $L = 60$ years. (a) For $R_0 = 5, 2, 1.5$ eradication is not possible even if 100% are vaccinated if the vaccine efficacy is less than 80%, 50%, and 33% (vertical dotted lines), respectively. (b) Eradication is not possible even if 100% are vaccinated if the vaccine efficacy is less than 33%, 60%, and 67%, when the duration of vaccine protection is lifelong, 75 years, and 60 years, respectively. Dotted lines show that the eradication fraction is the same ($p_h = 67\%$) for a vaccine with VE = 100%, and an average duration of protection of 60 years and a vaccine of 50% efficacy which protects for life.

Table 32.5 Types of vaccination strategy.

Type of vaccination strategy	Description	Example
Routine vaccination	Universal immunization of all members of a cohort of a given age to increase the vaccination coverage to high level. Because a cohort is only a fraction of the overall population, it takes several years before the population is immunized to the desired coverage [5].	The expanded program on immunization (EPI) and the Global Alliance for Vaccines and Immunization (GAVI) were created to achieve high vaccination coverage (>90% nationally) of children under 1 year of age in every district and country, against diseases such as tuberculosis, diphtheria, tetanus, pertussis, polio, and measles [47].
Mass vaccination	Immunization of a large segment of the population at one or more locations in a short interval of time in order to rapidly increase vaccination coverage and increase herd immunity [73,74]. It is used to limit mortality/morbidity in the setting of an existing or potential outbreak, especially if routine vaccination is absent or disrupted, to accelerate disease control when a new vaccine is introduce into routine immunization programs, and to meet international targets for eradication and mortality reduction [73,74].	Recent vaccination against H1N1. Such policy could be used to prevent potential bioterrorist attacks (e.g., with smallpox).
Ring vaccination	Immunization of a "ring" of all susceptible individuals in close contact with each infected/infectious cases or immunization of susceptible in a prescribed area around an outbreak.	Smallpox eradication campaign was initially based on a mass vaccination strategy to vaccinate more than 80% to achieve herd immunity. In 1967–1969, it moved to a containment and ring vaccination strategy, which required to diagnose and isolate suspected infectious cases as well as trace and vaccinate potential contacts of infected individuals before they developed symptoms and became infectious [27–30]
Pulse vaccination	Periodical repetitions of pulsed vaccinations of all individuals of selected age cohorts. At each vaccination time a constant fraction, f_c, of susceptible people is vaccinated. The name reflects the fact that all the vaccine doses are given over a much shorter period of time compared to the dynamics of the infection [76]. The key parameters to determine are the fraction to vaccinate at each pulse and the optimal pulsing period or inter-pulse interval. The maximum inter-pulse interval, for a homogeneous population with constant birth rate, in the absence of routine vaccination is $f_c \times A$, where f_c is the fraction vaccinated during a single pulse and A is the age at infection [75–78]. The objective is to reach children who are not immunized or only partially protected, or to boost immunity in those who have already been immunized. Thus, every child in the most susceptible age group is protected against infection at the same time, limiting transmission.	The Global Polio Eradication Initiative (GPEI), complements routine with pulse vaccination, known as National Immunization Days (NIDs) (i.e., 2 days one month apart), with the aim to immunize all children under 5 years of age, regardless of previous immunization status [40,77].

(Continued)

Table 32.5 Types of vaccination strategy. (*Continued*)

Type of vaccination strategy	Description	Example
Booster vaccination	Multiple vaccine doses offered during the life course of an individual in order to protect susceptible individuals because of an imperfect vaccine, where vaccines are only partially protective or have lost their vaccine immunity. A single-dose infant vaccination with an imperfect vaccine (VE < 100%, but lifelong) must protect vaccinees for a fraction of at least $((1 - 1/R_0) \times 1/VE)$ years of their average life expectancy, otherwise a booster may be required to be able to achieve eradication [5]. However, elimination or eradication may not always be possible even with a booster. The optimal strategy depends on the balance between the infant vaccination coverage, the rate at which booster is given, and the fraction of those receiving the booster doses who have previously been vaccinated [15].	Measles, mumps, and rubella vaccine (MMR): the first dose is given after 12 months and the second one between age 4 and 6 years.
Catch-up vaccination	Additional vaccination typically used when routine vaccination changes – such as new licensing approval for a vaccine or when the recommended age range at vaccination is expanded, or to protect those older than the cohort age of routine vaccination and increase herd immunity, especially when a new vaccine is introduced in a population.	In Australia the quadrivalent human papilloma virus (HPV) vaccine is routinely offered free to girls aged 12 and 13 years in a school-based program and to a catch-up group of 13–18-year-old girls [78].
Targeted vaccination	Program that aims to optimize resources by focusing on high-risk individuals or high transmission clusters in order to interrupt the chain of transmission. Theoretically, targeted approaches are particularly suited to control STIs because they are disproportionately transmitted by a small core group of individuals [1,5,26]. In reality, it is not always a practical solution because the target high-risk population has often already been infected by the time vaccination is offered (e.g. HPV).	Vaccines are currently available only against a few STIs (e.g., hepatitis B hepatitis A, human papilloma virus). HBV vaccination in the US was initially focused on high-risk individuals (e.g., contact with multiple/infected partners, injection-drug users). However, despite the availability, efficacy, and affordable HBV vaccine since 1981, its impact on disease has been modest because the uptake among high-risk individuals has remained low, partly because of the difficulties to gain access to these populations and because they are often reluctant to disclose their high-risk behaviors. High vaccination coverage, with subsequent declines in acute hepatitis B incidence among infants and adolescents, has been achieved since HBV vaccination has been included in routine infant immunization to prevent mother-to-child transmission.[a]

[a]www.cdc.gov/vaccines/vpd-vac/hepb/default.htm.

disease [24,35–41,46]. In models, these differences are mirrored by describing different modes of vaccine action [69–72]. A vaccine is said to have a "take-type" efficacy if a fraction VE_{take} of vaccinated individuals develops full protection against infection, while the remaining fraction $1 - VE_{take}$ remains totally susceptible. Alternatively, imperfect vaccine can confer a "degree-type" efficacy, which only partially reduces the susceptibility to infection of all vaccinated individuals by a fraction, VE_{degree}. More complicated modes of action allow for a combination of both efficacies [21]. Although, the eradication fraction is the same with either mode of action for a fixed vaccine efficacy (e.g., $p_h = 80\%$ at $VE_{take} = VE_{degree} = 75\%$), this aspect is nonetheless important because it influences the spread and endemic prevalence levels when coverage is suboptimal (i.e., coverage $< p_h$). For example, protecting 80% ($VE_{take} = 80\%$) of the population with a vaccine with 100% efficacy ($VE_{degree} = 100\%$) is better than protecting everybody ($VE_{take} = 100\%$) with a partially effective vaccine ($VE_{degree} = 80\%$) because with the latter vaccine every individual remains, albeit to a lesser extent, exposed to infection. Other vaccines, such as the HIV cytotoxic T-lymphocyte vaccine candidates, may also affect the course of disease and/or reduce infectiousness of vaccinated individuals with breakthrough infections [20].

For perfect vaccines that induce lifelong protection, it is better to vaccinate as soon as possible after the wane of maternally derived antibodies (roughly 6 months for most viruses) or for STIs, before the start of sexual debut, since it protects individuals for the majority of their susceptible life [5]. If the age at vaccination (V) is delayed, the eradication threshold increases (Table 32.4, Equation v and Figure 32.3d). However, when the infection risk and disease severity is age dependent and the vaccine of limited duration, determining the best age at vaccination and coverage requires more in-depth analysis to optimize program design and to avoid potentially negative impacts if susceptibility to serious infection increases with age where the average age at infection increases under the impact of mass vaccination [51,52].

Implementation

The full impact of vaccination on infection and disease can take many years to evolve following its introduction because of the time required to build up immunity in the population, especially in the situation of cohort targeted programs. Different vaccination strategies can be used to vaccinate susceptibles to the desired level of coverage (Table 32.5). The strategy or combination of strategies adopted depends on logistical constraints, the goal of the program (control, elimination, eradication, prevention of outbreaks), vaccine characteristics, epidemiology of infection, and how quickly coverage can be ramped up post the start of immunization [5,27, 28,73,74,77]. Routine cohort vaccination programs for children typically consist in the immunization of all members of specific age cohorts, and over time slowly build up the overall population vaccination coverage [1,5,47]. Mass vaccination across all age classes delivers immunization to a large segment of the population in a short time period, usually once, in order to rapidly increase coverage to accelerate disease control and to meet specific targets for elimination or for the mitigation of incidence and mortality reduction [5,28–31,73,74]. This approach can also be used prevent or mitigate outbreaks of emerging/re-emerging pathogens (e.g., H1N1) [73,74]. A pulse vaccination strategy, such as used by the global polio eradication initiative (GPEI), can replace or complement routine infant vaccination. It consists in vaccinating a fracsible of susceptibles over a very short period of time, on an "immunization day," at repeated intervals otherwise called inter-pulse intervals [5,75–77]. Although the smallpox eradication campaign was initially based on a mass vaccination strategy it has been argued that its success was due to the containment and ring vaccination strategy introduced in 1967–1969 [5,27–30]. However, mass vaccination may have paved the way for its success by increasing herd immunity to permit ring vaccination to work effectively in the final stages of eradication [5,29,30]. The approach was based on good diagnosis and subsequent isolation of suspected infectious cases. Potential contacts of infected individuals were traced and vaccinated before they developed symptoms and became infectious, to prevent further dissemination [5,29–31].

When the vaccine has imperfect efficacy (e.g., low efficacy, limited duration) additional vaccine doses, or boosters, can also be given over the life course of an individual to effectively immunize those in whom the vaccine may have failed or who were not reached by infant vaccination. A booster may be needed when an imperfect vaccine does not protect vaccinees for a sufficient fraction of their life expectancy. However, elimination and eradication may remain elusive even with a booster, if the vaccine is too poor and R_0 too high. This is especially the case if vaccine coverage is too low [5].

Cost-effectiveness analysis

Introducing new vaccines into national immunization programs presents many challenges for public health policy makers. New vaccines tend to be expensive as manufacturing companies need to recover research and development costs, which can be very large due to the need for very large phase III clinical trials. For many of the newer vaccines, such as human papilloma virus (HPV), the disease they prevent is less prevalent than the prevalence of childhood viral and bacterial infections so sales volumes are lower and therefore sometimes these vaccines are only purchased for populations in developed countries. Economic evaluation, such as cost-effectiveness analysis, is increasingly being used by government health departments in combination with mathematical modeling to inform and rationalize decisions about which vaccines to include in national programs and in the specific design of vaccination programs. Cost-effectiveness analysis provides an analytical framework to decide if a specific vaccine is worth introducing when compared with other uses of the same limited resources. Such analyses can also help decide who should be vaccinated, how many, and when [79].

In order to compare the health and economic impact of different interventions and to identify which interventions maximize the health of the population, results of cost-effectiveness analyses are usually presented as a cost-effectiveness ratio (CER)

[80]. This ratio measures the incremental cost of obtaining a unit of health benefit from vaccination compared to no vaccination (Equation 32.7) [80].

$$CER = \frac{\text{Net cost of vaccination}}{\text{Net health benefit}} \qquad (32.7a)$$

$$= \frac{(\text{Cost of vaccination} - \text{Cost offsets by preventing disease})}{\text{Gains in health by preventing disease}}$$

$$(32.7b)$$

The costs include elements such as the price of the vaccine, administration costs of vaccine delivery, physician visits, hospitalization, and treatment. The health benefits can be measured as cases prevented, deaths prevented, and life-years gained. However, in order to create a consistent basis of comparison of health benefits (across different diseases, populations, and studies) the most common measure of health benefits used in cost-effectiveness analysis is the quality-adjusted life-years (QALYs) gained [80]. The concept of QALYs was developed to simultaneously capture in a single measure gains from reduced morbidity and mortality (higher values reflecting better health) (details in legend of Figure 32.5). The QALYs gained following vaccination is the difference, over time, between the overall QALYs with and without vaccination. The disability-adjusted life years (DALYs) gained correspond to the sum of years of potential life lost due to premature mortality and the years of productive life lost due to disability, and are also used, mostly in analyses for developing countries.

When evaluating preventive vaccine against infectious diseases, two main methodological aspects of cost-effectiveness analyses require specific considerations, namely discounting and herd immunity [25,79].

Discounting

The comparisons of the health and economic impact of different interventions (e.g., vaccination versus no vaccination) must be made over a clearly defined time period. As different interventions produce different time profiles of costs and benefits, discounting techniques are used to convert and aggregate future costs and future health outcomes of interventions to their present value (PV)

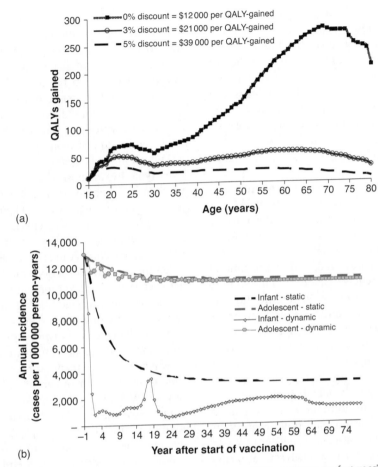

Figure 32.5 (a) Impact of the discount rate on the estimated QALYs-gained in a cohort of 100 000 girls vaccinated against HPV at 12 years of age (vaccine efficacy = 95%; average duration of vaccine protection = life). Results are adapted from Brisson *et al.* [82]. The concept of QALYs was developed to simultaneously capture in a single measure gains from reduced morbidity and mortality [80]. The measure assigns a quality of life-weight (utility), ranging from 0 (equivalent to death; some states may be considered worse than death and have a negative QALY) to 1 (optimal health) to health states [80]. This weight is then multiplied by the years of life spent in the health state [80]. The QALYs-gained following vaccination is the difference, over time, between the overall QALYs with and without vaccination. DALYs, originally developed by the WHO, are also commonly used, but mainly in developing countries. DALYs correspond to the sum of years of potential life lost due to premature mortality and the years of productive life lost due to disability. (b) Estimated varicella incidence over time by vaccine strategy (80% coverage, perfect vaccine) using a transmission dynamic and static model (e.g., cohort, Markov, or decision analysis). The impact of herd immunity on the incidence of infection is the difference between the dynamic and the static model. The extent of protection conferred by herd immunity depends on the amount of continuing infection in the community. Under the infant strategy (80% coverage), herd immunity (difference between the two models) is estimated to prevent 10 million cases of varicella over the first 80 years of vaccination in a country similar to England and Wales (50 million). On the other hand, under the adolescent strategy, the predicted number of cases of varicella over time is similar using the dynamic and static approaches. This is expected since the bulk of cases of varicella (85%) are in children under 11 years, thus vaccinating 11-year-olds has little effect on the overall force of infection of varicella (i.e., the risk of children getting chickenpox). Results adapted from Brisson and Edmunds *et al.* [25].

(Equation 32.8). Discounting consists of scaling down future costs and benefits to reduce their importance if they occur later in the future, and/or if the discount rate is higher. This reflects the fact that individuals, society, and health care payers prefer to receive dollars or health benefits sooner rather than later (what are called time preferences) [78–80]. The present value is calculated as follows:

$$PV = \sum_{t=0}^{w} O_t \left(1 + r\right)^{-t} \tag{32.8}$$

where PV is the present value, O_i is the future outcome of interest (e.g., cost, health outcome), R is the discount rate, and t is the timing of the outcome measurements over the time horizon of interest, w.

Due to the preventive nature of vaccination, costs of the program are incurred at the time of vaccination while benefits can occur in the short to long term post-immunization. Hence, the choice of discount rate can greatly influence results, more so for preventive than curative interventions. For example, discounting is particularly important when assessing the cost-effectiveness of HPV vaccination as the vaccine is given to young girls to prevent cervical cancer, which would typically occur 20 to 30 years post the acquisition of infection. A small decrease in discount rate (say, from 5% to 3%) can reverse the cost-effectiveness of HPV vaccination strategies from unattractive to attractive (Figure 32.5a) [82]. In situations where benefits occur in the medium to long term post-vaccination, higher discount rates make most preventive measures appear unattractive to government health departments.

Herd immunity externalities

A unique feature of infectious diseases is that following vaccination, the force of infection declines over time, producing herd immunity effects where fewer susceptibles will acquire infection than would be the case if no members of the population were immunized. In economic jargon this sort of effect is referred to as an externality. Currently two broad classes of models are typically used in economic evaluations of vaccination programs: (i) static models (i.e., cohort, Markov, or decision analysis) and (ii) transmission dynamics

models [81]. The key difference is that with static models, the force of infection is assumed to be constant over time ($\lambda(t) = k$) [1,25,81,83] whereas with transmission dynamic models, the force of infection depends on the prevalence of infection, and hence vaccine uptake, and can therefore vary over time (Equation 32.1a). Externalities can only be captured with the dynamic framework and this raises serious doubts about the value of static models, which are very widely used. The static framework typically underestimates the net benefit from vaccination especially as vaccination coverage rises to moderate or high levels (Figure 32.5b). This is because herd immunity effects are positive and prevent additional infections among non-vaccinees [84]. Negative effects can arise, as discussed earlier, when the incidence of serious morbidity rises with age such that some levels of immunization that act to increase the average age at infection also act to increase the number of cases of serious disease (e.g., rubella vaccines in Greece [56]). In these circumstances static models can overestimate the cost-effectiveness of vaccination programs. The magnitude of the over- or underestimation depends on how many transmissions are prevented by the program. If coverage, uptake, or vaccine efficacy is low, herd immunity effects are negligible and static and dynamic models produce similar results [25]. Although static models may be useful to rapidly estimate the worst-case scenario when herd immunity does not produce negative effects (e.g., shift in the age at infection where disease burden is greater), transmission dynamics models are preferable in all cost-effectiveness analyses evaluating prevention intervention against infectious diseases [82].

The application of mathematical models at different stages of vaccine development

Vaccine development is a lengthy and costly process, where many candidates need to be evaluated before the challenging stage of submission for licensing by the appropriate regulatory authority, such as the Food and Drug administration (FDA) [85–88]. The vaccine development process consists of five overlapping stages: (i) discovery and basic science, (ii) preclinical studies, (iii) clinical trials, (iv) product registration and licensing, and (v) production, manufacturing, and delivery (Figure 32.6) [8–87]. Typically, ten years or more are required for a single vaccine candidate to successfully complete the first three stages. The total cost to bring to licensure of a single vaccine candidate is estimated to lie between US $200 and $500 million as of 2009 [88] (Figure 32.6a). At the preclinical or clinical development stages, it is desirable to identify and pursue as early as possible the most promising candidates in terms of their potential public health impact and safety. This is not easy to accomplish since the full public health potential of vaccines cannot be estimated simply from the large double-blind individual randomized clinical control trials (I-RCT) that are typically used to test and progress vaccines through the different development stages [20]. By design, I-RCT can only estimate the direct effect of a vaccine in terms of reduction in the incidence of infection, morbidity, or mortality at the individual level among vaccines [20,69,72]. They cannot measure the potential indirect/herd effects among non-vaccinees, which depend on the balance between the vaccine characteristics and the target population, and the specific characteristics of a possible population-based vaccination program. Transmission dynamics models can help to evaluate the public health potential of vaccine candidates before they are licensed and made available on the market [20]. Of equal importance is their potential value in helping to design better trials that increase the chance of getting clear guidance on the likely efficacy and public health value of a candidate vaccine (Figure 32.6b).

Prior to evaluating a new vaccine candidate in a large I-RCT (i.e., phase IIb/III trials), models should be used to explore the potential population-level impact of the candidate assuming different characteristics (e.g., efficacy, duration of protection, mode of action) under a wide variety of settings and possible target populations in order to determine the minimum, most important, and "public-health relevant" characteristics that a vaccine must have to benefit populations as well as individuals. Once these public-health relevant vaccine characteristics

are identified, they should be used by vaccine developers for identifying the most promising candidates in the pipeline, and in clinical trials to determine the minimal vaccine efficacy that could be measured in the planned I-RCT and below which a vaccine would be of little public health use [20]. For example, Penny *et al.* [89] used a model to compare the population-level impact of potential pre-erythrocytic (PEV) and blood stage (BSV) theoretical malarial vaccine candidates on different outcomes. In terms of vaccine development, their analysis suggested a need for different vaccine types for different transmission settings, with PEV more likely to reduce mortality in low-transmission settings when compared with high-transmission settings. Their studies also indicated that the vaccine should have a minimum half-life of protection of 2–3 years to create a significant epidemiological effect [89].

It has recently been proposed that evidence from mathematical models and community-based randomized trial (C-RCTs[1]) should be used in tandem to factor the population-level and individual-level benefits and risks of vaccines into the licensing process [20]. Currently, new vaccines are approved for licensure based on their "good" benefit-to-risk ratio (not solely on their benefits) at the individual level only [90]. Compelling evidence of effectiveness in I-RCT under an intention-to-treat analysis with a good safety profile is usually sufficient to warrant licensure of a candidate vaccine [90]. However, vaccines aimed at healthy individuals need to demonstrate higher benefit-to-risk ratio than treatments for sick individuals, since higher risks are less acceptable for healthy than sick individuals with a poorer prognostic [20,90]. Since vaccines are usually administered to a larger fraction of a population than most drugs, a small risk can translate into a substantial number of serious adverse reactions, which may affect its acceptability in a population. Thus, ideally, the balance between individual-level benefits and the potential for adverse effects at the

---

[1] Although not possible with I-RCT, it is possible to measure the community-level impact of a vaccine empirically, through community randomized clinical trials (C-RCTs) [69,72].

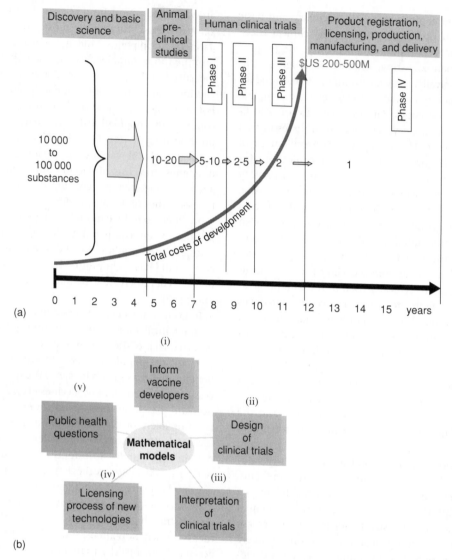

Figure 32.6 (a) Progression, and costs, of new vaccine through the different development stages [86–88] (see also ISOA/ARF Drug Development Tutorial at www.alzforum.org/drg/tut/ISOATutorial.pdf, accessed Feb 2012). (b) Use of transmission dynamics models at the different stages of vaccine development. Traditionally, transmission models have mostly been used to assist public health decisions at the fifth phase (v), when vaccines are already on the market. However, models can help evaluate the public-health potential of vaccine candidates before they are licensed in order to inform vaccine developers to pursue the most promising vaccine candidates (i); they can help at the licensing stage to decide if the candidate has any real public health value (iv); they can also help at the design stage to make sure trials are robustly designed and measure the important vaccine characteristics in order to get unequivocal results (ii); they can also help interpret trial results when there is a lot of uncertainty, heterogeneity in trial participants, and when the conditions of the trials are different than those assumed at the design stages (iii) [20].

population level (i.e., including positive and negative herd effects) should be formally evaluated and understood before licensing decisions are taken. A possible framework proposed by Boily *et al.* [20] can be summarized as follows. First, relevant authorities (e.g., FDA, WHO, National Institute for Health and Clinical Excellence [NICE]) would need to define precisely the public health criteria for what constitutes a useful vaccine at the population level. Following the completion of a large successful I-RCT (i.e., demonstrating some degree of vaccine efficacy), the potential population-level impact of the vaccine would be assessed using mathematical models and, together with the predefined public health criteria, these model results would be used to assess if a vaccine has any potential public health value in a specific setting (given the specific type and magnitude of protection conferred to vaccinated individuals in I-RCT). In combination with the strength of evidence from an I-RCT, modeling results could help decide if the vaccine should be licensed or rejected, or whether larger C-CRTs are warranted to estimate the indirect effects of the vaccine empirically before taking a licensing decision [20]. At present the licensing process could benefit greatly from more careful thought by health departments on the relevant and public health criteria for licensure of a vaccine for a defined infectious disease.

Transmission dynamics models provide a cost-effective and flexible framework to simulate and improve methodological aspects of trial design before implementation, to prevent flaws, and ensure that clear information emerges from these trials. Large I-RCTs of preventive interventions against infectious diseases are increasingly complex, costly, and challenging (Figure 32.6a). Many complex randomized controlled trials (I-RCT or C-RCT) have led to unexpected results that are often very difficult to interpret due to the nonlinear dynamic properties of infectious diseases transmission, nonadherence, loss to follow-up, and heterogeneous characteristics of patients and pathogens, which may all bias trial results (e.g., microbicide trials, STI treatment against HIV) [21,70,71,91–97]. For example, estimating the reduction in infectiousness (VE_i) of a prophylactic HIV vaccine among people

with breakthrough infections is much more complex than estimating a reduction in the risk of infection among susceptibles and it require innovative trial designs (e.g., partner studies) or the use of carefully chosen surrogate markers (e.g., HIV viral load among those who experience breakthrough infections) [20,95]. In addition, increasingly detailed information on the mechanisms of protection of vaccine over time is required to understand their full usefulness for individuals and populations. The dynamic simulation of clinical trials under various and heterogeneous conditions prior to implementation is an extremely useful tool for both methodological validation and identifying the ideal sites and populations in which to conduct trials [20,21, 93,94].

Discussion

In this chapter, we first presented some of the key concepts of infectious disease transmission and control by vaccination derived from relatively simple models of the transmission dynamics of infectious agents. Simple models are used to gain a general and intuitive understanding of key principles of the spread of infection in a population with time, age, and space, to identify the major epidemiologic forces acting on infectious agents. Of particular importance is their role in drawing attention to important gaps in knowledge, such as limited or no quantitative data on the key parameters that determine the typical course of infection and transmission between individuals. More complex models that capture relevant sources of heterogeneity, detailed contact patterns and age-dependencies are typically used when detailed information is available, when new hypotheses require testing (e.g., importance of heterogeneity of a given risk factor), to guide public health decisions, and to optimize vaccination programs in order to provide the greatest benefit to the population (effectiveness) in the most cost-effective manner. They have a special role in understanding counterintuitive situations where some levels of vaccination coverage can decrease the prevalence of infection but increase the incidence of serious disease such as in the case of rubella virus infection and the associated disease of congenital rubella in infants born to mothers who have acquired the infection during the first trimester of pregnancy [52].

Although traditionally models have mostly been used to address public health questions, they can be used more innovatively in a global initiative for vaccine research to inform vaccine development and licensing bodies about the characteristics that a vaccine should have to be of any public health use. Concomitantly, they also help assess which candidates in the pipeline are the most promising or provide the most benefits and least risk to individuals and populations. Political and media/public pressures advocating the development of effective vaccines and for the implementation of mass vaccination programs can be intense, especially in the context of major killer diseases such as malaria and HIV-1. In all such considerations it is vital to scientifically assess the possible public health impact of candidate vaccines within the licensing process [20]. This reduces the risks of wasting limited resources on vaccines of very restricted public health value. In the field of HIV prevention research, many large and costly clinical trials have produced negative or ambiguous results [96,97]. Dynamic clinical trials simulation is a cost-effective way to validate trial design and the statistical techniques employed to measure vaccine efficacy before the implementation of very costly trials [20, 21,71,93,94]. For example, modeling studies have been used to investigate the apparent discordant results from the Rakai and Mwanza community-based randomized trials of STI treatment to prevent HIV infection [91,92]. Needless to say, a better and faster understanding of both trial results would have been achieved if these mathematical modeling studies had been conducted prior to the launch of these trials to maximize the likelihood of a trial design that would most accurately measure intervention impact.

The degree of complexity required in a mathematical model of infectious disease transmission and vaccine impact is often the subject of debate but it should always be linked to the research question under consideration. The ideal model should be simple yet strive to represent reality as adequately as possible via capturing the key demographic, biological, and behavioral features necessary to address the question of interest. Due to the availability of increasingly powerful computers that permit large-scale simulation studies based on large populations where the individual is the basic unit of study, a current trend is for increased complexity in model design to represent the many complexities that influence transmission and vaccine uptake. Where data acquisition is good and parameter estimates of key epidemiologic features are available, it is now possible to use Bayesian techniques to fit models to epidemiologic data, improve model predictions, and better reflect the uncertainty of prediction based on uncertain parameter estimates [5,7,65,67,98]. Modelers are also increasingly "testing and validating" assumptions and trying to understand better the balance between simplicity and complexity that is required to address specific problems [67,99]. Simplicity yields the reward of analytical understanding – complexity can produce quantitative predictions and often increased trust from the public health professionals. What is certain, however, is that mathematical analysis will play an increasing role in vaccine development and public health delivery. Theory at present provides many insights of great value in the design of mass vaccination programs. As new vaccines are delivered for the more complex diseases, which have only partial efficacy and perhaps for only a short duration, models will be increasingly important in evaluating how much population-level impact will be achieved by a vaccine with defined properties. The most exciting area for future expansion is undoubtedly that of the simulation of vaccine clinical trial design [21,70].

References

1 Anderson RM, May RM. *Infectious Diseases of Humans: Dynamics and Control.* Oxford University Press, Oxford, 1991.

2 Dietz K, Heesterbeck JAP. Bernouilli was ahead of modern epidemiology. *Nature* 2000;**408**:513–14.

3 Blower S. An attempt at a new analysis of the mortality caused by smallpox and the advantages of

inoculation to prevent infection. *Rev Med Virol* 2004;**14**:275–88.

4   Begg NT, Gay NJ. Theory of infectious disease transmission and herd immunity. In A Balows, M Sussman (Eds) *Topley and Wilson's Microbiology and Microbial Infections*, 9th edn. Edward Arnold, London, 1997, vol 3, ch 10.

5   Keeling M, Rohani P. *Modeling Infectious Diseases in Humans and Animals*. Princeton University Press, Princeton, NJ, 2008.

6   Diekmann O, Heesterbeek JAP. *Mathematical Epidemiology of Infectious Diseases: Model Building, Analysis and Interpretation*. John Wiley & Sons, New York, 2000.

7   Grassly NC, Fraser C. Mathematical models of infectious disease transmission. *Nature Rev Microbiol* 2008;**6**:477–87.

8   Hamer WH. Epidemic diseases in England. *Lancet* 1906;**i**:733–9.

9   Ross R. Some a priori pathometric equations. *Br Med J* 1915;**1**:546–7.

10 Kermack WO, McKendrick AG. A contribution to the mathematical theory of epidemics. *Proc R Soc A* 1927;**115**:700–21.

11 Eames KTD, Read JM, Edmunds WJ. Epidemic prediction and control in weighted networks. *Epidemics* 2009;**1**:70–76.

12 Boily MC, Anderson RM. Sexual contact patterns between men and women and the spread of HIV-1 in urban centres in Africa. *IMA J Math Appl Med Biol* 1991;**8**(4):221–47.

13 Hens N, Ayele GM, Goeyvaerts N, *et al*. Estimating the impact of school closure on social mixing behaviour and the transmission of close contact infections in eight European countries. *BMC Infect Dis* 2009;**9**:187.

14 Ferguson NM, Donnelly CA, Anderson RM. Transmission intensity and impact of control policies on the foot and mouth epidemic in Great Britain. *Nature* 2001;**413**(6855):542–8.

15 Anderson RM, Fraser C, Ghani AC, *et al*. Epidemiology, transmission dynamics and control of SARS: the 2002–2003 epidemic. *Philos Trans R Soc Lond B Biol Sci* 2004;**359**(1447): 1091–105.

16 Riley S, Ferguson NM. Smallpox transmission and control: spatial dynamics in Great Britain. *Proc Natl Acad Sci U S A* 2006;**103**(33):12637–42.

17 White LF, Wallinga J, Finelli L, *et al*. Estimation of the reproductive number and the serial interval in early phase of the 2009 influenza A/H1N1 pandemic in the USA. *Influenza Other Respi Viruses* 2009;**3**(6):267–76.

18 Welte R, Trotter CL, Edmunds WJ, *et al*. The role of economic evaluation in vaccine decision making:

focus on meningococcal group C conjugate vaccine. *Pharmacoeconomics* 2005;**23**(9):855–74.

19 Walker DG, Hutubessy R, Beutels P. WHO Guide for standardisation of economic evaluations of immunization programmes. *Vaccine* 2010;**28**(11):2356–9.

20 Boily MC, Abu-Raddad L, Desai K, *et al*. Measuring the public-health impact of candidate HIV vaccines as part of the licensing process. *Lancet Infect Dis* 2008;**8**(3):200–207.

21 Desai KN, Boily MC, Masse BR, *et al*. Simulation studies of phase III clinical trials to test the efficacy of a candidate HIV-1 vaccine. *Epidemiol Infect* 1999;**123**(1):65–88.

22 Boily MC, Mâsse B. Mathematical models of disease transmission: a precious tool for the study of sexually transmitted diseases. *Can J Public Health* 1997;**88**(4):255–65.

23 Aron JL. Mathematical modeling: the dynamics of infection. In KE Nelson, CM Williams, NMH Graham (Eds) *Infectious Diseases Epidemiology: Theory and Practice*. Aspen, Frederick, MD, 2001, p. 151.

24 Fine P. Herd immunity: history, theory, practice. *Epidemiol Rev* 1993;**15**(2):265–300.

25 Brisson M, Edmunds WJ. Economic evaluation of vaccination programmes: the impact of herd-immunity. *Med Decis Making* 2003;**23**:76–82.

26 Garnett GP. Role of herd immunity in determining the effect of vaccines against sexually transmitted diseases. *J Infect Dis* 2005;**191**(Suppl 1):S97–106.

27 Aylward B, Hennessey KA, Zagaria N, *et al*. When is a disease eradicable? 100 years of lessons learned. *Am J Public Health* 2000;**90**:1515–20.

28 Aylward RB, Birmingham M. Eradicating pathogens: the human story. *Br Med J* 2005;**331**:1261–4.

29 Henderson DA. Eradication: lessons from the past. *Bull World Health Organ* 1998;**76**(Suppl 2):17–21.

30 Fenner F, Henderson DA, Arita I, Jezek Z, Ladnyi ID. *Smallpox and Its Eradication*. World Health Organization, Geneva, 1988, 1476 pp.

31 Miller M, Barrett S, Henderson DA. Control and eradication. In *Disease Control Priorities in Developing Countries*, 2nd edn. New York: Oxford University Press, 2006, pp. 1163–76.

32 Scherer A, McLean A. Mathematical models of vaccination. *Br Med Bull* 2002;**62**:187–99.

33 Orenstein WA, Hinman AR, Strebel PM. Eradicating measles: a feasible goal? *Pediatr Health* 2007; **1**(2):183–90.

34 Gay NJ. The theory of measles elimination: implications for the design of elimination strategies. *J Infect Dis* 2004;**189**(Suppl 1):S27–35.

35 Singh P, Das JK, Dutta PK. Eradicating polio: its feasibility in near future? *J Commun Dis* 2008;**40**(4): 225–32.

36 Chumakov K, Ehrenfeld E, Wimmer E, Agol VI. Vaccination against polio should not be stopped. *Nat Rev* 2007;**5**:952–8.

37 Arita I, Nakane M, Fenner F. Public health. Is polio eradication realistic? *Science* 2006;**312**:852–4.

38 Ehrenfeld E, Glass RI, Agol VI, *et al.* Immunisation against poliomyelitis: moving forward. *Lancet* 2008; **371**:1385–7.

39 Fine PEM, Carneiro AM. Transmissibility and persistence of oral polio vaccine viruses: implications for the global poliomyelitis eradication initiative. *Am J Epidemi* 1999;**150**(10):1001–21.

40 Heymann DL, Aylward RB. Eradicating polio. *N Engl J Med* 2004;**351**:1275–7.

41 Wassilak S, Orenstein W. Challenges faced by the global polio eradication initiative *Expert Rev Vaccines* 2010;**9**(5):447–9.

42 Grassly NC, Wenger J, Durrani S, *et al.* Protective efficacy of a monovalent oral type 1 poliovirus vaccine: a case-control study. *Lancet* 2007;**369**(9570):1356–62.

43 Grassly NC, Fraser C, Wenger J, *et al.* New strategies for the elimination of polio from India. *Science* 2006;**314**(5802):1150–53.

44 Kew OM, Wright PF, Agol VI, *et al.* Circulating vaccine-derived polioviruses: current state of knowledge. *Bull World Health Organ* 2004;**82**:16–23.

45 Kew OM, Morris-Glasgow V, Landaverde M, *et al.* Outbreak of poliomyelitis in Hispaniola associated with circulating type 1 vaccine-derived poliovirus. *Science* 2002;**296** (5566):356–9.

46 Eichner M, Dietz K. Eradication of poliomyelitis: when can one be sure that polio virus transmission has been terminated? *Am J Epidemiol* 1996;**143**(8): 816–22.

47 SAGE. Recommendations from the Strategic Advisory Group of Experts to the Department of Immunization, Vaccines and Biologicals. *Wkly Epidemiol Rec* 2005;**80**(2):11–18. Available at www.who.int/wer/2005/wer8002.pdf. Accessed Feb 2012.

48 John TJ. Vaccine-associated paralytic polio in India. *Bull WHO* 2002;**80** (11):917.

49 McLean AR, Anderson RM. Measles in developing countries. Part II. The predicted impact of mass vaccination. *Epidemiol Infect* 1988;**100**:419–42.

50 CDC. Rubella. In W. Atkinson, S Wolfe, J Hamborsky (Eds) *Centers for Disease Control and Prevention: Epidemiology and Prevention of Vaccine-Preventable Diseases*, 12th edn. Public Health Foundation, Washing-ton, DC, ch 18. Available at www.cdc.gov/vaccines/pubs/pinkbook/rubella.html. Accessed Feb 2012.

51 Anderson RM, Grenfell BT. Quantitative investigations of different vaccination policies for the control of congenital rubella syndrome (CRS) in the United Kingdom. *J Hyg (Lond)* 1986;**96**:305–33.

52 Anderson RM, May RM. Vaccination against rubella and measles – quantitative investigations of different policies. *J Hyg (Lond)* 1983;**90**:259–325.

53 Reef S, Redd S, Abernathy E, Icenogle J. Rubella. In SW Roush, L McIntyre, LM Baldy (Eds) *Manual for the Surveillance of Vaccine-Preventable Diseases*, 4th edn. Centers for Disease Control and Prevention, Atlanta, GA, 2008, ch 14. Available at www.cdc.gov/vaccines/pubs/surv-manual/chpt14-rubella.html. Accessed Feb 2012.

54 Miller E, Waight P, Gay N, *et al.* The epidemiology of rubella in England and Wales before and after the 1992 measles and rubella vaccination campaign: second joint report from the PHLS and the National Congenital Rubella Surveillance Programme. *Commun Dis Rep CDR Rev* 1993;**7**:R26–32.

55 Miller E, Waight P, Vurdien J, *et al.* Rubella surveillance to December 1992: second joint report from the PHLS and National Congenital Rubella Surveillance Programme. *Commun Dis Rep Rev* 1993;**3**:R35–40.

56 Panagiotopoulos T, Antoniadou I, Valassi-Adam E. Increase in congenital rubella occurrence after immunization in Greece: retrospective survey and systematic review. *Br Med J* 1999;**319**:1462–7.

57 Ukkonen P, von Bonsdorff CH. Rubella immunity and morbidity: effects of vaccination in Finland. *Scand J Infect Dis* 1988;**20**(3):255–9.

58 Ukkonen P. Rubella immunity and morbidity: impact of different vaccination programs in Finland 1979–1992. *Scand J Infect Dis* 1996;**28**(1):31–5.

59 Matter L, Germann D, Bally F, Schopfer K. Age-stratified seroprevalence of measles, mumps and rubella (MMR) virus infections in Switzerland after the introduction of MMR mass vaccination. *Eur J Epidemiol* 1997;**13**(1):61–6.

60 Farrington CP, Whitaker HJ. Estimation of effective reproduction numbers for infectious diseases using serological survey data. *Biostatistics* 2003;**4**(4): 621–32.

61 van Veen MG, Kramer MA, Op de Coul EL, *et al.* Disassortative sexual mixing among migrant populations in The Netherlands: a potential for HIV/STI transmission? *AIDS Care* 2009;**21**(6):683–91

62 Gregson S, Nyamukapa CA, Garnett GP, *et al.* Sexual mixing patterns and sex-differentials in teenage

exposure to HIV infection in rural Zimbabwe. *Lancet* 2002;**359**:1896–903.

63 Katz I, Low-Beer D. Why has HIV stabilized in South Africa, yet not declined further? Age and sexual behavior patterns among youth. *Sex Transm Dis* 2008;**35**(10):837–42.

64 Cauchemez S, Ferguson NM, Watchel C, *et al.* Closure of schools during an influenza pandemic. *Lancet Infectious Disease* 2009;**9**:473–81.

65 Cauchemez S, Temime L, Guillemot D, *et al.* Investigating heterogeneity in pneumococcal transmission: a Bayesian-MCMC approach applied to a follow-up of schools. *J Am Stat Assoc* 2006;**101**:946–58.

66 Greer AL, Tuite A, Fisman DN. Age, influenza pandemics and disease dynamics. *Epidemiol Infect* 2010; **22**:1–8.

67 Van de Velde N, Brisson M, Boily MC. Understanding differences in predictions of HPV vaccine effectiveness: a comparative model-based analysis. *Vaccine* 2010;**28**(33):5473-84.

68 Grenfell BT, Anderson RM. Pertussis in England and Wales: an investigation of transmission dynamics and control by mass vaccination. *Proc R Soc Lond B Biol Sci* 1989;**236**(1284):213–52.

69 Halloran ME. Overview of vaccine field studies: types of effects and designs. *J Biopharm Stat* 2006; **16**(4):415–27.

70 Boily MC, Mâsse BR, Desai K, Alary M, Anderson RM. Some important issues in the planning of phase III HIV vaccine efficacy trials. *Vaccine* 1999;**17**(7–8): 989–1004.

71 Haber M, Watelet L, Halloran ME. On individual and population effectiveness of vaccination. *Int J Epidemiol* 1995;**24**(6):1249–60.

72 Halloran ME, Longini IM Jr, Struchiner CJ. Design and interpretation of vaccine field studies. *Epidemiol Rev* 1999;**21**(1):73–88.

73 Heymann DL, Aylward RB. Mass vaccination: when and why. *Curr Top Microbiol Immunol* 2006;**304**: 1–16.

74 Grabenstein JD, Nevin RL. Mass immunization programs: principles and standards. *Curr Top Microbiol Immunol* 2006;**304**:31–51.

75 Agur Z, Cojocaru L, Mazor G, *et al.* Pulse mass measles vaccination across age cohorts. *Proc Natl Acad Sci U S A* 1993;**90**:11698–702.

76 d'Onofrio A. On pulse vaccination strategy in the SIR epidemic model with vertical transmission. *Appl Math Lett* 2005;**18**:729–32.

77 Grassly NC, Fraser C. Seasonal infectious diseases epidemiology. *Proc R Soc B* 2006;**273**:2541–50.

78 Fairley CK, Hocking JS, Gurrin LC, *et al.* Rapid decline in presentations of genital warts after the implementation of a national quadrivalent human papillomavirus vaccination programme for young women. *Sex Transm Infect* 2009;**85** (7):499–502.

79 Beutels P, Scuffham PA, MacIntyre CR. Funding of drugs: do vaccines warrant a different approach? *Lancet Infect Dis* 2008;**8**:727–33.

80 Drummond MF, O'Brien B, Stoddart GL, Torrance GW. *Methods for the Evaluation of Health Care Programmes.* Oxford University Press, New York, 1997.

81 Brisson M, Edmunds WJ. Impact of model, methodological and parameter uncertainty in the economic evaluation of vaccination programs. *Med Decis Making* 2006;**26**:434–46.

82 Brisson M, Van de Velde N, Boily MC. Economic evaluation of human papillomavirus vaccination in developed countries. *Public Health Genomics* 2009;**12**:343–51.

83 Edmunds WJ, Medley GF, Nokes DJ. Evaluating the cost-effectiveness of vaccination programmes: a dynamic perspective. *Stat Med* 1999;**18**:3263–82.

84 Trotter CL, Edmunds WJ. Reassessing the cost-effectiveness of meningococcal serogroup C conjugate (MCC) vaccines using a transmission dynamic model. *Med Decis Making* 2006;**26** (1):38–47.

85 International AIDS Vaccine Initiative. Uganda. Available at www.iavi.org/working-with-communities/country-programs/Pages/uganda.aspx. Accessed Feb 2012.

86 Ananthakrishnan R, Gona P. Pharmacological modeling and biostatistical analysis of new drugs. *Open Access J Clin Trials* 2010;**2**:59–82.

87 André FE. How the research-based industry approaches vaccine development and establishes priorities. *Dev Biol* 2002;**110**:25–9.

88 WHO. *The Initiative for Vaccine Research Strategic Plan: 2006–2009.* Available at www.path.org/vaccineresources/files/IVR_strategic_plan_2006_09.pdf. Accessed Feb 2012.

89 Penny MA, Maire N, Studer A, *et al.* What should vaccine developers ask? Simulation of the effectiveness of malaria vaccines. *PLoS One* 2008;**3**(9):e3193.

90 O'Neill R. A perspective on characterizing benefits and risks derived from clinical trials: can we do more? *Drug Inf J* 2008;**42** (3):235–45.

91 Orroth KK, Korenromp EL, White RG, *et al.* Higher risk behaviour and rates of sexually transmitted diseases in Mwanza compared to Uganda may help explain HIV prevention trial outcomes. *AIDS* 2003;**17**: 2653–60.

92 Boily MC, Lowndes CM, Alary M. Complementary hypothesis concerning the community sexually transmitted disease mass treatment puzzle in Rakai, Uganda. *AIDS* 2000;**14**:2583–92.

93 Mâsse BR, Boily MC, Dimitrov D, Desai K. Efficacy dilution in randomized placebo-controlled vaginal microbicide trials. *Emerg Themes Epidemiol* 2009;**6**:5.

94 McGowan I, Taylor DJ. Heterosexual anal intercourse has the potential to cause a significant loss of power in vaginal microbicide effectiveness studies. *Sex Transm Dis* 2010;**37**(6):361–4.

95 Datta S, Halloran ME, Longini IM. Augmented HIV vaccine trial design for estimating reduction in infectiousness and protective efficacy. *Stat Med* 1998;**17**: 185–200.

96 Padian NS, McCoy SI, Balkus JE, Wasserheit JN. Weighing the gold in the gold standard: challenges in HIV prevention research. *AIDS* 2010;**24**(5):621–35.

97 Grosskurth H, Gray R, Hayes R, *et al.* Control of sexually transmitted diseases for HIV-1 prevention: understanding the implications of the Mwanza and Rakai trials. *Lancet* 2000;**355**:1981–7.

98 Alkema L, Raftery AE, Brown T. Bayesian melding for estimating uncertainty in national HIV prevalence estimates. *Sex Transm Infect* 2008;**84**(Suppl 1):i11–16.

99 Penny WD, Stephan KE, Daunizeau J, *et al.* Comparing families of dynamic causal models. *PLoS Comput Biol* 2010;**6**(3):e1000709.

CHAPTER 33

Vaccine Safety

John Iskander[1], Claudia Vellozzi[2], Jane Gidudu[2], & Robert T. Chen[3]

[1]Office of the Associate Director for Science, [2]Division of Healthcare Quality Promotion, National Center for Emerging and Zoonotic Infectious Diseases, [3]Division of HIV/AIDS Prevention, National Center for HIV/AIDS, Viral Hepatitis, STD, and TB Prevention, Centers for Disease Control and Prevention (CDC), Atlanta, GA, USA

Immunizations are one of the most effective public health interventions in history. Vaccines can reduce morbidity and mortality in both developed and developing countries. Reported levels of vaccine-preventable diseases (VPD) in the United States are currently at historic lows [1]. Using measles containing vaccine (MCV) as a central tool, the global measles mortality reduction initiative has exceeded its target goals [2]. Vaccination programs may have additional benefits that extend beyond those vaccinated, as demonstrated by decreased carriage of pneumococcus and subsequent decreased disease levels in age groups not targeted for vaccination following introduction of pneumococcal conjugate vaccine [3]. However, vaccine safety has been a concern ever since Jenner's development of smallpox vaccination. Early opposition to smallpox vaccine was based on the perception that using the agent of a disease of cows (cowpox) to vaccinate humans might induce cow-like characteristics in recipients (William Atkinson, personal communication). During the 20th century, examples of the public health importance of vaccine safety monitoring have included the 1955 "Cutter incident," in which inadequately inactivated lots of polio vaccine from one of multiple manufacturers resulted in cases of paralytic polio, and the association of the 1976–1977 "swine flu" vaccine with an elevated risk of Guillain-Barré syndrome (GBS) [4,5].

Maximizing the public health benefits of vaccines requires relatively high and sustained vaccine coverage, so that herd immunity thresholds are achieved and susceptible individuals do not accumulate [6]. Paradoxically, it is just when vaccine benefits are most apparent and vaccine coverage is highest that vaccine safety concerns are most likely to arise in the general public and the media [7]. These concerns may arise partly because patients, parents, and health care providers no longer have any first-hand experience with VPD. People may be more likely to personally experience or know someone who has experienced an adverse event following immunization (AEFI) than they are to know someone who has had a VPD. By virtue of their absence, the diseases that vaccines prevent no longer serve as a reminder of the benefits of immunization. Loss of public confidence in vaccines is often followed by decreased coverage, leading to outbreaks of VPD, often with considerable morbidity and mortality [8]. This pattern has been observed in several countries, including Japan, the United Kingdom, and Nigeria. It is often only after return of wild-type disease that confidence in vaccination resumes and coverage rebounds, at the cost to society of preventable morbidity and mortality.

The ultimate purposes of monitoring vaccine safety are to protect public health, and improve the safety of vaccines and vaccination practices.

Vaccinology: Principles and Practice, First Edition. Edited by W. John W. Morrow, Nadeem A. Sheikh, Clint S. Schmidt and D. Huw Davies.
© 2012 Blackwell Publishing Ltd. Published 2012 by Blackwell Publishing Ltd.

Transparent reporting on vaccine safety on an on-going basis also has the potential to improve public and health care provider confidence in the safety of vaccines. In this chapter, we will outline the scientific framework for monitoring vaccine safety and will highlight recent case studies of global interest. Issues related to pre-licensure study of vaccine safety in clinical trials will be described briefly. Because a comprehensive review of all vaccine safety methodologies and specific contemporary issues under study is beyond the scope of this chapter, credible information resources, including websites, which provide updated information on emerging issues in vaccine safety, will be highlighted.

National regulatory authorities, such as the US Food and Drug Administration (FDA), are involved in testing of vaccines prior to their licensure. The need for such regulations in the United States was first identified due to tragic deaths after tetanus contamination of diphtheria antitoxins in the early 1900s. At a time when few remedies were available once an impure vaccine was administered, the Biologics Control Act of 1902 recognized the need to control the manufacturing facility as well as the safety and potency of the final vaccine products [9]. Subsequent regulations of vaccines and biologics have evolved along with changes in vaccinology, good manufacturing practices (GMP), and lessons learned from other mishaps such as the "Cutter incident," mentioned above [10]. Within the European Union (EU), the European Medicines Agency (EMA) is responsible for coordinating the evaluation, supervision, and pharmacovigilance of medicinal products in EU Member States, including vaccine safety (www.ema.europa.eu/ema/index.jsp?curl=pages/about_us/general/general_content_000106.jsp).

Safety evaluations are critical during the preclinical and investigational stages of a new candidate vaccine as they form the database needed for the eventual licensure application. If animal tests are successful, phase I human trials are undertaken to look for signs of gross toxicity in about ten human volunteers. Phase II trials (sometimes referred to as dose-ranging studies) in hundreds of volunteers evaluate the vaccine for more common adverse events. If the phase II results are acceptable,

phase III trials in 1000 to 10 000 subjects are undertaken. The phase III trial may need to be larger if a safety concern was previously demonstrated (e.g., rotavirus vaccine and intussusceptions) [11]. If phase III trials demonstrate the safety and the efficacy of the vaccine, then the FDA grants licensure of the vaccine to allow the sale and distribution of the product [12]. It is at this point that post-licensure monitoring of the vaccine, typically including mandated phase IV post-marketing studies conducted by industry, begins (e.g., pharmacovigilance for intussusceptions after the Rota Shield® vaccine) [13]. Review of post-licensure safety data from other countries already using current, prior, or biologically similar vaccines may also be relevant. The full vaccine safety lifecycle is illustrated schematically in Figure 33.1.

Several options are also available to enhance the current pre-licensure safety processes. To maximize comparability and interpretability of the adverse events monitored for safety assessment in clinical trials, internationally standardized Brighton Collaboration case definitions should be used [14,15]. Historically, clinical trials require the principal investigator to assess whether the observed adverse event might be causally related to the experimental vaccine. To minimize potential bias, analysis for nonrandom patterns of time intervals between vaccination exposure and adverse event onset can also be undertaken [16]. Historically, data safety monitoring boards (DSMB) are constituted separately for each clinical trial. This means that rarer adverse events seen across trials may be missed unless either a DSMB or the safety database for the candidate vaccine is collated across trials [13]. Furthermore, in our view, in addition to infectious disease experts, who typically comprise the members of DSMB for most vaccine trials, it is critical that DSMB be constituted with product safety and rare disease epidemiology expertise. Many new vaccines under development are targeted for use against diseases of high incidence in less developed settings. It will be important to improve the historically poorer safety surveillance infrastructures in such settings for clinical trials and post-licensure [17]. Finally, pharmacogenomics provides a valuable tool to understand the genetic basis of adverse events in the

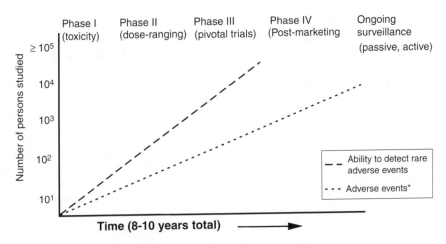

*Total number in safety database from pre- and post-licensure

Figure 33.1 Trial phases and post-licensure monitoring throughout the vaccine lifecycle.

new era of personalized medicine. The intensive clinical monitoring that occurs during trials provides a potential infrastructure for obtaining baseline data on vaccinated and control participants for comparison with subsequent incident cases of adverse reactions following licensure [18].

Overview of post-licensure monitoring

Comprehensive post-licensure monitoring of vaccines involves not only monitoring of safety, but also close attention to vaccine impact on disease levels, vaccine coverage, and vaccine supply. An example of such integrated surveillance is the European CDC's European Surveillance System (TESSy), which is used in monitoring available data on communicable diseases as well as the safety of vaccines. (http://ecdc.europa.eu/en/activities/surveillance/Pages/Surveillance_Tessy.aspx) The primary rationale for closely monitoring the safety of newly licensed vaccines, as well as established vaccines with new indications or recommendations, is that phase III clinical trials do not have the power to detect rare vaccine adverse events. Even the very largest trials [19], which have enrolled up to 70 000 participants, cannot detect vaccine adverse events (VAE) rarer than 1 in

10 000 vaccinees. Although rare side effects may halt vaccination programs on occasion [20], providers, public health officials, and others involved in providing vaccines should understand that some commonly used vaccines have known rare and potentially serious adverse effects; in these instances policy-making bodies have judged that the individual and community benefits of vaccination outweigh the established risks. For instance, MCV are associated with thrombocytopenia (which is typically self-limited and uncomplicated) in approximately 1 in 30 000 vaccinees [21].

Adverse reactions to vaccines may only emerge after extensive post-licensure use when rarer adverse outcomes may be identified. For example, the association of myopericarditis with the NYC BOH strain of smallpox vaccine in approximately 1 per 10 000 vaccinees was discovered long after global smallpox eradication was achieved, when the US undertook military and civilian smallpox vaccination programs in 2003 as part of bioterrorism preparedness activities [22]. This was likely partly due to the rareness of the finding but primarily because of the much more active safety monitoring measures undertaken for this mass vaccination program in the absence of wild disease [23].

Another key reason for post-licensure monitoring is that trials, regardless of their size, may exclude certain populations such as persons with underlying medical conditions, pregnant women, or premature infants [24]. Because vaccination recommendations, particularly for children, are often universal, the public health community has a duty to ensure the safety of new vaccines under conditions of everyday use and practice among diverse patient populations. Like other licensed medical products, vaccines may be subject to use outside of National Regulatory agencies' recommended age or risk group indications. This is referred to as "off label" use; monitoring off label vaccine usage may provide important vaccine safety information [25].

Comprehensive vaccine safety monitoring can ensure that the best safety data is available to inform immunization policies and recommendations for the safe and effective use of vaccines. Providers should be aware of recommendations for use of vaccines set forth by the advisory groups within their country of practice. The US Advisory Committee on Immunization Practices (ACIP) periodically publishes general immunization recommendations [26] and also publishes and posts online guidelines for use of specific vaccines in the United States [27]. As with any medical product, safety of vaccines should be rigorously scientifically assessed, and policy decisions should take into account evidence about both documented benefits and risks [28].

Beyond guidance for vaccine usage, activities of the US federal government concerning vaccine safety include licensure and regulation, surveillance, research, and provision of vaccine injury compensation. The National Childhood Vaccine Injury Act (NCVIA) of 1986 created the National Vaccine Injury Compensation Program (VICP). The VICP was established to ensure an adequate supply of vaccines, stabilize vaccine costs, and establish and maintain an accessible and efficient forum for individuals claiming to be injured by certain vaccines [29]. The VICP, which maintains a so-called Vaccine Injury Table (VIT), is a no-fault alternative to the traditional tort system for resolving vaccine injury claims that provides compensation to people found to be injured by certain vaccines. National immunization programs are increasingly incorporating such provisions as part of comprehensive vaccine safety risk management strategies [30].

The continued success of global immunization programs depends on a rigorous approach to vaccine safety. As global immunization coverage increases, the diseases prevented by vaccines are seen much less frequently. Therefore, communities pay increasing attention to the possibility of adverse events. With accelerated means of communication, local vaccine safety concerns are communicated rapidly to a global audience. The World Health Organization's (WHO) Global Advisory Committee on Vaccine Safety (GACVS) regularly reviews and publishes summary information regarding the safety of both new and established vaccines [31]. The GACVS, as the primary advisory body to the WHO for vaccine safety issues, plays a critical role in monitoring new safety issues and advising the WHO on safety aspects of vaccination policy. Beyond its well-established role of reviewing vaccine safety data, the GACVS also advises the WHO on issues such as strengthening national and regional vaccine safety monitoring and management capacity.

Overview of methodology and systems used to study vaccine safety

Unlike vaccine efficacy and effectiveness, vaccine safety cannot be measured directly; it can only be inferred from the relative absence of vaccine adverse events. All suspected reactions are referred to as adverse events following immunization or AEFI, a term which does not imply a causal relationship to vaccination but only refers to a temporal association of an event following vaccination. The term vaccine adverse event (VAE) may be used synonymously with AEFI. The lack of standard case definitions and guidelines for reporting specific AEFI has hindered the ability to compare vaccine safety data for different vaccines and vaccines used in different populations. The Brighton Collaboration (BC) is an international voluntary collaboration to enhance vaccine safety launched in 2000, whose first task was to develop standardized case definitions of AEFI. The BC consists of 2000 volunteers from more than 90 countries with expertise in vaccine safety, patient care, pharmaceuticals, regulatory affairs, public health, and vaccine delivery. The work of the BC constituted the first structured effort to develop standardized and internationally accepted case definitions for AEFI together with guidelines for collection, analysis, and publication of vaccine safety data. The general guidelines facilitate sharing and comparison of data on the safety of vaccines from different geographic locations and among vaccine safety professionals worldwide [14,32].

BC case definitions and guidelines are intended to enhance data comparability within and between clinical trials, surveillance systems, and epidemiologic studies. They neither provide a causal assessment of a given adverse event with immunization, nor do they establish criteria for management of patients. The case definitions are designed to define the levels of diagnostic certainty of reported AEFI. The case definitions are categorized by the levels of evidence available, which will differ based on whether it is gathered in prospective clinical trials or passive post-marketing surveillance, or whether it occurs in a developed or developing country [33]. The BC has defined common signs and symptoms such as fever and rash, as well as less common clinical entities such as aseptic meningitis and intussusceptions [34–37]. As of January 2010, a total of 28 case definitions have been completed and published; they are available for free download at https://brightoncollaboration.org/public/what-we-do/standards/case-definitions/available-definitions.html. The use of BC case definitions is recommended by key organizations in vaccine safety, including WHO, FDA, and EMA [38–40].

In the United States, there are three major complementary efforts in post-licensure monitoring: the Vaccine Adverse Events Reporting System (VAERS), the Vaccine Safety Datalink Project (VSD), and the Clinical Immunization Safety Assessment Network (CISA). Adverse event reporting systems for vaccines, often referred to as spontaneous reporting systems (SRS), are one of the primary ways in which vaccine safety is monitored. SRS are specialized public health surveillance or pharmacovigilance systems that have specific objectives as well as corresponding strengths and weaknesses [41]. Reporting suspected adverse reactions to vaccines to SRS is one of the key ways in which frontline health care providers can participate in improving the safety of vaccines. SRS can be used to identify vaccine safety hypotheses to be studied further by other systems, which are described later in this chapter.

VAERS, a national passive surveillance system that receives reports of AEFI for US licensed vaccines, has been jointly operated by CDC and FDA since 1990. Anyone can report to VAERS, and although events specified in the package insert as contraindications to future doses and adverse events listed in the Vaccine Injury Table are mandated for reporting, most reports are voluntary [41]. Manufacturers are required to report adverse events that they are aware of through reports from providers and review of the medical literature. Adverse event reports are classified by the US Code of Federal Regulations as serious if the report documents hospitalization, death, disability, and certain other categories of outcomes (e.g., congenital anomalies) [42]. Serious reports are subject to enhanced follow-up and clinical review. Regulatory designation of a report as "serious" does not imply a causal relationship to vaccination, nor does it necessarily indicate the medical severity of the event. A secure web-based version of the VAERS form has been available for online reporting by providers and the public since 2002. (www.vaers.hhs.gov).

VAERS has many strengths, including its national scope, ability to detect rare adverse events, and the capability of generating hypotheses about adverse events that can be studied more systematically in other vaccine safety systems. Published analyses of VAERS data may focus on specific vaccines or adverse events of interest, and may use descriptive epidemiologic and/or advanced signal detection techniques routinely used in pharmacovigilance [43,44]. VAERS is subject to the limitations of passive surveillance systems, including variable underreporting [45,46], reporting biases that may be related to publicity and/or the severity of the event, and, for individual reports, a general inability to assess causal relationship to vaccination [47]. The multiple system limitations in combination with the inherent complexity of the system and public availability of data make VAERS data subject to frequent misinterpretation [43].

In parallel with gradual but steady increases in vaccine dose distribution since the mid-1990s, there has been an increase in passive surveillance reports received by VAERS. The number of reports designated as serious by regulatory standards has also increased since the inception of the VAERS system, but has not increased as an overall percentage of reports [44]. The overall increase in reporting is likely attributable to multiple new vaccines, increased awareness and visibility of the system, and the ability for individuals to report electronically.

A variety of other SRS exist globally. Among the more well known are the United Kingdom's Yellow Card system, which, unlike VAERS, serves as a reporting mechanism for both therapeutic drugs and vaccines. The system has recently expanded the scope of who can report to it, and it has successfully supported introduction of new vaccines and mass vaccination campaigns [48,49]. The Canadian Adverse Event following Immunization Surveillance System (CAEFISS) is notable in that it has incorporated specific BC definitions into its reporting structure. In some countries such as Australia, annual summaries of data from reports to the SRS are published along with accompanying interpretive material [50].

A comparison between rates of specific adverse events in those who do and do not receive particular vaccines (or another appropriate comparison group) is necessary for comprehensive epidemiologic assessment of vaccine safety. VAERS and other SRS provide only a portion of this data, in part due to underreporting but also because these systems are limited to individuals who received the vaccine(s) and experienced adverse events. Unlike VAERS, the CDC-sponsored VSD includes denominator data (population of those vaccinated) and therefore can provide AEFI rates and appropriate comparison groups, and assess associations of vaccine with AEFIs. The VSD also conducts active vaccine safety surveillance for vaccine safety using a large linked database (LLDB), in which demographic, medical history, vaccination, medical outcome, and other clinical variables are linked

via a unique identifier. Diagnoses are identified using ICD-9 codes and can be validated using chart review [51].

Strengths of VSD include the ability to use a wide variety of study designs, including ascertainment of background incidence rates of outcomes of clinical interest, as well as its availability to conduct urgent studies [52]. Despite the fact that VSD covers approximately 3% of the US population, study of very rare events may require longer time periods for studies to achieve sufficient statistical power. Self-controlled case series methods allow for the comparison of events occurring at prespecified time periods before and after vaccination, thus allowing studies in situations of heavily vaccinated populations that control for potential biases and confounding [53]. A newly developed method in VSD called rapid cycle analysis (RCA) can provide near real-time active surveillance while maintaining the rigorous methodologic aspects of the VSD [54,55]. Historical or concurrent comparison groups are used for selected outcomes, based on the frequency of the outcome. Adverse events are selected for study in RCA on the basis of biologic properties of the vaccine, outcomes identified in pre-licensure data, and early data from VAERS or other SRS [55]. With active surveillance in the VSD comparisons can be made between rates of events in vaccinated and unvaccinated populations, or in vaccinated versus unvaccinated "person time." RCA supporting the safety of newly licensed adolescent and adult pertussis and rotavirus vaccines have been published [56,57].

Historically, most vaccines have been developed, produced, and first introduced in countries (primarily in North America and Europe) with considerable resources for evaluating safety in both clinical trials and post-marketing surveillance. Several other developed countries, including the UK and Denmark [58], already have LLDB to track vaccinations and clinical outcomes within their countries. However, vaccine manufacturing now occurs globally, with production in Brazil, China, India, and other countries. Some new vaccines are being introduced first in developing countries that lack extensive infrastructure for monitoring safety. The most recent example of this is rotavirus vaccine;

one product (Rotarix®, GlaxoSmithKline) has been introduced into the developing world (after extensive pre-licensure safety testing) before introduction in the United States or Europe.

Computer databases and technology exist in other countries that allow for the development of a Global Vaccine Safety DataNet (GVSD) [17]. Establishment of such a virtual network would greatly expand the geographic scope of current vaccine safety capacity. It also would allow results obtained in one country or region to be tested in additional populations, as well as provide additional statistical power for identifying rare adverse events. Furthermore, the development of data networks in locations that currently lack them will facilitate the local evaluation of safety issues or hypotheses in populations around the world [59]. This will be critical for vaccines in development, such as for prevention of malaria and tuberculosis, that may be introduced in the developing world but may not be used in the developed world, and may provide valuable information on the risk of adverse events whose occurrence rates differ by exposed population, or where the endemic rates of disease may affect the results of risk-benefit analyses. Any such endeavor would need to address data privacy concerns and follow published "best practices" for LLDB research [60].

Clinical vaccine safety research and practice

Although serious adverse events following vaccines are rare, they are concerning to patients or their parents as well as to vaccine providers, who may face complex medical decision making regarding future vaccinations after an AEFI. Building on successful models implemented in Australia and Italy [61,62], CISA, a network of six academic medical centers with expertise in immunization safety, was created to conduct rigorous clinical research on the pathophysiology or host risk factors underlying rare AEFI. CISA seeks to supply providers and the public with evidence-based guidelines when evaluating adverse events or considering vaccination of those at risk for adverse events. This national network of clinical sites can develop protocols to study rare events such as anaphylaxis [63], using sufficient number of subjects. Its goals are ultimately to be able to provide the evidence needed to safely vaccinate these individuals [64] or, if appropriate, defer further vaccine exposure. Future research directions might include exploration of genomic factors involved in beneficial and pathologic responses to vaccine [65,66].

Clinical health care providers who are involved in any aspect of vaccine delivery can participate actively in assuring the safety of vaccines and vaccination. Clinicians should observe the most current recommendations for vaccine storage, handling, and administration. Providers should routinely screen for and observe valid contraindications and precautions to immunization. The US NCVIA requires that a Vaccine Information Statement (VIS) be given to adult patients or to the parent/guardian of pediatric patients before administration of any dose of a universally recommended childhood vaccine. Providers are also subject to record-keeping requirements for vaccine administration, for example date of vaccination and lot number. Expanded clinician participation in vaccine safety reporting systems will improve AEFI surveillance and result in safer vaccines and improved recommendations for their use. Providers should report safety concerns to local or national public health authorities through established mechanisms. For newly licensed vaccines, attention to new recommendations in combination with reporting of vaccine adverse events to SRS or other designated reporting systems promotes optimal use of these potentially lifesaving products. In order to minimize the risk of injury to patients of all ages, clinicians should seek to prevent vaccine administration errors and post-vaccination syncope.

Vaccine administration errors are a type of preventable AEFI. These have been reviewed in the literature [67], and occasionally serious risk or harm may result from inadvertent substitution of various nonvaccine injectable products [68,69]. Other errors have been documented and include incorrect route of administration and use of age-inappropriate vaccine formulations. Although harm to patients rarely results, such errors can raise issues of vaccine effectiveness, which may require resource-intensive investigation [70]. Providers should adhere to standards for vaccine storage, handling, and administration [26], assure training in proper vaccine usage, and may also wish to participate in initiatives designed to decrease medical errors and improve patient safety.

Vasovagal syncope, a transient loss of postural tone and consciousness because of abnormal sympathetic reflex with spontaneous recovery, has been observed after medical procedures [71], including vaccination. Serious injury related to post-vaccination syncope can occur rarely. A review describing 107 reports of syncope-induced falls following vaccination indicated that more than 60% resulted in secondary injuries, including one fatality from intracranial hemorrhage in an adolescent boy aged 15 years [72]. To prevent injury from post-vaccination syncope, the CDC currently recommends that vaccine providers observe patients for 15 minutes after they are vaccinated, with continued observation for patients experiencing syncope or pre-syncope until the symptoms resolve [26]. Data from VAERS suggests that adolescents might be at greater risk for post-immunization syncope [73]. Additional research is needed to assess incidence and systematically evaluate adherence to the post-vaccination observation period and its efficacy in preventing syncope-related injuries.

Case studies

Safety surveillance for new vaccines involves coordinated surveillance and research efforts across systems. RotaTeq® vaccine, licensed in 2006, is approved in the United States for prevention of rotavirus disease. In 1999, RotaShield®, a different rotavirus vaccine, was withdrawn from the market after it was found to be causally associated with a type of bowel obstruction called intussusception. Based on possible concern with intussusception observed during pre-licensure trials, the package insert and ACIP recommendations noted it as an adverse event of special interest [74]. A small number of astute reporters to VAERS triggered two large studies that supported a causal association

[52,75] and led to withdrawal of RotaShield® [76], but also began a process that has resulted in development and licensure of new and safer rotavirus vaccines [77]. Results from published analyses to date indicate that the number of intussusceptions occurring following RotaTeq® is not greater than would be expected to occur by chance alone [78]. Monitoring via both VAERS and VSD is ongoing.

Human papillomavirus (HPV) is a major cause globally of cervical cancer, anogenital cancers, and genital warts. In 2006, a quadrivalent inactivated vaccine against HPV was licensed in the United States for 9–26-year-old females and recommended for use in adolescent and young adult women [79]. ACIP recommendations were accompanied by a systematic safety monitoring plan. Heavy attendant media publicity contributed to increased reporting to VAERS, as did the Weber effect, a phenomenon in which newly licensed products are associated with higher adverse event reporting rates [80]. A comprehensive review of available post-licensure data was conducted by the Global Advisory Committee on Vaccine Safety, which affirmed the vaccine's safety [81]. Subsequently published summaries of VAERS data conducted collaboratively by CDC and FDA vaccine safety and HPV subject matter experts found that while dose-adjusted adverse event reporting rates were higher than average for VAERS, the proportion of serious reports was less than 10%, and the most frequently reported events were consistent with pre-licensure data [82,83]. Potential safety outcomes identified from VAERS review that may require further study, including syncope and venous thromboembolism, are being systematically studied using VSD RCA. A bivalent HPV vaccine was licensed and recommended for use in the United States in 2009.

Vaccine safety monitoring is a critical component of any vaccination program to protect the public's health and maintain confidence in vaccination. During a large-scale vaccination campaign such as the one undertaken to prevent illness from the 2009 (H1N1) influenza virus, vaccine safety monitoring needs to be comprehensive, coordinated, and well communicated. In the United States, the influenza A (H1N1) 2009 monovalent vaccines were licensed and manufactured in the same manner as seasonal influenza vaccines; it was therefore anticipated that these vaccines would have safety profiles similar to seasonal influenza vaccines, which have been consistently safe [84]. However, during the 1976 swine influenza vaccination campaign, an unexpected increased risk of GBS was found to be associated with the vaccine [85]. In this context the US federal government (in collaboration with state and local health departments) implemented enhanced post-licensure vaccine safety monitoring to rapidly identify AEFI of potential concern following H1N1 vaccines [86].

Several federal agencies, departments, and private sector partners participated in 2009 (H1N1) monovalent vaccine safety monitoring. This new comprehensive approach was built upon the existing infrastructure, specifically VAERS and the VSD. Media outreach was used to educate providers and the public about VAERS and increase the quantity and quality of AEFI reporting. The Department of Defense (DoD), Indian Health Service (IHS), Department of Veterans Affairs (VA), and Centers for Medicare and Medicaid services (CMS) used their respective medical databases to implement the VSD/RCA model and contribute to active surveillance of H1N1 vaccine safety. Other CDC-supported systems included: active GBS case finding in a catchment area of the United States (~45 million persons) built on an existing CDC/state collaboration; active surveillance using an automated web-based algorithm designed and implemented by Johns Hopkins School of Public Health; and the Post-licensure Rapid Immunization Safety Monitoring (PRISM) system, a collaboration among managed care organizations, the National Vaccine Program Office, FDA, and Immunization Information Systems (IIS) providing data on up to 14 million additional persons to monitor vaccine safety.

As the frontline system, VAERS received the first adverse event reports following H1N1 vaccinations. The CDC and FDA reviewed reports daily and obtained and reviewed medical records for every serious report, searching for rare events or unusual patterns of reported events [87]. Within a few weeks following vaccine distribution, the VSD

and other systems accumulated both vaccine exposure data and appropriate comparison populations, using rapid sequential analysis to provide near-real time active surveillance [88]. All these systems worked together to detect possible vaccine safety concerns or "signals" and representatives met every two weeks to share data. Finally, an independent nongovernmental committee, the Vaccine Safety Risk Assessment Working Group (VSRAWG), was established to review data from all these systems every two weeks during the peak of the vaccination program and report their assessment of the safety of the H1N1 vaccines to the Department of Health and Human Services and the public. Results from this comprehensive effort to monitor H1N1 vaccine safety were to be used to inform vaccine recommendation and policy decisions if necessary. Any suggestion of an association of adverse event with the vaccine would be thoroughly studied but, depending on the strength of the signal, the procedures put in place allowed for policy decisions to be made ahead of definitive analyses, if warranted. At the time of this writing, unadjuvanted H1N1 monovalent vaccines have, as anticipated, proven to be as safe as seasonal influenza vaccines [89].

An international collaboration was also implemented during the 2009 H1N1 vaccination program. Data from many countries were shared on a regular basis (as often as weekly during peak vaccination efforts), mostly from SRS under the coordination and leadership of the WHO. This collaboration served as a platform to share methodologies, potential signals, and strategies for communicating with the public. This international collaboration has also led to the design of an international self-controlled case series [53] to assess the risk of GBS following immunization.

Approach to vaccine safety controversies

Recent high-profile vaccine safety issues have included the putative roles of the measles/mumps/rubella (MMR) vaccine and the preservative thimerosal in causing autism, as well as concerns about adjuvants in influenza and other vaccines in relationship to a variety of chronic disease outcomes [90]. While the work that led to the MMR controversy has been retracted [91] and replicated epidemiologic and laboratory research have consistently not supported hypothesized associations between vaccines and neurodevelopmental outcomes [92–94], several important lessons for future vaccine safety activities have emerged.

Regardless of the details of these or future vaccine safety "controversies," certain basic tenets apply. High-quality scientific study should be brought to bear upon the issue as rapidly as possible. Key research gaps should be identified and studied in a systematic manner [95]. Objective reviews of high-profile issues might need to be conducted, and expert groups need to be prepared to conduct updated analyses as new science emerges [96]. Because of resource limitations, study of issues of public concern must be balanced against the need for ongoing routine post-licensure surveillance. A recent example is the VSD case-control study, which found no link between pre- or postnatal thimerosal exposure and increased risk of autism; while time intensive, the study made use of both rigorous scientific methods and external policy oversight [97]. Risk communication should balance the need for clear information to protect public health while acknowledging areas where scientific information may be incomplete [98].

For particularly difficult or controversial issues involving vaccine safety, independent panels such as the VSRAWG implemented for influenza A (H1N1) 2009 monovalent vaccine may be convened to comprehensively review evidence and provide guidance to policy-making bodies and the public health and medical community, as well as recommendations for further research. The US Institute of Medicine has issued numerous reports concerning vaccine safety over the past two decades [99] but other types of systematic evidence reviews may be conducted as well. Expert meetings may also be convened, such as that held by the US National Vaccine Program Office at which evidence for a causal relationship between the first licensed rotavirus vaccine and intussusception was reviewed [100].

Summary

Medical and public health communities across the world will need to comprehensively address vaccine safety concerns in order to maintain high vaccine coverage and reap the full health and economic benefits of vaccination. Ideally this will involve a coordinated scientific and communications response. Clinicians should maintain awareness of vaccine safety issues, particularly those that have drawn considerable attention from the media, such as the thimerosal and MMR allegations, and should understand the most current scientific findings and be able to communicate these to concerned parents in a clear and empathic manner [101]. Providers should be aware of evidence-based elements of vaccine risk communication, including providing accurate information, maintaining trust in sources of information, keeping open lines of communication with parents who question use of vaccines, and referring patients to authoritative resources [102,103]. Clinicians who provide vaccines should be aware of and regularly access authoritative sources of current vaccine and vaccine safety information, such as the CDC, WHO, and the WHO-endorsed Vaccine Safety Net websites; patients seeking credible information should also be referred to these sites. Risk communication about vaccine safety will be an important tool in alleviating or mitigating some of the concerns that can affect the implementation of successful immunization programs around the world.

Relative to all other medical products, vaccines have a track record of being remarkably safe [104]. Ongoing measurable improvements have been a hallmark of vaccine safety science not only domestically but also globally [105], and such enhancements will need to continue as new vaccines and technologies are developed. History has taught us, counterintuitively, that the greatest scrutiny of vaccine safety will likely occur as the benefits of vaccines become most apparent. Several notable examples of post-licensure adverse event detection and subsequent actions (Table 33.1) reinforce the fact that absolute safety is not possible for any medical product, while also illustrating the increasing range of risk assessment and risk management

Table 33.1 Examples of post-licensure adverse event detection and risk management for vaccines.

Vaccine and year licensed	Adverse event (signal)	How detected	Key studies	Initial regulatory or policy action	Final resolution
Rotavirus (Rotashield®), 1999	Intussusception [37]	Reports to VAERS	VSD, national case-control	Suspension of vaccine use	Manufacturer withdrawal
Influenza (Nasalflu®), 2000–2001 influenza season	Bell's palsy [106]	Case reports to Swiss authorities	Case-control, case series	Suspension of vaccine distribution	Withdrawn from clinical use
Measles/mumps/rubella/varicella (ProQuad®), 2005	Increased risk for febrile seizure versus separate MMR/varicella vaccines	VSD RCA	VSD, manufacturer phase IV	Suspension of preference for MMRV by ACIP	Policy option (ACIP) to use MMRV or separate vaccines
Smallpox (Dryvax®), 2002	Myopericarditis [107]	Reports to US Military Vaccine Agency (MILVAX) and VAERS	Elevated in comparison with expected background rate in DMSS	Enhanced surveillance, education, and case management protocols	Myopericarditis monitoring for new smallpox vaccines; FDA approval subject to formal risk management plan

tools available to scientists, regulators, and policy makers.

The most prudent way forward is to maintain and strengthen safety monitoring infrastructure and expertise. An emerging model of an integrated regional approach to vaccine safety can be seen within the European Union (EU). The European Centers for Disease Control and Prevention (ECDC) has led the development of a group of eight EU Member States whose infrastructure and expertise will be used to monitor the safety of both routine and mass campaign (e.g., pandemic H1N1) vaccinations [108]. In Japan, recent leadership efforts have sought to create new policy structures (modeled on the ACIP) and improve vaccine post-licensure surveillance, which is currently achieved through a combination of reporting to manufacturers and efforts of various divisions of the Ministry of Health [109]. Continuing to build both surveillance and analytic research capacity worldwide will be crucial as vaccine safety expands into new scientific domains such as laboratory research [110].

The findings and conclusions in this chapter are those of the authors and do not necessarily represent the official position of the Centers for Disease Control and Prevention.

References

1 Roush SW, Murphy TV; Vaccine-Preventable Disease Table Working Group. Historical comparisons of morbidity and mortality for vaccine-preventable diseases in the United States. *JAMA* 2007;**298**(18): 2155–63.

2 Centers for Disease Control and Prevention (CDC). Global measles mortality, 2000–2008. *MMWR Morb Mortal Wkly Rep* 2009;**58**(47):1321–6.

3 Poehling KA, Talbot TR, Griffin MR, *et al.* Invasive pneumococcal disease among infants before and after introduction of pneumococcal conjugate vaccine. *JAMA* 2006;**295**(14):1668–74.

4 Offit PA. The Cutter incident, 50 years later. *N Engl J Med* 2005;**352**(14):1411–12.

5 Fineberg HV. Preparing for avian influenza: lessons from the "swine flu affair". *J Infect Dis* 2008;**197** (Suppl 1):S14–18.

6 Hutchins SS, Baughman AL, Orr M, *et al.* Vaccination levels associated with lack of measles transmission among preschool-aged populations in the United States, 1989–1991. *J Infect Dis* 2004;**189**:S108–15.

7 Chen RT. Vaccine risks: real, perceived and unknown. *Vaccine* 1999;**1717**(Suppl 3):S41–6.

8 Gangarosa EJ, Galazka AM, Wolfe CR, *et al.* Impact of anti-vaccine movements on pertussis control: the untold story. *Lancet* 1998;**351**(9099):356–61.

9 Baylor NW, Midthun K. Regulation and testing of vaccines. In S Plotkin, WA Orenstein (Eds) *Vaccines,* 5th edn. WB Saunders, Philadelphia, PA, 2008, pp. 1611–27.

10 Nathanson N, Langmuir AD. The Cutter incident. Poliomyelitis following formaldehyde-inactivated poliovirus vaccination in the United States during the Spring of 1955. II. Relationship of poliomyelitis to Cutter vaccine. 1963. *Am J Epidemiol* 1995;**142**(2): 109–40.

11 Heaton PM, Ciarlet M. Vaccines: the pentavalent rotavirus vaccine: discovery to licensure and beyond. *Clin Infect Dis* 2007;**45**(12):1618–24.

12 Ellenberg SS, Chen RT. The complicated task of monitoring vaccine safety. *Public Health Rep* 1997;**112**(1):10–20, discussion 21.

13 Rennels MB. The rotavirus vaccine story: a clinical investigator's view. *Pediatrics* 2000;**106**(1 Pt 1): 123–5.

14 Bonhoeffer J, Bentsi-Enchill A, Chen RT, *et al.* Guidelines for collection, analysis and presentation of vaccine safety data in pre- and post-licensure clinical studies. *Vaccine* 2009;**27**(16):2282–8.

15 WHO, UNICEF, World Bank. *State of the World's Vaccines and Immunization,* 3rd edn. World Health Organization, Geneva, 2009.

16 McClure DL, Glanz JM, Xu S, *et al.* Comparison of epidemiologic methods for active surveillance of vaccine safety. *Vaccine* 2008;**26**(26):3341–5.

17 Black S. Global Vaccine Safety DataNet meeting. *Expert Rev Vaccines* 2008;**7**(1):15–20.

18 Gurwitz D, Pirmohamed M. Pharmacogenomics: the importance of accurate phenotypes. *Pharmacogenomics* 2010;**11**(4):469–70.

19 Vesikari T, Giaquinto C, Huppertz HI. Clinical trials of rotavirus vaccines in Europe. *Pediatr Infect Dis J* 2006;**25**(1):S42–7.

20 Centers for Disease Control and Prevention (CDC). Suspension of rotavirus vaccine after reports of intussusception – United States, 1999. *MMWR Morb Mortal Wkly Rep* 2004;**53**(34):786–9; erratum in *MMWR Morb Mortal Wkly Rep* 2004;**53**(37):879.

21 France EK, Glanz J, Xu S, *et al.* Risk of immune thrombocytopenic purpura after measles-mumps-rubella immunization in children. *Pediatrics* 2008;**121**(3):e687–92.

22 Morgan J, Roper MH, Sperling L, *et al.* Myocarditis, pericarditis, and dilated cardiomyopathy after smallpox vaccination among civilians in the United States, January–October 2003. *Clin Infect Dis* 2008;**46**(Suppl 3):S242–50.

23 Casey CG, Iskander JK, Roper MH, *et al.* Adverse events associated with smallpox vaccination in the United States, January–October 2003. *JAMA* 2005;**294**(21):2734–43.

24 Klein NP, Massolo ML, Green J, *et al.* Risk factors for developing apnea after immunization in the neonatal intensive care unit. *Pediatrics* 2008;**121**(3):463–9.

25 Izurieta HS, Haber P, Wise RP, *et al.* Adverse events reported following live, cold-adapted, intranasal influenza vaccine. *JAMA* 2005;**294**(21):2720–5; erratum in: *JAMA* 2005;**294**(24):3092.

26 Kroger AT, Atkinson WL, Marcuse EK, *et al.* General recommendations on immunization: recommendations of the Advisory Committee on Immunization Practices (ACIP). *MMWR Recomm Rep* 2006;**55**(RR-15):1–48.

27 Smith JC, Snider DE, Pickering LK. Immunization policy development in the United States: the role of the Advisory Committee on Immunization Practices. *Ann Intern Med* 2009;**150**(1):45–9.

28 Halsey NA, Goldman L. Balancing risks and benefits: *primum non nocere* is too simplistic. *Pediatrics* 2001;**108**(2):466–7.

29 Evans G. Update on vaccine liability in the United States: presentation at the National Vaccine Program Office Workshop on strengthening the supply of routinely recommended vaccines in the United States, 12 February 2002. *Clin Infect Dis* 2006;**42**(Suppl 3):S130–7.

30 Evans G. Vaccine injury compensation programs worldwide. *Vaccine* 1999;**17**(Suppl 3):S25–35.

31 Global Advisory Committee on Vaccine Safety (GACVS); WHO secretariat. Global safety of vaccines: strengthening systems for monitoring, management and the role of GACVS. *Expert Rev Vaccines* 2009;**8**(6):705–16.

32 Bonhoeffer J, Bentsi-Enchill A, Chen RT, *et al.* Guidelines for collection, analysis and presentation of vaccine safety data in surveillance systems. *Vaccine* 2009;**27**(16):2289–97.

33 Kohl KS, Gidudu J, Bonhoeffer J, *et al.* The development of standardized case definitions and guidelines for adverse events following immunization. *Vaccine* 2007;**25**:5671–4.

34 Marcy SM, Kohl KS, Ron Dagan R, *et al.* Fever as an adverse event following immuniza-

tion: case definition and guidelines of data collection, analysis, and presentation. *Vaccine* 2004;**22**:551–6.

35 Beigel J, Kohl KS, Khuri-Bulos N, *et al.* Rash including mucosal involvement: case definition and guidelines for collection, analysis, and presentation of immunization safety data. *Vaccine* 2007;**25**:5697–706.

36 Tapiainen T, Prevots R, Izurieta HS, *et al.* Aseptic meningitis: case definition and guidelines for collection, analysis and presentation of immunization safety data. *Vaccine* 2007;**25**:5793–802.

37 Bines JE, Kohl KS, Forster J, *et al.* Acute intussusception in infants and children as an adverse event following immunization: case definition and guidelines of data collection, analysis, and presentation. *Vaccine* 2004;**22**:569–74.

38 WHO. WHO Consultation on Global Monitoring of Adverse Events following Immunization, 9–10 January 2006. *Wkly Epidemiol Rec* 2006;**81**(27):261–72.

39 Food and Drug Administration (FDA). Guidance for Industry. Toxicity Grading Scale for Healthy Adult and Adolescent Volunteers Enrolled in Preventive Vaccine Clinical Trials. Available at www.fda.gov/BiologicsBloodVaccines/GuidanceComplianceRegulatoryInformation/Guidances/Vaccines/ucm074775.htm. Accessed Feb 2012.

40 EMEA. Note for Guidance on the Clinical Evaluation of Vaccines. Committee for Human Medicinal Products (CHMP), May 17, 2005. Available at www.ema.europa.eu/docs/en_GB/document_library/Scientific_guideline/2009/09/WC500003875.pdf. Accessed Feb 2012.

41 Zhou W, Pool V, Iskander JK, *et al.* Surveillance for safety after immunization: Vaccine Adverse Event Reporting System (VAERS) – United States, 1991–2001. *MMWR Surveill Summ* 2003;**52**(1):1–24; erratum in *MMWR Morb Mortal Wkly Rep* 2003;**52**(6):113.

42 US Code of Federal Regulations, 21CFR600.80. Postmarketing reporting of adverse experiences. Available at www.accessdata.fda.gov/scripts/cdrh/cfdocs/cfcfr/CFRSearch.cfm?FR=600.80. Accessed Feb 2012.

43 Varricchio F, Iskander J, Destefano F, *et al.* Understanding vaccine safety information from the Vaccine Adverse Event Reporting System. *Pediatr Infect Dis J* 2004;**23**(4):287–94.

44 Iskander J, Pool V, Zhou W, *et al.* Data mining in the US using the Vaccine Adverse Event Reporting System. *Drug Saf* 2006;**29**(5):375–84.

45 Verstraeten T, Baughman AL, Cadwell B, *et al.* Enhancing vaccine safety surveillance: a capture-recapture analysis of intussusception after rotavirus vaccination. *Am J Epidemiol* 2001;**154**(11):1006–12.

46 Rosenthal S, Chen R. The reporting sensitivities of two passive surveillance systems for vaccine adverse events. *Am J Public Health* 1995;**85**(12):1706–9.

47 Iskander JK, Miller ER, Chen RT. The role of the Vaccine Adverse Event Reporting system (VAERS) in monitoring vaccine safety. *Pediatr Ann* 2004;**33**(9): 599–606.

48 Casiday RE, Cox AR. Restoring confidence in vaccines by explaining vaccine safety monitoring: is a targeted approach needed? *Drug Saf* 2006;**29**(12): 1105–9.

49 Ranganathan SS, Houghton JE, Davies DP, *et al.* The involvement of nurses in reporting suspected adverse drug reactions: experience with the meningococcal vaccination scheme. *Br J Clin Pharmacol* 2003;**56**(6):658–63.

50 Menzies R, Mahajan D, Gold MS, *et al.* Annual report: surveillance of adverse events following immunisation in Australia, 2008. *Commun Dis Intell* 2009;**33**(4):365–81.

51 Destefano F; Vaccine Safety Datalink Research Group. The Vaccine Safety Datalink project. *Pharmacoepidemiol Drug Saf* 2001;**10**(5):403–6.

52 Kramarz P, France EK, Destefano F, *et al.* Population-based study of rotavirus vaccination and intussusception. *Pediatr Infect Dis J* 2001;**20**(4):410–16.

53 Farrington P, Pugh S, Colville A, *et al.* A new method for active surveillance of adverse events from diphtheria/tetanus/pertussis and measles/mumps/rubella vaccines. *Lancet* 1995;**345**(8949):567–9.

54 Davis RL, Kolczak M, Lewis E, *et al.* Active surveillance of vaccine safety: a system to detect early signs of adverse events. *Epidemiology* 2005;**16**(3): 336–41.

55 Lieu TA, Kulldorff M, Davis RL, *et al.* Real-time vaccine safety surveillance for the early detection of adverse events. *Med Care* 2007;**45**(10 Suppl 2):S89–95.

56 Belongia EA, Irving SA, Shui IM, *et al.* Real-time surveillance to assess risk of intussusception and other adverse events after pentavalent, bovine-derived rotavirus vaccine. *Pediatr Infect Dis J* 2010; **29**(1):1–5.

57 Yih WK, Nordin JD, Kulldorff M, *et al.* An assessment of the safety of adolescent and adult tetanus-diphtheria-acellular pertussis (Tdap) vaccine, using active surveillance for adverse events in the Vaccine Safety Datalink. *Vaccine* 2009;**27**(32):4257–62.

58 Hviid A. Postlicensure epidemiology of childhood vaccination: the Danish experience. *Expert Rev Vaccines* 2006;**5**(5):641–9.

59 Ali M, Canh DG, Clemens JD, *et al.* The vaccine data link in Nha Trang, Vietnam: a progress report on the implementation of a database to detect adverse events related to vaccinations. *Vaccine* 2003;**21**(15): 1681–6.

60 Verstraeten T, DeStefano F, Chen RT, *et al.* Vaccine safety surveillance using large linked databases: opportunities, hazards and proposed guidelines. *Expert Rev Vaccines* 2003;**2**(1):21–9.

61 Zanoni G, Ferro A, Valsecchi M, *et al.* The "Green Channel" of the Veneto region as a model for vaccine safety monitoring in Italy. *Vaccine* 2005;**23** (17–18):2354–8.

62 Gold M, Goodwin H, Botham S, *et al.* Re-vaccination of 421 children with a past history of an adverse vaccine reaction in a special immunisation service. *Arch Dis Child* 2000;**83**(2):128–31.

63 Wood RA, Berger M, Dreskin SC, *et al.* An algorithm for treatment of patients with hypersensitivity reactions after vaccines. *Pediatrics* 2008;**122**(3): e771–7.

64 Rennels MB, Black S, Woo EJ, *et al.* Safety of a fifth dose of diphtheria and tetanus toxoid and acellular pertussis vaccine in children experiencing extensive, local reactions to the fourth dose. *C Pediatr Infect Dis J* 2008;**27**(5):464–5.

65 Klein NP, Fireman B, Enright A, *et al.* A role for genetics in the immune response to the varicella vaccine. *Pediatr Infect Dis J* 2007;**26**(4):300–305.

66 Ball R, Shadomy SV, Meyer A, *et al.* HLA type and immune response to *Borrelia burgdorferi* outer surface protein A in people in whom arthritis developed after Lyme disease vaccination. *Arthritis Rheum* 2009;**60**(4):1179–86.

67 Varricchio F, Reed J; VAERS Working Group. Follow-up study of medication errors reported to the vaccine adverse event reporting system (VAERS). *South Med J* 2006;**99**(5):486–9.

68 Varricchio F. Medication errors reported to the Vaccine Adverse Event Reporting System (VAERS). *Vaccine* 2002;**20**(25–26):3049–51.

69 Chang S, Pool V, O'Connell K, *et al.* Preventable mix-ups of tuberculin and vaccines: reports to the US Vaccine and Drug Safety Reporting Systems. *Drug Saf* 2008;**31**(11):1027–33.

70 Centers for Disease Control and Prevention (CDC). Inadvertent misadministration of meningococcal conjugate vaccine – United States, June–August

2005. *MMWR Morb Mortal Wkly Rep* 2006;**55**(37): 1016–17.

71 Oster LG, Sterner U, Lindahl IL. Physiologic responses in blood phobics. *Behav Res Ther* 1984;**22**: 109–17.

72 Woo EJ, Ball R, Braun MM. Fatal syncope-related fall after immunization. *Arch Pediatr Adolesc Med* 2005;**159**:1083.

73 Centers for Disease Control and Prevention (CDC). Syncope after vaccination – United States, January 2005–July 2007. *MMWR Morb Mortal Wkly Rep* 2008;**57**(17):457–60.

74 Centers for Disease Control and Prevention (CDC). Rotavirus vaccine for the prevention of rotavirus gastroenteritis among children. Recommendations of the Advisory Committee on Immunization Practices (ACIP). *MMWR Recomm Rep* 1999;**48**(RR-2): 1–20.

75 Murphy TV, Gargiullo PM, Massoudi MS, *et al.* Intussusception among infants given an oral rotavirus vaccine. *N Engl J Med* 2001;**344**(8):564–72; erratum in *N Engl J Med* 2001;**344**(20):1564.

76 Zanardi LR, Haber P, Mootrey GT, *et al.* Intussusception among recipients of rotavirus vaccine: reports to the vaccine adverse event reporting system. *Pediatrics* 2001;**107**(6):E97.

77 Patel MM, Haber P, Baggs J, *et al.* Intussusception and rotavirus vaccination: a review of the available evidence. *Expert Rev Vaccines* 2009;**8**(11):1555–64.

78 Haber P, Patel M, Izurieta HS, *et al.* Postlicensure monitoring of intussusception after RotaTeq vaccination in the United States, February 1, 2006, to September 25, 2007. *Pediatrics* 2008;**121**(6): 1206–12.

79 Markowitz LE, Dunne EF, Saraiya M, *et al.* Quadrivalent human papillomavirus vaccine: Recommendations of the Advisory Committee on Immunization Practices (ACIP). *MMWR Recomm Rep* 2007;**56**(RR-2): 1–24.

80 Hartnell NR, Wilson JP, Patel NC, *et al.* Adverse event reporting with selective serotonin-reuptake inhibitors. *Ann Pharmacother* 2003;**37**(10):1387–91.

81 World Health Organization. Global Advisory Committee on Vaccine Safety, 17–18 December 2008. *WHO Wkly Epidemiol Rec* 2009;**84**:37–40.

82 Slade BA, Leidel L, Vellozzi C, *et al.* Postlicensure safety surveillance for quadrivalent human papillomavirus recombinant vaccine. *JAMA* 2009;**302**(7): 750–57.

83 Wong C, Krashin J, Rue-Cover A, *et al.* Invasive and in situ cervical cancer reported to the vaccine adverse event reporting system (VAERS). *J Womens Health* 2010;**19**(3):365–70.

84 Vellozzi C, Burwen DR, Dobardzic A, *et al.* Safety of trivalent inactivated influenza vaccines in adults: background for pandemic influenza vaccine safety monitoring. *Vaccine* 2009;**27**(15):2114–20.

85 Schonberger LB, Bregman DJ, Sullivan-Bolyai JZ, *et al.* Guillain-Barre syndrome following vaccination in the National Influenza Immunization Program, United States, 1976–1977. *Am J Epidemiol* 1979;**110**(2):105–23.

86 Federal Immunization Task Force. *Federal Plans to Monitor Immunization Safety for the Pandemic 2009 H1N1 Influenza Vaccination Program*, 2009, pp. 1–20. Available at www.fda.gov/downloads/Advisory Committees/CommitteesMeetingMaterials/Blood VaccinesandOtherBiologics/VaccinesandRelated BiologicalProductsAdvisoryCommittee/UCM239499 .pdf. Accessed Feb 2012.

87 Centers for Disease Control and Prevention (CDC). Safety of influenza A (H1N1) 2009 monovalent vaccines – United States, October 1–November 24, 2009. *MMWR Morb Mortal Wkly Rep* 2009;**58**(48): 1351–6.

88 Greene SK, Kulldorff M, Lewis EM, *et al.* Near real-time surveillance for influenza vaccine safety: proof-of-concept in the Vaccine Safety Datalink Project. *Am J Epidemiol* 2010;**171**(2):177–88.

89 US Department of Health and Human Services. National Vaccine Advisory Committee (NVAC). Available at www.hhs.gov/nvpo/nvac, 2010. Accessed Feb 2012.

90 World Health Organization. Global Advisory Committee on Vaccine Safety, 17–18 June 2009. *WHO Wkly Epidemiol Rec* 2009;**84**:325–32.

91 Retraction – Ileal-lymphoid-nodular hyperplasia, non-specific colitis, and pervasive developmental disorder in children. *Lancet* 2010;**375**(9713): 445.

92 Hornig M, Briese T, Buie T, *et al.* Lack of association between measles virus vaccine and autism with enteropathy: a case-control study. *PLoS One* 2008;**3**(9):e3140.

93 Pichichero ME, Cernichiari E, Lopreiato J, *et al.* Mercury concentrations and metabolism in infants receiving vaccines containing thiomersal: a descriptive study. *Lancet* 2002;**360**(9347):1737–41.

94 Thompson WW, Price C, Goodson B, *et al.* Early thimerosal exposure and neuropsychological outcomes at 7 to 10 years. *N Engl J Med* 2007;**357**(13): 1281–92.

95 Payne DC, Franzke LH, Stehr-Green PA, *et al.* Development of the Vaccine Analytic Unit's research agenda for investigating potential adverse events associated with anthrax vaccine adsorbed. *Pharmacoepidemiol Drug Saf* 2007;**16**(1):46–54.

96 Meadows M. IOM report: no link between vaccines and autism. *FDA Consum* 2004;**38**(5):18–19.

97 Price CS, Thompson WW, Goodson B, *et al.* Prenatal and infant exposure to thimerosal from vaccines and immunoglobulins and risk of autism. *Pediatrics* 2010;**126**(4):656–64.

98 American Academy of Pediatrics. Thimerosal in vaccines: a joint statement of the American Academy of Pediatrics and the Public Health Service. *Neonatal Netw* 1999;**18**(6):65, 72.

99 Board on Health Promotion and Disease Prevention (HPDP), Institute of Medicine (IOM). Immunization Safety Review: Hepatitis B Vaccine and Demyelinating Neurological Disorders, 2002. Available at www.iom.edu/CMS/3793/4705/4435.aspx. Accessed Feb 2012.

100 Peter G, Myers MG; National Vaccine Advisory Committee; National Vaccine Program Office. Intussusception, rotavirus, and oral vaccines: summary of a workshop. *Pediatrics* 2002;**110**(6):e67.

101 Smith PJ, Kennedy AM, Wooten K, *et al.* Association between health care providers' influence on parents who have concerns about vaccine safety and vaccination coverage. *Pediatrics* 2006;**118**(5):e1287–92.

102 Hilton S, Petticrew M, Hunt K. Parents' champions vs. vested interests: who do parents believe about MMR? A qualitative study. *BMC Public Health* 2007;**7**:42.

103 Tenrreiro KN. Time-efficient strategies to ensure vaccine risk/benefit communication. *J Pediatr Nurs* 2005;**20**(6):469–76.

104 Jacobson RM, Zabel KS, Poland GA. The overall safety profile of currently available vaccines directed against infectious diseases. *Expert Opin Drug Saf* 2003;**2**(3):215–23.

105 Offit PA, Quarles J, Gerber MA, *et al.* Addressing parents' concerns: do multiple vaccines overwhelm or weaken the infant's immune system? *Pediatrics* 2002;**109**(1):124–9.

106 Mutsch M, Zhou W, Rhodes P, *et al.* Use of the inactivated intranasal influenza vaccine and the risk of Bell's palsy in Switzerland. *N Engl J Med* 2004;**350**(9):896–903.

107 Casey C, Vellozzi C, Mootrey GT, *et al.* Surveillance guidelines for smallpox vaccine (vaccinia) adverse reactions. *MMWR Recomm Rep.* 2006;**55**(RR-1):1–16.

108 Eurosurveillance editorial team. ECDC in collaboration with the VAESCO consortium to develop a complementary tool for vaccine safety monitoring in Europe. *Euro Surveill* 2009;**14**(39):pii: 19345.

109 Kamiya H, Okabe N. Leadership in Immunization: the relevance to Japan of the USA experience of the Centers for Disease Control and Prevention (CDC) and the Advisory Committee on Immunization Practices (ACIP). *Vaccine* 2009;**27**(11):1724–8.

110 Nachamkin I, Shadomy SV, Moran AP, *et al.* Antiganglioside antibody induction by swine (A/NJ/1976/H1N1) and other influenza vaccines: insights into vaccine-associated Guillain-Barré syndrome. *J Infect Dis.* 2008;**198**(2):226–33.

Index